Clinical Handbook of Rheumatology

Clinical Handbook of Rheumatology

Editor: Sullivan Princeton

AMERICAN
MEDICAL PUBLISHERS
www.americanmedicalpublishers.com

AMERICAN
MEDICAL PUBLISHERS
www.americanmedicalpublishers.com

Cataloging-in-Publication Data

Clinical handbook of rheumatology / edited by Sullivan Princeton.
p. cm.
Includes bibliographical references and index.
ISBN 978-1-63927-993-7
1. Rheumatology. 2. Joints--Diseases--Diagnosis. 3. Joints--Diseases--Treatment.
4. Connective tissues--Diseases--Diagnosis. 5. Connective tissues--Diseases--Treatment.
I. Princeton, Sullivan.
RC927 .C55 2023
616.723--dc23

American Medical Publishers,
41 Flatbush Avenue,
1st Floor, New York,
NY 11217, USA

ISBN 978-1-63927-993-7 (Hardback)

Contents

Preface

The world is advancing at a fast pace like never before. Therefore, the need is to keep up with the latest developments. This book was an idea that came to fruition when the specialists in the area realized the need to coordinate together and document essential themes in the subject. That's when I was requested to be the editor. Editing this book has been an honour as it brings together diverse authors researching on different streams of the field. The book collates essential materials contributed by veterans in the area which can be utilized by students and researchers alike.

Rheumatology refers to the medical specialty that focuses on the diagnosis and treatment of rheumatic diseases. It entails the study and treatment of conditions affecting the joints, as well as the ligaments, muscles and tendons that surround them. Rheumatic diseases are auto-immune and inflammatory conditions that include Lyme disease, dermatomyositis, vasculitis, sarcoidosis, arthritis, lupus erythematosus, etc. Rheumatology is also linked to soft tissue diseases, such as low back pain, olecranon bursitis and fibromyalgia. A variety of management techniques including occupational and physical therapy, rehabilitation, drug treatments and even surgery in extreme situations can be utilized for treating patients in rheumatology. Drug therapy includes opiates, antidepressants and anti-inflammatory medications. Patient care in rheumatology typically emphasizes on psychosocial interventions, patient education and self-management support. It also focuses on the physical components of the condition through assessments of physical health outcomes and biomarker review. This book unfolds the innovative aspects of rheumatology which will be crucial for the progress of this field in the future. It covers in detail some existent theories and clinical concepts revolving around this domain. Those with an interest in this field would find this book helpful.

Each chapter is a sole-standing publication that reflects each author´s interpretation. Thus, the book displays a multi-facetted picture of our current understanding of application, resources and aspects of the field. I would like to thank the contributors of this book and my family for their endless support.

Editor

1

Translation and cross-cultural adaptation of "Trapeziometacarpal Arthrosis Symptoms and Disability—TASD" into Brazilian Portuguese

Vinícius Alexandre de Souza Almeida*, Carlos Henrique Fernandes, Lia Miyamoto Meireles, Flavio Faloppa, Benno Ejnisman and Moises Cohen

Abstract

Background: Osteoarthritis is the most common form of hand arthritis and arthritis of the carpometacarpal joint of the thumb is a potentially limiting disease. There is no homogeneity in the evaluation of outcomes for the rhizarthrosis treatment. In an attempt to standardize the evaluation of results, some subjective questionnaires, non-specific, were used to evaluate rhizarthrosis. Trapeziometacarpal Arthrosis Symptoms and Disability (TASD) was described by Becker et al.with the purpose of evaluating symptom intensity and degree of disability, as to compare results after treatment. Our objective is to translate, validate and do the cultural adaptation of the questionnaire TASD into the Brazilian Portuguese.

Methods: The questionnaire was translated, with reverse translation. The translations were evaluated and synthesized by a committee, arriving at TASD-BR. Thirty-one patients with a diagnosis of rhizarthrosis answered the questionnaire. We evaluated, the internal consistency, reliability, agreement and ceiling and floor effect for validation.

Results: The questionnaires were translated and adapted according to defined protocols. The internal consistency, through Cronbach's α coefficient for TASD-BR, was 0.927. The questionnaire's reliability, through the Intraclass Correlation Coefficient, was also shown to be quite high, with κ = 0.961 (0.954–0.967). The agreement, measured through the Standard Error Measurement, remained with standardized values below 5%. There was no ceiling and floor effect.

Conclusion: Through specific methodology we consider TASD-BR translated and valid for the Brazilian Portuguese.

Keywords: Osteoarthritis, Surveys and questionnaires, Translation, Carpometacarpal joints, Reproducibility of Results

Background

Osteoarthritis is the most common form of hand arthri tis. It is a complex disorder that can be characterized in several subtypes such as interphalangeal arthrosis, nodular arthritis, erosive arthritis, and arthritis of the carpo metacarpal joint of the thumb, or rhizarthrosis [1, 2].

The handgrip mechanism depends mainly on the thumb. For the performance of this movement, besides the integrity and harmony of the tenar musculature, it is necessary to have adequate positioning and congruence of its joints, especially the carpometacarpal joint of the thumb [3].

Rhizarthrosis is a potentially limiting disease, which causes pain and decreases the capacity for work, leisure, physical activities, and daily activities with a consequent decrease in quality of life [4, 5]. However, the patient's symptoms do not always correspond to the radiographic findings. Radiographic variation or ultrasound exams showing joint degeneration may not correspond to functional or inflammatory limitations. This

*Correspondence: vinicius.asa@hotmail.com
Trauma and Orthopaedics Department, Federal University of Sao Paulo, São Paulo, Brazil

can disturb the management and the indications of treatment [1, 6].

There is no homogeneity in the evaluation of outcomes for the rhizarthrosis treatment. In a systematic review, 316 papers were evaluated, which found 65 instruments for outcome measures after some type of treatment [7]. This lack of standardization of measuring instruments can be a bias in the evaluation of clinical outcomes, and perhaps for this reason, no evidence of the superiority of one treatment over another is found [8].

In an attempt to standardize the evaluation of results, some subjective questionnaires, non-specific, were used to evaluate rhizarthrosis, without much success [7, 8]. We found in the literature three specific questionnaires for the evaluation of rhizarthrosis, all in English language. In 2007, the Nelson Score was described, which had little acceptance [9]. Also, specific to evaluate rhizarthrosis, the Thumb Disability Exam (TDX) questionnaire was described by Noback et al., with 20 questions [11]. At last, in 2016, Trapeziometacarpal Arthrosis Symptoms and Disability (TASD) was described by Becker et al.with the purpose of evaluating symptom intensity and degree of disability, as to compare results after treatment. It was the result of a summary done through information collected from doctors, patients and the literature. It was elaborated with 12 questions in 2 subdivisions, one of them with 7 items related to symptoms, and the other with 5 items related to the inability to perform activities [10].

The questions are answered considering what happened to the patient in the last two weeks. The "intensity of symptoms" was categorized on a scale of 1 (no symptoms) up to 5 (very intense symptoms), and the difficulty of performing activities was categorized on a scale of 1 (without difficulty) up to 5 (unable to do it), following the Likert scale [10]. The results obtained are transformed into a variable between 0 and 100, according the formula [10]:

$$Score - \left(\frac{N}{Q-B} - 1\right) * 25$$

where N is the total sum, Q is the number of total questions and B is the number of questions left blank, being a maximum of 2 to be considered valid. Thus, the higher the score, the greater the disability. This questionnaire are quick to fill out and easy to understand. In the original description, TASD showed good validity and reproducibility in relation to the specific symptoms and limitations of rhizarthrosis [10].

The translation and cultural adaptation process of questionnaires described in other languages is a common practice in the literature. The objective of this process is to make it possible to compare results through a homogeneous outcome, even in papers made in different cultural contexts [12]. Due to its characteristics, TDX has been translated and validated into Portuguese but we didn't find previous translations for TASD, in any other languages [11, 13]. Compared to TDX, the TASD questionnaire is easily and quickly for patients, therefore, the objective of this paper was to translate, do the cultural adaptation and validate the questionnaire "Trapeziometacarpal Arthrosis Symptoms and Disability Questionnarie (TASD)" into the Brazilian Portuguese.

Methods

This survey of translation, cultural adaptation and validation was carried out the postgraduate program in health sciences applied to sport and physical activity and at the hand surgery clinic at the University Hospital. The research was properly approved by the Research Ethics Committee. The authors of the original questionnaire authorized the translation process. All individuals who participated in the study filled out the informed consent form.

The translation and cultural adaptation were done following guidelines of Beaton et al. [14]. Initially, the translation into Brazilian Portuguese was done by two independent translators, one specialist in the medical field and the other specialist in languages. Both with Brazilian Portuguese as their native language. Two translations were achieved: T1 and T2. They were synthesized by an expert committee, reaching a T12 version in Brazilian Portuguese.

This T12 version was handed to two independent translators, different from the first ones, with English as their native language, and the reverse translation was done. So, we come to two reverse translations: BT1 and BT2. The experts committee composed of translators, orthopedists and physiotherapists, reviewed all documents, resolving discrepancies by consensus. The pre-test version of TASD-BR was completed.

The research was carried out using medical records of patients who were diagnosed with rhizarthrosis but had not been submitted to any surgical procedures between 2014 and 2017. We obtained a total of 69 patients, of whom 12 were excluded because of other pre-existing hand and wrist disorders. Out of the remaining 57 patients, 22 were excluded for not attending to phone calls and further 2 patients were excluded for declining to participate in a retest which was to be performed between 2 and 4 weeks after the first test. We therefore remained with 31 patients for the study. Out of these, 15 patients had a bilateral while 16 had a unilateral involvement, totaling 46 assessed hands.

The printed pre-test questionnaire was applied to the patients and completed without assistance. For patients with low education, the researcher, without direct interference, performed a reading. The same researcher made all the applications. The re-test was applied after 2 to 4 weeks, by e-mail or telephone contact, having the same researcher reading and filling out the questionnaire. In patients with bilateral disease, the questionnaire was performed for each hand.

Statistical analysis

The questionnaire validation process was done with the calculation of the psychometric variables. Internal consistency, a measure of the homogeneous relation of the items in the questionnaire, was calculated using Cronbach's α coefficient for each of the items, with $\alpha \geq 0.70$, as described by Streiner and Norman [15]. The ceiling and floor effect was considered when more than 15% of the interviewers reached the maximum (scored 95 or more) or minimum score (scored 5 or less). If this effect occurs, it is a sign of low content validity, and can unite different individuals in the same group, also harming reliability and responsiveness.

Reliability was assessed using the intraclass correlation coefficient (ICC) obtained through the test and re-test. We used the correlation classification scale according to Landis and Koch, through Cohen's kappa coefficient, κ, in which there is a variation from −1 to 1, where 1 means total agreement, −1 means total disagreement and zero means randomness [16]. Agreement was assessed using the standard error of measurement (SEM), which reflects the instrument intrinsic error. The SEM is calculated as the standard deviation of the differences between the scores of the two test and re-test sessions, divided by the square root of 2 [17, 18]. Construct Validity measures the relation of a new instrument with other instruments that theoretically assess similar hypotheses and concepts. It was verified by means of the linear correlation coefficient between Spearman ordinal variables in the translated questionnaires Trapeziometacarpal Arthrosis Symptoms and Disability (TASD-BR) and the Thumb Disability Exam (TDX-BR), considering good validity when the $\rho \geq 0.7$ coefficient [15, 17, 18].

The relation between the final score and the involvement of the dominant member was verified. The comparison was done using a paired t test. Correlations or significant differences were considered to be those in which the p value found was less than or equal to 0.05 [15].

Results

The questionnaire was applied to 31 patients, 29 answered the printed questionnaire individually and two patients with low education had the questionnaire read by a researcher. A total of 15 patients had bilateral involvement, and answered a questionnaire for each of the thumbs. A total of 46 questionnaires were taken.

In the population studied, 83.9% were women, 48.4% had the disease bilaterally, 32.2% only on the left and 19.4% only on the right. However, 90.3% had the right hand as dominant. Regarding the time of symptom beginning, 21.8% had symptoms less than 2 years, 43.4% between 2 and 10 years, and 34.8% more than 10 years.

The results of internal consistency, ceiling and floor effects, agreement and reliability are shown in Table 1. For the questionnaire, and even when separated by subdivisions "symptoms" and "ability to perform activities", high internal consistency was found ($\alpha > 0.70$), ceiling and floor notable effect were not observed, high confidence ($\kappa > 0.60$), and the agreement was considered as good (< 10%) or very good (< 5%) [15, 17, 18].

The construct validity was also shown to be high ($\rho = 0.893$, $p < 0.001$). Comparing the TASD-BR with the TDX-BR, previously translated, they demonstrate a linear relation, according to the dispersion graph in Fig. 1.

In 46 evaluated hands, 54.3% were non-dominant hands and 45.7% were dominant hands. The fact that the disease affects the dominant or non-dominant hand did not cause significant differences ($t = 0.34$; $p = 0.736$) (Fig. 2).

Patient related difficulties in completing the questionnaires, and the patients fill out once, without limit of

Table 1 Internal consistency, Floor and ceiling effects, reliability and agreement for the TASD questionnaire (n = 46)

	Cronbach's α	Floor/ceiling (in %)[a]	ICC – κ (IC95%)[b]	(SEM in %)[c]
TASD	0.927	4.3%/0%	0.961 (0.954–0.967)	3.87
Symptoms	0.919	2.2%/0%	0.966 (0.957–0.972)	3.68
Ability to perform activities	0.847	6.5%/2.2%	0.955 (0.942–0.965)	5.49

[a] Percentage of scores less than 5 or greater than 95

[b] ICC—Intraclass Correlation Coefficient

[c] SEM—Standard Error of Measurement

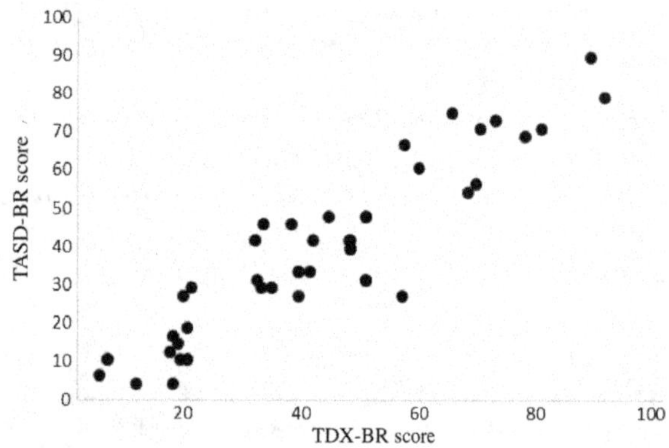

Fig. 1 Correlation between the patients' scores on the TDX-BR and TASD-BR questionnaires

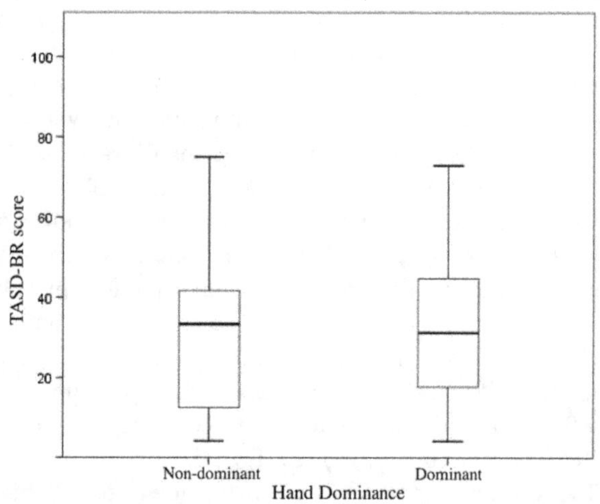

Fig. 2 Box diagram for TASD-BR score, in relation to the dominant or non-dominant hand

time or prior verification. All patients evaluated considered the questions clear and easy to understand. So the experts committee decided to not change the pre-test version and we concluded the final version of TASD-BR (Fig. 3).

Discussion

The diagnosis of rhizarthrosis is based on clinical signs and symptoms confirmed by imaging exams. The clinical condition of rhizarthrosis is characterized by progressive pain, limitation of pinch activities involving the thumb, edema at the base of the thumb, apparent angular deviation and crackling [19]. However, Baker et al. in reviewing the evidence-based literature observed that most of the patients with radiological images of rhizarthrosis are asymptomatic. The alterations found in the imaging exams do not always correspond to the clinical condition presented, that means, patients with typical alterations in the imaging exam may have mild symptoms or even be asymptomatic [20, 21].

Self-assessment questionnaires have been used in the literature to evaluate treatment results for different health problems. The translation and cultural adaptation to Brazilian Portuguese makes it possible to use these instruments in Brazil [22–24]. In search for a more specific tool, questionnaires have been described to evaluate the pain intensity and the functional limitation caused by rhizarthrosis. In 2007, the Nelson Score was described, which presents 10 questions about daily activities of living, with the objective of evaluating the surgical results of rhizarthrosis [9]. In 2016, the Thumb Disability Exam (TDX) was described, which consists of 20 questions. During the translation and validation process, it was considered reproducible for Brazilian Portuguese (TDX-BR), although difficulties in understanding some questions have been described, according to the translators [13]. In the description of the TASD, Becker et al.considered to be a simple and self-administered scoring system and was considered concise and useful in the evaluating of symptoms and disability related to rhizarthrosis [20]. In our paper, the application of the translated and validated TASD-BR to patients did not present any difficulty in understanding. We consider this questionnaire to be more concise and simpler, even though it maintains a good linear correlation with the TDX-BR. The time to complete the questionnaire was not measured, but because there are eight questions less than the TDX-BR, we deduce to be shorter.

Following the recommendations of Matsuo et al., we chose to keep the page in vertical format, as it facilitates understanding in the Brazilian socio-cultural context [25].

The method used to apply this questionnaire should be considered as a limitation factor. The first application was done personally with all the patients. The second application was carried out through telephone or e-mail contacts. We only had personal interviews with 2 patients who did not know how to read. This is used to prevent social exclusion of patients due to low education levels which could lead to reduction of the sample [26, 27]. Furthermore, many patients had financial limitations to move back to the hospital to a new evaluation. Since we never experienced or witnessed any difficulty in understanding the questionnaire during the first application, we considered that the second method of data collection could not result in significant results discrepancy.

For the TASD-BR questionnaire, and even when separated by subdivisions "symptoms" and "ability to perform activities", high internal consistency was found,

TASD-BR: Responda o Questionário com apenas uma alternativa:

Por favor, diga a intensidade dos seguintes sintomas:

1. Você sente dor na base dos seu polegar (próximo ao punho), sem atividades (mesmo quando não mexe o polegar)?
   1. NENHUMA
   2. LEVE
   3. MODERADA
   4. INTENSA
   5. MUITO INTENSA

2. Você sente dor na base dos seu polegar (próximo ao punho) durante atividades (quando mexe o polegar)?
   1. NENHUMA
   2. LEVE
   3. MODERADA
   4. INTENSA
   5. MUITO INTENSA

3. Você sente desconforto (incômodo) na base do polegar (próximo ao punho) quando aperta ou encosta em alguma coisa?
   1. NENHUM
   2. LEVE
   3. MODERADO
   4. INTENSO
   5. MUITO INTENSO

4. Você percebe inchaço (edema) na base do polegar (próximo ao punho)?
   1. NENHUM
   2. LEVE
   3. MODERADO
   4. INTENSO
   5. MUITO INTENSO

5. Você percebe Rigidez (endurecimento) na base do polegar (próximo ao punho) quando faz algum movimento?
   1. NENHUM (A)
   2. LEVE
   3. MODERADO (A)
   4. INTENSO (A)
   5. MUITO INTENSO (A)

6. Quanto você perdeu de movimento do polegar?
   1. NENHUM
   2. LEVE
   3. MODERADO
   4. INTENSO
   5. MUITO INTENSO

7. Você sente diminuição de força quando pega e segura algum objeto?
   1. NENHUMA
   2. LEVE
   3. MODERADA
   4. INTENSA
   5. MUITO INTENSA

Por favor avalie quanta dificuldade você tem ao fazer as seguintes atividades:

1. Abrir um pote ou garrafa com tampa de rosca apertada ou nova
   1. SEM DIFICULDADE
   2. UM POUCO DE DIFICULDADE
   3. DIFICULDADE MODERADA
   4. MUITA DIFICULDADE
   5. NÃO CONSEGUE FAZER

2. Virar uma chave (de uma porta)
   1. SEM DIFICULDADE
   2. UM POUCO DE DIFICULDADE
   3. DIFICULDADE MODERADA
   4. MUITA DIFICULDADE
   5. NÃO CONSEGUE FAZER

3. Girar a maçaneta redonda (do tipo bola) da porta
   1. SEM DIFICULDADE
   2. UM POUCO DE DIFICULDADE
   3. DIFICULDADE MODERADA
   4. MUITA DIFICULDAE
   5. NÃO CONSEGUE FAZER

4. Fechar o zíper (fecho-ecler)
   1. SEM DIFICULDADE
   2. UM POUCO DE DIFICULDADE
   3. DIFICULDADE MODERADA
   4. MUITA DIFICULDAE
   5. NÃO CONSEGUE FAZER

5. Segurar objetos grandes (copo, garrafa, livro, etc.)
   1. SEM DIFICULDADE
   2. UM POUCO DE DIFICULDADE
   3. DIFICULDADE MODERADA
   4. MUITA DIFICULDAE
   5. NÃO CONSEGUE FAZER

Fig. 3 TASD-BR final version

with $\alpha \geq 0.70$, and notable ceiling and floor effect were not observed. Internal consistency is the measurement property that assesses the ability of a questionnaire to measure a single concept using multiple items, or even evaluating it in subdivisions. Therefore, it is extremely important that this value is high, as they denote specificity in testing a construct.

We chose the interval of 2 to 4 weeks between the test and the re-test. This interval should be sufficient to avoid any change in symptoms or progression of the disease, neither for the patient to be able to remember the answers that he had answered in the previous questionnaire [18]. The questionnaire showed high reliability. Intraclass correlation coefficient (ICC) values greater than 0.60 are considered to be a good correlation. In our study, this value was $\kappa = 0.961$ (0.954–0.967). These values denote a high correlation between test and retest and demonstrate that the questionnaire is reliable in reproducing symptoms.

Agreement, measured using the SEM, was considered to be good (< 10%) or very good (< 5%). The questionnaire had a high correlation between the test and the retest, with $\kappa = 0.961$ (0.954–0.967). All variables maintained the same pattern when compared to the original questionnaire [10, 17, 18].

Construct Validity measures the relation of a new instrument with other instruments that theoretically assess similar hypotheses and concepts. As there was no description of a specific gold standard questionnaire for rhizarthrosis, the original TASD questionnaire maintained a linear correlation with The Disabilities of Arm Shoulder and Hand Score (DASH), Patient Health Questionnaire-9 (PHQ9) and Pain Self Efficacy Questionnaire (PSEQ) [10, 14]. In our research, the construct validity was measured by the correlation between the results of the TDX-BR questionnaire, previously translated [13]. A linear relation was found between the two questionnaires. This means that high scores on the TDX-BR must correlate with high scores on the TASD-BR, and vice versa. This correlation denotes efficiency in the two scores in measuring the same construct [15, 17, 18].

Although the disease was more prevalent in the non-dominant hand, the difference was not significant, and no correlation was found in the TASD-BR scores considering that. Thus, we conclude that this fact should not be considered as bias.

Conclusion

We consider the TASD questionnaire as translated into Brazilian Portuguese. The TASD-BR version is valid. Following consolidated guidelines, we have an objective instrument, which can be used in research related to rhizarthrosis in Brazil, in evaluating outcomes or diagnoses, with no need for authorization from the authors or training to apply.

Abbreviations

TASD: Trapeziometacarpal Arthrosis Symptoms and Disability; TASD-BR: Portuguese version of Trapeziometacarpal Arthrosis Symptoms and Disability; TDX: Thumb Disability Exam; ICC: Intraclass correlation coefficient; SEM: Standard error of measurement; TDX-BR: Portuguese version of Thumb Disability Exam; DASH: The Disabilities of Arm Shoulder and Hand Score; PHQ9: Patient Health Questionnaire-9; PSEQ: Pain Self Efficacy Questionnaire.

Acknowledgements

Not applicable

Authors' contributions

VASA did the interviews and applied the questionnaires to the participants, and was the major contributor in writing the manuscript. VASA, CHF and LMM where part of the experts committee. All authors read and approved the final manuscript.

References

1. Güven N, Dinçer F, Çetin A, et al. Hand strenght and dexterity in interphalangeal hand osteoarthritis and effects of osteophyte formations. Adv Rheumatol. 2020. https://doi.org/10.1186/s42358-020-00143-7.
2. Sacilotto NDC, Giorgi RDN, Vargas-Santos AB, et al. Real-rheumatoid arthritis in real life-study cohort: a sociodemographic profile of rheumatoid arthritis in Brazil. Adv Rheumatol. 2020. https://doi.org/10.1186/s42358-020-0121-5.
3. Hume MC, Gellman H, McKellop H, et al. Functional range of motion of the joints of the hand. J Hand Surg. 1990;15A(2):240–3.
4. Spaans AJ, Van Minnen LP, Kon M, et al. Conservative treatment of thumb base osteoarthritis: a systematic review. J Hand Surg. 2015;40(1):16–21.
5. Model Z, Liu AY, Kang L, et al. Evaluation of physical examination tests for thumb basal joint osteoarthritis. HAND. 2016;11(1):108–12.
6. Siviero P, Zambon S, Limongi F, et al. How hand osteoarthritis, comorbidity, and pain interact to determine functional limitation in older people: observations from the European Project on OSteoArthritis Study. Arthritis Rheumatol. 2016;68(11):2662–70.
7. Marks M, Schoones JW, Kolling C, et al. Outcome measures and their measurement properties for trapeziometacarpal osteoarthritis: a systematic literature review. J Hand Surg (European Volume). 2013;38(8):822–38.
8. Visser AW, Boyesen P, Haugen IK, et al. Instruments measuring pain, physical function, or Patient's global assessment in hand osteoarthritis: a systematic literature search. J Rheumatol. 2015. https://doi.org/10.3899/jrheum.141228.
9. Citron N, Hulme CE, Wardle N. A self-administered questionnaire for basal osteoarthritis of the thumb. J Hand Surg (European Volume). 2007;32(5):524–8.
10. Becker SJ, Teunis T, Ring D, et al. The trapeziometacarpal arthrosis symptoms and disability questionnaire: development and preliminary validation. HAND. 2016;11(2):197–205.
11. Noback PC, Lombardi JM, Seetharaman M, et al. Development and validation of a disease-specific questionnaire for basal joint arthritis. J Wrist Surg. 2017;6(02):126–33.
12. Guillemin F, Bombardier C, Beaton D. Cross-cultural adaptation of health-related quality of life measures: literature review and proposed guidelines. J Clin Epidemiol. 1993;46(12):1417–32.
13. Almeida VAS, Fernandes CH, Meireles LM, et al. Tradução e adaptação cultural do questionário "Thumb Disability Exam–TDX" para o português brasileiro. Revista Brasileira de Ortopedia. 2020. https://doi.org/10.1055/s-0040-1715508.
14. Beaton DE, Bombardier C, Guillemin F, Ferraz MB. Guidelines for the process of cross-cultural adaptation of self-report measures. Spine. 2000;25:3186–91.
15. Norman GR, Streiner DL. Biostatistics: the bare essentials. Shelton: PMPH-USA; 2008.

16. Landis JR, Koch GG. The measurement of observer agreement for categorical data. Biometrics. 1977. https://doi.org/10.2307/2529310.
17. Terwee CB, Bot SD, de Boer MR, et al. Quality criteria were proposed for measurement properties of health status questionnaires. J Clin Epidemiol. 2007;60(1):34–42.
18. Da Cunha RA, Hazime FA, da Silva Martins MC, et al. Translation, cross-cultural adaptation, and clinimetric testing of instruments used to assess patients with ankle sprain in the brazilian population. J Orthop Sports Phys Ther. 2016;46(12):1042–50.
19. Baker RH, Al-Shukri J, Davis TR. Evidence-based medicine: thumb basal joint arthritis. Plast Reconstr Surg. 2017;139(1):256e–66e.
20. Ladd AL, Messana JM, Berger AJ, et al. Correlation of clinical disease severity to radiographic thumb osteoarthritis index. J Hand Surg. 2015;40(3):474–82.
21. Becker SJ, Bruinsma WE, Guitton TG, et al. Interobserver agreement of the Eaton–Glickel classification for trapeziometacarpal and scaphotrapezial arthrosis. J Hand Surg. 2016;41(4):532–40.
22. Azevedo PM, Sanson ES, Skare TL, et al. The Brazillian version of the hand mobility in scleroderma (HAMIS) test: translation and validation. Adv Rheumatol. 2019. https://doi.org/10.1186/s42358-019-0093-5.
23. Carvalho GRD, Oliveira EAD, Rocha VTM, et al. Cross-cultural adaptation and reliability of the pain response to activity and position questionnaire. Adv Rheumatol. 2019. https://doi.org/10.1186/s42358-019-0098-0.
24. De Paula Costa RM, Cardinot TM, Mathias LNCDC, et al. Validation of the Brazilian version of the hip outcome score (HOS) questionnaire. Adv Rheumatol. 2018;58(1):1–8.
25. Matsuo RP, Fernandes CH, Meirelles LM, et al. Translation and cross-cultural adaptation of the 6-item Carpal Tunnel Syndrome Symptoms Scale and Palmar Pain Scale Questionnaire Into Brazilian Portuguese. Hand NY. 2016;11(2):168–72.
26. Fernandes CH, Neto JR, Meirelles LM, et al. Translation and cultural adaptation of the Brief Michigan Hand Questionnaire to Brazilian Portuguese language. HAND. 2014;9(3):370–4.
27. Oku EC, Andrade AP, Stadiniky SP, et al. Translation and cultural adaptation of the Modified-University of California at Los Angeles Shoulder Rating Scale to portuguese language. Rev Bras Reumatol. 2006;46(4):246–52.

2

Performance of 4 methods for screening of latent tuberculosis infection in patients with chronic inflammatory arthritis under TNFα inhibitors: A 24-month prospective study

Carina M. F. Gomes[1], Maria Teresa Terreri[2], Maria Isabel Moraes-Pinto[3] and Marcelo M. Pinheiro[4*]

Abstract

Background: The reactivation rate of tuberculosis in patients with chronic inflammatory arthritis (CIA) on TNFα inhibitors (TNFi) and baseline negative screening for latent tuberculosis infection (LTBI) is higher than in the general population.

Aim: To compare the performance of tuberculin skin test (TST), TST-Booster, ELISPOT (T-SPOT.TB) and QuantiFERON-TB Gold in tube (QFT-IT) to detect LTBI in patients with CIA on TNFi.

Patients and methods: A total of 102 patients with CIA [rheumatoid arthritis (RA), n = 40; ankylosing spondylitis (AS), n = 35; psoriatic arthritis (PsA), n = 7; and juvenile idiopathic arthritis (JIA), n = 20] were prospectively followed-up for 24 months to identify incident LTBI cases. Epidemiologic data, TST, T-SPOT.TB, QFT-IT and a chest X-ray were performed at baseline and after 6 months of LTBI treatment.

Results: Thirty six percent (37/102) of patients had positive TST or Interferon Gamma Release Assays (IGRAs) tests. Agreement among TST and IGRAs was moderate (k = 0.475; $p = 0.001$), but high between T-SPOT.TB and QFT-IT (k = 0.785; $p < 0.001$). During the 24-Month follow-up, 15 (18.5%) incident cases of LTBI were identified. In comparison to TST, the IGRAs increased the LTBI diagnosis power in 8.5% (95% CI 3.16–17.49). TST-Booster did not add any value in patients with negative TST at baseline. After 6-Month isoniazid therapy, IGRAs results did not change significantly.

Conclusions: Almost 20% of CIA patients had some evidence of LTBI, suggesting higher conversion rate after exposition to TNFi. TST was effective in identifying new cases of LTBI, but IGRAs added diagnostic power in this scenario. Our findings did not support the repetition of IGRAs after 6-Month isoniazid therapy and this approach was effective to mitigate active TB in 2 years of follow-up.

Keywords: Latent tuberculosis infection, Chronic inflammatory arthritis, TNFα inhibitors, IGRAs, Prospective cohort, Non-interventional trial

Introduction

TNFα inhibitors are important therapeutic agents used for the management of pain, inflammation, quality of life and function in patients with chronic inflammatory arthritis (CIA), including rheumatoid arthritis (RA) [1], psoriatic arthritis (PsA) [2], ankylosing spondylitis (AS) [3] and juvenile idiopathic arthritis (JIA) [4]. However,

*Correspondence: mpinheiro@uol.com.br
[4] Head of the Spondyloarthritis and Immunobiological Therapy Section, Rheumatology Division, Universidade Federal de Sao Paulo (Unifesp/EPM), Rua Leandro Dupré, 204, Conj. 74, Vila Clementino, São Paulo, SP CEP 04025-010, Brazil

these drugs, particularly the monoclonal inhibitors, are associated with an increased risk of reactivation of latent tuberculosis infection (LTBI) [5]. In this context, the clinical presentation of active tuberculosis (TB) occurs in the first 12 months of treatment with biolological drugs and some TB cases are severe, including extrapulmonary and miliary forms, which limit the clinical management of the underlying disease [6]. The pathophysiological mechanism is related to granuloma disorganization after TNFα inhibition in patients with latent forms or after re-exposure to *Mycobacterium tuberculosis* (*M. tuberculosis*) [6].

The incidence of active TB is approximately 3–9 times higher in patients on TNFα inhibitors than in the general population (86.9 cases per 100,000 person-years vs. 35.8 cases per 100,000 person-years, respectively) [7]. Therefore, different strategies have been developed to minimize the risk. Several guidelines have recommended to use tuberculin skin test (TST), as well as to assess epidemiological background and chest X-ray for diagnosing LTBI. If LTBI is identified, treatment is recommended. The LTBI treatment with isoniazid for 6 months was valid, safe, and efficient in patients with RA [8].

Moreover, active TB cases have been identified in patients with negative baseline LTBI test, particularly among those with AS [7]. Therefore, additional strategies, including the interferon gamma release assays (IGRAs), are necessary to better identify high-risk patients and to minimize the impact of incident TB cases. These tests were developed after the recognition of crucial role of IFN-gamma on cellular response against the *M. tuberculosis*, by specific targeting the peptides ESAT-6 and CFP-10, which are not present in the bacillus Calmette–Guérin (BCG) vaccine neither in most of the other non-tuberculous mycobacteria [9].

The aim of this study was to compare the performance of three methods for detecting LTBI, including TST, QuantiFERON-TB Gold in tube (QFT-IT) test and ELISPOT (T-SPOT.TB), in patients with active CIA on anti-TNFα therapy. In addition, we aimed to evaluate the TST-Booster phenomenon effectiveness in diagnosing LTBI, as well as to verify incident cases of mycobacterial infection in a 24-Month follow-up and to test the IGRA positivity after treatment with isoniazid for 6 months.

Patients and methods

A total of 102 patients with CIA classified according to classification criteria as RA [1], PsA [2], AS [3] and JIA [4] were selected and consecutively screened from Rheumatology and Paediatric Rheumatology Outpatients Clinic of the Federal University of São Paulo, Paulista School of Medicine (Universidade Federal de São Paulo/ Escola Paulista de Medicina, Unifesp/ EPM). All of them were on TNFα inhibitors for at least 6 months. However, 21 patients had previous positive TST and had been treated for LTBI according to local standard guidelines. Therefore, this study included 81 patients who were negative TST before starting TNFα inhibitors and were followed up for 24 months. Patients with active TB, previous neoplasms or other current infections were excluded.

Demographic data, medical history and concomitant medications were recorded. Disease activity was assessed using the Disease Activity Score (DAS28) [10] for RA, the Bath Ankylosing Spondylitis Disease Activity Index (BASDAI) for AS [11], the Psoriasis Area Severity Index (PASI) [12] for PsA and the Wallace criteria [13] for JIA. All participants answered a questionnaire about TB disease symptoms, including cough, weight loss, fever and sweating. Epidemiological data regarding personal, professional and family contact with TB, as well as BCG vaccination were also recorded. Chest X-rays were evaluated by a radiologist and by a rheumatologist, and tomography was performed, in case of disagreement between specialists. TST and IGRAs were conducted performed in this group of 81 patients with previous negative TST test before starting TNFα inhibitors.

TST was conducted via an intradermal inoculation of 0.1 mL (2 UT) of PPD-RT-23 (Statens Serum Institute, Denmark) on the left forearm, approximately 8 cm below the elbow crease. The results were read 72 h after inoculation by a trained nurse. TST was considered positive if the measured area of induration had a diameter larger than or equal to 5 mm. In case of negative results, a TST-Booster was performed, which consisted in repeating the TST in the contralateral forearm within 3 weeks after the first reading. TST-Booster was considered positive when the total area of induration was larger than 10 mm or whether the induration was 6 mm greater than the first TST measurement [14].

Blood samples were collected in the same visit along with TST and IGRAs. A 7 mL blood sample was collected from each patient: 3 mL were transferred to specific test tubes for use in the third generation QFT-IT system (Cellestis, Carnegie, Australia), and the remaining 4 mL were transferred to heparinized tubes for T-SPOT.TB (Oxford Immunitec, Abingdon, UK). All assays were performed according to the manufacturer's instructions.

In case of current contact with TB, chest X-ray suggestive alterations or positivity for TST, T-SPOT.TB or QFT-IT, but without evidence of active TB detected, patients were treated with isoniazid (10 mg/kg/day, maximum of 300 mg/day) for 6 months. After that, TST, T-SPOT.TB or QFT-IT were repeated and the patients were monitored for signs and symptoms of active TB during 24 months. Medical appointments occurred monthly during the first 6 months and quarterly thereafter. In addition, the LTBI tests (TST and IGRAs) were defined as modified if the status became from negative to positive or vice-versa after 6-Month of isoniazid treatment. In addition, the remaining 21 patients were clinically prospectively followed for 24 months to evaluate the active tuberculosis incidence.

Statistical analysis

Descriptive analyses were performed with demographic, anthropometric and clinical data for each CIA. Both baseline and current LTBI tests (after exposition to TNFα inhibitors), including TST, chest X-ray and epidemiology, were compared. The Kolmogorov–Smirnov test and Levine's test were used to test the normal data distribution. Categorical variables were compared using chi-square test and Fisher's exact test, when appropriate. Continuous variables with a non-normal distribution were compared using the Mann–Whitney test, whereas continuous variables with a normal distribution were compared using analysis of variance (ANOVA). The agreement between the tests was assessed using the kappa test. The qualitative results of the tests before and after the treatment of LTBI were compared using McNemar's test. The increment rate was calculated considering the percentage of cases detected by IGRAs methods (T-SPOT.TB or QFT-IT) but not by TST. All statistical analyses were performed using SPSS version 20.0 (IBM, USA). p value was set as 0.05.

Results

A total of 102 patients including 82 adults with CIA (40 with RA, 35 with AS and 7 with PsA) and 20 children with JIA were enrolled in this 24-month prospective study. RA patients had a predominance of women, while AS and PsA group had male predominance. The demographic and clinical data, including concomitant medication (conventional disease-modifying antirheumatic drugs [cDMARDs] and TNFα inhibitors) are shown in Table 1. Also, all tests to detect LTBI were performed before, as a recommended screening protocol by the Brazilian health authorities, and after TNFα inhibitors exposition, as research protocol design. The mean time interval since the introduction of these agents can be found in Table 1.

Table 1 Demographic and clinical data of patients treated with TNFα inhibitors

Parameter	JIA (n = 20)	RA (n = 40)	AS (n = 35)	PsA (n = 7)	*p* value
Age (years)	14.2 ± 7.2[a]	55.5 ± 9.3[c]	42.8 ± 9.9[b]	54.3 ± 6.7[c]	0.001
Female sex	12 (60%)	36 (90%)	10 (28.5%)	3 (42.9%)	0.001
Length of disease (years)	5.6 ± 3.3[a]	14.8 ± 8.2[b]	12.5 ± 7.7[b]	18.0 ± 7.9	0.001
Disease activity					
BASDAI			1.76 ± 1.51		
DAS28		2.86 ± 0.8			
PASI				2.68 ± 4.12	
Current medications					
Concomitant					
GC	1 (5%)	11 (27.5%)	0	0	0.001
Methotrexate	7 (35%)	17 (42.5%)	3 (8.6%)	5 (71.4%)	0.001
Leflunomide	7 (35%)	20 (50%)	0	1 (14.3%)	0.001
Sulfasalazine	0	0	4 (11.4%)	0	0.079
NSAIDs	2 (10%)	0	12 (34.3%)	0	0.001
CG	1 (5%)	11 (27.5%)	0	0	0.001
Cyclosporine	1 (5%)	0	0	0	0.267
Mesalazine	2 (10%)	0	0	0	0.07
Length of TNFi use to TNF inhibitorsα (years)	1.4 ± 1.1[a]	2.4 ± 1.9[a]	3.5 ± 1.6[b]	3.9 ± 1.9[b]	0.001
TNFα inhibitors					0.057
Adalimumab	5 (25%)	11 (27.5%)	7 (20%)	4 (57.2%)	
Etanercept	9 (45%)	22 (55%)	14 (40%)	0	
Infliximab	6 (30%)	7 (17.5%)	14 (40%)	3 (42.8%)	

Student's *t*-test, ANOVA; JIA, juvenile idiopathic arthritis; RA, rheumatoid arthritis; AS, ankylosing spondylitis; PsA, psoriatic arthritis; DAS-28, Disease Activity Score; BASDAI, Bath Ankylosing Spondylitis Disease Activity Index; PASI, Psoriasis Area Severity Index; NSAIDs, non-steroidal anti-inflammatory drugs; TNFi, TNF inhibitors; GC, glucocorticosteroids; (a) and (b) had different means according to Duncan's multiple comparison test (age and period of exposure) or (c) Dunnet's test at an overall level of significance of 5%

Despite living in an endemic country for TB, only twelve (11.8%) patients had consistent positive epidemiology. Three patients had chest X-ray abnormalities, including two with a calcified nodule (patient with RA, but negative for TST and IGRAs and another patient with AS, but positive for TST and IGRAs) and one with pulmonary fibrosis (patient with RA and negative for TST and IGRAs). RA, AS, PsA and JIA patients did not differ concerning to epidemiological data and chest X-ray findings. Regarding BCG, all children and adolescents with JIA had vaccine scar and BCG recorded on vaccination card. Although no adult patient had BCG vaccine recorded, a BCG scar was observed in more than 70% of patients with PsA and AS and 47% of RA patients (Table 2).

Patients with RA had lower TST positivity (30%) than those with AS (37.1%) and PsA (42.9%) ($p=0.017$). No patient with JIA had a positive TST. There was no significant difference regarding T-SPOT.TB and QFT-IT positivity among adult patients (31.7% and 22%, respectively). On the other hand, only one patient with JIA had a positive IGRA (T-SPOT.TB and QFT-IT). There was no association among the TNFα inhibitors and positivity of the 3 tests (TST, T-SPOT.TB and QFT-IT) (Table 3). TST-Booster was positive in only 3 patients (2 with AS and one with RA). These patients had baseline negative TST, but a positive IGRA in 2 of them (one for T-SPOT.TB and another one for QFT-IT), suggesting some agreement between TST-Booster and IGRA results. However, the TST-Booster did not add any value to identify LTBI.

Considering the 81 patients with negative TST pre-anti-TNFα screening, 10 of them (12.3%; 95% CI 6.1–21.5) became positive for TST after exposure to TNFα inhibitors. Among the remaining 71 patients, 6 had positive IGRAs [T-SPOT.TB, n = 6, 7.4% (95% CI 2.8–15.4); QFT-IT, n = 4, 4.9% (95% CI 1.4–12.1)] (Fig. 1). Four of them were positive for both QFT-IT and SPOT.TB.

Table 3 Positivity of TST, T-SPOT.TB and Quantiferon after treatment with TNFα inhibitors

LTBI tests	ADA (n = 27)	ETA (n = 45)	IFX (n = 30)	*p* value
TST	6 (22.2%)	14 (31.1%)	8 (26.7%)	0.75
T-SPOT.TB	4 (14.8%)	16 (35.6%)	7 (23.3%)	0.15
QFT-IT	3 (11.1%)	11 (24.4%)	5 (16.7%)	0.38

ADA, adalimumab; ETA, etanercept; IFX, infliximab; TST, tuberculin skin test; T-SPOT. TB, elispot; QFT-IT, quantiferon; LTBI, latent tuberculosis infection

The remaining 65 patients were negative for the 3 LTBI screening tests. However, patients with AS had moderate agreement between TST and IGRAs (kappa = 0.697; $p<0.01$), but 100% concordance between the T-SPOT.TB and QFT-IT. Similarly, total agreement between the T-SPOT.TB and QFT-IT was observed with JIA patients. The worst agreement was seen in patients with RA (TST and IGRAs: kappa = 0.294; T-SPOT.TB and QFT-IT: kappa = 0.632). Analysing only 35 AS patients, 22 of them had negative TST and IGRAs; 28 patients had negative QTF-IT and 25 had negative T-SPOT.TB. The Fig. 2 is showing only the 15 pacients who presented at least one positive test for LTBI. There was moderate agreement between the TST and IGRAs (kappa = 0.475; $p=0.001$) and high agreement between T-SPOT.TB and QFT-IT (kappa = 0.785, $p<0.001$).

In comparison to TST, IGRAs increased the diagnosis of LTBI in 8.5% (95% CI 3.16–17.49), particularly the T-SPOT.TB [8.5% for T-SPOT.TB (95% CI 3.16–7.49) vs. 5.6% (95% CI 1.56–13.8) for QFT-IT]. All patients with a positive QFT-IT test were also positive for T-SPOT.TB. In addition, all patients with a negative TST or T-SPOT.TB had also a negative QFT-IT.

Among the 81 patients who had a negative TST prior to TNFα therapy screening, 15 (18.5%) new cases of LTBI were identified after exposure to them. They were treated

Table 2 Clinical features and test results suggestive of latent tuberculosis infection in patients with chronic inflammatory arthritis after exposure to TNFα inhibitors

LTBI parameters	JIA (n = 20)	RA (n = 40)	AS (n = 35)	PsA (n = 7)	*p* value
BCG scar	20 (100%)	19 (47.5%)	27 (77.1%)	5 (71.4%)	0.001
Chest X-ray abnormalities	0	2 (5%)	1 (2.8%)	0	0.834
Positive TB epidemiology	0	7 (17.5%)	4 (11.4%)	1 (14.3%)	0.214
Positive TST	0	12 (30%)	13 (37.1%)	3 (42.9%)	0.017
Positive IGRA					
T-SPOT.TB	1 (5%)	14 (35%)	10 (28.6%)	2 (28.6%)	0.097
Quantiferon	1 (5%)	9 (22.5%)	7 (20%)	2 (28.6%)	0.277

JIA, juvenile idiopathic arthritis; RA, rheumatoid arthritis; AS, ankylosing spondylitis; PsA, psoriatic arthritis; BCG, Bacillus Calmette-Guérin, TB, tuberculosis, LTBI, latent tuberculosis infection; TST, tuberculin skin test; IGRA, interferon gamma release assay; T-SPOT.TB, Elispot

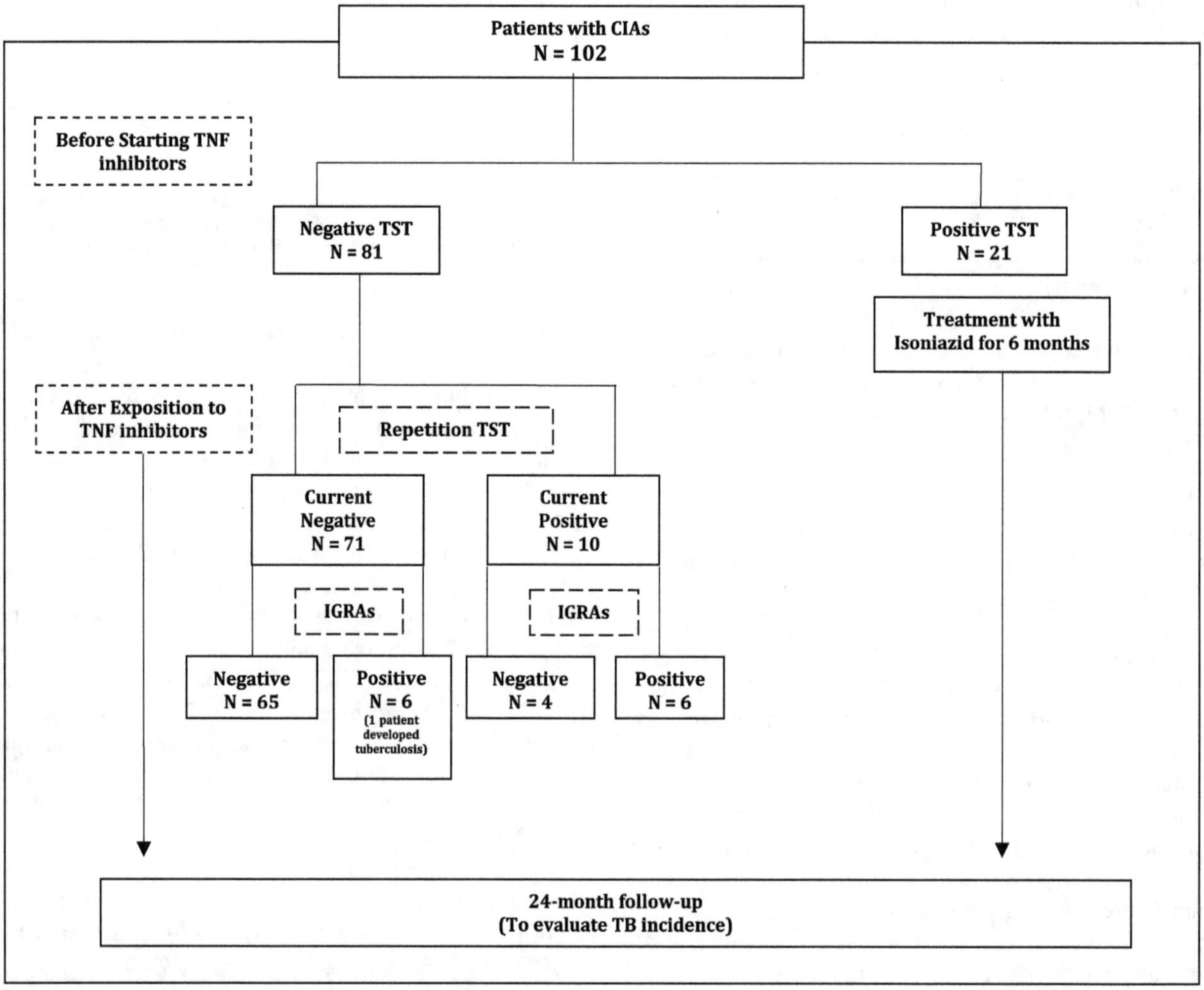

Fig. 1 Flowchart of TST and IGRAs after TNFα inhibitors introduction during a 24-Month follow-up, including a cross-sectional and other prospective phase

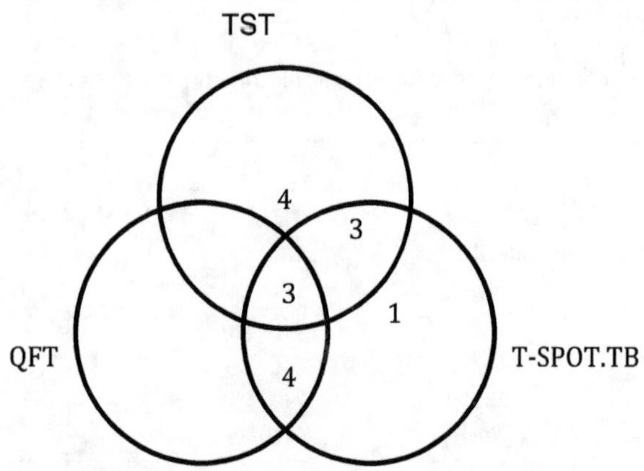

Fig. 2 Agreement among tests for LTBI screening

with isoniazid for 6 months and followed monthly. Considering that none of them had any symptom related to active TB, including fever, cough, weight loss and sweating, there was no withdrawal of TNFα-inhibitors after positive TST in patients on biological therapy.

After LTBI treatment with isoniazid, we observed some modifications of 3 tests results. For TST, 2/15 patients became negative; for T-SPOT.TB, 2/13 patients became negative. On the other hand, 4/15 patients changed QFT-IT status [3 became positive and one negative]. At least one LTBI screening test was positive after 6-Month treatment with isoniazid (Table 4). The observed modifications in IGRA results did not have any clinical implication in the management of patients. None of them developed active tuberculosis in 24 months.

From the group of patients with negative IGRAs and QFT-IT negative, during 24-Month follow-up, only 1 patient with AS had pleuropulmonary tuberculosis,

Table 4 Main outcomes and test results of new 15 patients with LTBI before and after treatment with isoniazid

Patient	Dx	TNF blocker	LT (years)	EPI	BCG	TST	Booster	ELISPOT	QFT	TST after	ELISPOT after	QFT after treatment
1	AS	ETA	3	–	+	10	NA	+	–	15	–	–
2	PsA	IFX	4	–	–	8	NA	+	+	7	+	+
3	AS	ETA	1	–	+	0	3	+	+	0	+	–
4*	AS	IFX	3	–	+	10	NA	+	+	0	+	+
5	AS	ADA	5	–	–	10	NA	+	–	10	Indet	–
6	RA	IFX	1	–	–	5	NA	+	+	20	+	+
7	RA	ETA	2	–	–	0	0	+	+	4	–	+
8	RA	ETA	1	+	+	16	NA	–	–	15	–	–
9	RA	IFX	2	–	+	9	NA	+	–	8	+	+
10	RA	ETA	3	–	+	15	NA	–	–	0	–	+
11	JIA	ETA	2	–	+	0	0	+	+	0	+	+
12	PsA	IFX	3	–	–	10	NA	–	–	8	Indet	–
13	AS	ADA	2	–	–	5	NA	–	–	5	–	–
14	RA	ETA	3	–	+	0	0	+	–	0	+	+
15	RA	ETA	1	+	+	4	10	+	+	4	+	+

* Patient diagnosed with pulmonary TB before and after treatment

RA, rheumatoid arthritis; AS, ankylosing spondylitis; PsA, psoriatic arthritis; JIA, juvenile idiopathic arthritis; TNF, tumor necrosis factor blockers; ADA, adalimumab; IFX, infliximab; ETA, etanercept; Dx, diagnosis; LT, length of treatment (in years); EPI, epidemiology; BCG, Bacillus Calmette-Guérin; TST, tuberculin skin test (in mm); QFT, Quantiferon, NA, not available; Indet, indeterminate

despite the fact that he had negative TST twice (before and after TNF-α inhibitors exposition), as well as negative IGRAs and PPD-Booster. He was on infliximab for 3 years and developed cough, fever and radiographic abnormalities (left upper lobe consolidation). Histopathological examination of lung specimen showed chronic granulomatous pleuritis with positive acid-fast bacilli, confirming pleuropulmonary TB. The TNFα blocker was withdrawn, and he was treated with rifampicin, isoniazid, pyrazinamide and ethambutol for 6 months with good outcome. Regarding the remaining 21 patients with previous LTBI treatment before starting TNF inhibitors, none of them had active TB during 24-Month follow-up.

None of clinical, laboratory or imaging parameters had a positive predictive value for changes or conversion of the LTBI tests in patients with CIA, including epidemiological data, joint disease activity, concomitant medications, type and length of use of TNFα inhibitors and vaccination with BCG.

Discussion

This study was the first to compare the efficacy of 3 approved tests for LTBI detection in adults and children with CIA who were on TNFα inhibitors and were treated with isoniazid. Our results showed that TST was efficient in identifying LTBI in an endemic region with moderate incidence of TB [7, 8]. In addition, 15 (18.5%) incident cases of LTBI were identified after using TNFα inhibitors and previous negative investigation, particularly in patients with RA. Interestingly, no cases of active TB were found in patients who had a positive TST and who received isoniazid before introduction of TNFα inhibitors, demonstrating high efficacy of LTBI treatment for 6 months. The positivity of LTBI screening was similar between TST and IGRAs in adult patients, regardless of CIA.

Recent meta-analysis demonstrated lower specificity and sensitivity (67% and 81%, respectively) of IGRAs in immunocompromised compared to immunocompetent patients (98.1 and 98%, respectively) when active TB diagnosis was considered as gold standard [15–18]. In contrast, we found no significant difference regarding IGRAs positivity after exposure to TNFα inhibitors.

Previous studies have highlighted that the negative predictive value for progression to TB in 2-Year follow-up was 97.8% for T-SPOT.TB and 99.8% for QFT-IT [9]. However, considering the lack of gold standard method for LTBI diagnosis and small number of active disease cases, it was not possible to calculate the specificity and sensitivity of these tests in our sampling. Besides, it is worth emphasizing that all LTBI new cases were treated with isoniazid in our study, by ethic reasons, minimizing the risk for TB disease progression. The only patient who developed active pulmonary TB over the 24-Month follow-up had negative TST and IGRAs at the time of evaluation. Interestingly, the 3 tests became positive at TB diagnosis, suggesting recent exposure to *M. tuberculosis*.

In our prospective study, no concomitant medication (cDMARDs, GC or TNFα inhibitors) hampered the results of the four tests for LTBI, showing that the release of IFN-γ was also not impaired. These results differ from previous studies, which found low frequency of TST positivity before anti-TNFα therapy, particularly in patients with RA treated with GC and conventional DMARDs [19, 20].

Although the clinical relevance of TST conversion from negative to positive results after exposure to TNFα inhibitors is still unknown, two main hypotheses could explain positivity increment. First of all, it can be related to new recent contact ("de novo" exposition) to *M. tuberculosis,* considering that the baseline TST was negative when tested 2 years before. Secondly, it might be associated with a "less immunocompromised status" caused by reduction of cDMARDs and GC dosage or an improvement of the cell response (a less anergic condition) after TNFα antagonists [21]. Moreover, none of these patients developed active disease during the 24-Month follow-up when the protocol was correctly followed. Lastly, it is important to emphasize that the possibility of false-positive results is low. However, future studies are necessary to confirm these hypotheses.

More recently, the increasing LTBI test conversion (13% for TST, 10% for T-SPOT.TB and 7% for QFT-IT; total = 30%) after 1 year of anti-TNFα therapy was also observed by Hatzara et al. [21]. Considering that 63% of the sample had positive TB epidemiology, the authors decided to conduct treatment with isoniazid for 9 months. No cases of active TB were observed after a mean of 27-Month follow-up. In addition, the TST-Booster phenomenon was 4 times more frequent than in our sample (11% vs. 3.6%, respectively), and the only risk factor associated with higher conversion rate was the previous exposure to TB (OR7.24; 95%CI 1.09–47.99; $p = 0.04$). Unexpectedly, infliximab had a significant protective role [21]. Our data supported for the first time that there is no need to withdraw the TNFα inhibitors after TST conversion, from negative to positive, in asymptomatic CIA patients on biological therapy, a new safety finding in this scenario.

Our initial hypothesis was that the TST-Booster could promote stimulation of cellular response and optimize the identification of more LTBI cases, which had not been identified by initial TST, related to attenuation of response due to disease activity itself or concomitant medication [14]. However, we could not confirm this hypothesis, due to the low rate of positive TST-Booster and an increment of TST positivity over time.

All these aspects contribute to the discussion regarding the best strategy for monitoring TB in patients exposed to TNFα antagonists. The latest recommendation from the American College of Rheumatology (ACR) has emphasized that patients with baseline negative TST or IGRA should perform them annually to identify new cases after exposition to TNFα inhibitors, even without evidence from robust randomized studies to support this decision [22]. In Brazil and other endemic areas, these recommendations should be applied because the exposure to mycobacteria is very common. In addition, considering the high TST positivity rate following exposure to TNFα inhibitors and the fact that the epidemiological data over time added little value to LTBI diagnosis, our data do not suggest the retesting of patients with negative initial screening for TST or IGRA could help to protect against active TB incident cases. Considering the 10%-increment in LTBI diagnosis with IGRAs, and the possibility of severe active TB disease development [7], we advise that, whenever possible, IGRAs might be performed. However, it is important to take into account the costs and availability of them in each epidemiological scenario, particularly after TNFα inhibitors exposition over time.

Furthermore, we found some interesting IGRA changes after treatment of LTBI with isoniazid. However, no patient with negative TST or SPOT.TB test became positive in 6-Month follow-up, which could suggest higher risk of TB disease. Surprisingly, the QFT-IT retest had an increment of positivity in 3 patients after the LTBI treatment, but without clinical relevance in 2-Year follow up. In contrast to Johnson et al. who found no significant differences in the qualitative and quantitative results of QFT-IT after treatment of LTBI in healthy subjects in South Africa, we observed some patients became positive for QFT-IT [23]. Moreover, a recent Brazilian study found no qualitative difference regarding IGRAs results in healthy children after LTBI treatment [24]. In Gambia, another study conducted in healthy subjects who had had contact with TB patients did not find quantitative or qualitative changes in T-SPOT.TB after LTBI treatment [25]. These data highlight that the repetition of IGRAs tests after the completion of therapy with isoniazid is not necessary for CIA patients treated with TNFα inhibitors.

Considering the prospective design and the requirement for patients to come to several appointments, it is worth mentioning that we obtained an excellent compliance, highlighting the main strength of our study. Another relevant question is the correct ethically management because all patients with some positive LTBI tests were treated with isoniazid and did not develop TB during 24-Month follow-up.

Our study has some limitations, particularly the lack of IGRA testing before starting TNFα blockers to better understand the conversion of LTBI tests after treatment. Also, we used the third generation QFT-IT system; using the now available fourth generation QFT-IT system, QFT results might be even better. Therefore, future studies are necessary to identify new biomarkers, including the ability to diagnose LTBI, greater power to predict the risk of active disease over time, as well as to differentiate active from latent disease and to indicate a favourable response to a specific treatment for mycobacteria.

Conclusion

Our results demonstrated as the main finding that approxi mately 20% of patients with CIAs had at least one positive test for LTBI during exposure to TNFα inhibitors. In adults, the TST was effective in identifying new cases of LTBI and the IGRAs added almost 10%-diagnostic power in this scenario. The TST-Booster did not provide additional infor mation compared to the other 3 methods. Given the high risk of TB in Brazil, our results suggest that in patients with CIA on TNFα inhibitors and with negative TST, the IGRAs may be a good strategy to identify LTBI cases and to mini mize the likelyhood of active disease during exposure to TNFα inhibitors.

Acknowledgements

The authors thank to Fundação de Amparo à Pesquisa do Estado de São Paulo (FAPESP 2011/02779-1) and Conselho Nacional de Desenvolvimento Científico e Tecnológico to MTT (CNPq 303752/2015-7).

Authors' contributions

CMFG performed the sample collection and processing, data analysis and drafted the manuscript. MTT participated in the design of the study, helped to data analysis and in drafting of the manuscript. MIdM-P participated in the design of the study, helped to data analysis and in drafting of the manuscript. MMP participated in the design of the study, helped to data analysis and in drafting of the manuscript. All authors read and approved the final manuscript.

Author details

[1]Rheumatology Division, Universidade Federal de Sao Paulo (Unifesp/EPM), São Paulo, Brazil. [2]Pediatric Rheumatology Unit, Department of Pediatrics, Universidade Federal de Sao Paulo (Unifesp/EPM), São Paulo, Brazil. [3]Pediatric Infectious Diseases Division, Department of Pediatrics, Universidade Federal de Sao Paulo (Unifesp/EPM), São Paulo, Brazil. [4]Head of the Spondyloarthritis and Immunobiological Therapy Section, Rheumatology Division, Universidade Federal de Sao Paulo (Unifesp/EPM), Rua Leandro Dupré, 204, Conj. 74, Vila Clementino, São Paulo, SP CEP 04025-010, Brazil.

References

1. Arnet FC, Edworthy SM, Bloch DA, McShane DJ, Fries JF, Cooper NS, et al. The American Rheumatism Association 1987 revised criteria for classification of rheumatoid arthritis. Arthritis Rheum. 1988;31:315–24.
2. Taylor W, Gladman D, Helliwell P, Marchesoni A, Mease P, Mielants H, et al. Classification criteria for psoriatic arthritis: development of new criteria from a large international study. Arthritis Rheum. 2006;54:2665–73.
3. Sieper J, Rudwaleit M, Baraliakos X, Brandt J, Braun J, Burgos-Vargas R, et al. The assessment of spondyloarthritis international society (ASAS) handbook: a guide to assess spondyloarthritis. Ann Rheum Dis. 2009;68(Suppl 2):ii1-44.
4. Petty RE, Southwood TR, Manners P, Baum J, Glass DN, Goldenberg J, et al. International league of associations for rheumatology classification of juvenile idiopathic arthritis: second revision, Edmonton, 2001. J Rheumatol. 2004;31:390–2.
5. Wallis RS, Broder MS, Wong JY, Hanson ME, Beenhouwer DO. Granulomatous infectious diseases associated with tumor necrosis factor antagonists. Clin Infect Dis. 2004;38:1261–5.
6. Brassard P, Kezouh A, Suissa S. Antirheumatic drugs and the risk of tuberculosis. Clin Infect Dis. 2006;43:717–22.
7. Gomes CM, Terreri MT, Moraes-Pinto MI, Barbosa C, Machado NP, Melo MR, et al. Incidence of active mycobacterial infections in Brazilian patients with chronic inflammatory arthritis and negative evaluation for latent tuberculosis infection at baseline—a longitudinal analysis after using TNFα blockers. Mem Inst Oswaldo Cruz. 2015;110:921–8.
8. Bonfiglioli KR, Ribeiro AC, Moraes JC, Saad CG, Souza FH, Calich AL, et al. LTBI screening in rheumatoid arthritis patients prior to anti-TNF treatment in an endemic area. Int J Tuberc Lung Dis. 2014;18:905–11.
9. Mazurek GH, Jereb J, Vernon A, LoBue P, Goldberg S, Castro K, et al. Updated guidelines for using interferon gamma release assays to detect *Mycobacterium tuberculosis* infection—United States, 2010. Centers for Disease Control and Prevention. MMWR Recomm Rep. 2010;59(RR-5):1–25.
10. Smolen JS, Breedveld FC, Eberl G, Jones I, Leeming M, Wylie GL, et al. Validity and reliability of the twenty-eight-joint count for the assessment of rheumatoid arthritis activity. Arthritis Rheum. 1995;38:38–43.
11. Garrett S, Jenkinson T, Kennedy LG, Whitelock H, Gaisford P, Calin A. A new approach to defining disease status in ankylosing spondylitis: the bath ankylosing spondylitis disease activity index. J Rheumatol. 1994;21:2286–91.
12. Fredriksson T, Pettersson U. Severe psoriasis—oral therapy with a new retinoid. Dermatologica. 1978;157:238–44.
13. Wallace CA, Ruperto N, Giannini E, Childhood Arthritis and Rheumatology Research Alliance, Pediatric Rheumatology International Trials Organization, Pediatric Rheumatology Collaborative Study Group. Preliminary criteria for clinical remission for select categories of juvenile idiopathic arthritis. J Rheumatol. 2004;31:2290–4.
14. Fuchs I, Avnon L, Freud T, Abu-Shakra M. Repeated tuberculin skin testing following therapy with TNF-alpha inhibitors. Clin Rheumatol. 2009;28:167–72.
15. Diel R, Goletti D, Ferrara G, Bothamley G, Cirillo D, Kampmann B, et al. Interferon-γ release assays for the diagnosis of latent Mycobacterium tuberculosis infection: a systematic review and meta-analysis. Eur Respir J. 2011;37:88–99.
16. Aichelburg MC, Rieger A, Breitenecker F, Pfistershammer K, Tittes J, Eltz S, et al. Detection and prediction of active tuberculosis disease by a whole-blood interferon-gamma release assay in HIV-1-infected individuals. Clin Infect Dis. 2009;48:954–62.
17. Tsiouris SJ, Coetzee D, Toro PL, Austin J, Stein Z, El-Sadr W. Sensitivity analysis and potential uses of a novel gamma interferon release assay for diagnosis of tuberculosis. J Clin Microbiol. 2006;44:2844–50.
18. Raby E, Moyo M, Devendra A, Pfistershammer K, Tittes J, Eltz S, et al. The effects of HIV on the sensitivity of a whole blood interferon gamma release assay in Zambian adults with active tuberculosis. PLoS ONE. 2008;3(6):e2489.
19. Callado MR, Lima JR, Nobre CA. Vieira WP [Low prevalence of reactive PPD prior to infliximab use: comparative study on a population sample of Hospital Geral de Fortaleza]. Rev Bras Reumatol. 2011;51:40–52.
20. Marques CDL, Duarte ALBP, Lorena VMB, de Souza JR, Souza W, Gomes YM, et al. Atenuate response to tuberculin skin test in the diagnosis of latent tuberculosis infection in patients with rheumatoid arthritis. Rev Bras Reumatol. 2009;42:121–31.
21. Hatzara C, Hadziynnis E, Kandili A, Tsikrika S, Minopetrou M, Georgiopoulos G, et al. Frequent conversion of tuberculosis screening tests during anti-tumor necrosis fator therapy in patients with rheumatic diseases. Ann Rheum Dis. 2015;74:1–6.
22. Singh JA, Furst DE, Bharat A, Curtis J, Kavanaugh A, Kremer J, et al. 2012 Update of the 2008 American College of Rheumatology (ACR) recommendations for the use of disease-modifying anti-rheumatic drugs and biologics in the treatment of rheumatoid arthritis (RA). Arthritis Care Res. 2012;64:625–39.
23. Johnson JL, Geldenhuys H, Thiel BA, Toefy A, Suliman S, Pienaar B, et al. Effect of isoniazid therapy for latent TB infection on QuantiFERON-TB gold in-tube responses in adults with positive tuberculin skin test results in a high TB incidence area: a controlled study. Chest. 2014;145:612–7.

24. Ferrarini MA, Spina FG, Weckx LY, Lederman HM, De Moraes-Pinto MI. Rate of tuberculosis infection in children and adolescents with household contact with adults with active pulmonary tuberculosis as assessed by tuberculin skin test and interferon-gamma release assays. Epidemiol Infect. 2016;144:712–23.
25. Adetifa IM, Ota MO, Jeffries DJ, Lugos MD, Hammond AS, Battersby NJ, et al. Interferon γ ELISPOT as a biomarker of treatment efficacy in latent tuberculosis infection: a clinical trial. Am J Respir Crit Care Med. 2013;187:439–45.

3

Recommendations of the Brazilian Society of Rheumatology for the use of JAK inhibitors in the management of rheumatoid arthritis

Karina Rossi Bonfiglioli[1*], Licia Maria Henrique da Mota[2], Ana Cristina de Medeiros Ribeiro[1], Adriana Maria Kakehasi[3], Ieda Maria Magalhães Laurindo[4], Rina Dalva Neubarth Giorgi[5], Angela Luzia Branco Pinto Duarte[6], Ana Paula Monteiro Gomides Reis[2], Mariana Peixoto Guimarães Ubirajara e Silva de Souza[7], Claiton Viegas Brenol[8], Geraldo da Rocha Castelar Pinheiro[9], Cleandro Pires de Albuquerque[2], Charlles Heldan de Moura Castro[10], Gustavo Luiz Behrens Pinto[11], Jose Fernando Verztman[12], Luciana Feitosa Muniz[13], Manoel Barros Bertolo[14], Maria Raquel da Costa Pinto[3], Paulo Louzada Júnior[15], Vitor Alves Cruz[16], Ivanio Alves Pereira[17], Max Vitor Carioca de Freitas[18], Bóris Afonso Cruz[19], Eduardo Paiva[20], Odirlei Monticielo[8], José Roberto Provenza[21] and Ricardo Machado Xavier[8]

Abstract

Rheumatoid arthritis (RA) is a chronic and autoimmune systemic inflammatory disease that can cause irreversible joint deformities, with increased morbidity and mortality and a significant impact on the quality of life of the affected individual. The main objective of RA treatment is to achieve sustained clinical remission or low disease activity. However, up to 40% of patients do not respond to available treatments, including bDMARDs. New therapeutic targets for RA are emerging, such as Janus kinases (JAKs). These are essential for intracellular signaling (via JAK-STAT) in response to many cytokines involved in RA immunopathogenesis. JAK inhibitors (JAKi) have established themselves as a highly effective treatment, gaining increasing space in the therapeutic arsenal for the treatment of RA. The current recommendations aim to present a review of the main aspects related to the efficacy and safety of JAKis in RA patients, and to update the recommendations and treatment algorithm proposed by the Brazilian Society of Rheumatology in 2017.

Introduction

Rheumatoid arthritis (RA) is a chronic and autoimmune systemic inflammatory disease characterized by involvement of the synovial membrane of peripheral joints. If not treated early and adequately, the disease can cause bone erosion and irreversible joint deformities, with increased morbidity and mortality and a significant impact on the quality of life of the affected individual [1]. RA affects up to 1% of the general population and is more common in women aged 40 to 60 years [2].

In the last 3 decades, there has been significant evolution in the management of patients with RA, with emphases on early diagnosis, rigorous monitoring of disease activity and goal-oriented treatment strategies. A better understanding of its pathophysiology has led to the development of new disease-modifying antirheumatic drugs (DMARDs), primarily biological DMARDs

*Correspondence: karina.bonfiglioli@hc.fm.usp.br

[1] Disciplina Reumatologia do Hospital das Clínicas, Faculdade de Medicina, Universidade de São Paulo (HC-FMUSP), Av. Dr. Arnaldo, 455 - 3° andar – Reumatologia, São Paulo, SP, CEP 01246-903, Brasil

(bDMARDs) and, more recently, targeted synthetic DMARDs (tsDMARDs). The treatment objectives remain reducing joint and systemic inflammation with the aims of inhibiting disease progression, preventing loss of functionality and preserving patient quality of life [3–5].

Despite the various therapeutic options available, there are patients who do not achieve the desired response (remission or low disease activity) due to an inadequate clinical response (primary failure) or loss of response (secondary failure) or drug toxicity [6].

According to the most recent recommendations of the Brazilian Society of Rheumatology (SBR, for its initials in Portuguese) [1] and the European Alliance of Associations for Rheumatology (EULAR) [7], the main objective of RA treatment is to achieve sustained clinical remission or, in cases where this is not possible, low disease activity. However, up to 40% of patients do not respond to available treatments, including bDMARDs [1, 7].

New RA therapeutic targets are emerging. Janus kinases (JAKs), enzimes involved in intracellular signaling (JAK-STAT pathway), are essential to the control of response of many cytokines involved in the immunopathogenesis of RA. Therefore, JAK inhibitors (JAKis) have shown efficacy in the treatment of RA [8]. JAKis currently approved for commercialization in Brazil include tofacitinib [9] (JAK1 and JAK3 inhibitor), baricitinib [10] (JAK1 and JAK2 inhibitor) and upadacitinib [11] (selective JAK1 inhibitor).

Objective

The objective of these recommendations is to present a review, directed to rheumatologists, of the main aspects related to the efficacy and safety of JAKis in RA patients and to update the recommendations and treatment algorithm proposed by the SBR in 2017 [1].

Method

This review followed a protocol developed by the members of the SBR Rheumatoid Arthritis Committee, who established questions based on real-life scenarios, that can be accessed in Additional files.

For the purposes of these recommendations, the following acronym and nomenclature system was adopted:

DMARDs	Disease-modifying antirheumatic drugs;
csDMARDs	Conventional synthetic disease-modifying antirheumatic drugs—methotrexate (MTX), leflunomide (LEF), sulfasalazine (SSZ) and hydroxychloroquine (HCQ);
tsDMARDs	Targeted synthetic disease-modifying antirheumatic drugs (JAK inhibitors)—baricitinib (BARI), tofacitinib (TOFA), upadacitinib (UPA), filgotinib (FILGO) and peficitinib (PEFI);
bDMARDs	Biological disease-modifying antirheumatic drugs—tumor necrosis factor (TNFα-i) inhibitors adalimumab (ADA), certolizumab (CTZ), etanercept (ETA), golimumab (GOLI) and infliximab (IFX) and drugs with other mechanisms of non-TNFα-i action, i.e., abatacept (ABA), rituximab (RTX) and tocilizumab (TCZ);
JAKi	Janus Kinase inhibitor
mTSS	Modified total Sharp score;
HAQ-DI	Health Assessment Questionnaire Disability Index;
NSAIDs	Nonsteroidal antiinflammatory drugs;
DAS28-CRP	Disease activity score 28/C-reactive protein.
DAS28-ESR	Disease activity score 28/erythrocyte sedimentation rate.
CDAI	Clinical Disease Activity Index.
SDAI	Simplified Disease Activity Index.
Remission	DAS28-CRP and/or DAS28-ESR < 2.6; and.
Low disease activity	DAS28-CRP and/or DAS28-ESR $\geq 2.6 < 3.2$.
RCT	Randomized controlled trial.

To answer the selected questions, systematic literature reviews (SLRs) were performed for each specific scenario.

Elements of study eligibility

The search for evidence was performed in virtual scientific information databases using search strategies specific to each question.

The searches in these databases were performed until the month corresponding to the completion and submission of these guidelines for publication, and a systematic review was performed in accordance with the Preferred Reporting Items for Systematic reviews and Meta-Analyses (PRISMA) guidelines [12].

The following data were extracted from the studies: name of the author and year of publication, population studied, methods of intervention and comparison, absolute number of events, and follow-up time.

The risk of bias in randomized clinical trials was analyzed based on the following criteria: randomization, blinded allocation, double blinding, losses, prognostic characteristics, presence of expected outcome, time to outcome, outcome measurement method, sample calculation, early interruption, and presence of other biases.

The measures used to express benefits and harms varied based on the outcomes and were expressed as continuous variables (mean and standard deviation) or categorical variables (absolute number of events). For continuous measures, the results reflect differences in means and standard deviation, and for categorical measures, the results reflect differences in risks and number needed to treat or produce harm, considering the number of patients. The confidence level was set at 95%. The results underwent meta-analysis when common outcomes among studies were observed.

The results of the included studies were aggregated and meta-analyzed using RevMan 5.4 software [13].

In addition, the quality of the evidence was scored as high, moderate, low or very low using the Grades of Recommendation, Assessment, Development, and Evaluation (GRADE) instrument [14], taking into account the risk of bias, the presence of inconsistencies, imprecise or indirect evidence in the meta-analysis of outcomes and the presence of publication bias.

The search strategies, selection process, characteristics and evaluation of the methodological quality of the included studies, as well as the synthesis of the results and quality of the evidence (based on GRADE), are available *online* as appendices.

Elaboration of recommendations

The process of drafting the recommendations relied on the participation of the SBR Rheumatoid Arthritis Committee, that included 27 rheumatologists from a panel of experts. Based on the SLR results for each clinical question as well as on the clinical experience of the experts, recommendations were elaborated and subjected to online voting.

The first step involved agreeing about the structure and content of each of the propositions, requiring 70% agreement for inclusion of the proposition. When this value was not attained, the propositions were reformulated and submitted to a new voting stage until 70% agreement was met. Subsequently, the level of agreement was established based on the content in the propositions: the panel of experts assigned a degree of agreement using a numerical scale from 0 ("strongly disagree") to 10 ("strongly agree") for each recommendation.

Results

A summary of the search and synthesis of the evidence for each SLR performed is presented below, based on the proposed clinical questions. In all scenarios, adult patients (>18 years old) who met the RA classification criteria of the American College of Rheumatology (ACR) of 1987 [15] or the 2010 ACR/EULAR criteria [16] were evaluated. All the details on the selection of studies, reasons for exclusion, list of excluded studies, and analysis of the quality of the evidence for the outcomes are available in the corresponding appendices of this publication.

Efficacy and safety of tsDMARDs (JAKis) under different scenarios

1. ***Are tsDMARDs (JAKis) safe and effective as a first-line treatment for RA patients? (ps.: treatment-naïve patients)***

A total of 403 studies were retrieved, individually accessed by title and/or abstract but only 3 were selected to support this evaluation. The reasons for exclusion and the list of excluded studies are available in the Additional file 1: Appendix 1 of this publication [17–19].

Evidence summary

The following evidence pertains to adult patients with recent onset RA (symptoms < 6 months) or established RA (symptoms ≥ 6 months), regardless of disease activity, who received a nontherapeutic dose or no csDMARDs/bDMARDs.

Results within 6 months

- TOFA (5 mg 12/12 h), BARI (4 mg/day) and UPA (15 or 30 mg/day), all in monotherapy, compared to MTX, led to a higher proportion of patients who achieved ACR (20%-50%-70%) and DAS28-ESR (remission and low activity) responses. There was also more significant improvement in functional capacity (measured by the HAQ-DI) in patients who received TOFA, BARI and UPA monotherapy. The quality of the evidence supporting these results is high.
- BARI (4 mg/day) monotherapy compared to BARI + MTX did not show superiority in any response criterion.

Results within 13 months

- BARI (4 mg/day) compared to MTX, both monotherapies, led to a higher proportion of patients who achieved an ACR response (20%-50%-70%) but not DAS28-ESR (remission or low activity). There was also more significant improvement in functional capacity, as measured by HAQ-DI. The quality of the evidence supporting this result is high.

- BARI (4 mg/day) monotherapy compared to BARI + MTX combined therapy showed no superiority in any response criterion.
- BARI (4 mg/day) + MTX combined therapy compared to MTX monotherapy led to a higher proportion of patients who achieved DAS28-ESR (remission and low activity). The quality of the evidence supporting this result is high.

Safety

- TOFA (5 mg 12/12 h) monotherapy and BARI (4 mg/day) monotherapy or in combination with MTX demonstrated acceptable safety compared to MTX monotherapy in the initial treatment of patients with active RA, based on assessments of severe adverse events (SAEs). The quality of the evidence supporting this result is high.
- MTX and UPA (15 mg/day) showed similar occurrences of SAEs. However, UPA at a dose of 30 mg/day had a higher risk of SAEs. The quality of the evidence supporting this result is moderate.

2. ***Are tsDMARDs (JAKis) safe and effective for the treatment of RA patients after csDMARD failure?***

The search for evidence resulted in a total of 1658 articles. After reading the titles and abstracts, 1581 studies were excluded. The full texts of 77 studies were accessed, of which 19 [20–38] were selected to support this evaluation. (Additional file 2: Appendix 2).

Evidence summary

The following evidence pertains to patients with moderate or high RA activity after DMARD failure, followed by treatment with a JAKi.

In monotherapy or in combination with MTX/other csDMARDs, or,

Compared with placebo in combination with MTX/other csDMARDs.

- TOFA (5 mg 12/12 h or 10 mg 12/12 h), alone or combined with MTX, improves ACR response outcomes (20%-50%-70%) and DAS28-ESR (remission and low activity). There was also improvement in functional capacity (measured by the HAQ-DI). The quality of evidence supporting this result is high.
- BARI (2 mg/day and 4 mg/day) monotherapy or combined with MTX led to a higher proportion of patients who achieved an ACR response (20%–50%–70%) and low disease activity and remission, as determined by DAS28-CRP and DAS28-ESR, in addition to significant improvement in functional capacity (as measured by the HAQ-DI). The quality of the evidence supporting this result is high/moderate.
- UPA (15 mg/day) monotherapy or combined with MTX led to a higher proportion of patients who achieved an ACR response (20–50–70) and low disease activity and remission, as determined by DAS28-CRP and DAS28-ESR. The quality of the evidence supporting this result is high/moderate.
- FILGO (100 mg/day and 200 mg/day) monotherapy led to a higher proportion of patients who achieved ACR 50, ACR 70, and low disease activity, as determined by DAS28-CRP and DAS28-ESR, with moderate quality of evidence. However, the quality of evidence for improvements in ACR 20 and the HAQ-DI score are moderate and low, respectively. PEFI (100 mg/day and 150 mg/day) as a monotherapy or combined with MTX led to a higher proportion of patients who achieved an ACR response (20–50–70), remission, as determined by DAS28-CRP and DAS28-ESR, and low disease activity, as determined by DAS28-CRP. The quality of the evidence supporting this result is low/very low.

Safety

All JAKis, alone or in combination with MTX, showed acceptable safety compared to placebo for patients with moderate or high RA after failure of regimens with different csDMARDs, as determined by analyzing SAEs. The quality of evidence for this outcome ranged from moderate to very low. To better understand/define the safety of JAKis, more phase 4 studies are needed.

3. ***Are tsDMARDs (JAKis) safe and effective for the treatment of RA patients after bDMARD failure?***

In the search for evidence, 58 studies were retrieved and individually assessed by title and/or abstract; 4 [39–42] references were selected for evaluation of their full texts. (Additional file 3: Appendix 3).

Evidence summary

The following evidence pertains to patients with a diagnosis of established RA who had an inadequate response to treatment with bDMARDs, followed by treatment with tsDMARDs (JAKis), either as a monotherapy or in combination with methotrexate or other csDMARDs, in comparison with placebo.

Results within 3 months

- TOFA, BARI, and FILGO led to a higher proportion of patients who achieved an ACR response (20%–50%–70%) in 3 months.
- UPA led to a higher proportion of patients who achieved ACR 20 and 50 responses in 3 months.
- TOFA led to a higher proportion of patients who reached low activity (DAS28-ESR) in 3 months.
- BARI led to a higher proportion of patients who achieved low activity and remission (DAS28-ESR) in 3 months.
- FILGO and UPA led to a higher proportion of patients who reached low activity (DAS28-CRP) in 3 months.
- There was improvement in functional capacity (measured by HAQ-DI) for all JAKis, in 3 months.
- The quality of the evidence supporting these results is high.

Safety

All JAKis, alone or in combination with MTX, after failure of bDMARDs, showed acceptable safety compared to placebo, as determined by analyzing SAEs. The quality of evidence supporting these results is high.

Effectiveness, safety and cost of tsDMARDs (JAKis) in relation to csDMARDs and bDMARDs

4. ***Are tsDMARDs (JAKis) more effective than csDMARDs in the treatment of RA?***

In the search for evidence, 1325 studies were retrieved and individually assessed by title and/or abstract, from which 42 references were selected for evaluation of their full texts. Of the 42 studies, 4 [17, 19, 43, 44] randomized clinical trials were selected to support this evaluation, i.e., JAKis (TOFA, BARI and UPA) compared with MTX. A flow diagram is provided in the online supplementary Additional file 4: Appendix 4.

Evidence summary

The following evidence pertains to adult patients who met the RA classification criteria of the ACR or ACR/EULAR 2010 and in whom the the use of JAKis (TOFA, BARI and UPA) and csDMARDs (MTX) was compared.

Results within 3–6 months

- UPA (15 mg/day and 30 mg/day) monotherapy, compared to MTX, led to a higher proportion of patients who achieved ACR 20% and 50% responses in 3 months. A higher proportion of patients also achieved clinical remission (DAS28-PCR) in 6 months. The quality of the evidence supporting this result is high.
- Compared with MTX, UPA (15 mg/day and 30 mg/day) after 6 months resulted in lower radiographic progression (Van der Heijde score) of RA. The quality of the evidence supporting this result is high.

Results within 6–12 months

- TOFA (5 mg 12/12 h and 10 mg 12/12 h), compared to MTX, both monotherapies, led to a higher proportion of patients who achieved an ACR (20–50%) response and low activity (DAS28-ESR). In 12 months, an ACR 70% response rate and remission, as determined by DAS28-ESR, were more frequent in patients who received TOFA. The quality of the evidence supporting this result is high.
- Compared with MTX, TOFA (5 mg 12/12 h and 10 mg 12/12 h) resulted in lower radiographic progression (modified Van der Heijde score) at 6 months. The quality of the evidence supporting this result is high.
- Compared to MTX, BARI (4 mg/day) monotherapy (or combined with MTX) led to a higher proportion of patients who achieved an ACR response (20%–50%–70%) and clinical remission (DAS28-ESR) at 6 and 12 months. The quality of the evidence supporting this result is high.
- Compared with MTX, BARI (4 mg/day) did not alter the risk of radiographic progression (Van der Heijde score). The quality of the evidence supporting this result is high.

Safety

- Compared with MTX monotherapy, TOFA (5 mg) monotherapy and BARI (4 mg) monotherapy or in combination with MTX demonstrated acceptable safety in the initial treatment of patients with active RA, as determined by analyzing SAEs. The quality of the evidence supporting this result is high.
- The adverse events resulting from treatment with MTX and UPA (15 mg/day) were similar, but there was a higher incidence of adverse events with 30 mg/day UPA. The quality of the evidence supporting this result is moderate.

5. ***Compared with bDMARDs, do tsDMARDs (JAKis) show evidence of greater efficacy for the treatment of RA?***

In the search for evidence, 1442 studies were retrieved and individually assessed by title and/or abstract, from which 33 references were selected for evaluation of their full texts. Of the 33 studies selected to support this evaluation, there were only 4 [45–48] randomized clinical trials that compared TOFA, BARI or UPA with ADA in combination with MTX. A flow diagram is provided in the Additional file 5: Appendix 5.

Evidence summary

The following evidence pertains to adult patients (>16 years) with recent onset RA (symptoms<6 months) and established RA (symptoms≥6 months), regardless of disease activity, in whom the use of JAKis as a monotherapy or in combination with MTX was compared with the use of bDMARDs alone or combined with MTX.

Results within 6 months

- Compared to ADA+MTX, TOFA (5 mg 12/12 h) as a monotherapy did not led to different ACR 20%, ACR 50%, and ACR 70% outcomes and was inferior to ADA+MTX regarding low activity outcomes (DAS28-ESR).
- TOFA (10 mg 12/12 h) was superior to ADA+MTX combined therapy with respect to ACR 70% outcomes; there was no difference between the treatments for the other outcomes. The quality of the evidence supporting this result is moderate.
- UPA (15 mg/day) combined with MTX, compared to ADA+MTX, led to a higher proportion of patients who achieved ACR 20% and 50% responses. The quality of the evidence supporting this result is moderate.
- Compared with ADA+MTX, UPA (15 mg/day) combined with MTX did not reduce the risk of radiographic progression (mTSS). The quality of the evidence supporting this result is moderate.

Results within 12 months

- Compared with ADA+MTX, TOFA (5 mg 12/12 h) as a monotherapy did not alter ACR 20%, 50%, and 70% outcomes and resulted in lower low activity and remission outcomes (DAS28-VHS) at 12 months.
- BARI (4 mg/day) combined with MTX, compared to ADA+MTX, led to a higher proportion of patients who achieved ACR 20% and 50% responses, with no difference for ACR 70% outcomes, remission and low activity (DAS28-PCR). The quality of the evidence supporting this result is moderate.
- Compared with ADA+MTX, BARI (4 mg/day) combined with MTX reduced the risk of radiographic progression (mTSS) at 6 and 12 months. The quality of the evidence supporting this result is moderate.

Safety

- The rate of SAEs at 6 and 12 months was higher in patients who used BARI than in those who used ADA. There was no difference in SAEs when comparing those for TOFA or UPA with ADA at the 6-month follow-up. The quality of the evidence supporting this result is moderate.

6. ***Is there evidence of better cost-effectiveness for DMARDs (JAKis) compared with csDMARDs?***

In the search for evidence, 203 studies were retrieved and individually assessed by title and/or abstract, from which 16 references were selected for full text evaluation. Of the 16 studies, only 2 were selected to support this evaluation [49, 50]. A flow diagram is provided in the online supplementary Additional file 6: Appendix 6.

Evidence summary

In patients with moderate to severe active RA, tsDMARDs (JAKis), compared with csDMARDs, were cost-effective in patients with inadequate responses to biological therapy.

The literature, however, lacks studies that evaluate whether tsDMARDs are cost-effective when compared with csDMARDs after failure with another csDMARD. Future studies are needed to evaluate this scenario.

7. ***Is there evidence of better cost-effectiveness for tsDMARDs (JAKis) compared with bDMARDs?***

Studies were evaluated for risk of bias using the Critical Appraisal Skills Program—CASP (economic) evaluation checklist [1]. In the search for evidence, 203 studies were retrieved and individually assessed by title and/or abstract, of which 16 references were selected for full text evaluation. Of the 16 studies, only 6 were selected to support this evaluation [51–57]. Supporting material is available online in the supplementary Additional file 7: Appendix 7.

Evidence summary

- Compared with the use of biological therapies (ADA, ETA, CERTOLI, RITUXI, ABATA and TOCILI), the use of JAKis (BARI and TOFA combined or not with MTX) is cost-effective in patients with active, moderate to severe RA, with inadequate response to csDMARDs or anti-TNF bDMARDs.

- Future studies are needed to evaluate the cost-effectiveness of JAKis compared to that of DMARDs in the Brazilian scenario, as well as the cost-effectiveness of other JAKis.

8. ***Is there evidence for vaccination effectiveness against herpes zoster (HZ) before starting treatment with JAKis?***

Evidence indicates that the use of JAKis is accompanied by a higher risk of infection by HZ [58, 59].

In the search for evidence, 1909 studies were retrieved and individually assessed by title and/or abstract, from which 19 references were selected for full text evaluation. Finally, in regard to the eligibility criteria, 4 studies were included [60–63]; the reasons for exclusion are found in the online supplementary Additional file 8: Appendix 8.

Evidence summary

- The efficacy of the live attenuated HZ vaccine (LZV) is questionable in patients using JAKis, especially in combination with MTX. The quality of the evidence supporting this result is moderate.
- Therapy with TOFA has no negative impact on the established immune response after vaccination with LZV. The quality of the evidence supporting this result is moderate.
- Therapy with TOFA has no impact on the incidence of HZ during patient follow-up after LZV vaccination. The quality of the evidence supporting this result is moderate

9. ***Is there evidence of a higher risk of venous thromboembolic events (VTEs) related to JAKi treatment?***

In the search for evidence, 1541 studies (RCT) were retrieved and individually assessed by title and/or abstract, from which 30 references were selected for full text evaluation. Of the 30 studies, 10 were selected to support this evaluation [64–73] (Fig. 1). The reasons for exclusion and the list of excluded studies, as well as the description of the included studies, are available in the Additional file 9: Appendix 9.

Evidence summary

The following evidence pertains to adult patients with RA who used tsDMARDs (JAKis) as a monotherapy or in combination with MTX or other csDMARDs.

- There was no significant increase in the risk of VTE.
- The use of low doses of JAKi seemed to offer a lower risk of VTE than high doses. The quality of the evidence supporting this result is high.

Safety of JAKi in light of recent warnings

Although the present SLR has not shown unexpected findings regarding safety within each of the questions that guided the search, the authors considered necessary to discuss some recent data not covered in the SLR search period.

On Oral Surveillance study [74], the prespecified non-inferiority criteria for the co-primary endpoints of major adverse cardiovascular events (MACE) and malignancies (excluding non-melanoma skin cancer), were not met for the primary comparison of the combined tofacitinib doses (5 mg twice daily and 10 mg twice daily) to TNF inhibitors (either etanercept 50 mg once weekly or adalimumab 40 mg every other week).

However, despite this trial wrapping in July 2020,, its full results have been submitted but not yet published. Updates on this subject can be accessed at clinicaltrials.gov (https://clinicaltrials.gov/ct2/show/results/NCT02092467).

In February 2021, a new "Food and Drug Administration" (FDA) warning regarding tofacitinib was issued [75]. FDA warned providers of an increased cardiovascular and cancer risk among older patients (> 50 years), compared with TNF-inhibitors. These warning has been based on interim and preliminary results from the ORAL Surveillance study [74].

In September 2021, FDA updated this previous warning, concluding that there is an increased risk of serious heart-related events such as heart attack or stroke, cancer, blood clots and death related with Tofacitinib. Based on that conclusion, required "Boxed warning" addings and revisions for all JAKi, including these findings and limiting all approved uses to certain patients who have not responded or cannot tolerate one or more TNF blockers [75].

European Medicines Agency (EMA) has also recommended an update to the product information for tofacitinib, and uttered a reminding to healthcare professionals to carefully evaluate a patient's individual benefit-risk profile when deciding to prescribe or continue the treatment [76].

Considering clinical aspects of the patients included in the post-marketing trial, who presented not only advanced age, but also other risk factors for unfavorable outcomes, we suggest taking into account the risk–benefit ratio when considering prescription of JAKi. For

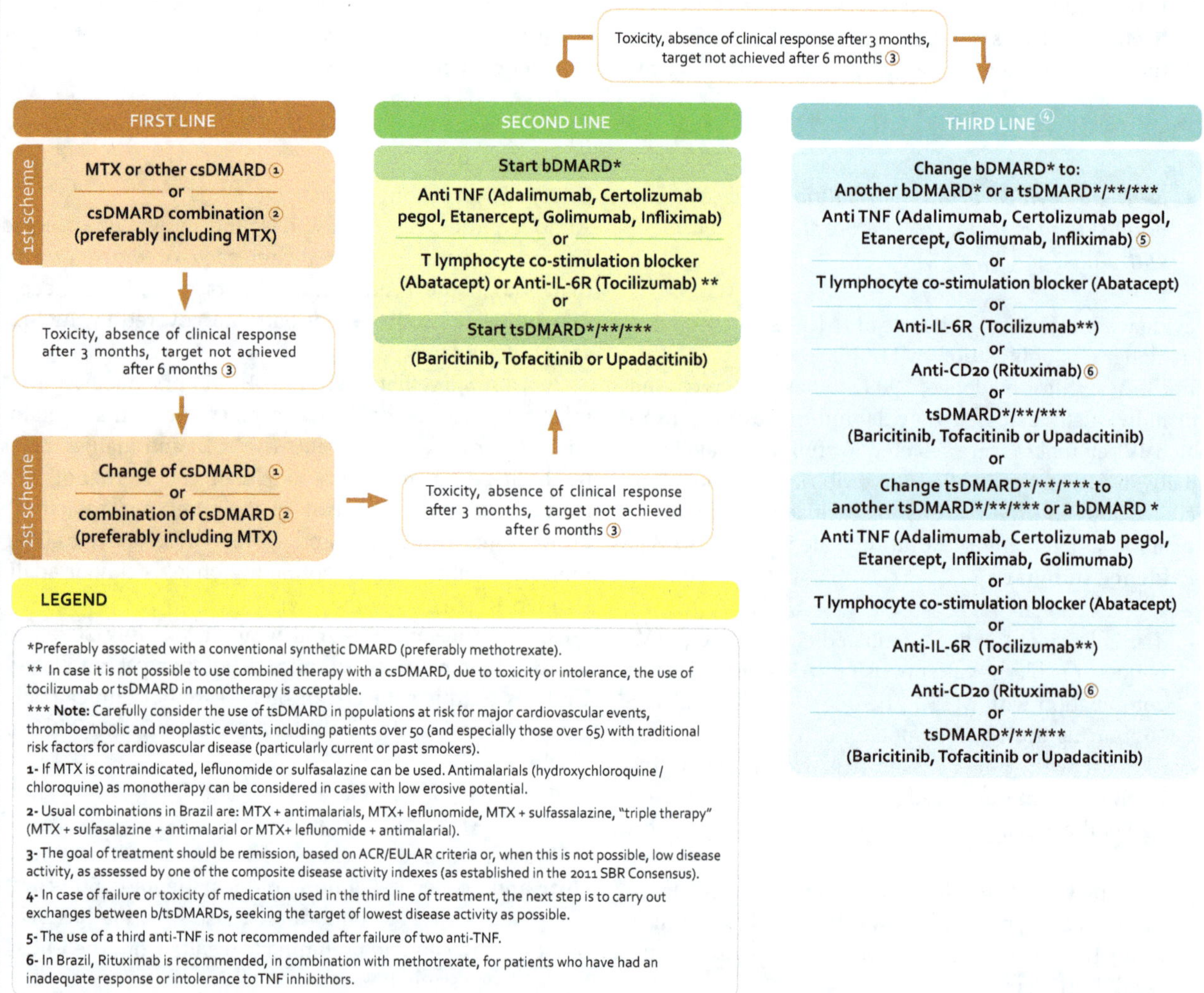

Fig. 1 Updated flowchart of RA treatment in Brazil

patients already receiving JAKi, strict surveillance of those who meet the high-risk profile is recommended.

Also taking into account the recent data, the SBR RA committee decided to re-vote recommendations 5 and 9 (see Table 1), and a warning note was included for JAKi prescription, as it follows:

Recommendation 5: After failure of 2 csDMARD regimens, a bDMARD or a tsDMARD can be used, preferably combined with a csDMARD. Note: Carefully consider the use of tsDMARD in populations at risk for major cardiovascular events, thromboembolic and neoplastic events, including patients over 50 (and especially those over 65) with traditional risk factors for disease cardiovascular (particularly current or past smokers).

Recommendation 9: In case of failure of a bDMARD as initial treatment, a second bDMARD or a tsDMARD can be used. Note: Carefully consider the use of **tsDMARD** in risk groups for major cardiovascular events, thromboembolic and neoplastic events, including patients over 50 (and especially those over 65) with traditional risk factors for cardiovascular disease (particularly current or past smokers).

Update of general assumptions and recommendations of the SBR committee on rheumatoid arthritis

Based on the data previously presented and the voting process described, the RA Commission updated the therapeutic recommendations for RA in relation to the previous document [1]. Table 1 summarizes the general assumptions and recommendations of the SBR Rheumatoid Arthritis Committee for pharmacological treatment of RA in Brazil. The ones included in the present recommendations (5, 8, 9, 10 and 12) are highlighted in Table 1.

Table 1 General assumptions and recommendations of the SBR for the drug treatment of RA in Brazil

General assumptions
1. The treatment of RA patients should preferably have a multidisciplinary approach, coordinated by a rheumatologist Degree of agreement: 9.9
2. Treatment of RA patients should include guidance on lifestyle, strict control of comorbidities and vaccination card updates Degree of agreement: 9.9
3. The treatment of RA patients should be based on decisions shared between patients and physicians, after clarification about their disease and available therapeutic options Degree of agreement: 10
4. The goal of treatment is a persistent state of clinical remission or, when this is not possible, low disease activity Degree of agreement: 9.9
SBR recommendations for drug treatment of RA
Recommendation 1: First-line treatment should be performed with csDMARDs as soon as the diagnosis of RA is established Degree of agreement: 9.9
Recommendation 2: Methotrexate should be the first-choice csDMARD Degree of agreement: 9.8
Recommendation 3: The combination of 2 or more csDMARDs, preferably including methotrexate, can be used as a first-line treatment Degree of agreement: 9.6
Recommendation 4: After failure of first-line methotrexate therapy, subsequent strategies include combination with another csDMARD, combination with 2 csDMARDs or exchanging MTX for another csDMARD as a monotherapy Degree of agreement: 9.6
Recommendation 5: After failure of 2 csDMARD regimens, a bDMARD or a tsDMARD can be used, preferably combined with a csDMARD **Note:** Carefully consider the use of tsDMARD in populations at risk for major cardiovascular events, thromboembolic and neoplastic events, including patients over 50 (and especially those over 65) with traditional risk factors for cardiovascular disease (particularly current or past smokers).Degree of agreement: 8.6
Recommendation 6: The different bDMARDs combined with methotrexate have similar efficacy; therefore, the choice should take into account the particularities of each medication in terms of safety and cost Degree of agreement: 9.6
Recommendation 7: The combination of b/tsDMARDs and methotrexate is preferred over the use of b/tsDMARDs as monotherapy. If monotherapy is necessary, consider preferentially the use of tocilizumab or tsDMARDs Degree of agreement: 9.1
Recommendation 8: The different tsDMARDs have a similar efficacy profile; therefore, the choice should take into account the particularities of each medication in terms of safety and cost. Degree of agreement: 9.7
Recommendation 9: In case of failure of a bDMARD as initial treatment, a second bDMARD or a tsDMARD can be used **Note:** Carefully consider the use of tsDMARD in populations at risk for major cardiovascular events, thromboembolic and neoplastic events, including patients over 50 (and especially those over 65) with traditional risk factors for cardiovascular disease (particularly current or past smokers).Degree of agreement: 9.0
Recommendation 10: In case of failure of a tsDMARD, another tsDMARD or a bDMARD may be used Degree of agreement: 9.4
Recommendation 11: Corticosteroids, preferably in low doses, for the shortest possible time, should be considered in periods of disease activity, after evaluating the relationship between risk and benefit Degree of agreement: 9.7
Recommendation 12: The possibility of reduction, dose spacing or eventual discontinuation of bDMARDs or tsDMARDs can be considered in patients who are in persistent remission (6 to 12 months of remission), especially when the patient is using a tsDMARD Degree of agreement: 9.2

Recommendations included in this update: 5, 8, 9, 10 and 12

RA: rheumatoid arthritis; *DMARDs*: disease-modifying antirheumatic drugs; *csDMARDs*: conventional synthetic disease-modifying antirheumatic drugs—methotrexate, leflunomide, sulfasalazine and hydroxychloroquine; *tsDMARDs*: targeted synthetic disease-modifying antirheumatic drugs—baricitinib, tofacitinib and upadacitinib; *bDMARDs*: biological disease-modifying antirheumatic drugs; *bDMARDs*: biological disease-modifying antirheumatic drugs that include: tumor necrosis factor inhibitor (TNFi), i.e., adalimumab, certolizumab, etanercept, golimumab and infliximab, and drugs with other non-TNFi mechanisms of action, i.e., abatacept, rituximab and tocilizumab; *NSAIDs*: nonsteroidal antiinflammatory drugs; *Remission*: remission according to ACR/EULAR criteria

Flowchart for drug treatment of rheumatoid arthritis

Figure 1 summarizes the updated flowchart for drug treatment of RA in Brazil proposed by the RA Commission of the SBR.

Conclusions

Important advances in the management of RA patients are leading a better patient prognosis. Rheumatologists, as specialist, are most familiar with the range of drugs available and their indications and adverse effects and are essential in the evaluation and treatment of patients diagnosed with RA.

The appropriate allocation of healthcare resources, especially in a country of continental dimensions and with a growing population, such as Brazil, conducts to access to drugs and appropriate technologies for the treatment of various conditions. These recommendations took into account, in addition to issues of safety, efficacy and cost, the experience of specialists in the management of RA, considering specific characteristics of Brazil, such as the availability of drugs and the socioeconomic level of the population.

Because the pace of knowledge acquisition in this field of science and the rise of new medications that are being analyzed for approval by Brazilian regulatory agencies, we recommend updating these guidelines every 2 years.

Supplementary Information

Additional file 1. PICO 1 - Are tsDMARD (JAK inhibitors) effective and safe for the treatment ofRA patients in 1st line of treatment? (NOTE: "naive" or treatment-naive patients).

Additional file 2. PICO 2 - Are tsDMARD (JAK inhibitors) effective and safe for the treatment ofRA patients after csdmard failure?.

Additional file 3. PICO 3 - Are tsDMARD (JAK inhibitors) effective and safe for the treatment ofRA patients after bDMARD failure?.

Additional file 4. PICO 4 - Are tsDMARD (JAK inhibitors) more effective for the treatment ofpatients with RA, compared to csDMARD?.

Additional file 5. PICO 5 - Are tsDMARD (JAK inhibitors) more effective for the treatment ofpatients with RA compared to bDMARD?.

Additional file 6. PICO 6 – Is there any evidence of better cost-effectiveness of tsDMARD (JAKinhibitors) compared to csDMARD?.

Additional file 7. PICO 7 – Is there any evidence of better cost-effectiveness of tsDMARD (JAKinhibitors) compared to bDMARD?.

Additional file 8. PICO 8 - Is there any evidence for herpes zoster vaccination eficcacybefore starting tsDMARD (JAK inhibitor) treatment?.

Additional file 9. PICO 9 - Is there evidence of an increased risk of thromboembolic events related to treatment withMMCDsae (JAK inhibitors)?.

Acknowledgements

The authors wish to acknowledge the researcher Wanderley Bernardo, who is responsible for the systematic review—presented in detail in the supplementary material, funded by the Brazilian Society of Rheumatology.

Authors' contributions

All authors made substantial contributions to the acquisition of data, have been involved in drafting the manuscript or revising it critically for important intellectual content, gave final approval of the version to be published and have participated sufficiently in the work to take public responsibility for appropriate portions of the content; and agreed to be accountable for all aspects of the work in ensuring that questions related to the accuracy or integrity of any part of the work are appropriately investigated and resolved. All authors read and approved the final manuscript.

Competing interests

Karina Rossi Bonfiglioli: Personal fees and/or non-financial support from Pfizer, Abbvie, Roche, Novartis, Boheringer-Ingelheim. Financial competing interest: none. Non-financial competing interest: none. Licia Maria Henrique da Mota: Has received personal or institutional support from Abbvie, Janssen, Pfizer and Roche; has delivered speeches at events related to this work and sponsored by Abbvie, Boheringer- Ingelheim, Janssen, Pfizer, Roche, Sandoz, Lilly and UCB. Financial competing interest: none. Non-financial competing interest: none. Ana Cristina de Medeiros Ribeiro: No conflicts declared. Adriana Maria Kakehasi: Research funds: CNPq, SBR, FAPEMIG Support for Scientific Events: Abbvie, BMS, Janssen Lecture Fees: UCB, Janssen, Pfizer, Roche, BMS Clinical research: Roche, Pfizer Advisory board: Janssen, Roche, BMS, Pfizer. Angela Luzia Branco Pinto Duarte: Lecture Fees: Janssen, BMS. Rina Dalva Neubarth Giorgi: Has received consulting fees,speaking fees and support for international congresses from: Roche,Pfizer,Bristol-Myers-Squibb, UCB Pharma, Eli-Lilly, AbbVie, Novartis, Amgen, Biogen and Janssen. Ieda Maria Magalhães Laurindo: Consultants for Abbvie,Amgen, Boehring-Ingelheim, Bristol, GSK, Janssen, Lilly, Pfizer and UCB; has received personal or institutional support from Abbvie, Bristol, Janssen, Lilly, Pfizer, UCB; has delivered speeches at events related to this work and sponsored by Abbvie, Bristol, Janssen, Lilly, Pfizer, Roche and UCB. Financial competing interest: none. Non-financial competing interest: none. Mariana Peixoto Guimarães Ubirajara e Silva de Souza: Suport for Research, Scientific Events, Lecture: UCB, Abbvie, BMS, Novartis, Pfizer, Amgen, Sandoz, Roche. Ana Paula Monteiro Gomides: Assistance for participation in events: Pfizer. Claiton Viegas Brenol: Has participated in clinical and/or experimental studies related to this work and sponsored by the PI (Abbvie, BMS, Janssen, Pfizer and Roche); has received personal or institutional support from the PI (Abbvie, BMS, Janssen, Pfizer and Roche); has delivered speeches at events related to this work and sponsored by the PI (Abbvie, Janssen, Pfizer and Roche). Financial competing interest: none. Non-financial competing interest: none. Geraldo da Rocha Castelar Pinheiro: No conflicts declared. Charlles Heldan de Moura Castro: No conflicts declared. Cleandro Pires de Albuquerque: Personal fees and/or non-financial support from Pfizer, Abbvie, AstraZeneca, Janssen, Bristol-Myers-Squibb, Roche, Novartis and UCB, outside the submitted article. Gustavo Luiz Behrens Pinto: Personal fees and/or non-financial support from Abbvie, Janssen, Roche and Novartis, outside the submitted article. Jose Fernando Verztman: personal fees and/or non-financial support from Pfizer, Abbvie, Roche, Novartis, Janssen, Lilly. Financial competing interest: none. Non-financial competing interest: none. Luciana Feitosa Muniz: No conflicts declared. Manoel Barros Bertolo: Has participated in clinical and/or experimental studies related to this work and sponsored by the PI (Roche); has delivered speeches at events related to this work and sponsored by the PI (Abbvie, Pfizer). Financial competing interest: none. Non-financial competing interest: none. Maria Raquel da Costa Pinto: Support in Congresses: UCB, Roche, Janssen, Bristol, Pfizer, Boheringer. Advisory Board: Janssen. Paulo Louzada Júnior: Sponsored by: Bristol-Myers Squibb, UCB, Pfizer Board Participation: Pfizer. Vitor Alves Cruz: Support in Congresses: UCB, Jansen, Abbvie and Pfizer. Ivanio Alves Pereira: Has received personal fee for lectures from Abbvie, Janssen, Pfizer and Roche; has delivered speeches at events related to this work and sponsored by Abbvie, Boheringer- Ingelheim, Janssen, Pfizer, Roche, Sandoz, Lilly and UCB. Financial competing interest: none. Non-financial competing interest: none. Max Vitor Carioca de Freitas: Speaker at events related to this work and sponsored by Abbvie, Novartis, Roche, Pfizer and UCB. Managing Partner of Integrare Therapeutics. Bóris Afonso Cruz: Support for Scientific Events and Lecture Fees: Abbvie, BMS, Janssen, Novartis, Pfizer, Roche. Eduardo Paiva: No conflicts declared. Odirlei Monticielo: Lectures and consultancies: Abbvie, APSEN, BMS, GSK, Janssen, Lilly, Novartis, Pfizer, Roche, UCB. José Roberto Provenza: No conflicts declared. Ricardo Machado Xavier: Lectures, consultancies: Abbvie, BMS, GSK, Janssen, Lilly, Novartis, Pfizer, Roche, UCB Clinical trials: Abbvie, UCB, Pfizer, GSK, Lilly.

Author details

[1]Disciplina Reumatologia do Hospital das Clínicas, Faculdade de Medicina, Universidade de São Paulo (HC-FMUSP), Av. Dr. Arnaldo, 455 - 3° andar – Reumatologia, São Paulo, SP, CEP 01246-903, Brasil. [2]Serviço de Reumatologia do Hospital, Universitário de Brasília (HUB/UnB), Brasília, Brazil. [3]Serviço de Reumatologia, Universidade Federal de Minas Gerais (UFMG), Belo Horizonte, Brazil. [4]Disciplina de Reumatologia, Universidade Nove de Julho (UNINOVE), São Paulo, Brazil. [5]Serviço de Reumatologia, Hospital do Servidor Público Estadual de São Paulo (HSPE-IAMSPE), São Paulo, Brazil. [6]Universidade Federal

de Pernambuco (UFPE), Recife, Brazil. [7]Santa Casa de Belo Horizonte (MG), Belo Horizonte, Brazil. [8]Hospital de Clínicas de Porto Alegre, Universidade Federal do Rio Grande do Sul (HCPA/UFRGS), Porto Alegre, Brazil. [9]Universidade do Estado do Rio de Janeiro (UERJ), Rio de Janeiro, Brazil. [10]Escola Paulista de Medicina, Universidade Federal de São Paulo, São Paulo, Brazil. [11]Universidade Federal da Bahia (UFBA), Salvador, Brazil. [12]Hospital Federal dos Servidores do Estado do RJ, Rio de Janeiro, Brazil. [13]Hospital Regional de Sobradinho (DF), Brasília, Brazil. [14]Disciplina de Reumatologia, Faculdade de Ciências Médicas, Universidade Estadual de Campinas, Campinas, Brazil. [15]Disciplina de Reumatologia, Faculdade de Medicina de Ribeirão Preto, Universidade de São Paulo (USP-RP), Ribeirão Preto, Brazil. [16]Disciplina de Reumatologia, Faculdade de Medicina, Universidade Federal de Goiás, Goiânia, Brazil. [17]Serviço de Reumatologia do Hospital Universitário, Universidade Federal de Santa Catarina-UFSC, Florianópolis, Brazil. [18]Universidade de Fortaleza - UNIFOR, Fortaleza, Brazil. [19]Pulsus – Belo Horizonte (MG), Belo Horizonte, Brazil. [20]Disciplina de Reumatologia, Universidade Federal do Paraná (UFPR), Curitiba, Brazil. [21]Disciplina de Reumatologia da Pontifícia, Universidade Católica de Campinas, PUC-Campinas, Campinas, Brazil.

References

1. Mota LMHD, Kakehasi AM, Gomides APM, et al. 2017 recommendations of the Brazilian Society of Rheumatology for the pharmacological treatment of rheumatoid arthritis. Adv Rheumatol. 2018;58(1):2. https://doi.org/10.1186/s42358-018-0005-0.
2. Alamanos Y, Voulgari PV, Drosos AA. Incidence and prevalence of rheumatoid arthritis, based on the 1987 American College of Rheumatology-criteria: a systematic review. Semin Arthritis Rheum. 2006;36:182–8.
3. Emery P, Salmon M. Early rheumatoid arthritis: time to aim for remission? Ann Rheum Dis. 1995;54:944–7.
4. Kavanaugh A. Economic consequences of established rheumatoid arthritis and its treatment. Best Pract Res Clin Rheumatol. 2007;21:929–42.
5. Klarenbeek NB, Allaart CF, Kerstens PJ, Huizinga TW, Dijkmans BA. The BeSt story: on strategy trials in rheumatoid arthritis. Curr Opin Rheumatol. 2009;21:291–8.
6. Ghabri S, Binard A, Pers YM, Maunoury F, Caro JJ. Economic evaluation of sequences of biological treatments for patients with moderate-to-severe rheumatoid arthritis and inadequate response or intolerance to methotrexate in France. Value Health. 2020;23(4):461–70. https://doi.org/10.1016/j.jval.2019.12.003.
7. Smolen JS, Landewé RBM, Bijlsma JWJ, et al. EULAR recommendations for the management of rheumatoid arthritis with synthetic and biological disease-modifying antirheumatic drugs: 2019 update. Ann Rheum Dis. 2020;79(6):685–99. https://doi.org/10.1136/annrheumdis-2019-216655.
8. Angelini J, Talotta R, Roncato R, et al. JAK-inhibitors for the treatment of rheumatoid arthritis: a focus on the present and an outlook on the future. Biomolecules. 2020;10(7):E1002. https://doi.org/10.3390/biom10071002.
9. Bula Tofacinib, Aug, 10, 2020.
10. Bula Bariticinite Aug, 10, 2020.
11. Bula Upadacitinib.
12. Moher D, Shamseer L, Clarke M, Ghersi D, Liberati A, Petticrew M, Shekelle P, Stewart LA. Preferred Reporting Items for Systematic Review and Meta-Analysis Protocols (PRISMA-P) 2015 statement. Syst Rev. 2015;4(1):1. https://doi.org/10.1186/2046-4053-4-1.
13. Review Manager (RevMan) [Computer program]. Version 5.4. Copenhagen: The Nordic Cochrane Center, The Cochrane Collaboration, 2014.
14. GRADEpro GDT: GRADEpro Guideline Development Tool [Software]. McMaster University, 2015 (developed by Evidence Prime, Inc.). gradepro.org.
15. Arnett FC, Edworthy SM, Bloch DA, McShane DJ, Fries JF, Cooper NS, et al. The American Rheumatism Association 1987 revised criteria for the classification of rheumatoid arthritis. Arthritis Rheum. 1988;31:315–24.
16. Aletaha D, Neogi T, Silman AJ, et al. 2010 Rheumatoid arthritis classification criteria: an American College of Rheumatology/European League Against Rheumatism collaborative initiative. Arthritis Rheum. 2010;62(9):2569–81. https://doi.org/10.1002/art.27584.
17. Lee EB, Fleischmann R, Hall S, Wilkinson B, Bradley JD, Gruben D, et al. Tofacitinib versus methotrexate in rheumatoid arthritis. N Engl J Med. 2014;19(370):2377–86.
18. Fleischmann R, Schiff M, van der Heijde D, Ramos-Remus C, Spindler A, Stanislav M, et al. Baricitinib, methotrexate, or combination in patients with rheumatoid arthritis and no or limited prior disease-modifying antirheumatic drug treatment. Arthritis Rheumatol. 2017;69:506–17.
19. van Vollenhoven R, Takeuchi T, Pangan AL, et al. Efficacy and safety of upadacitinib monotherapy in methotrexate-naïve patients with moderately to severely active rheumatoid arthritis (SELECT-EARLY): a randomized, double-blind, active-comparator, multi-center, multi-country trial [published online ahead of print, 2020 Jul 8]. Arthritis Rheumatol. 2020. https://doi.org/10.1002/art.41384.
20. Li Z, Hu J, Bao C, Li X, Xu J, Spindler A, et al. SAT0218 Efficacy and safety of baricitinib in mtx-ir patients with rheumatoid arthritis: 52 week results from a phase 3 study (RA-BALANCE). Ann Rheum Dis. 2018;77(Suppl 2):969.
21. Tanaka Y, Takeuchi T, Yamaoka K, Oribe M, Kawano M, Zhou Y, et al. SAT0257 a phase 2b/3 randomised, placebo-controlled, double-blind study of upadacitinib, a selective jak1 inhibitor, in japanese patients with active rheumatoid arthritis and inadequate response to conventional synthetic dmards. Ann Rheum Dis. 2018;77(Suppl 2):991.
22. Burmester GR, Kremer JM, Van den Bosch F, Kivitz A, Bessette L, Li Y, et al. Safety and efficacy of upadacitinib in patients with rheumatoid arthritis and inadequate response to conventional synthetic disease-modifying anti-rheumatic drugs (SELECT-NEXT): a randomised, double-blind, placebo-controlled phase 3 trial. Lancet. 2018;391(10139):2503–12.
23. Dougados M, van der Heijde D, Chen YC, Greenwald M, Drescher E, Liu J, et al. Baricitinib in patients with inadequate response or intolerance to conventional synthetic DMARDs: results from the RA-BUILD study. Ann Rheum Dis. 2017;76(1):88–95.
24. Taylor PC, Keystone EC, van der Heijde D, Weinblatt ME, Del Carmen ML, Reyes Gonzaga J, et al. Baricitinib versus placebo or adalimumab in rheumatoid arthritis. N Engl J Med. 2017;376(7):652–62.
25. Tanaka Y, Emoto K, Cai Z, Aoki T, Schlichting D, Rooney T, et al. Efficacy and safety of baricitinib in japanese patients with active rheumatoid arthritis receiving background methotrexate therapy: a 12-week, double-blind, randomized placebo-controlled study. J Rheumatol. 2016;43(3):504–11.
26. Keystone EC, Taylor PC, Drescher E, Schlichting DE, Beattie SD, Berclaz PY, et al. Safety and efficacy of baricitinib at 24 weeks in patients with rheumatoid arthritis who have had an inadequate response to methotrexate. Ann Rheum Dis. 2015;74(2):333–40.
27. Westhovens R, Taylor PC, Alten R, Pavlova D, Enríquez-Sosa F, Mazur M, et al. Filgotinib (GLPG0634/GS-6034), an oral JAK1 selective inhibitor, is effective in combination with methotrexate (MTX) in patients with active rheumatoid arthritis and insufficient response to MTX: results from a randomised, dose-finding study (DARWIN 1). Ann Rheum Dis. 2017;76(6):998–1008.
28. Kavanaugh A, Kremer J, Ponce L, Cseuz R, Reshetko OV, Stanislavchuk M, et al. Filgotinib (GLPG0634/GS-6034), an oral selective JAK1 inhibitor, is effective as monotherapy in patients with active rheumatoid arthritis: results from a randomised, dose-finding study (DARWIN 2). Ann Rheum Dis. 2017;76(6):1009–19.
29. Takeuchi T, Tanaka Y, Tanaka S, Kawakami A, Iwasaki M, Katayama K, et al. Efficacy and safety of peficitinib (ASP015K) in patients with rheumatoid arthritis and an inadequate response to methotrexate: results of a phase III randomised, double-blind, placebo-controlled trial (RAJ4) in Japan. Ann Rheum Dis. 2019;78(10):1305–19.
30. Kivitz AJ, Gutierrez-Ureña SR, Poiley J, Genovese MC, Kristy R, Shay K, et al. Peficitinib, a JAK inhibitor, in the treatment of moderate-to-severe rheumatoid arthritis in patients with an inadequate response to methotrexate. Arthritis Rheumatol. 2017;69(4):709–19.
31. Fleischmann R, Mysler E, Hall S, Kivitz AJ, Moots RJ, Luo Z, et al. Efficacy and safety of tofacitinib monotherapy, tofacitinib with methotrexate, and adalimumab with methotrexate in patients with rheumatoid arthritis (ORAL Strategy): a phase 3b/4, double-blind, head-to-head, randomised controlled trial. Lancet. 2017;390(10093):457–68.
32. van der Heijde D, Tanaka Y, Fleischmann R, Keystone E, Kremer J, Zerbini C, et al. Tofacitinib (CP-690,550) in patients with rheumatoid arthritis receiving methotrexate: twelve-month data from a twenty-four-month phase III randomized radiographic study. Arthritis Rheum. 2013;65(3):559–70.
33. van Vollenhoven RF, Fleischmann R, Cohen S, Lee EB, García Meijide JA, Wagner S, et al. Tofacitinib or adalimumab versus placebo in rheumatoid arthritis. N Engl J Med. 2012;367(6):508–19.
34. Kremer JM, Cohen S, Wilkinson BE, Connell CA, French JL, Gomez-Reino J,

et al. A phase IIb dose-ranging study of the oral JAK inhibitor tofacitinib (CP-690,550) versus placebo in combination with background metho trexate in patients with active rheumatoid arthritis and an inadequate response to methotrexate alone. Arthritis Rheum. 2012;64(4):970–81.

35. Tanaka Y, Suzuki M, Nakamura H, Toyoizumi S, Zwillich SH. Phase II study of tofacitinib (CP-690,550) combined with methotrexate in patients with rheumatoid arthritis and an inadequate response to methotrexate. Arthritis Care Res (Hoboken). 2011;63(8):1150–8.
36. Smolen JS, Pangan AL, Emery P, Rigby W, Tanaka Y, Vargas JI, et al. Upadacitinib as monotherapy in patients with active rheumatoid arthritis and inadequate response to methotrexate (SELECT-MONOTHERAPY): a randomised, placebo-controlled, double-blind phase 3 study. Lancet. 2019;393(10188):2303–11.
37. Genovese MC, Smolen JS, Weinblatt ME, Burmester GR, Meerwein S, Camp HS, et al. Efficacy and safety of ABT-494, a selective JAK-1 inhibitor, in a phase IIb study in patients with rheumatoid arthritis and an inadequate response to methotrexate. Arthritis Rheumatol. 2016;68(12):2857–66.
38. Fleischmann R, Pangan AL, Song IH, Mysler E, Bessette L, Peterfy C, et Upadacitinib versus placebo or adalimumab in patients with rheumatoid arthritis and an inadequate response to methotrexate: results of a phase III, double-blind, randomized controlled trial. Arthritis Rheumatol. 2019;71(11):1788–800.
39. Burmester GR, Blanco R, Charles-Schoeman C, Wollenhaupt J, Zerbini C, Benda B, et al. Tofacitinib (CP-690,550) in combination with methotrexate in patients with active rheumatoid arthritis with an inadequate response to tumor necrosis factor inhibitors: a randomized phase 3 trial. Lancet. 2013;9(381):451–60.
40. Genovese MC, Kremer J, Zamani O, Ludivico C, Krogulec M, Xie L, Beattie SD, et al. Baricitinib in patients with refractory rheumatoid arthritis. N Engl J Med. 2016;31(374):1243–52.
41. Genovese MC, Fleischmann R, Combe B, Hall S, Rubbert-Roth A, Zhang Y, et al. Safety and efficacy of upadacitinib in patients with active rheumatoid arthritis refractory to biologic disease-modifying anti-rheumatic drugs (SELECT-BEYOND): a double-blind, randomized controlled phase 3 trial. Lancet. 2018;23(391):2513–24.
42. Genovese MC, Kalunian K, Gottenberg JE, Mozaffarian N, Bartok B, Matzk ies F, et al. Effect of filgotinib vs. placebo on clinical response in patients with moderate to severe rheumatoid arthritis refractory to disease-modifying antirheumatic drug therapy: the FINCH 2 randomized clinical trial. JAMA. 2019;322:315–25.
43. Conaghan PG, Østergaard M, Bowes MA, Wu C, Fuerst T, van der Heijde D, Irazoque-Palazuelos F, Soto-Raices O, Hrycaj P, Xie Z, Zhang R. Comparing the effects of tofacitinib, methotrexate and the combination, on bone marrow oedema, synovitis and bone erosion in methotrexate-naive, early active rheumatoid arthritis: results of an exploratory randomized MRI al. study incorporating semiquantitative and quantitative techniques. Ann Rheum Dis. 2016;75(6):1024–33.
44. Fleischmann R, Schiff M, van der Heijde D, Ramos-Remus C, Spindler A, Stanislav M, Zerbini CA, Gurbuz S, Dickson C, de Bono S, Schlichting D. Baricitinib, methotrexate, or combination in patients with rheumatoid arthritis and no limited prior disease—modifying antirheumatic drug treatment. Arthritis & Rheumatology. 2017;69(3):506–17.
45. Fleischmann R, Mysler E, Hall S, Kivitz AJ, Moots RJ, Luo Z, DeMasi R, Soma K, Zhang R, Takiya L, Tatulych S. Efficacy and safety of tofacitinib monotherapy, tofacitinib with methotrexate, and adalimumab with methotrexate in patients with rheumatoid arthritis (ORAL Strategy): a phase 3b/4, double-blind, head-to-head, randomised controlled trial. The Lancet. 2017;390(10093):457–68.
46. Fleischmann R, Pangan AL, Song IH, Mysler E, Bessette L, Peterfy C, Durez P, Ostor AJ, Li Y, Zhou Y, Othman AA. Upadacitinib versus placebo or adalimumab in patients with rheumatoid arthritis and an inadequate response to methotrexate: results of a phase iii, double-blind, randomized controlled trial. Arthritis Rheumatol. 2019;71(11):1788–800.
47. Hall S, Nash P, Rischmueller M, Bossingham D, Bird P, Cook N, Witcombe D, Soma K, Kwok K, Thirunavukkarasu K. Tofacitinib, an oral Janus Kinase inhibitor: pooled efficacy and safety analyses in an Australian rheumatoid arthritis population. Rheumatol Ther. 2018;5(2):383–401.
48. Taylor PC, Keystone EC, van der Heijde D, Weinblatt ME, del Carmen ML, Reyes Gonzaga J, Yakushin S, Ishii T, Emoto K, Beattie S, Arora V. Baricitinib versus placebo or adalimumab in rheumatoid arthritis. N Engl J Med. 2017;376(7):652–62.
49. Jansen JP, Incerti D, Mutebi A, Peneva D, MacEwan JP, Stolshek B, Kaur P, Gharaibeh M, Strand V. Cost-effectiveness of sequenced treatment of rheumatoid arthritis with targeted immune modulators. J Med Econ. 2017;20(7):703–14.
50. Wehler E, Boytsov N, Nicolay C, Herrera-Restrepo O, Kowal S. A Budget impact and cost per additional respond analysis for baricitinib for the treatment of moderate-to-severe rheumatoid arthritis in patients with an inadequate response to tumor necrosis factor inhibitors in the USA. Pharmacoeconomics. 2020;38(1):39–56.
51. Critical Appraisal Skills Programme. CASP economic evaluation checklist.
52. Chen DY, Hsu PN, Tang CH, Claxton L, Valluri S, Gerber RA. Tofacitinib in the treatment of moderate-to-severe rheumatoid arthritis: a cost-effectiveness analysis compared with adalimumab in Taiwan. J Med Econ. 2019;22(8):777–87.
53. Claxton L, Jenks M, Taylor M, Wallenstein G, Mendelsohn AM, Bourret JA, Singh A, Moynagh D, Gerber RA. An economic evaluation of tofacitinib treatment in rheumatoid arthritis: modeling the cost of treatment strategies in the United States. J Manag Care Spec Pharm. 2016;22(9):1088–102.
54. Lee MY, Park SK, Park SY, Byun JH, Lee SM, Ko SK, Lee EK. Cost-effectiveness of tofacitinib in the treatment of moderate to severe rheumatoid arthritis in South Korea. Clin Ther. 2015;37(8):1662–76.
55. Navarro F, Martinez-Sesmero JM, Balsa A, Peral C, Montoro M, Valderrama M, Gómez S, de Andrés-Nogales F, Casado MA, Oyagüez I. Cost-effectiveness analysis of treatment sequences containing tofacitinib for the treatment of rheumatoid arthritis in Spain. Clin Rheumatol. 2020;17:1–2.
56. Schlueter M, Finn E, Díaz S, Dilla T, Inciarte-Mundo J, Fakhouri W. Cost-effectiveness analysis of baricitinib versus adalimumab for the treatment of moderate-to-severe rheumatoid arthritis in Spain. ClinicoEconomics Outcomes Res: CEOR. 2019;11:395.
57. Van De Laar CJ, Voshaar MA, Fakhouri WK, Zaremba-Pechmann L, De Leonardis F, De La Torre I, Van De Laar MA. Cost-effectiveness of a JAK1/JAK2 inhibitor vs a biologic disease-modifying antirheumatic drug (bDMARD) in a treat-to-target strategy for rheumatoid arthritis. ClinicoEconomics Outcomes Res: CEOR. 2020;12:213.
58. Curtis JR, Xie F, Yun H, et al. Real-world comparative risks of herpes virus infections in tofacitinib and biologic-treated patients with rheumatoid arthritis. Ann Rheum Dis. 2016;75:1843–7.
59. Winthrop KL, Curtis JR, Lindsey S, et al. Herpes zoster and tofacitinib: clinical outcomes and the risk of concomitant therapy. Arthritis Rheumatol. 2017;69(10):1960–8.
60. Calabrese LH, Abud-Mendoza C, Lindsey SM, Lee SH, Tatulych S, Takiya L, et al. Live zoster vaccine in patients with rheumatoid arthritis treated with tofacitinib with or without methotrexate, or adalimumab with methotrexate: a post hoc analysis of data from a phase IIIb/IV randomized study. Arthritis Care Res (Hoboken). 2020;72:353–9.
61. Winthrop KL, Wouters AG, Choy EH, Soma K, Hodge JA, Nduaka CI, et al. The safety and immunogenicity of live zoster vaccination in patients with rheumatoid arthritis before starting tofacitinib: a randomized phase II trial. Arthritis Rheumatol. 2017;69:1969–77.
62. Winthrop KL, Wouters A, Choy EH, Chen C, Biswas P, Wang L, et al. Long-term effectiveness of live herpes zoster vaccine in patients with rheumatoid arthritis subsequently treated with tofacitinib. Ann Rheum Dis. 2020;79:669–71.
63. Stevens E, Weinblatt ME, Massarotti E, Griffin F, Emani S, Desai S. Safety of the zoster vaccine recombinant adjuvanted in rheumatoid arthritis and other systemic rheumatic disease patients: a single center's experience with 400 patients. ACR Open Rheumatol. 2020. https://doi.org/10.1002/acr2.11150.
64. Fleischmann R, Kremer J, Cush J, et al. Placebo-controlled trial of tofacitinib monotherapy in rheumatoid arthritis. N Engl J Med. 2012;367(6):495–507. https://doi.org/10.1056/NEJMoa1109071.
65. van Vollenhoven RF, Fleischmann R, Cohen S, et al. Tofacitinib or adalimumab versus placebo in rheumatoid arthritis [published correction appears in N Engl J Med. 2013 Jul 18;369(3):293]. N Engl J Med. 2012;367(6):508–19. https://doi.org/10.1056/NEJMoa111207
66. Burmester GR, Blanco R, Charles-Schoeman C, et al. Tofacitinib (CP-690,550) in combination with methotrexate in patients with active rheumatoid arthritis with an inadequate response to tumour necrosis fac tor inhibitors: a randomised phase 3 trial. Lancet. 2013;381(9865):451–60. https://doi.org/10.1016/S0140-6736(12)61424-X.
67. Genovese MC, Fleischmann R, Combe B, et al. Safety and efficacy of upadacitinib in patients with active rheumatoid arthritis refractory to biologic disease-modifying anti-rheumatic drugs (SELECT-BEYOND): a double-

blind, randomised controlled phase 3 trial. Lancet. 2018;391(10139):2513–24. https://doi.org/10.1016/S0140-6736(18)31116-4.

68. Burmester GR, Kremer JM, Van den Bosch F, et al. Safety and efficacy of upadacitinib in patients with rheumatoid arthritis and inadequate response to conventional synthetic disease-modifying anti-rheumatic drugs (SELECT-NEXT): a randomised, double-blind, placebo-controlled phase 3 trial. Lancet. 2018;391(10139):2503–12. https://doi.org/10.1016/S0140-6736(18)31115-2.
69. Fleischmann R, Pangan AL, Song IH, et al. Upadacitinib versus placebo or adalimumab in patients with rheumatoid arthritis and an inadequate response to methotrexate: results of a phase III, double-blind, randomized controlled trial. Arthritis Rheumatol. 2019;71(11):1788–800. https://doi.org/10.1002/art.41032.
70. Tanaka Y, Emoto K, Cai Z, Aoki T, Schlichting D, Rooney T, Macias W. Efficacy and safety of baricitinib in japanese patients with active rheumatoid arthritis receiving background methotrexate therapy: a 12-week, double-blind, randomized placebo-controlled study. J Rheumatol. 2016;43(5):998. https://doi.org/10.3899/jrheum.150613.C1.
71. Dougados M, van der Heijde D, Chen YC, et al. Baricitinib in patients with inadequate response or intolerance to conventional synthetic DMARDs: results from the RA-BUILD study [published correction appears in Ann Rheum Dis. 2017 Sep;76(9):1634]. Ann Rheum Dis. 2017;76(1):88–95. https://doi.org/10.1136/annrheumdis-2016-210094.
72. Taylor PC, Keystone EC, van der Heijde D, et al. Baricitinib versus placebo or adalimumab in rheumatoid arthritis. N Engl J Med. 2017;376(7):652–62. https://doi.org/10.1056/NEJMoa1608345.
73. Genovese MC, Kalunian K, Gottenberg JE, et al. Effect of filgotinib vs placebo on clinical response in patients with moderate to severe rheumatoid arthritis refractory to disease-modifying antirheumatic drug therapy: the FINCH 2 randomized clinical trial [published correction appears in JAMA. 2020 Feb 4;323(5):480]. JAMA. 2019;322(4):315–25. https://doi.org/10.1001/jama.2019.9055.
74. https://clinicaltrials.gov/ct2/show/results/NCT02092467. Last checked in 30 Sept 2021.
75. https://www.fda.gov/drugs/drug-safety-and-availability/fda-requires-warnings-about-increased-risk-serious-heart-related-events-cancer-blood-clots-and-death. Last checked in 30 Sept 2021.
76. https://www.ema.europa.eu/en/news/meeting-highlights-pharmacovigilance-risk-assessment-committee-prac-7-10-june-2021. Last checked in 30 Sept 2021.

4

Brazilian Society of Rheumatology 2020 guidelines for psoriatic arthritis

Sueli Carneiro[1*], Penelope Esther Palominos[2], Sônia Maria Alvarenga Anti[3], Rodrigo Luppino Assad[4], Rafaela Silva Guimarães Gonçalves[5], Adriano Chiereghin[6], Andre Marun Lyrio[7], Antônio Carlos Ximenes[8], Carla Gonçalves Saad[9], Célio Roberto Gonçalves[9], Charles Lubianca Kohem[2], Cláudia Diniz Lopes Marques[5], Cláudia Goldenstein Schainberg[9], Eduardo de Souza Meirelles[9], Gustavo Gomes Resende[10], Lenise Brandao Pieruccetti[11], Mauro Waldemar Keiserman[12], Michel Alexandre Yazbek[13], Percival Degrava Sampaio-Barros[9], Ricardo da Cruz Lage[10], Rubens Bonfiglioli[7], Thauana Luíza Oliveira[14], Valderílio Feijó Azevedo[15], Washington Alves Bianchi[16], Wanderley Marques Bernardo[9], Ricardo dos Santos Simões[17], Marcelo de Medeiros Pinheiro[14] and Cristiano Barbosa Campanholo[18]

Abstract

Psoriatic arthritis (PsA) is a chronic and systemic immune disease characterized by inflammation of peripheral and/or axial joints and entheses in patients with psoriasis (PsO). Extra-articular and extracutaneous manifestations and numerous comorbidities can also be present. These recommendations replace the previous version published in May 2013. A systematic review of the literature retrieved 191 articles that were used to formulate 12 recommendations in response to 12 clinical questions, divided into 4 sections: diagnosis, non-pharmacological treatment, conventional drug therapy and biologic therapy. These guidelines provide evidence-based information on the clinical management for PsA patients. For each recommendation, the level of evidence (highest available), degree of strength (Oxford) and degree of expert agreement (interrater reliability) are reported.

Keywords: Psoriatic arthritis, Spondyloarthropathies, Inflammation, Treatment, Guideline

Introduction

Psoriatic arthritis (PsA) is defined as chronic inflammatory arthropathy associated with psoriasis (PsO), with an equal distribution between men and women. A meta-analysis of 28 studies regarding the frequency of PsA in the general population of several countries found an incidence of 83 cases per 100.000 person-years and an estimated prevalence of 133 cases per 100.000 people [1].

It is estimated that one in 3 or 4 patients with Pso will also have PsA [2, 3].

*Correspondence: sueli@hucff.ufrj.br
[1] Universidade Federal do Rio de Janeiro (UFRJ), Rua Farme de Amoedo, 140/601. Ipanema, Rio de Janeiro, RJ CEP 22420-020, Brazil

The diagnosis of PsA is clinical, based on anamnesis, physical examination and imaging tests. Classification criteria can be used to homogenize patients and are valuable for scientific communication and clinical studies.

Regarding anamnesis and physical examination, some findings suggest the presence of PsA even in the absence of PsO: inflammatory arthropathy with involvement of the distal interphalangeal joints (DIP), asymmetric arthritis, nail lesions such as pitting and onycholysis, dactylitis and family history of PsO [4].

Bone and cartilage destruction with the pathological formation of new bone is one of the most striking aspects of PsA. Radiographs of peripheral joints may show bone loss with eccentric erosions and decreased joint space as well as new bone formation characterized by periostitis, enthesophytes or bone ankylosis [5]. In the axial skeleton, the changes associated with PsA include unilateral or bilateral sacroiliitis and bulky paramarginal vertical syndesmophytes (or parasyndesmophytes). Magnetic resonance imaging (MRI) may reveal focal erosions, synovitis and bone marrow edema in the peripheral and/or axial skeleton, particularly in entheses. Ultrasound (US) can identify synovitis, tenosynovitis, increased blood flow, enthesophytes and early erosive disease [5].

The treatment of PsA aims to achieve a state of remission, defined as complete resolution of signs and symptoms of inflammatory activity depending on the clinical judgment of the specialist or a Disease Activity index for PSoriatic Arthritis (DAPSA) score £ 4 or fulfillment the 7 Minimal Disease Activity (MDA) criteria, also called very low disease activity (VLDA). When remission cannot be achieved, a state of minimal disease activity may be acceptable and is defined as a DAPSA score between 4 and 14 points or fulfillment of at least 5 of the 7 MDA criteria. When there is axial involvement, metrics proposed for axial spondyloarthritis, i.e., Bath Ankylosing Spondylitis Disease Activity Index (BASDAI) £ 4 or Ankylosing Spondylitis Disease Activity Score with C-Reactive Protein (ASDAS-CRP) £ 1.3, are recommended [6–8]. These strategies are expected to optimize the function and improve the well-being of patients, prevent structural damage and minimize disease and treatment complications [9] (Tables 1, 2, 3 and 4).

The impact of the disease on pain, function, quality of life and structural damage should be evaluated. In addition, inflammation may influence other commonly related clinical conditions, such as cardiovascular disease, uveitis, inflammatory bowel disease and others.

Therapeutic decisions must be individualized and shared between the patient and physician, reflecting patient preferences based on adequate information [6, 9].

Table 2 MDA criteria for the evaluation of inflammatory disease activity [7, 198]

When meeting at least 5 of the 7 criteria	
1. Painful joint count	≤ 1
2. Swollen joint count	≤ 1
3. PASI ≤ 1 or BSA	≤ 3
4. VAS for pain by the patient	≤ 15
5. VAS for overall activity by the patient	≤ 20
6. HAQ	≤ 0.5
7. Pain points in entheses	≤ 1

MDA: minimal disease activity; BSA: body surface area; HAQ: health assessment questionnaire; PASI: psoriasis area severity index; VAS: visual analog scale

* Patients who meet 7 of the 7 criteria are considered to have very low inflammatory activity and are considered to be in remission

Drug choice may be influenced by factors such as disease activity, structural damage, concomitant clinical conditions and previously used therapies [6–10].

Ideally, patients should be evaluated regularly, with treatment adjusted as needed.

The objective of these guidelines is to provide evidence-based information on the clinical management of patients with PsA, including diagnosis, treatment and prognosis for rheumatologists, specialists in related fields, clinicians and other health professionals who deal directly with these patients.

This version replaces the previous guidelines published on May 26, 2013 [11].

Methods

A systematic literature review was conducted by a group of experts of the Brazilian Medical Association. Keywords defined according to the PICO strategy (Patient | Intervention | Comparison | Result) were used to search for records in the following databases: MEDLINE,

Table 1 DAPSA criteria for the evaluation of inflammatory disease activity [7, 197]

Domain	Rating
VAS Pain	0 to 10
GDA (Pt)	0 to 10
Painful joints	68
Swollen joints	66
CRP	mg/dL
DAPSA	**Simple sum**
DAPSA ≤ 4	Activity = Remission
DAPSA > 4–14	Activity = Low
DAPSA > 14–28	Activity = Moderate
DAPSA > 28	Activity = High

DAPSA: Disease Activity index for Psoriatic Arthritis; VAS: visual analog scale; GDA (Pt): patient global disease assessment; CRP: C-reactive protein

Table 3 BASDAI assessment criteria for axial inflammatory activity in spondyloarthritis [8, 199]

BASDAI	
1. How would you describe the overall level of fatigue/tiredness you have experienced?	0 to 10 (none to intense)
2. How would you describe the overall level of AS neck, back or hip pain you have had?	0 to 10 (none to intense)
3. How would you describe the overall level of pain/swelling in joints other than neck, back, hips you have had?	0 to 10 (none to intense)
4. How would you describe the overall level of discomfort you have had in any areas tender to touch or pressure?	0 to 10 (none to intense)
5. How would you describe the overall level of morning stiffness you have had from the time you wake up?	0 to 10 (none to intense)
6. How long does your morning stiffness last from the time you wake up?	0 to 10 (0 to 2 or more hours)
BASDAI = [(Q5 + Q6)/2 + (Q1 + Q2 + Q3 + Q4)]/5	
BASDAI < 4	Inactive or low-activity disease
BASDAI from 4 to 10	Active disease

BASDAI: Bath Ankylosing Spondylitis Disease Activity Index = mean of the values of questions 5 and 6 plus the values of questions 1 to 4, divided by 5

Table 4 ASDAS-CRP evaluation criteria for axial inflammatory activity in spondyloarthritis [8, 200, 201]

ASDAS-CRP							
1. Overall back pain (BASDAI question 2)							
2. Global patient assessment							
3. Peripheral pain/inflammation (BASDAI question 3)							
4. Duration of morning stiffness (BASDAI question 6)							
5. C-reactive protein (CRP) in mg/l [or erythrocyte sedimentation rate (ESR)]							
$ASDAS_{CRP}$	**0.12 X overall back pain**	+	**0.06 X duration of morning stiffness**	+	**0.07 X Peripheral pain/ inflammation**	+	**0.58 X Ln(CRP + 1)**
$ASDAS_{CRP} < 1.3$	Activity = Inactive						
$1.3 \leq ASDAS_{CRP} < 2.1$	Activity = Low disease activity						
$2.1 \leq ASDAS_{CRP} < 3.5$	Activity = High						
$ASDAS_{CRP} > 3.5$	Activity = Very high						

ASDAS-CRP: Ankylosing Spondylitis Disease Activity Score with C-Reactive Protein

EMBASE, SciELO/LILACS and the Cochrane Library, from March 1st, 2012, to December 31st, 2019.

After conducting the systematic literature review there were added some relevant studies published until December 31st 2020, including the validation study of the Portuguese version of the TOronto Psoriatic Arthritis Screen II (TOPAS-II), two pivotal randomized clinical trial that approved guselkumab and upadacitinib for the treatment of PsA, and two other head-to-head clinical trials studies comparing IL-17 inhibitors (secukinumab and ixekizumab) with adalimumab.

The target population included patients with joint, axial and entheseal musculoskeletal inflammatory pain according to the 2006 Classification of Psoriatic Arthritis (CASPAR) criteria [12] (Table 5). Studies were selected and used to formulate 12 recommendations, answering 12 clinical questions, which were divided into 4 sections: diagnosis, nonpharmacological treatment, conventional therapy and biologic therapy. For each recommendation, the level of evidence (highest available) and the degree of strength (Oxford Center for Evidence-Based Medicine Level of Evidence) [12–16] were reported. The degree of expert agreement

Table 5 Classification criteria for psoriatic arthritis [12]

Presence of established inflammatory joint disease	
(arthritis, enthesitis, axial) and at least 3 points	Points
Current skin psoriasis OR	2 or
History of psoriasis OR	1 or
Family history of psoriasis	1
Dactylitis	1
Nail dystrophy	1
Negative rheumatoid factor	1
Juxta-articular bone neoformation	1

Sensitivity 0.914; Specificity 0.987

Table 6 Guidelines of the Brazilian Society of Rheumatology for the diagnosis and treatment of psoriatic arthritis with their respective level of evidence, strength of recommendation and degree of agreement among experts (interrater reliability), 2020

	Question/Recommendation	Level of evidence	Strength of recommendation	Degree of agreement
1	What are the criteria for considering that an individual has psoriatic arthritis?			
	The diagnosis of PsA should be based on clinical and imaging criteria, and the CASPAR should be used for disease classification	1A	A	0.97
	The use of PsA screening questionnaires in patients with PsO is recommended, with preference for those that have already been validated in the Brazilian population, such as the PASE, PEST and TOPAS-II	1A	A	0.94
2	Is there a correlation between skin, nail and osteoarticular manifestations in psoriatic arthritis?			
	All patients with PsO should be evaluated for the presence of musculoskeletal manifestations, and those with involvement of the nails, intergluteal region, scalp or of extensive areas are at higher risk for musculoskeletal involvement	2B	B	0.94
3	What are the comorbidities most associated with psoriatic arthritis?			
	The most frequent comorbidities in patients with PsA, such as metabolic syndrome, atherosclerosis, cardiovascular disease, mood disorders, inflammatory bowel disease, osteoporosis and uveitis, should be screened and managed	2B	B	0.96
4	Is there evidence of benefits of exercise in the treatment of psoriatic arthritis?			
	Aerobic and resistance exercises should be individually prescribed to improve functional capacity, pain and quality of life	1B	A	0.97
5	What is the evidence for the use of corticosteroids in patients with psoriatic arthritis?			
	The use of intra-articular corticosteroid injection is recommended for localized, mono- or oligoarticular disease, especially in patients who are unresponsive to systemic treatment	2C	B	0.95
	Due to the lack of quality data on the efficacy of the use of systemic corticosteroids in PsA and the known adverse effects, their long-term use is not recommended	5	D	0.94
6	What is the evidence for the use of nonsteroidal antiinflammatory drugs (NSAIDs) in patients with psoriatic arthritis?			
	The use of NSAIDs is recommended as a symptomatic treatment in patients with peripheral arthritis	1B	A	0.95
	The use of NSAIDs is recommended as a symptomatic treatment in patients with enthesitis, dactylitis and axial manifestations	5	D	0.96
	As there is no evidence of a difference in efficacy among NSAIDs*, the choice of the drug should be based on the physician's familiarity with the drug and individual patient preference, respecting the concomitant clinical conditions**	*1B**5	B	0.96
7	What is the evidence for the use of conventional DMARDs in the treatment of psoriatic arthritis?			
	The use of methotrexate (MTX) is recommended as the first option among cDMARDs for the treatment of peripheral articular and skin involvement in PsA*, preferably at doses higher than 15 mg/week and subcutaneously**.	*1B **5	B	0.93
	If MTX is not available, cyclosporine, leflunomide or sulfasalazine should be used in patients with peripheral arthritis	2B	B	0.93
	There is NO scientific evidence of the use of cDMARDs in axial disease and limited evidence for enthesitis	5	D	0.89
8	When are biologic DMARDs or targeted synthetic DMARDs indicated for the treatment of PsA?			
	A bDMARD should be initiated in patients with PsA and peripheral arthritis who remain with active disease despite the use of a cDMARD, preferably MTX, for at least 3 months	1B	A	0.95
	In the case of failure or inability to use a bDMARD, a tsDMARD can be used	1B	B	0.95
	The use of a bDMARD is recommended for patients with PsA and axial manifestations who remain with active disease despite the use of 2 classes of NSAIDs, in full dose, for at least 30 days each	1B	B	0.92
9	Is there a difference in the efficacy of biologic DMARDs and targeted synthetic DMARDs in the treatment of PsA?			
	For the treatment of peripheral arthritis, dactylitis and enthesitis, the use of any of the following drugs is recommended: anti-TNFs (adalimumab, certolizumab pegol, etanercept, golimumab and infliximab), anti-IL-17 (ixekizumab and secukinumab), anti-IL-12/23 (ustekinumab) and anti-IL-23 (guselkumab)	1B	A	0.98

Table 6 (continued)

	Question/Recommendation	Level of evidence	Strength of recommendation	Degree of agreement
	The choice of drug should take into account patient preference (in regard to the route of administration and frequency of use, for example), concomitant clinical conditions, medical history (e.g., history of tuberculosis, fungal infections, and herpes zoster), cost, availability in the health system and presence of extra-articular manifestations of PsA	5	D	0.99
	In patients with axial manifestations, the use of anti-TNF and anti-IL-17 drugs is preferentially recommended	1B	B	0.98
	In patients with PsA and severe PsO, anti-IL-23, anti-IL-17, and anti-IL-12/23 drugs are preferentially recommended over anti-TNFs	1B	A	0.95
	In patients with recurrent uveitis, the use of anti-TNF monoclonal antibodies is recommended	1B	B	0.99
	In patients with concomitant active Crohn's disease, the use of IFX, ADA, CTZ, and UST is preferentially recommended	1B	B	0.98
	In patients with concomitant active ulcerative colitis, the use of IFX, ADA, GOL, UST or TOF is preferentially recommended	1B	B	0.98
10	Is there a difference in the safety of biologic DMARDs in the treatment of PsA?			
	Screening and treatment of latent tuberculosis infection (LTBI) or disease is recommended before the use of any immunobiologic and JAK inhibitor	2B	B	0.98
	In general, the biologics used for the treatment of PsA have similar safety profiles, and the particularities inherent to the cytokine to be inhibited should be considered	1B	B	0.96
	The use of anti-TNFs in patients with demyelinating disease or class III or IV heart failure is not recommended	4	C	0.99
	The use of JAK inhibitors in patients with disseminated or recurrent herpes zoster is not recommended	1B	A	0.99
	The use of IL-17 inhibitors in patients with a history of severe or recurrent fungal infections is not recommended	1B	A	0.98
11	Is there evidence for the use of conventional DMARDs combined with biologic DMARDs or target synthetic DMARDs?			
	Regarding monoclonal anti-TNF biologics, the concomitant use of MTX is recommended to increase survival, although there is no evidence of increased efficacy	*2B **1B	B	0.88
	Regarding non-anti-TNF biologics or tsDMARDs, there is no evidence of increased efficacy or survival with the concomitant use of cDMARDs	1B	A	0.97
12	Is there evidence for switching biologic and small-molecule DMARDs in patients with psoriatic arthritis?			
	In patients with PsA and bDMARD failure, switching to any other immunobiologic agent or to JAK inhibitors is recommended, with no differences between drugs, and the most relevant manifestations of the disease and concomitant clinical conditions should be considered	*1B **5	B	0.96
	When the therapeutic failure of an anti-TNF agent is attributed to skin inflammatory activity, switching to drugs with another mechanism of action, such as anti-IL23, anti-IL17 or anti-IL-12/23 agents, can be evaluated	1B	B	0.95
	When the therapeutic failure of an anti-TNF agent is attributed to serious adverse events, especially infections, switching to drugs with another mechanism of action, such as anti-IL-17, anti-IL-12/23, and anti-IL23 drugs or CTLA4 inhibitors	2B	B	0.98
	If there is a preference for oral medication or contraindications to injectable medications, the use of tofacitinib may be considered	5	D	0.96

(interrater reliability) was determined by the Delphi method [17] through an anonymous online survey. Table 6 summarizes these recommendations, and Fig. 1 shows a guidance algorithm for the management of PsA.

The results are presented, whenever possible, in absolute values, followed by a measure of the effect size to highlight the clinical significance or practical relevance. In the comparisons between treated and untreated individuals (placebo), the number needed to treat (NNT) or the number needed to harm (NNH) and the respective confidence intervals (95% CI) were calculated using a normal approximation, which is the most accepted statistical method. The data from each study used to define these intervals are available from the authors. In comparisons between paired means (before and after treatment), the effect size was calculated using the Cohen method (difference between the means divided by the standard deviation) [18]. Effect sizes were considered small when they ranged from 0.2 to 0.4, medium when they ranged from 0.4 to 0.8 and large when they were greater than 0.8 [19].

Clinical questions

What are the criteria for considering that an individual has psoriatic arthritis?

Diagnosis

The CASPAR is internationally accepted and has a sensitivity of 91% and specificity of 99% [12]. In this classification, individuals with established inflammatory joint disease (peripheral, axial or entheseal) are classified as having PsA if their points add up to 3 or more from the following categories (Table 5):

- PsO skin lesions: present/current (2 points) or previous (1 point) or family history of PsO (1 point);
- Nail lesions (onycholysis or pitting): 1 point;
- Current dactylitis, defined as whole-digit edema or a history of dactylitis: 1 point;
- Negative rheumatoid factor: 1 point; and
- Juxta-articular new bone neoformation: defined as poorly defined ossification near the joint margins (but excluding osteophyte formation) on plain radiographs of the hands or feet: 1 point.

  Questionnaires and survey instruments were developed to assist clinicians and dermatologists in the early identification of cases of PsA among patients with PsO: CONTEST [20, 21], TOPAS-II [22, 23], PURE-4 (Psoriatic arthritis UnclutteRed screening Evaluation-4) [24], SiPAS (Simple Psoriatic Arthritis Screening) [25], PASE (Psoriatic Arthritis Screening Evaluation) [23, 26–28], PEST (Psoriasis Epidemiology Screening Tool) [23, 28, 29], and EARP (Early Psoriatic Arthritis Screening Questionnaire) [23, 28, 30, 31].

The CONTEST instrument was developed from the PASE, PEST and TOPAS. Studies comparing the CONTEST and PEST questionnaires found no significant differences in efficacy between them [20, 32]. Considering that the PEST is shorter and simpler than the CONTEST, the use of the latter has become unfeasible in clinical practice [20, 32]. However, a recent systematic review with meta-analysis showed the EARP had better accuracy (sensitivity and specificity = 0.85 each) for PsA screening among psoriasis patients when compared to other self-administered tools (PASE, TOPAS, PEST) including 2280 references and 130 for the final analysis [31].

The TOPAS-II considers images of PsO, joint inflammation and dactylitis, improving doctor-patient agreement, being a useful tool to identify PsA in patients with PsO and to track PsO in the general population [22, 23, 33].

Further evidence is needed to recommend the routine use of the SiPAS and PURE-4 questionnaires [24, 25].

To date, only the PASE, PEST and TOPAS-II questionnaires have been translated into Portuguese and validated in the Brazilian population [33–35]. The Portuguese version of the PEST is available free of charge through the app of the Group for Research and Assessment of Psoriasis and Psoriatic Arthritis (GRAPPA) [35].

The sensitivity and specificity of the instruments vary according to the studied population (Table 7).

Recommendation

The diagnosis of PsA should be based on clinical and imaging criteria, and the CASPAR criteria should be used for disease classification. **Level of evidence: 1A; Strength of recommendation: A; Degree of agreement: 0.97.**

The use of PsA screening questionnaires in patients with PsO is recommended, with preference for those

(See figure on next page.)

Fig. 1 Algorithm proposed by the Brazilian Society of Rheumatology for the management of psoriatic arthritis patients, 2020. **cDMARDs**: conventional disease-modifying antirheumatic drugs; **MTX**: methotrexate; **LFN**: leflunomide; **SSZ**: sulfasalazine; **CSP**: cyclosporine; **NSAIDs**: nonstreroidal antiinflammatory drugs; **DAPSA**: Disease Activity Index for Psoriatic Arthritis; **MDA**: minimal disease activity; **VLDA**: very low disease activity; **BASDAI**: Bath Ankylosing Spondylitis Disease Activity Index; **ASDAS**: Ankylosing Spondylitis Disease Activity Score; **bDMARDs**: biologic disease-modifying antirheumatic drugs; **tsDMARDs** targeted synthetic disease modifying antirheumatic drugs; **TNFi:** TNF-alpha inhibitor; **ADA**: adalimumab, **CTZ**: certolizumab pegol; **ETN**: etanercept; **GOL**: golimumab; **IFX**: infliximab; **IL-17i**: IL-17 inhibitor; **IXE**: ixekizumab; **SEC**: secukinumab; **IL-12/23i:** IL-12/23 inhibitors; **UST**: ustekinumab; **IL-23i**: IL-23 inhibitor; **GUS**: guselkumab; **ABA**: abatacept; **TOF**: tofacitinib. **1**. Analgesics, NSAIDs and intra-articular corticosteroid infiltrations can be used in all stages, when necessary. **2**. Preferably use TNFi or IL-17i if there are axial manifestations; IL-23i or IL-17i or IL-12/23i if significant psoriasis; monoclonal TNFi if recurrent uveitis; TNFi (IFX, ADA, CTZ) or IL-12/23i if concomitant active Crohn's disease; TNFi (IFX, ADA, GOL) or IL-12/23i or JAKi (TOF) if concomitant active ulcerative colitis. **3**. Preferably use IL-17i if significant psoriasis; monoclonal TNFi if recurrent uveitis; TNFi (IFX, ADA, CTZ) if concomitant active Crohn's disease; TNFi (IFX, ADA, GOL) if concomitant active ulcerative colitis

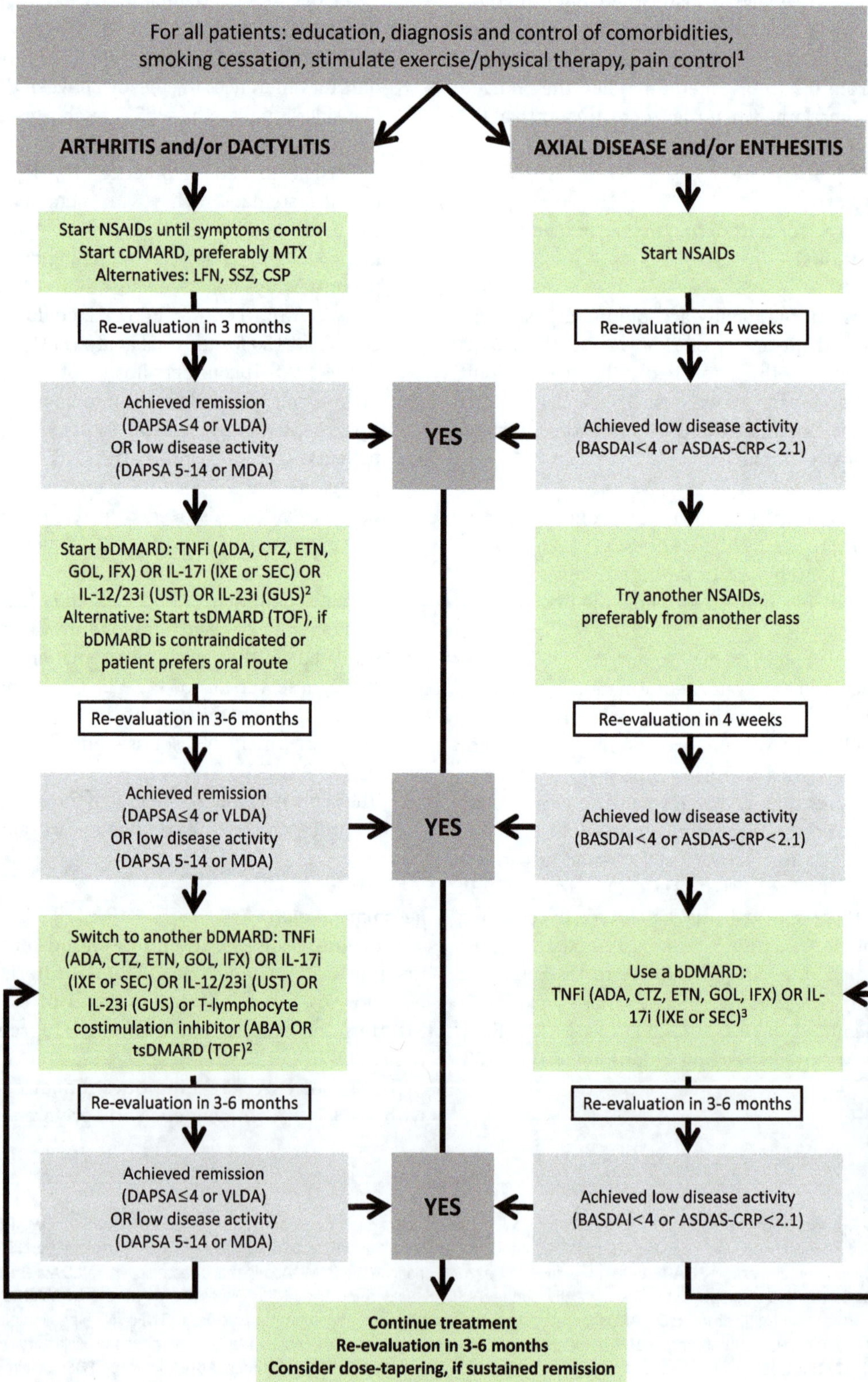

Fig. 1 (See legend on previous page.)

Table 7 Description of sensitivity, specificity and area under the curve (AUC) of the main PsA screening questionnaires

Authors	Questionnaires evaluated	Number of participants	Sensitivity	Specificity	AUC
Coates et al., 2018 [31]	CONTEST/ PEST	159	PEST 0.72 CONTEST 0.65	PEST 0.60 CONTEST 0.53	PEST 0.76 CONTEST 0.71
Coates et al., 2016 [20]	CONTEST/CONTESTjt X PEST	191	CONTEST 0.76 CONTESTjt 0.76 PEST 0.65	CONTEST 0.56 CONTESTjt 0.53 PEST 0.53	CONTEST 0.69 CONTESTjt 0.70 PEST 0.60
Duruoz et al., 2018 [32]	TOPAS II X CASPAR	150	TOPAS II 0.95	TOPAS II 0.98	TOPAS II 0.99
You et al., 2015 [27]	PASE X Rheumatologist (based on CASPAR and Moll and Wright)	148	PASE 0.77	PASE 0.82	PASE 0.79
Karreman et al., 2017 [28]	PEST X PASE X EARP X CASPAR	420	PEST 0.68 PASE 0.59 EARP 0.87	PEST 0.71 PASE 0.66 EARP 0.34	PEST 0.71 PASE 0.64 EARP0.68
Audureau et al., 2018 [24]	PURE-4 X CASPAR	168	PURE-4 0.85	PURE-4 0.83	PURE-4 0.87
Salaffi et al., 2018 [25]	SiPAS X CASPAR	202	SiPAS 0.79	SiPAS 0.87	SiPAS 0.60
Iragorri et al., 2019 [31]	PASE X TOPAS X PEST X EARP	15,208	PASE 0.66 ToPAS 0.74 PEST 0.66 EARP 0.85	PASE 0.82 ToPAS 0.79 PEST 0.83 EARP 0.78	PASE 0.68 ToPAS 0.65 PEST 0.85 EARP 0.85

CASPAR = Classification Criteria for Psoriatic Arthritis; CONTEST = Comparison of 3 screening tools to detect psoriatic arthritis in patients with psoriasis; CONTESTjt = CONTEST with the addition of a joint manikin; EARP = Early Psoriatic Arthritis Screening Questionnaire; PASE = Psoriatic Arthritis Screening Evaluation; PAQ = Psoriasis and Arthritis Questionnaire; PASQ = Psoriasis and Arthritis Screening Questionnaire; PEST = Psoriasis Epidemiology Screening Tool; PURE-4 = Psoriatic arthritis UnclutteRed screening Evaluation; SiPAS = Simple Psoriatic Arthritis Screening; TOPAS = Toronto Psoriatic Arthritis Screen

that have already been validated in the Brazilian population, such as the PASE, PEST and TOPAS-II. **Level of evidence: 1A; Strength of recommendation: A; Degree of agreement: 0.94.**

Is there a correlation between skin, nail and osteoarticular manifestations in psoriatic arthritis?

Correlations

Musculoskeletal involvement occurs simultaneously with or after the onset of PsO skin lesions in 82–87% of cases, while arthritis precedes the skin picture in 13–18% of patients [36–38].

A retrospective cohort study that included 1593 patients with PsO showed a higher incidence rate of PsA over time in patients with scalp lesions [hazard ratio (HR) = 3.89; 95%CI 2.18–6.94] and intergluteal/perianal lesions [HR = 2.35 (95%CI 1.32–4.19)] [39]. Two other cross-sectional studies that included 1928 and 459 patients with PsO also showed an increased prevalence of PsA in patients with scalp lesions (90.2% vs. 76.4%, $p = 0.001$ and 87% vs. 72%, $p = 0.0237$, respectively) [38, 40].

The duration and extent of skin disease assessed by affected body surface area (BSA) were associated with a higher chance of developing PsA [odds ratio (OR) = 7.42 (95%CI 3.86–14.25) and OR = 3.34 (95%CI 2.40–4.65), respectively] [41]. A greater number of skin sites affected by PsO also increases the risk of PsA by 2.24 (95%CI 1.23–4.08) [39].

Nail involvement in patients with PsO predisposing to musculoskeletal involvement was demonstrated in 1 cohort study [39] and in 13 cross-sectional studies [38, 40, 42–52]. The retrospective cohort [39] showed a higher incidence rate of PsA over time in patients with PsO and nail dystrophy [HR = 2.93; 95%CI 1.68–5.12] [39]. An increased risk of PsA in patients with nail PsO was observed in 12 of the 13 cross-sectional studies that evaluated this association [38, 40, 42–52] (OR = 2.92; 95%CI 2.34–3.64), although with a significant level of heterogeneity ($I^2 = 66\%$; $p = 0.0005$). The case–control study did not observe such a relationship (OR = 1.16; 95%CI 0.46–2.92) [53].

Eight small cross-sectional studies published between 1985 and 2010 specifically evaluated the link between nail PsO and DIP impairment [37, 49, 52, 54–57]. Of these, 5 showed a significant association between nail PsO and DIP involvement [37, 49, 52, 54, 55].

Recommendation

All patients with PsO should be evaluated for the presence of musculoskeletal manifestations. Those with involvement of the nails, intergluteal region, or scalp or extensive areas are at higher risk for musculoskeletal involvement. **Level of evidence: 2B; Strength of recommendation: B; Degree of agreement: 0.94.**

What are the comorbidities most associated with psoriatic arthritis?
Concomitant clinical conditions

The coexistence of clinical conditions associated with PsA, such as obesity, metabolic syndrome, cardiovascular disease (CVD), uveitis, inflammatory bowel disease, and mood disorders, has been reported. More than half of patients have at least 1 comorbidity that can negatively impact quality of life.

Obesity

The prevalence of obesity in patients with PsA is approximately 30–37% [58–60], and the incidence in these patients is 1.8–10.1% higher than that in control groups (NNH: 55–10) [60, 61]; when compared to patients with PsO without arthritis, there is a 3.5% increase ($p < 0.05$) in the incidence of obesity (NNH: 32) [58].

In addition, obesity seems to influence the therapeutic response in PsA. Obese individuals were less likely to achieve a therapeutic response based on the MDA criterion [obesity grade I with HR = 3.98; 95%CI 1.96–8.06, $p < 0.001$, and obesity grade II with HR = 5.4; 95%CI 3.09–9.43, $p < 0.001$] [62]. Intervention studies showed that weight loss increased the chance of achieving MDA [5–10% weight loss with OR = 3.75; 95%CI 1.36–10.36, $p = 0.011$ and ≥ 10% with OR = 6.67; 95%CI 2.41–18.41, $p < 0.001$] [63].

Metabolic syndrome

Approximately 40.6–44% of patients with PsA present metabolic syndrome* [64, 65], with an increased incidence of 5.24% ($p < 0.05$) compared to patients with other spondyloarthritis (NNH: 19) [66], 15.9% compared to patients with rheumatoid arthritis (NNH: 6) [66] and 22.9% ($p < 0.05$) compared to patients with PsO without arthritis (NNH: 4) [67]. A high prevalence of CVD risk factors was observed among metabolic syndrome components such as arterial hypertension, elevated waist circumference and triglycerides [64], as defined by the National Cholesterol Education Program Adult Treatment Panel III (NCEP-ATPIII) criteria.

Hypertension

Hypertension has a prevalence of 33.6–38.7% in patients with PsA [58, 60, 68]. In these patients, there was an increase of 2.3–11.8% ($p < 0.05$) compared to control patients (NNH: 14–8) [60, 68].

In addition, patients with PsA compared to those with PsO without arthritis have a 17.5% increased incidence ($p < 0.05$) of hypertension (NNH: 6) [58].

A longer disease duration may result in a higher risk of hypertension. Older patients with PsA for longer than 2 years have a higher risk of hypertension than patients in the early phase of the disease [increase of 22.9–49.3% ($p < 0.05$) (NNH: 4–2) vs. increase of 22.8–26.6% ($p < 0.05$) (NNH: 4)] [69].

Diabetes

The prevalence of diabetes in patients with PsA is 11.5–13.6% [58, 60, 69]. Compared to control patients, patients with PsA have increased rates, by 3.2–2.6–2.51% ($p < 0.05$), of diabetes (NNH: 31–38–40) [60, 61, 70].

Patients with PsA, when compared to patients with PsO without arthritis, have increased rates, by 5.3% ($p < 0.05\%$) of type II diabetes (NNH: 19) [58]. Patients with a later age of onset of PsO symptoms and shorter time interval until diagnosis of PsA have a higher risk of diabetes [(2.4% increase ($p < 0.05$) (NNH: 42)] than do patients with PsA established for more than 2 years [69].

Hyperlipidemia

The prevalence of hyperlipidemia in patients with PsA is 17.5–20.7% [58, 60]. Such patients showed an increased risk, by 1.71–4.1–13.87% ($p < 0.05$), of hyperlipidemia when compared to controls (NNH: 58–24–7) [60, 61, 66].

Patients with PsA, compared to patients with PsO without arthritis, have an increased rate, by 6.2%, (– < 0.05%) of hyperlipidemia (NNH: 16) [58].

The LDL level, which is a risk factor for atherosclerosis, was significantly higher in patients with PsA than in patients without PsA (9.0 ± 10.7 vs. 2.9 ± 4.7 mg/dL; $p < 0.05$) [58].

Atherosclerosis/coronary artery disease

Systemic inflammation in PsA extends beyond the skin and joints. Recent studies highlight the increased risk of atherosclerotic disease and consequently major cardiovascular adverse events (combined outcome of myocardial infarction, stroke and cardiovascular death) in patients with PsA.

Patients with PsA have a 22.9–32% increased incidence of atherosclerosis ($p < 0.05$) compared to controls (NNH: 4–3) [71, 72]. Linear regression analysis comparing a cohort of patients with PsA with and without metabolic syndrome to non-PsO/PsA controls showed no correlation between atheromatous plaques and metabolic syndrome but rather a correlation with PsA alone [B = 0.865 (0.236–1.493), $p = 0.008$] [72].

Cardiovascular disease

Compared to control patients without PsA, patients with PsA showed a 3.2–7.5% increase ($p < 0.05$) in the prevalence of CVD risk (NNH: 31–13) [61, 73], and when compared to patients with PsO without arthritis, the risk of CVD increased by 4.9% ($p < 0.05$) (NNH: 20) [58].

Depression and/or anxiety

Compared to control patients matched for age, sex, geographic region and year of follow-up, patients with PsA had a 5.4% increased incidence ($p < 0.05$) for depression (NNH: 18) and 3.0% increased incidence ($p < 0.05$) for anxiety (NNH: 33) [61]. When compared to patients with PsO without arthritis, the incidence of depression and/or anxiety increased by 11.4% (p = 0.0001) (NNH: 9) [58].

Osteoporosis

Patients with PsA, compared to control patients matched for age, sex, geographic region and year of follow-up, had a 1% increased incidence ($p < 0.05$) of osteoporosis (OP) (NNH: 100) [61].

Compared to control patients, patients with PsA have a high probability of OP (OR = 4.04; 95%CI 3.80–4.29, $p < 0.0001$) and a consequent increased risk of fracture (OR = 3.41; 95%CI 2.94–3.96, $p < 0.0001$) [74].

When the OP prevalence were compared among PsA and PsO patients, no differences were observed (3.5% vs. 2.9%; 95%CI 0.18–1.70, $p = 0.56$) (multivariate model adjusted for age, sex, education level, PsO duration, current smoking, Psoriasis Area and Severity Index (PASI) score, use of immunobiologics, methotrexate (MTX) and nonsteroidal antiinflammatory drugs (NSAIDs), CVD, hypertension, and gastrointestinal disease) [58].

Uveitis

Uveitis is a comorbidity that may be present in 7% of patients with PsA, unilaterally and bilaterally, with a similar distribution of anterior and posterior presentations and insidious onset in 19% of patients, occurring, on average, 9 years after the diagnosis of arthritis [75].

Patients with PsA, when compared to patients with PsO without arthritis, have an incidence of uveitis of 0.9–1.2% ($p < 0.05$) (NNH: 111–83) [61, 76].

Inflammatory bowel disease

Compared to controls, patients with PsA exhibited an increased risk for Cronh's disease (0.7–0.82%, $p < 0.05$; NNH: 142–117) and ulcerative colitis (0.38–0.6%, $p < 0.05$; NNH: 264–167) [61, 77].

Recommendation

The most frequent comorbidities in patients with PsA, such as metabolic syndrome, atherosclerosis, cardiovascular disease, mood disorders, inflammatory bowel disease, osteoporosis and uveitis, should be managed routinely in the clinical practice. **Level of evidence: 2B; Strength of recommendation: B; Degree of agreement: 0.96.**

Nonpharmacological treatment

Few studies have evaluated the benefit of exercise in patients with PsA [10, 78–80]. The results obtained for individuals with other inflammatory arthropathies [80] have been extrapolated for patients with PsA. Exercise can influence the inflammatory activity of PsA, as well as aerobic capacity and muscle strength, in addition to assisting in weight loss, which in turn was associated with a better response to treatment with immunobiologics [62, 81].

Is there evidence for benefits of physical exercise in the treatment of psoriatic arthritis?

Three studies [78–80, 82] with adequate scientific methodology provided specific evidence of exercise practice in PsA. The interventions studied were resistance exercises and high-intensity interval training (HIIT) [78, 80]. The outcomes analyzed were pain [78, 79], fatigue [78], strength [79], functional capacity [79], disease activity [78, 79], quality of life [79], maximum oxygen consumption (VO_2 max) [80], fat percentage [80] and body mass index [80].

Impact on aerobic capacity

Compared to a control group, patients subjected to HIIT training (3 times per week for 11 weeks) showed significant improvement in VO_2 max ($p < 0.001$); however, there was no significant difference in the following outcomes: fat percentage ($p = 0.14$) or body mass index ($p = 0.11$) [80].

Impact on disease activity

Compared to a control group, patients performing resistance exercises (twice a week for 12 weeks) showed significant improvement in their functional capacity [Health Assessment Questionnaire—Spondyloarthritis (HAQ-S), $p = 0.048$)], disease activity [BASDAI, $p = 0.038$], pain [Short-Form 36 (SF-36), $p = 0.017$] and general health (SF-36, $p = 0.002$) at the end of the protocol [79].

Compared to a control group, patients who performed HIIT training (3 times per week for 11 weeks) showed significant improvement in fatigue at a 12-week evaluation ($p = 0.005$), but there was no improvement regarding pain ($p = 0.47$) or disease activity using different metrics [Patient Global Assessment (PGA), $p = 0.85$; Disease Activity Score in 44 joints (DAS44), $p = 0.22$; ASDAS-CRP, $p = 0.42$; high sensitivity C-reactive protein (hs-CRP), $p = 0.67$)] [78]. When re-evaluated 6 months after the end of training, no benefit was observed for any of the analyzed outcomes.

Recommendation

Aerobic and resistance exercises should be individually prescribed to improve functional capacity, pain and quality of life. **Level of evidence: 1B; Strength of recommendation: A; Degree of agreement: 0.97.**

Drug treatment

NSAIDs, corticosteroids and conventional disease-modifying antirheumatic drugs (cDMARDs).

Corticosteroids (CSs) can be used as adjuvant treatment for disease [83]. Few randomized, double-blind, placebo-controlled clinical trials with NSAIDs have been conducted in PsA patients with peripheral involvement. As a therapeutic option for axial disease, NSAIDs have also not been specifically studied; therefore, measures and outcomes developed for ankylosing spondylitis (AS) have been accepted.

The drugs methotrexate (MTX), cyclosporine (CSP), leflunomide (LFN) and sulfasalazine (SSZ) are cDMARDs and have been used for several years to control the inflammatory process, modify disease progression, achieve remission and inhibit/reduce structural damage in PsA [84]. Most studies with these drugs evaluated their effects in patients with peripheral presentation and not with axial involvement.

What is the evidence for the use of corticosteroids in patients with psoriatic arthritis?

Local corticosteroid use

Intra-articular CSs injection (triamcinolone and methylprednisolone) at doses of 5–80 mg can be performed in inflamed joints, such as interphalangeal, knee and hip joints of patients with PsA. The probability of achieving an adequate clinical response in 3 months was 41.6%, but there may be recurrence in 25.5% of cases after 1 year [83].

Systemic CS use

The systemic use of CSs in patients with PsA has not been well studied. Nevertheless, these drugs have been prescribed, with caution, due to possible worsening of skin involvement, for PsA in 24.4–30% of cases [85]. In addition, specialists contraindicate the use of systemic CSs for the treatment of PsO, except in very special cases, and chronic use must be avoided [86].

Recommendation

The use of intra-articular CS injection is recommended for localized, mono- or oligoarticular disease, especially for patients who do not respond to systemic treatment. **Level of evidence: 2C; Strength of recommendation: B; Degree of agreement: 0.95.**

Due to the lack of quality data on the efficacy of the use of systemic CSs in PsA and the known adverse effects, their long-term use is not recommended. **Level of evidence: 5; Strength of recommendation: D; Degree of agreement: 0.94.**

What is the evidence for the use of nonsteroidal anti-inflammatory drugs (NSAIDs) in patients with psoriatic arthritis?

Peripheral arthritis

Short-term studies (2–4 weeks) show clinical scores improvement, including pain, joint swelling, morning stiffness and pain intensity [87, 88].

Small trials comparing different NSAIDs reported improvements regarding clinical parameters, pain and functional evaluations but were not able to demonstrate efficacy differences [89–91].

Axial disease

In patients with mild axial symptoms (inflammatory low back pain without functional loss or radiographic progression), the use of NSAIDs can reduce pain and improve stiffness [92]. Two prospective randomized studies, 1 with celecoxib (selective COX-2 inhibitor) [93] and 1 with diclofenac (nonselective NSAID) [94], evaluated radiographic inhibition in patients with AS, comparing the continuous and on-demand use of the drug over 2 years. In the study with celecoxib, less radiographic progression was observed in the continuous use group than in the on-demand group [93] ($p=0.002$), and a post-hoc analysis showed that this reduction was greater in patients with evidence of inflammatory activity (erythrocyte sedimentation rate (ESR) and CRP) [95]. In the study with diclofenac, this difference was not observed [94] ($p=0.39$). Thus, the decision to use NSAIDs continuously or not may vary depending on symptom severity, patient preferences and concomitant comorbidities, particularly gastrointestinal, renal and cardiovascular comorbidities.

Enthesitis

There are no adequately designed clinical studies that evaluate the effect of NSAIDs on enthesitis [96], but based on clinical experience and expert opinion, NSAIDs may be the first-line treatment in these cases [9].

Dactylitis

There are no clinical studies evaluating the use of NSAIDs in cases of dactylitis, but in daily practice, NSAIDs are the most commonly prescribed medications [97].

The evidence that the use of NSAIDs can trigger or exacerbate PsO is weak and based on case reports [98–100]. A single case–control study found a greater chance of exacerbation of skin lesions in patients who recently used NSAIDs (OR 3.7; 95%CI 1.6–7.1) [101]. The possibility should be considered that skin lesion exacerbation occurs simultaneously with arthritis, and thus, there is a potential bias in the observed associations [98–101]. The NSAIDs already described as potential triggers of PsO skin lesions are indomethacin [98], phenylbutazone [99], ibuprofen [100], diclofenac and naproxen [101].

Recommendation The use of NSAIDs is recommended as a symptomatic treatment in cases of peripheral arthritis **Level of evidence: 1B; Strength of recommendation: A; Degree of agreement: 0.95**, enthesitis **Level of evidence: 5; Strength of recommendation: D; Degree of agreement: 0.96**, dactylitis **Level of evidence: 5 Strength of recommendation: D; Degree of agreement: 0.96**, and axial manifestations **Level of evidence: 5; Strength of recommendation: D; Degree of agreement: 0.96.**

There is no evidence of a difference in efficacy among NSAIDs. **Level of evidence: 1B, Strength of recommendation: B; Degree of agreement: 0.96.**

The choice of the drug should be based on the physician's familiarity with the drug and the patient's individual preference, respecting the concomitant clinical conditions **Level of evidence: 5; Strength of recommendation: B; Degree of agreement: 0.96.**

What is the evidence for the use of conventional DMARDs in the treatment of psoriatic arthritis?

Methotrexate (MTX)

MTX is one of the most widely used cDMARDs worldwide for the treatment of PsA, [102, 103] despite few clinical trials evaluating its effectiveness [104] and controversial clinical evidence.

A study in which patients were administered MTX at a dose of 2.5–5.0 mg every 12 h for 3 consecutive days for 12 weeks showed, compared to patients who did not use it, no benefit in relation to swelling, morning stiffness, pain, or joint involvement, but there was a reduction in the physician-rated evaluated severity score [105].

In another open-label, prospective, randomized study with 35 patients with recent-onset oligoarticular PsA, the use of intramuscular MTX 10 mg/week combined with NSAIDs was compared with the use of NSAIDs for 3 months. Significant improvement ($p<0.05$) was observed regarding the number of painful and swollen joints, ESR, visual analog scale (VAS) for pain and physician global assessment in both groups. A comparison between groups showed significant superiority in terms of number of painful and swollen joints in those on MTX. After this period, the placebo group received MTX, for a duration of 6 months, and comparisons between the groups at the end of 6 months showed no significant differences [106].

The Methotrexate In Psoriatic Arthritis (MIPA) study showed that after 6 months, oral MTX at a dose of 15 mg/week was not superior to NSAIDs for reducing painful and swollen joints, as evaluated by the Psoriatic Arthritis Response Criteria (PsARC) (OR = 1.77; 95%CI 0.97–3.23), DAS-28 (OR = 1.70; 95%CI 0.90–3.17) and American College of Rheumatology 20% improvement criteria (ACR20) (OR = 2.00; 95%CI 0.65–6.22), although there were significant improvements in the following outcomes: patient ($p=0.03$) and physician ($p<0.001$) global assessment and skin scores ($p=0.02$) [107].

The TIght COntrol of inflammation in early Psoriatic Arthritis (TICOPA) study, an open-label, randomized controlled, parallel group trial with 206 patients evaluated, for 48 weeks, the target-based model for the treatment of patients with early PsA. The evaluations were performed every 4 weeks, with MTX dose escalation (15, 20, 25 mg/week) and subsequent combination with other cDMARDs as needed to achieve the MDA response. Patients undergoing target-based treatment showed better results than patients receiving standard therapy, with a greater probability of achieving ACR20 (OR = 1.91; 95%CI 1.03–3.55, $p=0.039$), ACR50 (OR = 2.36; 95%CI 1.25–4.47, $p=0.008$), ACR70 (OR = 2.64; 95%CI 1.32–5.26, $p=0.006$) and ≥ 75% PASI improvement (PASI75) (OR = 2.92; 95% CI 1.51–5.65, $p=0.001$) [108].

In a double-blind study, 851 patients with PsA were randomly allocated at a 1:1:1 ratio into 3 treatment arms: subcutaneous (sc) MTX 20 mg/week monotherapy, etanercept (ETN) 50 mg/week monotherapy, and MTX 20 mg/week + ETN 50 mg/week combination therapy; an evaluation at week 24 found that the ACR20 (50.7% vs. 60.9% vs. 65.0%, respectively) and MDA (22.9% vs. 35.9% vs. 35.7%, respectively) responses were significantly higher in patients who received ETN monotherapy vs. MTX monotherapy (ACR20, $p=0.029$ and MDA $p=0.005$) and in patients who received combination therapy vs. MTX monotherapy (ACR20, $p=0.005$ and MDA $p=0.005$). Patients in the 2 ETN groups showed less radiographic progression at week 48 than did patients who received MTX monotherapy [109]. Thus, although the results for MTX monotherapy had been inferior to those observed for ETN, ACR20 was achieved by 50% and MDA by 23% of patients who received MTX monotherapy, and thus, it could be an initial approach for patients with peripheral disease.

Cyclosporine (CSP)

A multicenter, randomized, open, controlled trial evaluated 99 patients with PsA (1:1:1) treated with CSP (3–5 mg/kg/day) or SSZ (2 g/day) for 6 months, both combined with symptomatic therapy (NSAIDs, analgesics and/or prednisone ≤ 5 mg/d), or treated with symptomatic therapy alone. There was a significant difference regarding pain reduction (VAS) in the CSP versus SSZ and symptomatic therapy groups ($p < 0.05$). There was also a greater reduction of swollen joints number ($p = 0.05$), painful joints ($p = 0.01$), joint pain/sensitivity score ($p = 0.002$), spondylitis functional index ($p = 0.002$), and patient and physician global assessments, in favor of CSP versus symptomatic therapy. In the comparison between SSZ and symptomatic therapy, there was a reduction only in the spondylitis functional index in the SSZ group ($p = 0.03$) [110].

A small, open-label, controlled and randomized prospective study evaluated 35 patients with PsA treated with CSP (3–5 mg/kg/day) or MTX (7.5–15 mg/week) and found that after 12 months, the medications had similar benefits regarding improvements in joint pain/swelling, morning stiffness, grip strength, CRP and inflammatory disease activity based on patient and physician global assessments [111].

An open, non-randomized, prospective 12-month study compared patients who received CSP (2.5–3.75 mg/kg/day), adalimumab (ADA) (40 mg 14/14 days) or a combination of both; a PsARC response was observed in 65%, 85% and 95% of patients, and an ACR50 response was observed in 36%, 69% and 87% of patients on the 3 different therapeutic regimens, respectively [112], demonstrating the benefit of CSP, the superiority of the immunobiologic ADA relative to CSP, and synergism, with better response when CSP is used in combination with the immunobiologic ADA [113].

Leflunomide (LFN)

A double-blind, randomized, placebo-controlled study evaluated the use of LFN (100 mg/day for 3 days followed by 20 mg/day) in 190 patients with PsA and observed a 29.2% increase in PsARC response (NNT: 3), 16.3% increase in ACR20 response (NNT: 6) and improvement in HAQ functional capacity, with a reduction of 0.19 [113]. In the same study, clinical improvements in skin lesions, as assessed by the PASI75, were significantly higher in the LFN group (17.4% vs. 7.8%, $p = 0.048$). The main adverse events observed were diarrhea and increased transaminases in the LFN group [113].

An observational cohort study was conducted to evaluate the efficacy and safety of LFN alone or in combination with MTX in patients with PsA. Of 85 patients, 43 (50.6%) used LFN alone, and 42 (49.4%) received combined LFN and MTX therapy. Thirty patients (16 LFN and 14 LFN + MTX) discontinued treatment due to toxicity. Of the 55 patients who continued using the drugs, there was a $\geq 40\%$ reduction in the count of actively inflamed joints in 38%, 48% and 56% at 3, 6 and 12 months, respectively. PASI75 was reached by 19% of patients at 3 and 6 months and by 32% at 12 months. Those who received MTX were more likely to achieve a PASI50 response [114].

Sulfasalazine (SSZ)

A multicenter, prospective, double-blind, randomized, placebo-controlled study compared the efficacy and tolerability of SSZ in patients with PsA and, after 24 weeks, showed only a reduction in pain, as measured by VAS, without differences in other outcomes, including morning stiffness, affected joints number or the Ritchie joint index [115].

Two other studies, with short-term follow-up and a reduced number of patients, demonstrated a minimal effect of SSZ when compared to placebo in relation to pain, morning stiffness and global disease activity assessment [116, 117].

Recommendation The use of methotrexate (MTX) is recommended as the first choice among cDMARDs for the treatment of skin and peripheral joint involvement in PsA **Level of evidence: 1B**, preferably at doses higher than 15 mg/week and subcutaneously. **Level of evidence: 5 Strength of recommendation: B; Degree of agreement: 0.93.**

If MTX is not available or cannot be used regarding safety issues, CSP, LFN or SSZ could be used in cases of peripheral arthritis **Level of evidence: 2B; Strength of recommendation: B; Degree of agreement: 0.93.**

There is NO scientific evidence for using cDMARDs in patients with axial involvement, as well as there is limited evidence for enthesitis. **Level of evidence: 5; Strength of recommendation: D; Degree of agreement: 0.89.**

Treatment of PsA with immunobiologics and targeted synthetic drugs In addition to the drugs commercially available in Brazil at the time of the systematic literature review (December 2019), guselkumab (approved in 2020 for PsA) [118, 119] and direct comparison studies also published in 2020 [120, 121] were included.

1. Biologic DMARDs (bDMARDs)
    - Tumor necrosis factor inhibitors (TNFi): monoclonal antibodies (infliximab, adalimumab, golimumab, certolizumab pegol) and soluble receptor (etanercept)
    - Interleukin-17 inhibitors (IL17i)/anti-IL17 (secukinumab and ixekizumab)
    - Interleukin-12/23 inhibitors (IL12/23i)/anti-IL2/23 (ustekinumab)
    - Interleukin 23 inhibitors/anti-IL23 (guselkumab)
    - T-lymphocyte costimulation inhibitor (abatacept)

2. Targeted synthetic or small-molecule DMARDs (tsDMARDs)
   - Janus kinase 1 and 3 inhibitor (JAKi) (tofacitinib)

Phase 3 clinical studies with different bDMARDs (abatacept [122], adalimumab [123], certolizumab [124], etanercept [125, 126], golimumab [127], infliximab [128], ixekizumab [129], secukinumab [130, 131], ustekinumab [132], guselkumab [118, 119], and tsDMARDs (tofacitinib [133]) and a meta-analysis demonstrated the superiority of these drugs relative to control groups (patients using NSAIDs and/or cDMARDs) for skin (PASI) and joint outcomes [Health Assessment Questionnaire-Disability Index (HAQ-DI) and ACR20, ACR50 and ACR70 efficacy criteria)].

When are biologic DMARDs or targeted synthetic DMARDs indicated for the treatment of PsA?

bDMARDs should be initiated in patients with PsA and peripheral arthritis who present with active disease despite the use of at least one cDMARD (preferably MTX) for a minimum period of 3 months. Active disease can be defined by the presence of any of the following conditions: peripheral arthritis, spinal inflammation, enthesitis, dactylitis or skin or nail lesion due to PsO and/or extra-articular manifestations such as uveitis or inflammatory bowel disease. Active disease can also be defined using measures that evaluate peripheral joint involvement, such as the DAPSA or MDA (Tables 1 and 2), and axial involvement, such as the BASDAI or ASDAS-CRP (Tables 3 and 4).

Although evidence regarding the efficacy of MTX in PsA is controversial and is based on studies with low methodological quality and using low doses of the drug [109, 133, 134], a course of MTX $\geq$ 15 mg/week for at least 3 months should be attempted before switching treatment to a bDMARD. The tsDMARD tofacitinib can be used in patients with peripheral arthritis in cases of failure of at least 1 bDMARD for a minimum of 3–6 months or when a bDMARD cannot be used.

For PsA with axial involvement, a bDMARD should be started after failure with at least 2 NSAIDs, preferably from different classes, used for a minimum period of 30 days each. This recommendation is based on studies conducted in patients with axial spondyloarthritis because there is still no consensus regarding axial PsA, and the first study that recruited patients with these characteristics did not include in their inclusion criteria imaging tests that confirmed this diagnosis [8, 135].

Recommendation

A bDMARD should be initiated in patients with PsA and peripheral arthritis who remain with active disease despite the use of cDMARD, preferably MTX, for at least 3 months. **Level of evidence: 1B; Strength of recommendation: A. Degree of agreement: 0.95.**

In the case of failure or inability to use a bDMARD, a tsDMARD can be used. **Level of evidence: 1B; Strength of recommendation: B. Degree of agreement: 0.95.**

The use of a bDMARD is recommended in patients with PsA and axial manifestations who remain with active disease despite the use of 2 classes of NSAIDs, in full dose, for at least 30 days each. **Level of evidence: 1B; Strength of recommendation: B; Degree of agreement: 0.92.**

Is there a difference in the efficacy of biologic DMARDs and targeted synthetic DMARDs in the treatment of PsA?

Abatacept (ABA)

In a clinical study, patients with PsA and previous failure of cDMARDs and/or anti-TNFs were randomly assigned to receive placebo, ABA 3 mg/kg, ABA 10 mg/kg or ABA at 2 doses, 30 mg/kg followed by 10 mg/kg. When the general population was analyzed (with and without previous use of anti-TNF) at 6 months of follow-up, there was an increase in the proportion of patients who achieved an ACR20 response with intravenous ABA treatment (NNT: 5) at the 30/10 mg/kg dose (23%) and (NNT: 4) at the of 10 mg/kg dose (29%). The was no difference in the ACR20 response between the 3 mg/kg dose and placebo. The ACR50/70 responses at 6 months were studied only as an exploratory analysis, and the authors described that the proportions of patients who achieved ACR50 and ACR70 were numerically higher among those receiving ABA compared to placebo: the difference was greater in the group receiving 10 mg/kg, with 25% of these achieving ACR50 and 13% achieving ACR70 [122].

Another randomized clinical trial compared sc ABA 125 mg weekly with placebo, evaluating the proportion of patients who achieved ACR20 at week 24: 39.4%, ABA versus 22.3%, placebo ($p < 0.001$); this efficacy was maintained at the 52nd week [136]. There was no significant difference in the proportion of patients in the ABA and placebo groups who achieved ACR50 and ACR70. The proportion of patients who achieved clinically significant improvements in the HAQ-DI at week 24 (decrease of at least 0.35 points compared to baseline) was evaluated: although numerically more patients achieved this outcome in the ABA group, there was no significant difference between the ABA and placebo groups (31.0% versus 23.7%, $p = 0.097$) [136].

Adalimumab (ADA)

In adult patients with moderate to severe active PsA, treatment with sc ADA 40 mg every 14 days increased the proportion of patients who achieved ACR20 (NNT: 2) by week 24 by 42% [123]. After 48 weeks, 56%, 44%

and 30% of patients who received ADA achieved ACR20, ACR50 and ACR70 responses, respectively [137].

When compared to placebo at week 24 in the ADEPT study, ADA had the following effects:

- increased the proportion of patients who achieved a clinically significant decrease in the HAQ-DI (decrease at least 0.3 points) by 23.6% (NNT: 4) at week 24 [138]; and
- increased the proportion of patients with complete resolution of HAQ-DI (HAQ-DI = zero) by 20.9% (NNT: 5) [138].

At 2 years of follow-up, in the same study, the percentages of patients who achieved ACR20, ACR50, and ACR70 responses were 57.3%, 42.7% and 29.9%, respectively. A full functional response (HAQ-DI = zero) was achieved by 38.5% of patients, and the proportion of patients who reached the clinically significant decrease for the HAQ-DI was 47.6% [138].

In another study, treatment with 40 mg ADA in alternating weeks for 24 weeks resulted in 65%, 43% and 27% of patients achieving ACR 20/50/70 responses, respectively [139].

Certolizumab (CTZ)

In 1 study, patients with PsA were randomly assigned to 1 of 3 groups: placebo, 200 mg of CTZ every 2 weeks or 400 mg of CTZ every 4 weeks [124]. Patients with previous anti-TNF therapy were not excluded. CTZ therapy resulted in the following:

- 27.6% increase (NNT: 4) in the proportion of patients who achieved ACR20 in week 12 (with the dose of 400 mg every 4 weeks) [124];
- 33.7% increase (NNT: 3) in the proportion of patients who achieved ACR20 in week 12 (with the dose of 200 mg every 2 weeks) [124].

Etanercept (ETN)

Compared to placebo, the treatment of patients with active PsA with ETN 25 mg twice a week for 12 weeks increased the ACR20 response by 60% (NNT: 2) and increased the functional response by 29% (NNT: 3) [125].

In another study, patients with PsA and an inadequate response to NSAIDs were treated with ETN 25 mg twice a week, with the following results compared to placebo:

- at week 12, the ACR20 response increased by 44% (NNT: 2) [125]; and
- at week 24, functional improvement (HAQ) increased by 48% (NNT: 2) [125].

These results were maintained long term: the ACR20 response in patients using ETN was 64% at 12 months [140].

Another study evaluated outcomes reported by patients and found that in patients with PsA treated with ETN 25 mg twice a week, 47.2% exhibited improvements in the HAQ-DI at 24 weeks, with 41.2% of patients showing a full response (HAQ-DI = zero) at 48 weeks [141].

Golimumab (GOL)

In the GO-REVEAL study, among patients diagnosed with PsA and with inadequate response to cDMARDs and NSAIDs treated with GOL 50 mg or 100 mg every 4 weeks, 42% and 36% achieved an ACR20 response at 14 and 20 weeks, respectively, regardless of combined treatment with MTX [127]. At week 24, patients treated with GOL 50 and 100 mg had better physical function scores than did patients who received placebo [142].

With GOL, a sustained clinical response was maintained at 2 years; at week 104, 63%, 46% and 29% of patients receiving GOL 50 mg every 4 weeks achieved ACR20, ACR50 and ACR70 responses, respectively [143]. A sustained clinical response was also maintained at 5 years (62.8% with an ACR20 response, 43.4% with an ACR50 response and 30.8% with an ACR70 response with a dose of 50 mg every 4 weeks) [144].

Patients with PsA diagnosed at least 6 months prior and who were naive to biologic treatment received intravenous GOL at a dose of 2 mg/kg at weeks 0 and 4 and thereafter every 8 weeks. At week 24, compared to placebo, GOL treatment resulted in the following:

- 52.5% increase in the ACR20 response (NNT: 2) [145];
- 47.2% increase in the ACR50 response (NNT: 2) [145]; and
- a greater decrease in HAQ compared to baseline (−0.63 vs. − 0.14; $p<0.05$) [145].

Guselkumab (GUS)

GUS was superior to placebo in a phase 2 clinical trial, with 58% of patients with PsA receiving 100 mg GUS on weeks 0 and 4 and every 8 weeks thereafter, achieving ACR20 on week 24; in comparison, 18% of patients receiving placebo achieved the same outcome (NNT = 3) [146].

A randomized, double-blind, phase 3 clinical trial that studied the efficacy of guselkumab in patients with PsA with previous failure of cDMARDs used the proportion of patients who achieved ACR20 at week 24 as an outcome. This study showed that GUS was superior to placebo: 33% of patients in the placebo group achieved ACR20 at week 24, and 64% of patients who received GUS every 4 weeks (NNT = 3) and 64% of those who received GUS at weeks 0 and 4 and every 8 weeks thereafter (NNT = 3) achieved ACR20 at week 24 [119]. At week 24, patients using GUS also showed a greater decrease in the HAQ-DI compared to baseline than did patients receiving placebo [119].

Infliximab (IFX)

The results of the IMPACT 1 study showed that among patients with a diagnosis of PsA established for more than 6 months, with cDMARD treatment failure, and with peripheral polyarthritis treated with IFX 5 mg/kg on weeks 0, 2, 6 and 14, 55% achieved an ACR20 response in week 16 (NNT: 2), 46% achieved an ACR50 response (NNT: 2), and 29% achieved an ACR70 response (NNT: 3) [128].

In the IMPACT 2 study, which evaluated patients with the same profile described above, the following results were reported for the infliximab 5 mg/kg group compared to the placebo group at week 24:

- higher ACR20 (38%; NNT: 2), ACR50 (37%; NNT: 3), ACR70 (25%; NNT: 4) response rates [147]; and
- 32% increase (NNT: 3) in the proportion of patients who achieved a clinical response (HAQ) [147].

After 2 years of follow-up, the ACR20, ACR50 and ACR70 response rates in the IFX group were 45%, 45% and 35%, respectively [148].

Ixekizumab (IXE)

Patients with PsA who never received biologic therapy were randomly assigned to 1 of 4 groups administered the following subcutaneous injections: placebo (N = 106), IXE 80 mg every 2 weeks (N = 103), IXE 80 mg every 4 weeks (N = 107) or ADA (active control) 40 mg once every 2 weeks (N = 101). Both IXE regimens included an initial dose of 160 mg. The primary objective was to compare the proportion of patients in the placebo and IXE groups who achieved ACR20 at week 24. The study had no objective nor the power to compare ADA and IXE. At week 24, IXE, compared to placebo, increased the proportion of patients who achieved ACR20 by 31.9% (NNT: 3) at the dose given every 2 weeks and by 27.7% (NNT: 4) at the dose given every 4 weeks [129]. At weeks 12 and 24, functional disability improved significantly with both IXE dosages compared to placebo [129].

Secukinumab (SEC)

In a phase 3 study to evaluate the efficacy and safety of SEC (75, 150 and 300 mg) in patients with PsA, the ACR20 response after 24 weeks was 54% with 300 mg SEC, 51% with 150 mg SEC, 29% with 75 mg SEC and 15% with placebo [131].

In a randomized, double-blind clinical trial, SEC (75 and 150 mg) was compared to placebo in patients with active PsA previously treated with cDMARDs or anti-TNFs. The following ACR20 response rates were observed at week 24: 50% and 50.5% in the SEC 150 and 75 mg groups and 17.3% in the placebo group. Improvements were maintained until week 54 [131].

Patients with active PsA were treated with SEC 300 mg, 150 mg, 75 mg or placebo at weeks 0, 1, 2, 3, and 4 and every 4 weeks thereafter [149]. At week 24 in the general study population (with or without previous use of anti-TNFs), the following were observed:

- compared to placebo, SEC 300 mg increased the proportion of patients who achieved ACR20 by 38.7% (NNT: 3) [149]; and
- compared to placebo, SEC 150 mg increased the proportion of patients who achieved ACR20 by 35.7% (NNT: 3) [149].

Among the patients who previously used anti-TNFs, only those who received SEC 300 mg had outcomes that were significantly different from those for patients in the placebo group, with SEC 300 mg increasing the proportion of patients who achieved ACR20 (31.2% increase, NNT: 4), ACR 50 (18.7% increase, NNT: 6) and ACR70 (15.2% increase, NNT: 7) [149].

Regarding functional improvement at week 24 (measured by the decrease in HAQ-DI score from baseline), both SEC 150 and 300 mg were more effective than placebo in patients who had not previously used anti-TNFs, and the 300 mg dose was more effective than placebo in patients who previously used anti-TNFs [149].

Tofacitinib (TOF)

One study evaluated the efficacy of oral TOF 5 mg twice daily and 10 mg twice daily versus placebo in patients with prior cDMARDs failure, using sc ADA 40 mg every 2 weeks as an active comparator. At 3 months, in the group that received TOF 10 mg twice daily, 28% (NNT: 4) of patients achieved an ACR20 response and 30% (NNT: 3) achieved an ACR50 response, and patients who received TOF had better functional outcomes than those who received placebo (decrease in HAQ-DI of − 0.4 with TOF vs. − 0.18 with placebo; $p < 0.05$) [133].

Ustekinumab (UST)

In patients with active PsA, treatment with UST increased the ACR20, ACR50 and ACR70 response rates by 28% (NNT: 4), 18% (NNT: 6) and 11% (NNT: 9), respectively, at the 12th week of follow-up [132].

At week 12, in the UST group, there was a 25% increase (NNT: 4) in the proportion of patients who achieved clinically significant improvement on the HAQ (decrease of at least 0.3 points) [132].

Another study showed that UST increased the proportion of patients who achieved an ACR20 response by 23.6% at week 24 (NNT: 4) [150]. In a subgroup of patients previously treated with anti-TNFs, efficacy was also observed; at week 24, the following results were obtained (UST versus placebo): ACR20, 35.6% vs 14.5% and mean change in HAQ-DI compared to baseline, − 0.13 versus 0.0 [150].

At week 52, UST efficacy was maintained, with 38.9% of patients achieving ACR20 and with a mean change of − 0.13, compared to baseline, on the HAQ-DI [150].

Direct comparison studies involving anti-IL17 and anti-TNF immunobiologics A randomized, multicenter, nonblind clinical trial compared IXE versus ADA in patients with PsA and previous cDMARD failure; the evaluator of the primary outcome was blinded, but patients and investigators were not blinded. The primary outcome in this study was a composite outcome: proportion of patients who simultaneously achieved ACR50 and PASI100. Regarding the simultaneous outcome ACR50 + PASI100, IXE was superior to ADA (36% IXE vs. 28%; $p = 0.036$). When only the articular outcome was evaluated (ACR50), there was no significant difference between the 2 drugs (51% IXE vs. 47% ADA). When only the cutaneous outcome (PASI100) was analyzed, IXE generated a better response than ADA (60% IXE vs. 47% ADA) [120].

A randomized double-blind clinical trial compared SEC with ADA and used the proportion of patients who achieved ACR20 at week 52 as the primary outcome. This study did not demonstrate the superiority of SEC over ADA for the primary outcome (67% SEC vs. 62% ADA), but treatment with SEC was associated with a higher drug retention rate [121].

There are no direct comparison studies among the TNFa inhibitors, but an indirect evaluation showed no clinically relevant efficacy difference [151, 152].

A direct comparison of anti-TNF and anti-IL-17 drugs showed no difference between the classes regarding their efficacy in musculoskeletal symptoms, but anti-IL-17 drugs were superior for the treatment of skin manifestations of PsO [120, 121].

No direct comparison studies involving drugs with other mechanisms of action, such as ABA (T-lymphocyte co-stimulation inhibitor) and GUS (anti-IL-23), were available at the time these recommendations were performed.

During the implementation of these recommendations, the results of the first direct comparison of a Janus kinase 1 inhibitor (upadacitinib, UPA) and ADA were presented [153]; the results indicated the superiority of upadacitinib 30 mg compared to ADA in achieving ACR20 at week 12. In addition, MDA was more achieved by PsA patients with prior inadequate response or intolerance to at least one b-DMARD taking UPA 15 mg/ day than placebo at week 24 (28.9% vs. 2.8%, $p < 0.001$). However, the study (SELECT PSA1) had not yet been published at the time of publication of these recommendations and the drug upadacitinib was not commercially available for the treatment of PsA in Brazil.

Recommendation For the treatment of peripheral arthritis, dactylitis and enthesitis, the use of any of the following drugs is recommended: anti-TNFs (adalimumab, certolizumab pegol, etanercept, golimumab and infliximab), anti-IL-17 (ixekizumab and secukinumab), anti-IL-12/23 (ustekinumab) and anti-IL-23 (guselkumab). **Level of evidence: 1B; Strength of recommendation: A; Degree of agreement: 0.98.**

The choice of drug and mechanism of action should take into account patient preference (in regard to the route of administration and frequency of use, for example), concomitant clinical conditions, medical history (e.g., history of tuberculosis, fungal infections, and herpes zoster), cost, availability in the health system and presence of extra-articular manifestations of PsA. **Level of evidence: 5; Strength of recommendation: D; Degree of agreement: 0.99.**

In patients with axial manifestations, the use of anti-TNF and anti-IL-17 drugs is preferentially recommended. **Level of evidence: 1B; Strength of recommendation: B; Degree of agreement: 0.98.**

In patients with PsA and severe PsO, anti-IL-23, anti-IL-17, and anti-IL-12/23 drugs are preferentially recommended over anti-TNFs. **Level of evidence: 1B; Strength of recommendation: A; Degree of agreement: 0.95.**

In patients with recurrent uveitis, the use of anti-TNF monoclonal antibodies is recommended. **Level of evidence: 1B; Strength of recommendation: B; Degree of agreement: 0.99.**

In patients with concomitant active Crohn's disease, the use of IFX, ADA, CTZ, and UST is preferentially recommended. **Level of evidence: 1B; Strength of recommendation: B; Degree of agreement: 0.98.**

In patients with concomitant active ulcerative colitis, the use of IFX, ADA, GOL, UST or TOF is preferentially recommended. **Level of evidence: 1B; Strength of recommendation: B; Degree of agreement: 0.98.**

Is there a difference in the safety of biologic DMARDs in the treatment of PsA?

Tuberculosis

TNF is part of the type I immune response and plays an important role in the host defense against intracellular pathogens, such as mycobacteria, and it is essential for granuloma formation. TNF inhibitor treatment was associated with several reported cases of TB [154–158].

In contrast, to date, there has been no report of latent tuberculosis infection (LTBI) reactivation in patients using anti-IL17, and in UST phase III trials, of the 167 patients with LTBI before treatment, only 1 patient who did not receive treatment with isoniazid experienced LTBI reactivation [159]. There are still not enough data on GUS to draw conclusions.

There is clearly a lower risk of LTBI activation in patients using non-TNF biologics. However, there is no contraindication to the use of anti-TNFs in patients with LTBI, but treatment with these agents should preferably be started 30 days after the start of treatment for LBTI.

Candidiasis

Interleukin-17 is part of the type 17 immune response and plays a role in the defense against fungal infections. The number of *Candida* infectious events was higher in patients treated with anti-IL17 than in those treated with placebo [120, 121].

In direct comparison studies of anti-IL-17 versus anti-TNF, as expected, a higher rate of *Candida* infections was identified in patients using anti-IL-17 (SPIRIT H2H: 2.5% IXE vs. 0.7% ADA; EXCEED: 4% SEC vs. 2% ADA) [120, 121].

In general, when a patient develops oral and/or esophageal candidiasis, this event usually occurs during the induction period; the use of the biologic should be continued, and concomitant treatment with oral systemic antifungals should be administered. Notably, disseminated candidiasis has not been observed to date.

Demyelinating disease

Although there is a lack of evidence supporting a causal relationship between TNF blockade and the onset of demyelinating diseases, a 0.02–0.2% incidence rate for demyelinating disorders has been described in patients undergoing treatment with these agents [160–167].

The use of anti-TNF therapy should be avoided in patients with a family history or occurrence of multiple sclerosis or other demyelinating diseases [168, 169].

To date, there are no reports of worsening or onset of demyelinating diseases in patients treated using IL-17 and IL-12/23 inhibitors, suggesting that their use is safe in these patients (23, 24) [170, 171]. Regarding the use of anti-IL-23, there are not sufficient data to provide recommendations.

Herpes zoster

A higher incidence of herpes zoster was observed among patients with PsA who used TOF than among those who received placebo [172] and among those who used ADA [133].

General serious adverse events and discontinuation due to adverse events

Regarding serious adverse events and the treatment discontinuation rate due to adverse events, there is no apparent difference among biologic classes in pivotal studies or in indirect comparison studies [129–131, 149, 173–175].

Studies comparing IXE and ADA reported that adverse events were more frequent in patients who received IXE (69.6% IXE vs. 61.1% ADA). However, ADA was associated with more serious adverse events (3.5% IXE vs. 8.5% ADA). In addition, there was no significant difference in the drug discontinuation rate due to serious or nonserious adverse events [120].

Another randomized double-blind study that compared SEC to ADA did not find a difference in the proportion of patients presenting general adverse events (77% SEC vs. 79% ADA) or serious adverse events (8% SEC vs. 7% ADA). Patients using ADA had more hypersensitivity reactions (9% SEC vs. 14% ADA), and the discontinuation rate due to adverse events was higher in the ADA group: 3.5% (SEC) vs. 7% (ADA) [121].

Recommendation

Screening and treatment of LTBI or active disease is recommended before using any immunobiologics and JAK inhibitors. **Level of evidence: 2B; Strength of recommendation: B; Degree of agreement: 0.98.**

In general, the biologics used for the treatment of PsA have similar safety profiles, and the particularities inherent to the cytokine to be inhibited should be considered. **Level of evidence: 5; Strength of recommendation: B; Degree of agreement:**

Degree of agreement: 0.96

The use of anti-TNFs in patients with demyelinating disease or class III or IV heart failure is not recommended. **Level of evidence: 4; Strength of recommendation: C; Degree of agreement: 0.99.**

The use of JAK inhibitors in patients with history of disseminated or recurrent herpes zoster is not recommended. **Level of evidence: 1B; Strength of recommendation: A; Degree of agreement: 0.99.**

The use of IL-17 inhibitors in patients with a history of severe or recurrent fungal infections is not recommended. **Level of evidence: 1B; Strength of recommendation: A; Degree of agreement: 0.98.**

Is there evidence for the use of conventional DMARDs combined with biologic DMARDs or target synthetic DMARDs?

To date, there was no difference in efficacy between monotherapy with bDMARDs and combined therapy with bDMARDs and MTX. Pivotal studies on anti-TNF agents for the treatment of PsA allowed patients receiving MTX at the beginning of the study to continue or stop using MTX, and similar clinical responses were observed between patients who received combined therapy with MTX and those who received anti-TNF monotherapy [123, 124, 126, 127, 176]. The SEAM-PsA study (Study of Etanercept and Methotrexate in Combination or as Monotherapy in Subjects with Psoriatic Arthritis), comparing MTX monotherapy vs. ETN monotherapy vs. MTX combined with ETN, evaluated patients with early PsA and observed that combined therapy was not superior to anti-TNF therapy alone but that both were superior to MTX monotherapy [177]. Observational studies found higher percentages of patients with PsA receiving MTX combined with anti-TNFs than receiving anti-TNF monotherapy. Similar to clinical trials, data obtained from registers such as SSTA (South Swedish Arthritis Treatment Group Register) and NOR-DMARD (NORwegian DMARD Register) showed that combined therapy with MTX did not influence the therapeutic response [178' 179]. A small benefit of the concomitant use of MTX and anti-TNFs was observed in the ACR20 response rate in patients in the DANBIO (DANish BIOlogics Registry) [180] and in the ACR20/50/70 outcomes in the ADA arm of the SPIRIT H2H study [120].

Regarding the drug retention rate, studies results are divergent. In the SSTA registry, there was better retention of bDMARDs with concomitant use of MTX due to the lower occurrence of adverse events [6], and in the NOR-DMARD registry and British Society for Rheumatology Biologics Register (BSRBR), higher retention was observed for patients treated with IFX and ADA who received MTX concomitantly, which was not observed for patients treated with ETN [179, 181]. The Analyses of the COnsortium of Rheumatology Researchers of North America (CORRONA) registry showed no difference in anti-TNF persistence between patients on combined therapy and monotherapy (32.4 vs. 30.8 months, $p=0.73$); however, when anti-TNF agents (ADA, ETN, IFX) were analyzed separately, the concomitant use of MTX increased IFX persistence [180, 182]. Thus, outcomes may depend on the anti-TNF agent evaluated and possible anti-drug antibody formation. Immunogenicity in response to anti-TNF therapy may result in lower serum drug concentrations, loss of therapeutic response and shorter drug survival [22, 23]. The concomitant use of MTX may reduce the formation of anti-drug antibodies [147, 180, 182].

Studies of UST, SEC and IXE [129, 183] showed no differences between patients who received MTX and those who did not [130, 131, 150, 184]. No data were reported in the studies on TOF [133, 172] and GUS [118, 119, 180].

Recommendation

Regarding monoclonal anti-TNF biologics, the concomitant use of MTX is recommended to increase drug survival, **Level of evidence: 2B; Strength of recommendation: B,** although there is no evidence of increased efficacy **Level of evidence: 1B; Strength of recommendation: A. Degree of agreement: 0.88.**

Regarding tsDMARDs or biologics other than anti-TNF, there is no evidence of increased efficacy or drug survival with concomitant use of cDMARDs. **Level of evidence: 1B; Strength of recommendation: A. Degree of agreement: 0.97.**

Is there evidence for switching biologic and small-molecule DMARDs in patients with psoriatic arthritis?

Treatment switch in patients with PsA occurs due to therapeutic failure, which may be due to inefficacy, adverse events, difficulties in accessing the drug or inability to administer it [131, 133, 149, 150, 183, 185–188].

Approximately 30 to 50% of patients with PsA discontinue anti-TNFs during the first year of treatment due to adverse events or inefficacy. Throughout follow-up, it has been found that treatment effectiveness decreases [11, 189].

The literature does not present evidence for all possible switches, but with more use experience, data accumulate that support the eventual need for replacements.

When the reason for switching from an anti-TNF drug to a second anti-TNF drug was the occurrence of adverse events, an adequate response was observed in 60% of patients, while in patients in whom the switch was due to primary failure, the response rates varied between 20 and 80%, and lower rates were related to a third anti-TNF drug [185–191].

The drug retention rate tends to decrease with time of use: it is lower with the second agent and even lower with a third agent [192, 193].

Recommendation

In patients with PsA and failure to bDMARD, switching to any other immunobiologic agent or to JAK inhibitors is recommended, with no differences between drugs **Level of evidence: 1B**, and the most relevant manifestations of the disease and concomitant clinical conditions should be considered **Level of evidence: 5; Strength of recommendation: B. Degree of agreement: 0.96.**

When the therapeutic failure of an anti-TNF agent is attributed to skin inflammatory activity, switching to drugs with another mechanism of action, such as anti-IL23, anti-IL17 or anti-IL-12/23 agents, can be evaluated. **Level of evidence: 1B; Strength of recommendation: B. Degree of agreement: 0.95.**

When the therapeutic failure of any anti-TNF agent is attributed to serious adverse events, especially infections, switching to drugs with another mechanism of action, such as anti-IL-17, anti-IL-12/23, and anti-IL23 agents or selective costimulation modulator, can be considered. **Level of evidence: 2B; Strength of recommendation: B; Degree of agreement: 0.98.**

If there is a preference for oral medication or contraindications to injectable medications, the use of tofacitinib may be considered. **Level of evidence: 5; Strength of recommendation: D; Degree of agreement: 0.96.**

Conclusions

The recommendations presented here bring together the current scientific evidence for doctors and other health professionals involved in the care of patients with psoriatic disease.

These guidelines considered the current criteria, therapeutic efficacy, safety and critical evaluation and experience of a panel of experts in the standardization of the clinical management of PsA.

However, the autonomy of professionals to choose the best approach among the different therapeutic options is respected and ensured. But it is necessary to take into account some factors that must be remembered when monitoring the treatment, such as:

1. Some DMARDs used in PsA treatment can impact untreated HBV and HCV. Patients should be screened for HBV and HCV prior to therapy initiation. Seek gastroenterology/hepatology input regarding the use of antivirals when initiating patients with active or past HBV on therapy. [194]
2. Biological therapy, especially TNFi, increased the risk of developing TB. Screening and treatment of LTBI or active disease is recommended before using any immunobiologics and JAK inhibitors. [195]
3. Many csDMARDs as well as bDMARDs and JAKi are associated with an increased risk for nonmelanoma skin cancer. Patients should be counseled to undergo full skin assessment annually [196].

Although the objective of this guideline has not included the questioning on therapeutic management after clinical remission in PsA patients, the most recent evidence has supported the tapering approach of cDMARDs and bDMARDs, according to the opinion of the physician and based on the validated instruments for measuring the disease activity.

Abbreviations

ACR: American College of Rheumatology; ASAS: Assessment of Spondyloarthritis International Society; ASDAS-PCR: Ankylosing Spondylitis Disease Activity Score with C Reactive Protein level; BASDAI: Bath Ankylosing Spondylitis Activity Index; BASFI: Bath Ankylosing Spondylitis Functional Index; BSA: Body surface área; CASPAR: Classification criteria for psoriatic arthritis; CORRONA: Consortium of Rheumatology Researchers of North America Registry; CRP: C reactive protein; CVD: Cardiovascular disease; DAPSA: Disease activity in psoriatic arthritis; DAS 28: Disease activity score in 28; DAS44: Disease activity score in 44 joints; bDMARD: Biologic disease-modifying antirheumatic drugs; cDMARD: Conventional disease-modifying antirheumatic drugs; tsDMARD: Targeted synthetic disease-modifying antirheumatic drugs; EARP: Early psoriatic arthritis screening questionnaire; ESR: Erithrocyte sedimentation rate; HAQ: Health assessment questionnaire; HAQ-S: HAQ modified for the Spondyloarthropathies; HIIT: High intensity interval training; MDA: Minimal disease activity; NSAIDs: Nonsteroidal anti-inflammatory drugs; NNH: Number need to harm; NNT: Number need to treat; PASE: Psoriatic arthritis screening evaluation; PASI: Psoriasis Area and severity index; hs-CRP: High sensitivity C reactive protein; PGA: Patient's global assessment; PGA: Physician global assessment; PEST: Psoriasis epidemiology screening tool; PsA: Psoriatic arthritis; PsARC : Psoriatic arthritis response criteria; PsO: Psoriasis; TOPAS-II: Toronto psoriatic arthritis screen-2nd version; VAS: Visual analogue scale; VLDA: Very low disease activity.

Author details

[1]Universidade Federal do Rio de Janeiro (UFRJ), Rua Farme de Amoedo, 140/601. Ipanema, Rio de Janeiro, RJ CEP 22420-020, Brazil. [2]Universidade Federal Do Rio Grande Do Sul (UFRS), Porto Alegre, Brazil. [3]Hospital Do Servidor Público Do Estado de São Paulo, São Paulo, Brazil. [4]Universidade de São Paulo (USP), Ribeirão Preto, São Paulo, Brazil. [5]Universidade Federal de Pernambuco (UFPE), Recife, Brazil. [6]Pontifícia Universidade Católica de Sorocaba (PUC), Sorocaba, Brazil. [7]Pontifícia Universidade Católica de Campinas (PUC), Campinas, Brazil. [8]Hospital Estadual Geral de Goiania (HGG), Goiânia, Brazil. [9]Universidade de São Paulo (USP), São Paulo, Brazil. [10]Universidade Federal de Minas Gerais (UFMG), Belo Horizonte, MG, Brazil. [11]Hospital Heliópolis, São Paulo, Brazil. [12]Pontifícia Universidade Católica de Porto Alegre (PUC), Porto Alegre, Brazil. [13]Universidade Estadual de Campinas (UNICAMP), Campinas, Brazil. [14]Universidade Federal de São Paulo (UNIFESP), São Paulo, Brazil. [15]Universidade Federal do Paraná (UFPR), Curitiba, Paraná, Brazil. [16]Santa Casa de Misericórdia do Rio de Janeiro (SCM), Rio de Janeiro, Brazil. [17]Associação Médica Brasileira, Conselho Federal de Medicina (AMB/CFM), São Paulo, Brazil. [18]Santa Casa de Misericórdia de São Paulo (SCM), São Paulo, Brazil.

References

1. Scotti L, Franchi M, Marchesoni A, Corrao G. Prevalence and incidence of psoriatic arthritis: a systematic review and meta-analysis. Semin Arthritis Rheum. 2018;48(1):28–34. https://doi.org/10.1016/j.semarthrit.2018.01.003.
2. Alinaghi F, Calov M, Kristensen LE, et al. Prevalence of psoriatic arthritis in patients with psoriasis: a systematic review and meta-analysis of observational and clinical studies. J Am Acad Dermatol. 2019;80(1):251–65. https://doi.org/10.1016/j.jaad.2018.06.027.
3. Ranza R, Carneiro S, Qureshi AA, et al. Prevalence of psoriatic arthritis in a large cohort of Brazilian patients with psoriasis. J Rheumatol. 2015;42(5):829–34. https://doi.org/10.3899/jrheum.140474.
4. Scarpa R, Cosentini E, Manguso F, et al. Clinical and genetic aspects of psoriatic arthritis "sine psoriasis." J Rheumatol. 2003;30(12):2638–40.

5. Poggenborg RP, Østergaard M, Terslev L. Imaging in psoriatic arthritis. Rheum Dis Clin North Am. 2015;41(4):593–613. https://doi.org/10.1016/j.rdc.2015.07.007.
6. Gossec L, Smolen JS, Ramiro S, et al. European League Against Rheumatism (EULAR) recommendations for the management of psoriatic arthritis with pharmacological therapies: 2015 update. Ann Rheum Dis. 2016;75(3):499–510. https://doi.org/10.1136/annrheumdis-2015-208337.
7. Mease PJ. Measures of psoriatic arthritis: tender and Swollen Joint Assessment, Psoriasis Area and Severity Index (PASI), Nail Psoriasis Severity Index (NAPSI), Modified Nail Psoriasis Severity Index (mNAPSI), Mander/Newcastle Enthesitis Index (MEI), Leeds Enthesitis Index (LEI), Spondyloarthritis Research Consortium of Canada (SPARCC), Maastricht Ankylosing Spondylitis Enthesis Score (MASES), Leeds Dactylitis Index (LDI), Patient Global for Psoriatic Arthritis, Dermatology Life Quality Index (DLQI), Psoriatic Arthritis Quality of Life (PsAQOL), Functional Assessment of Chronic Illness Therapy-Fatigue (FACIT-F), Psoriatic Arthritis Response Criteria (PsARC), Psoriatic Arthritis Joint Activity Index (PsAJAI), Disease Activity in Psoriatic Arthritis (DAPSA), and Composite Psoriatic Disease Activity Index (CPDAI). Arthritis Care Res (Hoboken). 2011;63(Suppl 11):S64-85. https://doi.org/10.1002/acr.20577.
8. Resende GG, Meirelles ES, Marques CDL, Chiereghin A, Lyrio AM, Ximenes AC, Saad CG, Gonçalves CR, Kohem CL, Schainberg CG, Campanholo CB, Bueno Filho JSS, Pieruccetti LB, Keiserman MW, Yazbek MA, Palominos PE, Goncalves RSG, Lage RDC, Assad RL, Bonfiglioli R, Anti SMA, Carneiro S, Oliveira TL, Azevedo VF, Bianchi WA, Bernardo WM, Pinheiro MM, Sampaio-Barros PD. The Brazilian Society of Rheumatology guidelines for axial spondyloarthritis—2019. Adv Rheumatol. 2020;60(1):19. https://doi.org/10.1186/s42358-020-0116-2.
9. Coates LC, Kavanaugh A, Mease PJ, et al. Group for research and assessment of psoriasis and psoriatic arthritis 2015 treatment recommendations for psoriatic arthritis. Arthritis Rheumatol. 2016;68(5):1060–71. https://doi.org/10.1002/art.39573.
10. Singh JA, Guyatt G, Ogdie A, et al. Special article: 2018 American College of Rheumatology/National Psoriasis Foundation Guideline for the Treatment of Psoriatic Arthritis. Arthritis Rheumatol. 2019;71(1):5–32. https://doi.org/10.1002/art.40726.
11. Carneiro S, Azevedo VF, Bonfiglioli R, et al. Recommendations for the management and treatment of psoriatic arthritis. Rev Bras Reumatol. 2013;53:227–41.
12. Taylor W, Gladman D, Helliwell P, et al. Classification criteria for psoriatic arthritis: development of new criteria from a large international study. Arthritis Rheum. 2006;54(8):2665–73. https://doi.org/10.1002/art.21972
13. Guyatt GH, Oxman AD, Vist GE, et al. GRADE: an emerging consensus on rating quality of evidence and strength of recommendations. BMJ. 2008;336(7650):924–6. https://doi.org/10.1136/bmj.39489.470347.AD.
14. Andrews J, Guyatt G, Oxman AD, et al. GRADE guidelines: 14. Going from evidence to recommendations: the significance and presentation of recommendations. J Clin Epidemiol. 2013;66(7):719–25. https://doi.org/10.1016/j.jclinepi.2012.03.013.
15. Andrews JC, Schünemann HJ, Oxman AD, et al. GRADE guidelines: 15. Going from evidence to recommendation-determinants of a recommendation's direction and strength. J Clin Epidemiol. 2013;66(7):726–35. https://doi.org/10.1016/j.jclinepi.2013.02.003.
16. Howick J, Chalmers I, Glasziou P, Greenhalgh T, Heneghan C, Liberati A, Moschetti I, Phillips B, Thornton H; OCEBM Levels of Evidence Working Group. The Oxford 2011 Levels of Evidence. Oxford Centre for Evidence-Based Medicine. 2011. www.cebm.ox.ac.uk/resources/levels-of-evidence/ocebm-levels-of-evidence
17. Hasson F, Keeney S, McKenna H. Research guidelines for the Delphi survey technique. J Adv Nurs. 2000;32(4):1008–15.
18. Cohen J. Statistical power analysis for the behavioral sciences. 2nd ed. Hillsdale: Lawrence Erlbaum Associates; 1988.
19. Nakagawa S, Cuthill IC. Effect size, confidence interval and statistical significance: a practical guide for biologists [published correction appears in Biol Rev Camb Philos Soc. 2009 Aug;84(3):515]. Biol Rev Camb Philos Soc. 2007;82(4):591–605. https://doi.org/10.1111/j.1469-185X.2007.00027
20. Coates LC, Savage L, Waxman R, Moverley AR, Worthington S, Helliwell PS. Comparison of screening questionnaires to identify psoriatic arthritis in a primary-care population: a cross-sectional study. Br J Dermatol. 2016;175(3):542–8. https://doi.org/10.1111/bjd.14604.
21. Coates LC, Aslam T, Al Balushi F, et al. Comparison of three screening tools to detect psoriatic arthritis in patients with psoriasis (CONTEST study) [published correction appears in Br J Dermatol. 2013 Jun;168(6):1376. Burden-The, E [corrected to Burden-Teh, Esther]]. Br J Dermatol. 2013;168(4):802–807. https://doi.org/10.1111/bjd.12190
22. Tom BD, Chandran V, Farewell VT, Rosen CF, Gladman DD. Validation of the Toronto psoriatic arthritis screen version 2 (ToPAS 2). J Rheumatol. 2015;42(5):841–6. https://doi.org/10.3899/jrheum.140857.
23. Mishra S, Kancharla H, Dogra S, Sharma A. Comparison of four validated psoriatic arthritis screening tools in diagnosing psoriatic arthritis in patients with psoriasis (COMPAQ Study). Br J Dermatol. 2017;176(3):765–70. https://doi.org/10.1111/bjd.14929.
24. Audureau E, Roux F, Lons Danic D, et al. Psoriatic arthritis screening by the dermatologist: development and first validation of the "PURE-4 scale." J Eur Acad Dermatol Venereol. 2018;32(11):1950–3. https://doi.org/10.1111/jdv.14861.
25. Salaffi F, Di Carlo M, Luchetti MM, et al. A validation study of the Simple Psoriatic Arthritis Screening (SiPAS) questionnaire to screen psoriasis patients for psoriatic arthritis. Clin Exp Rheumatol. 2018;36(1):127–35.
26. Husni ME, Meyer KH, Cohen DS, Mody E, Qureshi AA. The PASE questionnaire: pilot-testing a psoriatic arthritis screening and evaluation tool. J Am Acad Dermatol. 2007;57(4):581–7. https://doi.org/10.1016/j.jaad.2007.04.001.
27. You HS, Kim GW, Cho HH, et al. Screening for psoriatic arthritis in Korean psoriasis patients using the psoriatic arthritis screening evaluation questionnaire. Ann Dermatol. 2015;27(3):265–8. https://doi.org/10.5021/ad.2015.27.3.265.
28. Karreman MC, Weel AEAM, van der Ven M, et al. Performance of screening tools for psoriatic arthritis: a cross-sectional study in primary care. Rheumatology (Oxford). 2017;56(4):597–602. https://doi.org/10.1093/rheumatology/kew410.
29. Ibrahim GH, Buch MH, Lawson C, Waxman R, Helliwell PS. Evaluation of an existing screening tool for psoriatic arthritis in people with psoriasis and the development of a new instrument: the Psoriasis Epidemiology Screening Tool (PEST) questionnaire. Clin Exp Rheumatol. 2009;27(3):469–74.
30. Tinazzi I, Adami S, Zanolin EM, et al. The early psoriatic arthritis screening questionnaire: a simple and fast method for the identification of arthritis in patients with psoriasis. Rheumatology (Oxford). 2012;51(11):2058–63. https://doi.org/10.1093/rheumatology/kes187.
31. Iragorri N, Hazlewood G, Manns B, Danthurebandara V, Spackman E. Psoriatic arthritis screening: a systematic review and meta-analysis. Rheumatology (Oxford). 2019;58(4):692–707. https://doi.org/10.1093/rheumatology/key314.PMID:30380111;PMCID:PMC6434376.
32. Coates LC, Savage LJ, Chinoy H, et al. Assessment of two screening tools to identify psoriatic arthritis in patients with psoriasis. J Eur Acad Dermatol Venereol. 2018;32(9):1530–4. https://doi.org/10.1111/jdv.14971.
33. Gonçalves RSG, Pereira GA, de Andrade LE, Martins THF, Junior JOA, Carvalho JB, Mariz HA, Dantas AT, Duarte ALBP. Validation of the Toronto Psoriatic Arthritis Screen II (ToPAS II) questionnaire in a Brazilian population. Clin Rheumatol. 2021;40(5):1889–92. https://doi.org/10.1007/s10067-020-05509-2.
34. Costa CZ, Goldenstein-Schainberg C, Carneiro S, Rodrigues JJ, Romiti R, Barros TBM, et al. Semantic and psychometric validation of the Brazilian Portuguese version (PASE-P) of the psoriatic arthritis screening and evaluation questionnaire. PLoS ONE. 2018;13(10):e0205486. https://doi.org/10.1371/journal.pone.0205486.
35. Mazzotti NG, Palominos PE, Bredemeier M, Kohem CL, Cestari TF. Cross-cultural validation and psychometric properties of the Brazilian Portuguese version of the Psoriasis Epidemiology Screening Tool (PEST-bp). Arch Dermatol Res. 2020;312(3):197–206. https://doi.org/10.1007/s00403-019-02013-9.
36. Gladman DD, Shuckett R, Russell ML, Thorne JC, Schachter RK. Psoriatic arthritis (PSA)—an analysis of 220 patients. Q J Med. 1987;62(238):127–41.
37. Jones SM, Armas JB, Cohen MG, Lovell CR, Evison G, McHugh NJ. Psoriatic arthritis: outcome of disease subsets and relationship of joint disease to nail and skin disease. Br J Rheumatol. 1994;33(9):834–9. https://doi.org/10.1093/rheumatology/33.9.834.
38. Yang Q, Qu L, Tian H, et al. Prevalence and characteristics of psoriatic arthritis in Chinese patients with psoriasis. J Eur Acad Dermatol Venereol. 2011;25(12):1409–14. https://doi.org/10.1111/j.1468-3083.

2011.03985.x.
39. Wilson FC, Icen M, Crowson CS, McEvoy MT, Gabriel SE, Kremers HM. Incidence and clinical predictors of psoriatic arthritis in patients with psoriasis: a population-based study [published correction appears in Arthritis Rheum. 2010 Apr;62(4):574]. Arthritis Rheumil. 2009;61(2):233–239. doi:https://doi.org/10.1002/art.24172
40. Zanolli MD, Wikle JS. Joint complaints in psoriasis patients. Int J Dermatol. 1992;31(7):488–91. https://doi.org/10.1111/j.1365-4362.1992.tb02696.x.
41. Ogdie A, Langan S, Love T, et al. Prevalence and treatment patterns of psoriatic arthritis in the UK. Rheumatology (Oxford). 2013;52(3):568–75. https://doi.org/10.1093/rheumatology/kes324.
42. Love TJ, Gudjonsson JE, Valdimarsson H, Gudbjornsson B. Psoriatic arthritis and onycholysis—results from the cross-sectional Reykjavik psoriatic arthritis study. J Rheumatol. 2012;39(7):1441–4. https://doi.org/10.3899/jrheum.111298.
43. Gladman DD, Chandran V. Observational cohort studies: lessons learnt from the University of Toronto Psoriatic Arthritis Program. Rheumatology (Oxford). 2011;50(1):25–31. https://doi.org/10.1093/rheumatology/keq262.
44. Soltani-Arabshahi R, Wong B, Feng BJ, Goldgar DE, Duffin KC, Krueger GG. Obesity in early adulthood as a risk factor for psoriatic arthritis. Arch Dermatol. 2010;146(7):721–6. https://doi.org/10.1001/archdermatol.2010.141.
45. Reich K, Krüger K, Mössner R, Augustin M. Epidemiology and clinical pattern of psoriatic arthritis in Germany: a prospective interdisciplinary epidemiological study of 1511 patients with plaque-type psoriasis. Br J Dermatol. 2009;160(5):1040–7. https://doi.org/10.1111/j.1365-2133.2008.09023.x.
46. Jamshidi F, Bouzari N, Seirafi H, Farnaghi F, Firooz A. The prevalence of psoriatic arthritis in psoriatic patients in Tehran. Iran Arch Iran Med. 2008;11(2):162–5.
47. Salvarani C, Lo Scocco G, Macchioni P, et al. Prevalence of psoriatic arthritis in Italian psoriatic patients. J Rheumatol. 1995;22(8):1499–503.
48. Stern RS. The epidemiology of joint complaints in patients with psoriasis. J Rheumatol. 1985;12(2):315–20.
49. Soy M, Karaca N, Umit EU, Bes C, Piskin S. Joint and nail involvement in Turkish patients with psoriatic arthritis. Rheumatol Int. 2008;29(2):223–5. https://doi.org/10.1007/s00296-008-0686-5.
50. Eder L, Law T, Chandran V, et al. Association between environmental factors and onset of psoriatic arthritis in patients with psoriasis. Arthritis Care Res (Hoboken). 2011;63(8):1091–7. https://doi.org/10.1002/acr.20496.
51. Maejima H, Taniguchi T, Watarai A, Katsuoka K. Evaluation of nail disease in psoriatic arthritis by using a modified nail psoriasis severity score index. Int J Dermatol. 2010;49(8):901–6. https://doi.org/10.1111/j.1365-4632.2009.04452.x.
52. Love TJ, Gudjonsson JE, Valdimarsson H, Gudbjornsson B. Small joint involvement in psoriatic arthritis is associated with onycholysis: the Reykjavik Psoriatic Arthritis Study. Scand J Rheumatol. 2010;39(4):299–302. https://doi.org/10.3109/03009741003604559.
53. Thumboo J, Uramoto K, Shbeeb MI, et al. Risk factors for the development of psoriatic arthritis: a population based nested case control study. J Rheumatol. 2002;29(4):757–62.
54. Scarpa R, Soscia E, Peluso R, et al. Nail and distal interphalangeal joint in psoriatic arthritis. J Rheumatol. 2006;33(7):1315–9.
55. Cohen MR, Reda DJ, Clegg DO. Baseline relationships between psoriasis and psoriatic arthritis: analysis of 221 patients with active psoriatic arthritis. Department of Veterans Affairs Cooperative Study Group on Seronegative Spondyloarthropathies. J Rheumatol. 1999;26(8):1752–1756
56. Moghaddassi M, Shahram F, Chams-Davatchi C, Najafizadeh SR, Davatchi F. Different aspects of psoriasis: analysis of 150 Iranian patients. Arch Iran Med. 2009;12(3):279–83.
57. Scarpa R, Manguso F, Oriente A, Peluso R, Atteno M, Oriente P. Is the involvement of the distal interphalangeal joint in psoriatic patients related to nail psoriasis? Clin Rheumatol. 2004;23(1):27–30. https://doi.org/10.1007/s10067-003-0817-z.
58. Husted JA, Thavaneswaran A, Chandran V, et al. Cardiovascular and other comorbidities in patients with psoriatic arthritis: a comparison with patients with psoriasis. Arthritis Care Res (Hoboken). 2011;63(12):1729–35. https://doi.org/10.1002/acr.20627.
59. Bhole VM, Choi HK, Burns LC, et al. Differences in body mass index among individuals with PsA, psoriasis, RA and the general population. Rheumatology (Oxford). 2012;51(3):552–6. https://doi.org/10.1093/rheumatology/ker349.
60. Jafri K, Bartels CM, Shin D, Gelfand JM, Ogdie A. Incidence and management of cardiovascular risk factors in psoriatic arthritis and rheumatoid arthritis: a population-based study. Arthritis Care Res (Hoboken). 2017;69(1):51–7. https://doi.org/10.1002/acr.23094.
61. Kaine J, Song X, Kim G, Hur P, Palmer JB. Higher incidence rates of comorbidities in patients with psoriatic arthritis compared with the general population using U.S. Administrative claims data. J Manag Care Spec Pharm. 2019;25(1):122–132. https://doi.org/10.18553/jmcp.2018.17421
62. Di Minno MN, Peluso R, Iervolino S, et al. Obesity and the prediction of minimal disease activity: a prospective study in psoriatic arthritis. Arthritis Care Res (Hoboken). 2013;65(1):141–7. https://doi.org/10.1002/acr.21711.
63. Di Minno MN, Peluso R, Iervolino S, et al. Weight loss and achievement of minimal disease activity in patients with psoriatic arthritis starting treatment with tumour necrosis factor α blockers. Ann Rheum Dis. 2014;73(6):1157–62. https://doi.org/10.1136/annrheumdis-2012-202812.
64. Haroon M, Gallagher P, Heffernan E, FitzGerald O. High prevalence of metabolic syndrome and of insulin resistance in psoriatic arthritis is associated with the severity of underlying disease. J Rheumatol. 2014;41(7):1357–65. https://doi.org/10.3899/jrheum.140021.
65. Özkan SG, Yazısız H, Behlül A, Gökbelen YA, Borlu F, Yazısız V. Prevalence of metabolic syndrome and degree of cardiovascular disease risk in patients with Psoriatic Arthritis [published correction appears in Eur J Rheumatol. 2017 Dec;4(4):307]. Eur J Rheumatol. 2017;4(1):40–45. https://doi.org/10.5152/eurjrheum.2017.16052
66. Haque N, Lories RJ, de Vlam K. Comorbidities associated with psoriatic arthritis compared with non-psoriatic spondyloarthritis: a cross-sectional study. J Rheumatol. 2016;43(2):376–82. https://doi.org/10.3899/jrheum.141359.
67. Raychaudhuri SK, Chatterjee S, Nguyen C, Kaur M, Jialal I, Raychaudhuri SP. Increased prevalence of the metabolic syndrome in patients with psoriatic arthritis. Metab Syndr Relat Disord. 2010;8(4):331–4. https://doi.org/10.1089/met.2009.0124.
68. Ahmed N, Prior JA, Chen Y, Hayward R, Mallen CD, Hider SL. Prevalence of cardiovascular-related comorbidity in ankylosing spondylitis, psoriatic arthritis and psoriasis in primary care: a matched retrospective cohort study. Clin Rheumatol. 2016;35(12):3069–73. https://doi.org/10.1007/s10067-016-3362-2.
69. Khraishi M, MacDonald D, Rampakakis E, Vaillancourt J, Sampalis JS. Prevalence of patient-reported comorbidities in early and established psoriatic arthritis cohorts. Clin Rheumatol. 2011;30(7):877–85. https://doi.org/10.1007/s10067-011-1692-7.
70. Costa L, Caso F, Del Puente A, Di Minno MN, Peluso R, Scarpa R. Incidence of malignancies in a cohort of psoriatic arthritis patients taking traditional disease modifying antirheumatic drug and tumor necrosis factor inhibitor therapy: an observational study. J Rheumatol. 2016;43(12):2149–54. https://doi.org/10.3899/jrheum.160542.
71. Han C, Robinson DW Jr, Hackett MV, Paramore LC, Fraeman KH, Bala MV. Cardiovascular disease and risk factors in patients with rheumatoid arthritis, psoriatic arthritis, and ankylosing spondylitis. J Rheumatol. 2006;33(11):2167–72.
72. Szentpetery A, Healy GM, Brady D, et al. Higher coronary plaque burden in psoriatic arthritis is independent of metabolic syndrome and associated with underlying disease severity. Arthritis Rheumatol. 2018;70(3):396–407. https://doi.org/10.1002/art.40389.
73. Li L, Hagberg KW, Peng M, Shah K, Paris M, Jick S. Rates of cardiovascular disease and major adverse cardiovascular events in patients with psoriatic arthritis compared to patients without psoriatic arthritis. J Clin Rheumatol. 2015;21(8):405–10. https://doi.org/10.1097/RHU.0000000000000306.
74. Kathuria P, Gordon KB, Silverberg JI. Association of psoriasis and psoriatic arthritis with osteoporosis and pathological fractures. J Am Acad Dermatol. 2017;76(6):1045–53. https://doi.org/10.1016/j.jaad.2016.11.046.
75. Paiva ES, Macaluso DC, Edwards A, Rosenbaum JT. Characterisation of uveitis in patients with psoriatic arthritis. Ann Rheum Dis.

2000;59(1):67–70. https://doi.org/10.1136/ard.59.1.67

76. Bengtsson K, Forsblad-d'Elia H, Lie E, et al. Are ankylosing spondylitis, psoriatic arthritis and undifferentiated spondyloarthritis associated with an increased risk of cardiovascular events? A prospective nationwide population-based cohort study. Arthritis Res Ther. 2017;19(1):102. https://doi.org/10.1186/s13075-017-1315-z.
77. Zohar A, Cohen AD, Bitterman H, et al. Gastrointestinal comorbidities in patients with psoriatic arthritis. Clin Rheumatol. 2016;35(11):2679–84. https://doi.org/10.1007/s10067-016-3374-y.
78. Thomsen RS, Nilsen TIL, Haugeberg G, Bye A, Kavanaugh A, Hoff M. Impact of High-intensity interval training on disease activity and disease in patients with psoriatic arthritis: a randomized controlled trial. Arthritis Care Res (Hoboken). 2019;71(4):530–7. https://doi.org/10.1002/acr.23614.
79. Roger-Silva D, Natour J, Moreira E, Jennings F. A resistance exercise pro gram improves functional capacity of patients with psoriatic arthritis: a randomized controlled trial. Clin Rheumatol. 2018;37(2):389–95. https://doi.org/10.1007/s10067-017-3917-x.
80. Thomsen RS, Nilsen TIL, Haugeberg G, Bye A, Kavanaugh A, Hoff M. Effect of high-intensity interval training on cardiovascular disease risk factors and body composition in psoriatic arthritis: a randomised controlled trial. RMD Open. 2018;4(2):e000729. https://doi.org/10.1136/rmdopen-2018-000729.
81. Al-Mutairi N, Nour T. The effect of weight reduction on treatment outcomes in obese patients with psoriasis on biologic therapy: a randomized controlled prospective trial. Exp Opin Biol Ther. 2014;14(6):749–56. https://doi.org/10.1517/14712598.2014.900541.
82. Baillet A, Zeboulon N, Gossec L, et al. Efficacy of cardiorespiratory aerobic exercise in rheumatoid arthritis: meta-analysis of randomized controlled trials. Arthritis Care Res (Hoboken). 2010;62(7):984–92. https://doi.org/10.1002/acr.20146.
83. Eder L, Chandran V, Ueng J, et al. Predictors of response to intra-articular steroid injection in psoriatic arthritis. Rheumatology (Oxford). 2010;49(7):1367–73. https://doi.org/10.1093/rheumatology/keq102.
84. Kingsley GH, Scott DL. Assessing the effectiveness of synthetic and biologic disease-modifying antirheumatic drugs in psoriatic arthritis—a systematic review. Psoriasis (Auckl). 2015;5:71–81. https://doi.org/10.2147/PTT.S52893.
85. Soriano ER, McHugh NJ. Therapies for peripheral joint disease in psoriatic arthritis. A systematic review. J Rheumatol. 2006;33(7):1422–30.
86. Grassi W, De Angelis R, Cervini C. Corticosteroid prescribing in rheumatoid arthritis and psoriatic arthritis. Clin Rheumatol. 1998;17(3):223–6. https://doi.org/10.1007/BF01451052.
87. Sarzi-Puttini P, Santandrea S, Boccassini L, Panni B, Caruso I. The role of NSAIDs in psoriatic arthritis: evidence from a controlled study with nimesulide. Clin Exp Rheumatol. 2001;19(1 Suppl 22):S17–20.
88. Kivitz AJ, Espinoza LR, Sherrer YR, Liu-Dumaw M, West CR. A comparison of the efficacy and safety of celecoxib 200 mg and celecoxib 400 mg once daily in treating the signs and symptoms of psoriatic arthritis. Semin Arthritis Rheum. 2007;37(3):164–73. https://doi.org/10.1016/j.semarthrit.2007.03.004.
89. Lassus A. A comparative pilot study of azapropazone and indomethacin in the treatment of psoriatic arthritis and Reiter's disease. Curr Med Res Opin. 1976;4(1):65–9. https://doi.org/10.1185/03007997609109283.
90. Lonauer G, Wirth W. Kontrollierte Doppelblindstudie zur Uberprüfung der Wirksamkeit und Verträglichkeit von Acemetacin und Indometacin bei der Behandlung der Arthritis psoriatica [Controlled double blind study on the effectiveness and adverse effects of acemetacin and indomethacin in the treatment of psoriatic arthritis]. Arzneimittelforschung. 1980;30(8A):1440–4.
91. Leatham PA, Bird HA, Wright V, Fowler PD. The run-in period in trial design: a comparison of two non-steroidal anti-inflammatory agents in psoriatic arthropathy. Agents Actions. 1982;12(1–2):221–4. https://doi.org/10.1007/BF01965150.
92. van der Heijde D, Baraf HS, Ramos-Remus C, et al. Evaluation of the efficacy of etoricoxib in ankylosing spondylitis: results of a fifty-two-week, randomized, controlled study. Arthritis Rheum. 2005;52(4):1205–15. https://doi.org/10.1002/art.20985.
93. Wanders A, Heijde D, Landewé R, et al. Nonsteroidal antiinflammatory drugs reduce radiographic progression in patients with ankylosing spondylitis: a randomized clinical trial. Arthritis Rheum. 2005;52(6):1756–65. https://doi.org/10.1002/art.21054
94. Sieper J, Listing J, Poddubnyy D, et al. Effect of continuous versus on-demand treatment of ankylosing spondylitis with diclofenac over 2 years on radiographic progression of the spine: results from a randomised multicentre trial (ENRADAS). Ann Rheum Dis. 2016;75(8):1438–43. https://doi.org/10.1136/annrheumdis-2015-207897.
95. Kroon F, Landewé R, Dougados M, van der Heijde D. Continuous NSAID use reverts the effects of inflammation on radiographic progression in patients with ankylosing spondylitis. Ann Rheum Dis. 2012;71(10):1623–9. https://doi.org/10.1136/annrheumdis-2012-201370.
96. Sakkas LI, Alexiou I, Simopoulou T, Vlychou M. Enthesitis in psoriatic arthritis. Semin Arthritis Rheum. 2013;43(3):325–34. https://doi.org/10.1016/j.semarthrit.2013.04.005.
97. Rose S, Toloza S, Bautista-Molano W, Helliwell PS, GRAPPA Dactylitis Study Group. Comprehensive treatment of dactylitis in psoriatic arthritis. J Rheumatol. 2014;41(11):2295–300. https://doi.org/10.3899/jrheum.140879.
98. Katayama H, Kawada A. Exacerbation of psoriasis induced by indomethacin. J Dermatol. 1981;8(4):323–7. https://doi.org/10.1111/j.1346-8138.1981.tb02551.x.
99. Reshad H, Hargreaves GK, Vickers CF. Generalized pustular psoriasis precipitated by phenylbutazone and oxyphenbutazone. Br J Dermatol. 1983;109(1):111–3. https://doi.org/10.1111/j.1365-2133.1983.tb04000.x.
100. Ben-Chetrit E, Rubinow A. Exacerbation of psoriasis by ibuprofen. Cutis. 1986;38(1):45.
101. Cohen AD, Bonneh DY, Reuveni H, Vardy DA, Naggan L, Halevy S. Drug exposure and psoriasis vulgaris: case-control and case-crossover studies. Acta Derm Venereol. 2005;85(4):299–303. https://doi.org/10.1080/00015550510032823.
102. Kvien TK, Heiberg, Lie E, et al. A Norwegian DMARD register: prescriptions of DMARDs and biological agents to patients with inflammatory rheumatic diseases. Clin Exp Rheumatol. 2005;23(5 Suppl 39):S188-S194.
103. Theander E, Husmark T, Alenius GM, et al. Early psoriatic arthritis: short symptom duration, male gender and preserved physical functioning at presentation predict favourable outcome at 5-year follow-up. Results from the Swedish Early Psoriatic Arthritis Register (SwePsA). Ann Rheum Dis. 2014;73(2):407-413. https://doi.org/10.1136/annrheumdis-2012-20197
104. Jones G, Crotty M, Brooks P. Interventions for psoriatic arthritis. Cochrane Database Syst Rev. 2000;(3):CD000212. https://doi.org/10.1002/14651858.CD000212
105. Willkens RF, Williams HJ, Ward JR, et al. Randomized, double-blind, placebo controlled trial of low-dose pulse methotrexate in psoriatic arthritis. Arthritis Rheum. 1984;27(4):376–81. https://doi.org/10.1002/art.1780270403.
106. Scarpa R, Peluso R, Atteno M, et al. The effectiveness of a traditional therapeutical approach in early psoriatic arthritis: results of a pilot randomised 6-month trial with methotrexate. Clin Rheumatol. 2008;27(7):823–6. https://doi.org/10.1007/s10067-007-0787-7.
107. Kingsley GH, Kowalczyk A, Taylor H, et al. A randomized placebo-controlled trial of methotrexate in psoriatic arthritis. Rheumatology (Oxford). 2012;51(8):1368–77. https://doi.org/10.1093/rheumatology/kes001.
108. Coates LC, Navarro-Coy N, Brown SR, et al. The TICOPA protocol (TIght COntrol of Psoriatic Arthritis): a randomised controlled trial to compare intensive management versus standard care in early psoriatic arthritis. BMC Musculoskelet Disord. 2013;14:101. https://doi.org/10.1186/1471-2474-14-101.
109. Mease PJ, Gladman DD, Collier DH, et al. Etanercept and methotrexate as monotherapy or in combination for psoriatic arthritis: primary results from a randomized, controlled phase III trial. Arthritis Rheumatol. 2019;71(7):1112–24. https://doi.org/10.1002/art.40851.
110. Salvarani C, Macchioni P, Olivieri I, et al. A comparison of cyclosporine, sulfasalazine, and symptomatic therapy in the treatment of psoriatic arthritis. J Rheumatol. 2001;28(10):2274–82.
111. Spadaro A, Riccieri V, Sili-Scavalli A, Sensi F, Taccari E, Zoppini A. Comparison of cyclosporin A and methotrexate in the treatment of psoriatic arthritis: a one-year prospective study. Clin Exp Rheumatol. 1995;13(5):589–93.
112. Karanikolas GN, Koukli EM, Katsalira A, et al. Adalimumab or cyclosporine as monotherapy and in combination in severe psoriatic arthritis: results from a prospective 12-month nonrandomized unblinded

clinical trial. J Rheumatol. 2011;38(11):2466–74. https://doi.org/10.3899/jrheum.110242.
113. Kaltwasser JP, Nash P, Gladman D, et al. Efficacy and safety of leflunomide in the treatment of psoriatic arthritis and psoriasis: a multinational, double-blind, randomized, placebo-controlled clinical trial. Arthritis Rheum. 2004;50(6):1939–50. https://doi.org/10.1002/art.20253.
114. Asiri A, Thavaneswaran A, Kalman-Lamb G, Chandran V, Gladman DD. The effectiveness of leflunomide in psoriatic arthritis. Clin Exp Rheumatol. 2014;32(5):728–31.
115. Combe B, Goupille P, Kuntz JL, Tebib J, Lioté F, Bregeon C. Sulphasalazine in psoriatic arthritis: a randomized, multicentre, placebo-controlled study. Br J Rheumatol. 1996;35(7):664–8. https://doi.org/10.1093/rheumatology/35.7.664.
116. Fraser SM, Hopkins R, Hunter JA, Neumann V, Capell HA, Bird HA. Sulphasalazine in the management of psoriatic arthritis. Br J Rheumatol. 1993;32(10):923–5. https://doi.org/10.1093/rheumatology/32.10.923.
117. Gupta AK, Grober JS, Hamilton TA, et al. Sulfasalazine therapy for psoriatic arthritis: a double blind, placebo controlled trial. J Rheumatol. 1995;22(5):894–8.
118. Deodhar A, Helliwell PS, Boehncke WH, et al. Guselkumab in patients with active psoriatic arthritis who were biologic-naive or had previously received TNFα inhibitor treatment (DISCOVER-1): a double-blind, randomised, placebo-controlled phase 3 trial [published correction appears in Lancet. 2020 Apr 4;395(10230):1114]. Lancet. 2020;395(10230):1115–1125. https://doi.org/10.1016/S0140-6736(20)30265-8
119. Mease PJ, Rahman P, Gottlieb AB, et al. Guselkumab in biologic-naive patients with active psoriatic arthritis (DISCOVER-2): a double-blind, randomised, placebo-controlled phase 3 trial [published correction appears in Lancet. 2020 Apr 4;395(10230):1114]. Lancet. 2020;395(10230):1126–1136. https://doi.org/10.1016/S0140-6736(20)30263-4.
120. Mease PJ, Smolen JS, Behrens F, et al. A head-to-head comparison of the efficacy and safety of ixekizumab and adalimumab in biological-naïve patients with active psoriatic arthritis: 24-week results of a randomised, open-label, blinded-assessor trial. Ann Rheum Dis. 2020;79(1):123–31. https://doi.org/10.1136/annrheumdis-2019-215386.
121. McInnes IB, Behrens F, Mease PJ, et al. Secukinumab versus adalimumab for treatment of active psoriatic arthritis (EXCEED): a double-blind, parallel-group, randomised, active-controlled, phase 3b trial [published correction appears in Lancet. 2020 May 30;395(10238):1694]. Lancet. 2020;395(10235):1496–1505. https://doi.org/10.1016/S0140-6736(20)30564-X
122. Mease P, Genovese MC, Gladstein G, et al. Abatacept in the treatment of patients with psoriatic arthritis: results of a six-month, multicenter, randomized, double-blind, placebo-controlled, phase II trial. Arthritis Rheum. 2011;63(4):939–48. https://doi.org/10.1002/art.30176.
123. Mease PJ, Gladman DD, Ritchlin CT, et al. Adalimumab for the treatment of patients with moderately to severely active psoriatic arthritis: results of a double-blind, randomized, placebo-controlled trial. Arthritis Rheum. 2005;52(10):3279–89. https://doi.org/10.1002/art.21306.
124. Mease PJ, Fleischmann R, Deodhar AA, et al. Effect of certolizumab pegol on signs and symptoms in patients with psoriatic arthritis: 24-week results of a Phase 3 double-blind randomised placebo-controlled study (RAPID-PsA). Ann Rheum Dis. 2014;73(1):48–55. https://doi.org/10.1136/annrheumdis-2013-203696.
125. Mease PJ, Goffe BS, Metz J, VanderStoep A, Finck B, Burge DJ. Etanercept in the treatment of psoriatic arthritis and psoriasis: a randomised trial. Lancet. 2000;356(9227):385–90. https://doi.org/10.1016/S0140-6736(00)02530-7.
126. Mease PJ, Kivitz AJ, Burch FX, et al. Etanercept treatment of psoriatic arthritis: safety, efficacy, and effect on disease progression. Arthritis Rheum. 2004;50(7):2264–72. https://doi.org/10.1002/art.20335
127. Kavanaugh A, McInnes I, Mease P, et al. Golimumab, a new human tumor necrosis factor alpha antibody, administered every four weeks as a subcutaneous injection in psoriatic arthritis: Twenty-four-week efficacy and safety results of a randomized, placebo-controlled study [published correction appears in Arthritis Rheum. 2010 Aug;62(8):2555]. Arthritis Rheum. 2009;60(4):976–986. https://doi.org/10.1002/art.24403
128. Antoni CE, Kavanaugh A, Kirkham B, et al. Sustained benefits of infliximab therapy for dermatologic and articular manifestations of psoriatic arthritis: results from the infliximab multinational psoriatic arthritis controlled trial (IMPACT) [published correction appears in Arthritis Rheum. 2005 Sep;52(9):2951]. Arthritis Rheum. 2005;52(4):1227–1236. https://doi.org/10.1002/art.20967
129. Mease PJ, van der Heijde D, Ritchlin CT, et al. Ixekizumab, an interleukin-17A specific monoclonal antibody, for the treatment of biologic-naive patients with active psoriatic arthritis: results from the 24-week randomised, double-blind, placebo-controlled and active (adalimumab)-controlled period of the phase III trial SPIRIT-P1. Ann Rheum Dis. 2017;76(1):79–87. https://doi.org/10.1136/annrheumdis-2016-209709.
130. Mease PJ, McInnes IB, Kirkham B, et al. Secukinumab inhibition of interleukin-17A in patients with psoriatic arthritis. N Engl J Med. 2015;373(14):1329–39. https://doi.org/10.1056/NEJMoa1412679.
131. McInnes IB, Mease PJ, Kirkham B, et al. Secukinumab, a human anti-interleukin-17A monoclonal antibody, in patients with psoriatic arthritis (FUTURE 2): a randomised, double-blind, placebo-controlled, phase 3 trial. Lancet. 2015;386(9999):1137–46. https://doi.org/10.1016/S0140-6736(15)61134-5.
132. Gottlieb A, Menter A, Mendelsohn A, et al. Ustekinumab, a human interleukin 12/23 monoclonal antibody, for psoriatic arthritis: randomised, double-blind, placebo-controlled, crossover trial [published correction appears in Lancet. 2009 Apr 18;373(9672):1340] [published correction appears in Lancet. 2010 Nov 6;376(9752):1542]. Lancet. 2009;373(9664):633–640. https://doi.org/10.1016/S0140-6736(09)60140-9
133. Mease P, Hall S, FitzGerald O, et al. Tofacitinib or adalimumab versus placebo for psoriatic arthritis. N Engl J Med. 2017;377(16):1537–50. https://doi.org/10.1056/NEJMoa1615975.
134. Wilsdon TD, Whittle SL, Thynne TR, Mangoni AA. Methotrexate for psoriatic arthritis. Cochrane Database Syst Rev. 2019;1(1):CD012722. https://doi.org/10.1002/14651858.CD012722.pub2
135. Baraliakos X, Coates L, Gossec L, Jeka S, Mera A, Schulz B, Rissler M, Das Gupta A, Perella C, Pournara E. Secukinumab Improves Axial Manifestations in Patients with Psoriatic Arthritis and Inadequate Response to NSAIDs: Primary Analysis of Phase 3 Trial [abstract]. Arthritis Rheumatol. 2019; 71 (suppl 10). https://acrabstracts.org/abstract/secukinumab-improves-axial-manifestations-in-patients-with-psoriatic-arthritis-and-inadequate-response-to-nsaids-primary-analysis-of-phase-3-trial/. Accessed 11 Aug 2021
136. Mease PJ, Gottlieb AB, van der Heijde D, et al. Efficacy and safety of abatacept, a T-cell modulator, in a randomised, double-blind, placebo-controlled, phase III study in psoriatic arthritis. Ann Rheum Dis. 2017;76(9):1550–8. https://doi.org/10.1136/annrheumdis-2016-210724
137. Gladman DD, Mease PJ, Ritchlin CT, et al. Adalimumab for long-term treatment of psoriatic arthritis: forty-eight week data from the adalimumab effectiveness in psoriatic arthritis trial. Arthritis Rheum. 2007;56(2):476–88. https://doi.org/10.1002/art.22379.
138. Mease PJ, Ory P, Sharp JT, et al. Adalimumab for long-term treatment of psoriatic arthritis: 2-year data from the Adalimumab Effectiveness in Psoriatic Arthritis Trial (ADEPT). Ann Rheum Dis. 2009;68(5):702–9. https://doi.org/10.1136/ard.2008.092767.
139. Genovese MC, Mease PJ, Thomson GT, et al. Safety and efficacy of adalimumab in treatment of patients with psoriatic arthritis who had failed disease modifying antirheumatic drug therapy [published correction appears in J Rheumatol. 2007 Jun;34(6):1439]. J Rheumatol. 2007;34(5):1040–1050. Erratum in: J Rheumatol. 2007;34(6):1439.
140. Mease PJ, Kivitz AJ, Burch FX, et al. Continued inhibition of radiographic progression in patients with psoriatic arthritis following 2 years of treat ment with etanercept. J Rheumatol. 2006;33(4):712–21.
141. Mease PJ, Woolley JM, Singh A, Tsuji W, Dunn M, Chiou CF. Patient-reported outcomes in a randomized trial of etanercept in psoriatic arthritis. J Rheumatol. 2010;37(6):1221–7. https://doi.org/10.3899/jrheum.091093
142. Kavanaugh A, McInnes IB, Krueger GG, et al. Patient-reported outcomes and the association with clinical response in patients with active psoriatic arthritis treated with golimumab: findings through 2 years of a phase III, multicenter, randomized, double-blind, placebo-controlled trial. Arthritis Care Res (Hoboken). 2013;65(10):1666–73. https://doi.org/10.1002/acr.22044
143. Kavanaugh A, McInnes IB, Mease PJ, et al. Clinical efficacy, radio graphic and safety findings through 2 years of golimumab treatment

in patients with active psoriatic arthritis: results from a long-term extension of the randomised, placebo-controlled GO-REVEAL study. Ann Rheum Dis. 2013;72(11):1777–85. https://doi.org/10.1136/annrheumdis-2012-202035.
144. Kavanaugh A, McInnes IB, Mease P, et al. Clinical efficacy, radiographic and safety findings through 5 years of subcutaneous golimumab treatment in patients with active psoriatic arthritis: results from a long-term extension of a randomised, placebo-controlled trial (the GO-REVEAL study). Ann Rheum Dis. 2014;73(9):1689–94. https://doi.org/10.1136/annrheumdis-2013-204902.
145. Kavanaugh A, Husni ME, Harrison DD, et al. Safety and efficacy of intravenous golimumab in patients with active psoriatic arthritis: results through week twenty-four of the GO-VIBRANT study. Arthritis Rheumatol. 2017;69(11):2151–61. https://doi.org/10.1002/art.40226.
146. Deodhar A, Gottlieb AB, Boehncke WH, et al. Efficacy and safety of guselkumab in patients with active psoriatic arthritis: a randomised, double-blind, placebo-controlled, phase 2 study. Lancet. 2018;391(10136):2213–24. https://doi.org/10.1016/S0140-6736(18)30952-8.
147. Kavanaugh A, Krueger GG, Beutler A, et al. Infliximab maintains a high degree of clinical response in patients with active psoriatic arthritis through 1 year of treatment: results from the IMPACT 2 trial. Ann Rheum Dis. 2007;66(4):498–505. https://doi.org/10.1136/ard.2006.058339.
148. Antoni CE, Kavanaugh A, van der Heijde D, et al. Two-year efficacy and safety of infliximab treatment in patients with active psoriatic arthritis: findings of the Infliximab Multinational Psoriatic Arthritis Controlled Trial (IMPACT). J Rheumatol. 2008;35(5):869–76.
149. Kavanaugh A, McInnes IB, Mease PJ, et al. Efficacy of subcutaneous secukinumab in patients with active psoriatic arthritis stratified by prior tumor necrosis factor inhibitor use: results from the randomized placebo-controlled FUTURE 2 study. J Rheumatol. 2016;43(9):1713–7. https://doi.org/10.3899/jrheum.160275.
150. Ritchlin C, Rahman P, Kavanaugh A, et al. Efficacy and safety of the anti-IL-12/23 p40 monoclonal antibody, ustekinumab, in patients with active psoriatic arthritis despite conventional non-biological and biological anti-tumour necrosis factor therapy: 6-month and 1-year results of the phase 3, multicentre, double-blind, placebo-controlled, randomised PSUMMIT 2 trial. Ann Rheum Dis. 2014;73(6):990–9. https://doi.org/10.1136/annrheumdis-2013-204655.
151. Lu C, Wallace BI, Waljee AK, Fu W, Zhang Q, Liu Y. Comparative efficacy and safety of targeted DMARDs for active psoriatic arthritis during induction therapy: a systematic review and network meta-analysis. Semin Arthritis Rheum. 2019;49(3):381–8. https://doi.org/10.1016/j.semarthrit.2019.06.001.
152. Strand V, Elaine Husni M, Betts KA, Song Y, Singh R, Griffith J, Beppu M, Zhao J, Ganguli A. Network meta-analysis and cost per responder of targeted Immunomodulators in the treatment of active psoriatic arthritis. BMC Rheumatol. 2018;12(2):3. https://doi.org/10.1186/s41927-018-0011-1.
153. Mease PJ, Lertratanakul A, Anderson JK, Papp K, Van den Bosch F, Tsuji S, Dokoupilova E, Keiserman M, Wang X, Zhong S, McCaskill RM, Zueger P, Pangan AL, Tillett W. Upadacitinib for psoriatic arthritis refractory to biologics: SELECT-PsA 2. Ann Rheum Dis. 2020;80(3):312–20. https://doi.org/10.1136/annrheumdis-2020-218870.
154. Desai SB, Furst DE. Problems encountered during anti-tumour necrosis factor therapy. Best Pract Res Clin Rheumatol. 2006;20(4):757–90. https://doi.org/10.1016/j.berh.2006.06.002.
155. Gómez-Reino JJ, Carmona L, Angel Descalzo M; Biobadaser Group. Risk of tuberculosis in patients treated with tumor necrosis factor antagonists due to incomplete prevention of reactivation of latent infection. Arthritis Rheum. 2007;57(5):756–761. https://doi.org/10.1002/art.22768
156. Culver EL, Travis SP. How to manage the infectious risk under anti-TNF in inflammatory bowel disease. Curr Drug Targets. 2010;11(2):198–218. https://doi.org/10.2174/138945010790310009.
157. Mariette X, Vencovsky J, Lortholary O, et al. The incidence of tuberculosis in patients treated with certolizumab pegol across indications: impact of baseline skin test results, more stringent screening criteria and geographic region. RMD Open. 2015;1(1):e000044. https://doi.org/10.1136/rmdopen-2014-000044.
158. Kay J, Fleischmann R, Keystone E, et al. Five-year safety data from 5 clinical trials of subcutaneous golimumab in patients with rheumatoid arthritis, psoriatic arthritis, and ankylosing spondylitis. J Rheumatol. 2016;43(12):2120–30. https://doi.org/10.3899/jrheum.160420.
159. Tsai TF, Ho V, Song M, et al. The safety of ustekinumab treatment in patients with moderate-to-severe psoriasis and latent tuberculosis infection. Br J Dermatol. 2012;167(5):1145–52. https://doi.org/10.1111/j.1365-2133.2012.11142.x.
160. Bernatsky S, Renoux C, Suissa S. Demyelinating events in rheumatoid arthritis after drug exposures. Ann Rheum Dis. 2010;69(9):1691–3. https://doi.org/10.1136/ard.2009.111500.
161. Bruè C, Mariotti C, Rossiello I, Saitta A, Giovannini A. Demyelinizing neurological disease after treatment with tumor necrosis factor-α antagonists. Case Rep Ophthalmol. 2016;7(2):345–53. https://doi.org/10.1159/000447086.
162. Ryu YS, Park SH, Kim JM, et al. A case of leukoencephalopathy associated with adalimumab-treated rheumatoid arthritis and a review of literature. Rheumatol Int. 2012;32(11):3481–5. https://doi.org/10.1007/s00296-011-2216-0.
163. Kameda T, Dobashi H, Kittaka K, et al. A case of rheumatoid arthritis complicated by demyelination in both cerebral cortex and spinal cord during etanercept therapy. Mod Rheumatol. 2008;18(4):399–402. https://doi.org/10.1007/s10165-008-0062-z.
164. Tanno M, Nakamura I, Kobayashi S, Kurihara K, Ito K. New-onset demyelination induced by infliximab therapy in two rheumatoid arthritis patients. Clin Rheumatol. 2006;25(6):929–33. https://doi.org/10.1007/s10067-005-0097-x.
165. Al Saieg N, Luzar MJ. Etanercept induced multiple sclerosis and transverse myelitis. J Rheumatol. 2006;33(6):1202–4.
166. Pfueller CF, Seipelt E, Zipp F, Paul F. Multiple sclerosis following etanercept treatment for ankylosing spondylitis. Scand J Rheumatol. 2008;37(5):397–9. https://doi.org/10.1080/03009740802136164.
167. Kunzmann S, Warmuth-Metz M, Girschick HJ. Cerebral demyelination in association with TNF-inhibition therapy in a 5-year-old girl with aseptic meningitis as the first symptom of Still's disease. Scand J Rheumatol. 2005;34(1):76–8. https://doi.org/10.1080/03009740510017887.
168. Ding T, Ledingham J, Luqmani R, et al. BSR and BHPR rheumatoid arthritis guidelines on safety of anti-TNF therapies. Rheumatology (Oxford). 2010;49(11):2217–9. https://doi.org/10.1093/rheumatology/keq249a.
169. Marchesoni A, Olivieri I, Salvarani C, et al. Recommendations for the use of biologics and other novel drugs in the treatment of psoriatic arthritis: 2017 update from the Italian Society of Rheumatology. Clin Exp Rheumatol. 2017;35(6):991–1010.
170. Segal BM, Constantinescu CS, Raychaudhuri A, et al. Repeated subcutaneous injections of IL12/23 p40 neutralising antibody, ustekinumab, in patients with relapsing-remitting multiple sclerosis: a phase II, double-blind, placebo-controlled, randomised, dose-ranging study. Lancet Neurol. 2008;7(9):796–804. https://doi.org/10.1016/S1474-4422(08)70173-X.
171. Havrdová E, Belova A, Goloborodko A, et al. Activity of secukinumab, an anti-IL-17A antibody, on brain lesions in RRMS: results from a randomized, proof-of-concept study. J Neurol. 2016;263(7):1287–95. https://doi.org/10.1007/s00415-016-8128-x.
172. Gladman D, Rigby W, Azevedo VF, et al. Tofacitinib for Psoriatic Arthritis in Patients with an Inadequate Response to TNF Inhibitors. N Engl J Med. 2017;377(16):1525–36. https://doi.org/10.1056/NEJMoa1615977.
173. Ruyssen-Witrand A, Perry R, Watkins C, et al. Efficacy and safety of biologics in psoriatic arthritis: a systematic literature review and network meta-analysis. RMD Open. 2020;6:e001117. https://doi.org/10.1136/rmdopen-2019-001117.
174. Bilal J, Riaz IB, Kamal MU, Elyan M, Sudano D, Khan MA. A systematic review and meta-analysis of efficacy and safety of novel interleukin inhibitors in the management of psoriatic arthritis. J Clin Rheumatol. 2018;24(1):6–13. https://doi.org/10.1097/RHU.0000000000000583.
175. Wu D, Yue J, Tam LS. Efficacy and safety of biologics targeting interleukin-6, -12/23 and -17 pathways for peripheral psoriatic arthritis: a network meta-analysis. Rheumatology (Oxford). 2018;57(3):563–71. https://doi.org/10.1093/rheumatology/kex452
176. Antoni C, Krueger GG, de Vlam K, et al. Infliximab improves signs and symptoms of psoriatic arthritis: results of the IMPACT 2 trial. Ann Rheum Dis. 2005;64(8):1150–7. https://doi.org/10.1136/ard.2004.032268.
177. Mease PJ, Gladman DD, Samad AS, et al. Design and rationale of the

study of etanercept and methotrexate in combination or as monotherapy in subjects with psoriatic arthritis (SEAM-PsA). RMD Open. 2018;4(1):e000606. https://doi.org/10.1136/rmdopen-2017-000606.
178. Kristensen LE, Gülfe A, Saxne T, Geborek P. Efficacy and tolerability of anti-tumour necrosis factor therapy in psoriatic arthritis patients: results from the South Swedish Arthritis Treatment Group register. Ann Rheum Dis. 2008;67(3):364–9. https://doi.org/10.1136/ard.2007.073544.
179. Fagerli KM, Lie E, van der Heijde D, et al. The role of methotrexate co-medication in TNF-inhibitor treatment in patients with psoriatic arthritis: results from 440 patients included in the NOR-DMARD study. Ann Rheum Dis. 2014;73(1):132–7. https://doi.org/10.1136/annrheumdis-2012-202347.
180. Glintborg B, Østergaard M, Dreyer L, et al. Treatment response, drug survival, and predictors thereof in 764 patients with psoriatic arthritis treated with anti-tumor necrosis factor α therapy: results from the nationwide Danish DANBIO registry. Arthritis Rheum. 2011;63(2):382–90. https://doi.org/10.1002/art.30117.
181. Saad AA, Ashcroft DM, Watson KD, et al. Efficacy and safety of anti-TNF therapies in psoriatic arthritis: an observational study from the British Society for Rheumatology Biologics Register [published correction appears in Rheumatology (Oxford). 2017 Apr 1;56(4):672–673]. Rheumatology (Oxford). 2010;49(4):697–705. https://doi.org/10.1093/rheumatology/kep423
182. Mease PJ, Collier DH, Saunders KC, Li G, Kremer JM, Greenberg JD. Comparative effectiveness of biologic monotherapy versus combination therapy for patients with psoriatic arthritis: results from the Corrona registry. RMD Open. 2015;1(1):e000181. https://doi.org/10.1136/rmdopen-2015-000181.
183. Nash P, Kirkham B, Okada M, et al. Ixekizumab for the treatment of patients with active psoriatic arthritis and an inadequate response to tumour necrosis factor inhibitors: results from the 24-week randomised, double-blind, placebo-controlled period of the SPIRIT-P2 phase 3 trial. Lancet. 2017;389(10086):2317–27. https://doi.org/10.1016/S0140-6736(17)31429-0.
184. McInnes IB, Kavanaugh A, Gottlieb AB, et al. Efficacy and safety of ustekinumab in patients with active psoriatic arthritis: 1 year results of the phase 3, multicentre, double-blind, placebo-controlled PSUMMIT 1 trial. Lancet. 2013;382(9894):780–9. https://doi.org/10.1016/S0140-6736(13)60594-2.
185. Coates LC, Cawkwell LS, Ng NW, et al. Sustained response to long-term biologics and switching in psoriatic arthritis: results from real life experience. Ann Rheum Dis. 2008;67(5):717–9. https://doi.org/10.1136/ard.2007.082925.
186. Fagerli KM, Lie E, van der Heijde D, et al. Switching between TNF inhibitors in psoriatic arthritis: data from the NOR-DMARD study. Ann Rheum Dis. 2013;72(11):1840–4. https://doi.org/10.1136/annrheumdis-2012-203018.
187. Favalli EG, Becciolini A, Carletto A, et al. Efficacy and retention rate of adalimumab in rheumatoid arthritis and psoriatic arthritis patients after first-line etanercept failure: the FEARLESS cohort. Rheumatol Int. 2020;40(2):263–72. https://doi.org/10.1007/s00296-019-04416-3.
188. Kristensen LE, Lie E, Jacobsson LT, et al. Effectiveness and feasibility associated with switching to a second or third TNF inhibitor in patients with psoriatic arthritis: a cohort study from Southern Sweden. J Rheumatol. 2016;43(1):81–7. https://doi.org/10.3899/jrheum.150744.
189. Simard JF, Arkema EV, Sundström A, et al. Ten years with biologics: to whom do data on effectiveness and safety apply? Rheumatology (Oxford). 2011;50(1):204–13. https://doi.org/10.1093/rheumatology/keq326.
190. Haberhauer G, Strehblow C, Fasching P. Observational study of switching anti-TNF agents in ankylosing spondylitis and psoriatic arthritis versus rheumatoid arthritis. Wien Med Wochenschr. 2010;160(9–10):220–4. https://doi.org/10.1007/s10354-010-0795-0
191. Soubrier AS, Bele-Philippe P, Cortet B, et al. Treatment response, drug survival and safety of anti-tumour necrosis factor α therapy in 193 patients with psoriatic arthritis: a twelve-year "real life" experience. Joint Bone Spine. 2015;82(1):31–7. https://doi.org/10.1016/j.jbspin.2014.08.001.
192. Gomez-Reino JJ, Carmona L; BIOBADASER Group. Switching TNF antagonists in patients with chronic arthritis: an observational study of 488 patients over a four-year period. Arthritis Res Ther. 2006;8(1):R29. https://doi.org/10.1186/ar1881
193. Saad AA, Ashcroft DM, Watson KD, et al. Persistence with anti-tumour necrosis factor therapies in patients with psoriatic arthritis: observational study from the British Society of Rheumatology Biologics Register. Arthritis Res Ther. 2009;11(2):R52. https://doi.org/10.1186/ar2670.
194. Snast I, Atzmony L, Braun M, Hodak E, Pavlovsky L. Risk for hepatitis B and C virus reactivation in patients with psoriasis on biologic therapies: a retrospective cohort study and systematic review of the literature. J Am Acad Dermatol. 2017;77(1):88–97
195. Soare A, Gheorghiu AM, Aramă V, Bumbăcea D, Dobrotă R, Oneaţă R, Pintilie S, Milicescu M, Ancuţa I, Martin A, Sasu M, Ciofu C, Macovei L, Stoica V, Bojincă M, Mihai C. Risk of active tuberculosis in patients with inflammatory arthritis receiving TNF inhibitors: a look beyond the baseline tuberculosis screening protocol. Clin Rheumatol. 2018;37(9):2391–7. https://doi.org/10.1007/s10067-017-3916-y.
196. Fagerli KM, Kearsley-Fleet L, Mercer LK, Watson K, Packham J, Symmons DPM, Hyrich KL. Malignancy and mortality rates in patients with severe psoriatic arthritis requiring tumour-necrosis factor alpha inhibition: results from the British Society for Rheumatology Biologics Register. Rheumatology (Oxford). 2019;58(1):80–5. https://doi.org/10.1093/rheumatology/key241.
197. Michelsen B, Sexton J, Smolen JS, Aletaha D, Krogh NS, van der Heijde D, Kvien TK, Hetland ML. Can disease activity in patients with psoriatic arthritis be adequately assessed by a modified Disease Activity index for PSoriatic Arthritis (DAPSA) based on 28 joints? Ann Rheum Dis. 2018;77(12):1736–41. https://doi.org/10.1136/annrheumdis-2018-213463.
198. Coates LC, Fransen J, Helliwell PS. Defining minimal disease activity in psoriatic arthritis: a proposed objective target for treatment. Ann Rheum Dis. 2010;69(1):48–53. https://doi.org/10.1136/ard.2008.102053.
199. Popescu C, Trandafir M, Badica A, Morar F, Predeteanu D. Ankylosing spondylitis functional and activity indices in clinical practice. J Med Life. 2014;7(1):78–83.
200. Zochling J. Measures of symptoms and disease status in ankylosing spondylitis: ankylosing Spondylitis Disease Activity Score (ASDAS), Ankylosing Spondylitis Quality of Life Scale (ASQoL), Bath Ankylosing Spondylitis Disease Activity Index (BASDAI), Bath Ankylosing Spondylitis Functional Index (BASFI), Bath Ankylosing Spondylitis Global Score (BAS-G), Bath Ankylosing Spondylitis Metrology Index (BASMI), Dougados Functional Index (DFI), and Health Assessment Questionnaire for the Spondylarthropathies (HAQ-S). Arthritis Care Res (Hoboken). 2011;63(Suppl 11):S47-58. https://doi.org/10.1002/acr.20575.
201. Machado PM, Landewé R, Heijde DV. Assessment of SpondyloArthritis international Society (ASAS). Ankylosing Spondylitis Disease Activity Score (ASDAS): 2018 update of the nomenclature for disease activity states. Ann Rheum Dis. 2018;77(10):1539–1540. doi: https://doi.org/10.1136/annrheumdis-2018-213184

5

Correlation and agreement between physical and ultrasound examination after a training session dedicated to the standardization of synovitis assessment in rheumatoid arthritis patients

Gerardo Quintana-López[1,2,3*], Kevin Maldonado-Cañón[1], Jorge Bruce Flórez-Suárez[1], Paul Méndez-Patarroyo[1,3], Paola Coral-Alvarado[1,3] and Enrique Calvo[4]

Abstract

Objectives: Assessing disease activity in rheumatoid arthritis (RA) patients requires comprehensive quantification of tender and swollen joints. We aimed to evaluate the correlation and agreement between rheumatologists after a training session dedicated to the standardization of synovitis assessment and compare its performance with a reference imaging modality such as musculoskeletal ultrasonography (MSUS).

Methods: In this cross-sectional study, a total of 28 and 10 joints in RA patients were evaluated by physical examination and ultrasound (US), respectively. After participating in a training session, individual joint assessment for tenderness and swelling was performed by three rheumatologists. MSUS examination was performed separately by an experimented radiologist in a standardized manner, evaluating findings according to the Outcome Measures in Rheumatology Clinical Trial (OMERACT) guidelines.

Results: A total of 80 RA patients were included, with a mean Disease Activity Score based on 28 joints (DAS28)-ESR of 4.02. The interobserver overall agreement and concordance rate in a total of 2240 joints assessed was 81.7% (k = 0.449, $p < 0.0001$) for tender joints and 66% (k = 0.227, $p < 0.0001$) for swollen joints. The overall concordance rate was fair (Fleiss' kappa = 0.21, $p = 0.027$) with an overall agreement of 67.18% yet, more joints were found to be swollen by the US assessment, compared to the physical examination (43% vs 39%).

Conclusion: In our study population, joint tenderness showed better interobserver agreement, correlation, and concordance rate than joint swelling. When comparing the US assessment to the physical examination, a fair overall concordance rate supports the need for the implementation of training sessions dedicated to standardization in rheumatology clinics.

Keywords: Physical examination, Rheumatoid arthritis, Synovitis, Ultrasonography

Introduction

Rheumatoid arthritis (RA) is a chronic systemic autoimmune disease characterized by hyperplasia and inflammation of synovial tissue with subsequent bone erosion and loss of joint space with a noteworthy

*Correspondence: gquintanal@unal.edu.co

[1] Reumavance Group, Rheumatology Section, Department of Internal Medicine, Fundación Santa Fe de Bogotá University Hospital, Carrera 7 No. 117-15, 110111 Bogota, Colombia

association on functionality and quality of life [1]. In order to assess disease activity in RA patients, there is not an individual parameter to be used. It is thus necessary to achieve a comprehensive approach through the use of several individual clinical and or laboratory parameters and to develop quantitative indexes to be used in daily clinical practice by rheumatology health professionals [2–4].

Among the most commonly used methods, the Disease Activity Score (DAS), and its modified version, DAS28, are based on a tender and swollen joint count, combined with other parameters such as a patient global health assessment [4, 5]. Joint tenderness assessments estimate the patient's response to potentially painful stimulation. On the other hand, joint swelling assessment measures synovial inflammation or effusion recognized by fluid displacement. The examination technique should include exerting continuous and direct pressure on an affected joint with the thumb and index fingers until the examiner's nail bed turns pale; this compares with a pressure of approximately 4 kg/cm^2 [6, 7].

Although tender and swollen joint counts are considered fundamental parameters to estimate disease activity, its assessment is not as straightforward as assumed, thus exhibiting certain potential disadvantages. Amongst the prevailing concerns are poor reproducibility and substantial interobserver variability [6, 8]. One of the reasonable explanations could be the training and clinical experience gap among practitioners; therefore, finding a feasible solution through standardization.

Historically, training sessions focused on standardization of all DAS28 parameters assessment have been proposed, and once applied, have shown to provoke a substantial reduction regarding the variation between examiners [6–8]. The entire medical and nursing staff who will be assessing RA patients should be trained regularly (at least once every year) and should be trained together, allowing discussion about current standard procedures. There has been proposed as well the use of ultrasonography to demonstrate active synovitis in case of disagreement [6].

Prognostic factors, treatment decisions, monitoring, and complications are defined based on disease activity, thus consequently on a reliable tender and swollen joint count for each RA patient [9]. The aim of this study was to evaluate the correlation and agreement between rheumatologists after a training session dedicated to the standardization of synovitis assessment and compare its performance with a reference imaging modality such as musculoskeletal ultrasonography (MSUS).

Materials and methods

Patients

Patients were recruited from an outpatient clinic based in the Rheumatology Department at Fundación Santa Fe de Bogotá University Hospital, Colombia. Stratified random sampling was conducted, selecting patients with different disease activity states (according to the most recent clinical record) from a previously established ongoing cohort of 820 patients. The sample size was calculated for the desired correlation coefficient of 0.6, a population correlation coefficient of 0.8, a power of 0.8, and a confidence interval of 0.95. All those who were invited to participate fulfilled the 2010 ACR/European League Against Rheumatism (EULAR) classification criteria [10] and were at least 18 years old. Those who had a history of trauma, septic arthritis, joint replacement or synovectomy, joint deformity, and or crystal arthropathy were excluded.

The following data were registered at baseline: age, gender, treatment, erythrocyte sedimentation rate (ESR), C-reactive protein (CRP), rheumatoid factor (RF), global health assessed by the patient (GH), Clinical Disease Activity Index (CDAI), and Simplified Disease Activity Index (SDAI).

Training session dedicated to standardization

Our planned training session was structured to focus on standardization of the tenderness and swelling assessment of 28 joints (bilateral shoulders, elbows, wrists, knees, metacarpophalangeal (MCP), and interphalangeal (PIP)).

Three rheumatologists, with 10, 13, and 15 years of experience in clinical examination of RA patients, attended three sessions (separated by 1–2 weeks). Each session was divided into three steps: (1) individual joint assessment was performed by each rheumatologist (blinded to both clinical and other rheumatologist's data), (2) 20-min discussion on practice observations, difficulties, limitations, and facilitating factors during the physical examination, in order to reach agreement on uniform criteria and technique, and (3) joint individual reassessment based on the unified criteria. On the third session, disease activity indexes (DAS28-ESR, SDAI, and CDAI) were calculated individually by each rheumatologist.

Ultrasound assessment

Twenty minutes after the last training session's third step, each patient was instructed to proceed to the ultrasound (US) assessment room. The US examination was performed by a radiologist with 15 years of experience and training in musculoskeletal radiology (blinded to physical examinations' data) on 10 joints (bilateral wrists, and 2nd to 5th MCPs), using a GE (General Electric) LOGICQ E ultrasound machine with a 6–13 Hz multifrequency linear transducer. Findings were systematically graded according to the Outcome Measures in Rheumatology Clinical Trial (OMERACT) guidelines, evaluating synovitis as synovial hypertrophy defined by an abnormal nondisplaceable and poorly compressible hypoechoic intraarticular tissue [11]. PIPs joins were considered as potential confounders due to the eventual overlapping of tenosynovitis, therefore were not assessed.

Synovitis grading was conducted based on a scoring method initially introduced by Szkudlarek et al., widely used for studies of this kind [12–14] and currently supported by the EULAR-OMERACT ultrasound taskforce [15, 16] (0 = absence of synovial thickening, 1 (mild) = minimal synovial thickening, filling the angle between the periarticular bones, without bulging over the line linking tops of the corresponding bones, 2 (moderate) = synovial thickening bulging over the line linking tops of the periarticular bones but without extension along the bone diaphysis, 3 (severe) = severe synovial thickening bulging over the line linking tops of the periarticular bones and with extension to at least one bone diaphysis). Normal distances between bone and joint capsule were acknowledged based on average population values proposed by Schmidt et al. [17].

Table 1 Clinical and demographic characteristics for all patients

Characteristics	Values (n = 80)
Age, years	55.3 (8.6)
Female, n (%)	68 (85)
Disease duration (years)	11.56 (7.93)
Positive RF, n (%)	71 (88)
ESR (mm/h)	19.32 (5.6)
CRP (mg/dL)	5.6 (12)
DAS28-ESR	4.02 (1.12)
SDAI	24.4 (8.59)
CDAI	18.7 (9.01)
Number of DMARDs	
1, n (%)	15 (18%)
≥ 2, n (%)	58 (72%)
bDMARD use, n (%)	16 (20)
Oral glucocorticoid use, n (%)	27 (33)
TJC-28, median	9
SJC-28, median	5

Values are the mean (SD) unless otherwise indicated

RF, rheumatoid factor; ESR, erythrocyte sedimentation rate; CRP, C-reactive protein; DAS28-ESR, Disease Activity Score based on 28 joint count and ESR; SDAI, Simplified Disease Activity Index; CDAI, Clinical Disease Activity Index; DMARDs, disease-modified anti-rheumatic drug; bDMARD, biological disease-modified anti-rheumatic drug; TJC, tender joint count; SJC, swollen joint count

Statistical analysis

Statistical analysis was performed using STATA software, version 15.0. Descriptive analysis was presented for continuous variables with central tendency measures as mean and standard deviation (SD) or as the median and interquartile range (IQR) for normally or nonnormally distributed data, respectively. For dichotomous variables, data were presented with percentages and absolute values.

Interobserver agreement and concordance were calculated through Cohen's kappa (between two observers considering all the possible pairs, i.e., Observer A vs B, observer A vs C, observer B vs C), Fleiss' kappa (between the three observers), and percentage of an overall agreement (percentage of observed exact agreements). The relative strength of agreement was described according to the following ranges of kappa (k) coefficients: < 0.00 = poor, 0.00–0.20 = slight, 0.21–0.40 = fair, 0.41–0.60 = moderate, 0.61–0.80 = substantial, and 0.81–1.00 = almost perfect [18]. Linear correlation coefficients (Pearson correlation coefficient) were also calculated for tender and swollen joint counts.

Results

Patient characteristics

The demographic and clinical characteristics of the 80 selected patients are illustrated in Table 1. The majority of them were women (85%), mean age was 55.3 years, with 71 (88%) being seropositive for RF. The mean (± SD) DAS28-ESR, SDAI, and CDAI were 4.02 ± 1.12 (moderate activity), 24.4 ± 8.59, and 18.7 ± 9.01, respectively. All our patients received disease-modifying antirheumatic drugs (DMARDs) treatment, corresponding to mono, ≥ 2 DMARD, and biological (b) DMARD therapy in 18%, 72%, and 20% of cases. Twenty-seven (33%) patients were receiving oral glucocorticoid therapy (daily dose of 5–10 mg (prednisone equivalent)).

Interobserver correlation and agreement

A total of 2240 joints (i.e., 28 joints in 80 patients) were evaluated through physical examination. Compared with tenderness, swelling assessment showed a slight strength of agreement with lower percentage of overall agreement and concordance rates (66% and Fleiss kappa = 0.227; 95% CI 0.203–0.250, $p < 0.0001$ vs 81.7% and Fleiss kappa = 0.449; 95% CI 0.403–0.493, $p < 0.0001$) (see Table 2).

The linear correlation coefficient (Spearman's correlation coefficient) was calculated, taking all the possible pairs (observer A–B, observer A–C, observer B–C), thus having an overall correlation coefficient of 0.81 and 0.431 for swollen and tender joints, respectively.

Table 2 Interobserver agreement and concordance for physical examination (PE) tenderness and swelling assessment

Joint	Inter-observer agreement and concordance							
	PE tenderness assessment				PE swelling assessment			
	Fleiss kappa	95% CI	*p* value	Count	Fleiss kappa	95% CI	*p* value	Count
Right shoulder	0.521	0.494–0.652	< 0.0001	83	0.249	0.124–0.322	0.0001	27
Left shoulder	0.446	0.198–0.546	< 0.0001	64	0.134	0.092–0.184	0.018	23
Right elbow	0.4	0.308–0.537	< 0.0001	71	0.146	0.092–0.287	0.012	69
Left elbow	0.403	0.258–0.446	< 0.0001	64	0.245	0.166–0.392	0.0001	79
Right wrist	0.392	0.263–0.548	< 0.0001	78	0.121	0.007–0.168	0.030	123
Left wrist	0.325	0.261–0.419	< 0.0001	72	0.042	− 0.192 to 0.234	0.259	145
Right MCP1	0.394	0.326–0.551	< 0.0001	50	− 0.166	− 0.178 to 0.151	0.995	134
Right MCP2	0.298	0.225–0.362	< 0.0001	53	0.13	0.109–0.140	0.023	158
Right MCP3	0.282	0.153–0.323	< 0.0001	49	0.218	0.070–0.292	0.0004	109
Right MCP4	0.297	0.235–0.379	< 0.0001	33	0.397	0.376–0.476	< 0.0001	53
Right MCP5	0.379	0.236–0.477	< 0.0001	36	0.306	0.272–0.387	< 0.0001	63
Left MCP1	0.304	0.187–0.394	< 0.0001	44	0.094	0.024–0.148	0.073	95
Left MCP2	0.444	0.391–0.619	< 0.0001	36	0.262	0.133–0.314	< 0.0001	110
Left MCP3	0.382	0.323–0.453	< 0.0001	41	0.27	0.268–0.334	< 0.0001	69
Left MCP4	0.315	0.086–0.375	< 0.0001	32	0.177	0.059–0.232	0.003	45
Left MCP5	0.353	0.183–0.569	< 0.0001	26	0.217	0.172–0.266	0.0004	71
Right PIP1	0.299	0.050–0.367	< 0.0001	22	0.128	0.087–0.227	0.023	53
Right PIP2	0.353	0.310–0.379	< 0.0001	28	0.042	0.015–0.094	0.258	95
Right PIP3	0.351	0.312–0.486	< 0.0001	30	− 0.017	− 0.102 to 0.113	0.603	118
Right PIP4	0.232	0.111–0.250	< 0.0001	28	0.074	0.037–0.117	0.126	82
Right PIP5	0.396	0.294–0.431	< 0.0001	26	0.245	0.091–0.318	0.244	48
Left PIP1	0.165	0.018–0.304	< 0.0001	21	0.02	− 0.203 to 0.242	0.376	39
Left PIP2	0.167	0.085–0.299	< 0.0001	24	− 0.061	− 0.236 to 0.2	0.827	50
Left PIP3	0.298	0.196–0.368	< 0.0001	35	0.077	− 0.071 to 0.219	0.116	101
Left PIP4	0.185	0.018–0.267	< 0.0001	31	0.121	0.056–0.197	0.030	74
Left PIP5	0.339	0.270–0.573	< 0.0001	18	0.113	0.041–0.267	0.040	46
Right knee	0.476	0.318–0.530	< 0.0001	48	0.428	0.295–0.525	< 0.0001	58
Left knee	0.379	0.350–0.471	< 0.0001	57	0.214	0.038–0.362	0.0005	62
Overall agreement (%)	0.449 (81.7%)	0.403–0.493	< 0.0001		0.227 (66%)	0.203–0.250	< 0.0001	

MCP, metacarpophalangeal; PIP, proximal interphalangeal

Agreement and concordance between physical and US examination

What is interesting in Table 3 is that, from the then joints assessed by both methods, there has been a slight relative increase in the number of swollen joints through US examination (345 of 800 joints assessed by US (43%)), when compared to physical examination (946 of 2400 joints assessed by our three rheumatologist (39%)). Concordance strength of agreement was fair and ranged from Fleiss kappa 0.168–0.264. Likewise, the k coefficients between physical and US examination in the left MCP5 joint (k = 0.168, *p* 0.06) followed by left MCP4 (k = 0.177, *p* 0.053) joint stand out as the lowest values. By contrast, k coefficient in wrist was slightly higher (k = 0.241 (*p* 0.007) and k = 0.213 (*p* 0.023)). The percentage of overall agreement and

Table 3 Agreement and concordance between physical and US examination swelling assessment

Joint	Overall agreement (%)	Fleiss kappa	*p* value
Right wrist	62.5	0.241	0.007
Left wrist	63.7	0.213	0.022
Right MCP 2	60.0	0.195	0.040
Right MCP 3	66.2	0.264	0.009
Right MCP 4	69.6	0.197	0.039
Right MCP 5	70.9	0.244	0.014
Left MCP 2	62.5	0.244	0.011
Left MCP 3	67.5	0.228	0.019
Left MCP 4	77.5	0.177	0.053
Left MCP 5	71.2	0.168	0.06

MCP, metacarpophalangeal; PIP, proximal interphalangeal

concordance rate was 67.18% and k = 0.210; (p 0.027), respectively.

Discussion

As explained in the introduction, it is clear that training sessions focused on the standardization of joint assessment techniques play a pivotal role in understanding the reliability of quantitative indexes daily used in RA patients. We aimed to evaluate the correlation and agreement between rheumatologists after such a training session and compare its performance with a reference imaging modality, namely, MSUS, to find a reasonable approach on behalf of the inevitable high intra- and inter-observer variability described in the literature.

Contrary to expectations, despite the fact that all three participating rheumatologists attended the proposed training sessions, interobserver variability among them was still present. The wide range of perceived concordance rates suggests that the assessment of some individual joints may be particularly challenging on their own, thereby showing specific difficulties during standardization, with possible attribution to an underlying long and comprehensive learning process.

In terms of overall interobserver agreement and concordance rates, as well as of overall correlation, our findings propose that tenderness assessment was more homogenous than swelling assessment. A possible explanation for these results may be the fact that joint tenderness is inferred solely by the patient's response, while that of joint swelling by physicians' technique and interpretation of findings.

The importance of training sessions focused on standardization was first stated by Scott et al. in 1996 [19], whose findings suggested a considerably increased sensitivity of measurement for both tender and swollen joints and a reduction in the mean coefficient of variation for the number of swollen joints (82% vs 59%) after a 60-min training session based on the EULAR handbook for joint evaluation. Unlike Scott et al., on a multicentric cohort study evaluating standardization based on the aforementioned EULAR handbook, Grunke et al. [20] stated that even when consistency and variability significantly improved, the mean number of tender, as well as swollen joints decreased. Nonetheless, a reference imaging modality was not used.

In addition, clinical experience plays an essential part as recently proposed by El-Hadidi et al. [21] where after a consensus on joint assessment, the interobserver agreement was calculated to compare an experienced rheumatology professor (30 years of experience) with a young Rheumatology fellow (3 years of training). Although a high correlation between professor and candidate was described, specific results on joint assessment correlation are similar to ours, showing a more robust correlation regarding tender joints compared to that of swollen joints.

When compared to MUSC, as previously stated, agreement and concordance were slightly lower for swelling assessment. This discrepancy could be attributed to the mean age of our patients (55 years); it seems possible that the older the patient, the more frequent synovial thickening and incipient joint deformities, thus being confounding for not only MSUS but also for PE assessment. Moreover, it is important to consider what has been widely held by recent reports, that is, the trend towards higher agreement and concordance rates regarding swollen joints count [22, 23]. These data must be interpreted with caution because of the use of the OMERACT synovitis definition and its implications of considering even a minimal amount of intraarticular tissue as an abnormal finding of synovial hypertrophy, thereby involving a potential overestimation.

It could be argued that the average age and the duration and activity of the disease could contribute to the differences between physical examination and US; nevertheless, those patients with joint deformity were excluded. It is relevant to bear in mind that, in those populations with a poorly controlled- and a longer- disease, joint assessment either by physical examination or by ultrasound remains a challenge when considering joint surface irregularities. It supports the pivotal role of conventional radiography as the first choice for the evaluation of structural changes such as erosions.

The limitations of this study include firstly the absence of power Doppler ultrasonographic assessment due to timing issues on behalf of the vast number of evaluated joints; prior studies have noted the role of power Doppler US in detecting subclinical and residual synovitis when assessing synovial vascularity, although, it was beyond the scope of our work to evaluate such conditions. Secondly, we did not count on another radiologist with sufficient experience in MSUS to be considered as a second evaluator; additionally, the US evaluation performed by a radiologist and not an articular US rheumatologist might be considered as a source of uncertainty; nonetheless, the vast experience, as well as the specific MSUS training of our radiologist, support the internal validity of the assessments. Very little was found in the literature on the question of performance differences between those scenarios (radiologist vs. rheumatologist), remaining as an intriguing issue for future research, especially for low and middle-income countries where training for such medical sub-specialties is not as frequent.

Thirdly, the absence of early RA patients, as well as of patients in clinical remission, and finally, that we did not report pretraining session joint count results in order to propose a variability improvement. The latter consideration must be handled with care when considering that this decision was based on the fact that pretraining session correlation and agreement scores were certainly variable, close to the null value, and even negative. Taking this into consideration, the gain of the stated training session was to revert such tendency and yet turn it to positive values, even though the kappa coefficients were in the range of slight to moderate. It is worth mentioning that when adding more than two observers to the calculations, the slightest discrepancy substantially lowers the statistical estimator; thus, an adjusted threshold must be taken when interpreting such results. Finally, a reasonable approach could be to hypothesize that the increase in the total swollen joint count through US examination would have a substantial implication in the categorization of the activity of the disease; nevertheless, even when it was beyond our scope, we trust that future research on this behalf will rise as a natural progression of this work.

Conclusions

Taken together, our findings indicate that joint tenderness assessment had a better interobserver agreement and concordance rate, moreover a higher overall correlation coefficient than joint swelling. The evidence from our results suggests a fair overall concordance rate when comparing the US examination to the physical examination, thus supporting the need for the implementation of training sessions dedicated to standardization in rheumatology clinics to guarantee reliability in identifying tender and swollen joints within rheumatologists.

Acknowledgements

Not applicable.

Authors' contributions

GQ-L: Conceptualization, methodology, formal analysis, investigation, writing-original draft preparation, writing-review and editing. KM-C: Writing-original draft preparation, writing-review and editing. JBF-S: writing-original draft preparation, writing-review and editing. PM-P: Conceptualization, methodology, investigation. PC-A: Conceptualization, methodology, investigation. EC: Investigation. All authors read and approved the final manuscript.

Author details

[1]Reumavance Group, Rheumatology Section, Department of Internal Medicine, Fundación Santa Fe de Bogotá University Hospital, Carrera 7 No. 117-15, 110111 Bogota, Colombia. [2]Department of Internal Medicine, School of Medicine, Universidad Nacional de Colombia, Bogota, Colombia. [3]Department of Internal Medicine, School of Medicine, Universidad de Los Andes, Bogota, Colombia. [4]Department of Radiology, School of Medicine, Universidad Nacional de Colombia, Bogota, Colombia.

References

1. McInnes IB, Schett G. The pathogenesis of rheumatoid arthritis. N Engl J Med. 2011;365:2205–19.
2. Backhaus M, Kamradt T, Sandrock D, Loreck D, Fritz J, Wolf KJ, et al. Arthritis of the finger joints: a comprehensive approach comparing conventional radiography, scintigraphy, ultrasound, and contrast-enhanced magnetic resonance imaging. Arthritis Rheum. 1999;42:1232–45.
3. Naredo E, Bonilla G, Gamero F, Uson J, Carmona L, Laffon A. Assessment of inflammatory activity in rheumatoid arthritis: a comparative study of clinical evaluation with grey scale and power Doppler ultrasonography. Ann Rheum Dis. 2005;64:375–81.
4. Van der Heijde D, Van't Hof M, Van Riel P, et al. Development of a disease activity score based on judgment in clinical practice by rheumatologists. J Rheumatol. 1993;20:579–81.
5. Prevoo MLL, Van't Hof MA, Kuper HH, et al. Modified disease activity scores that include twenty-eight-joint counts. Development and validation in a prospective longitudinal study of patients with rheumatoid arthritis. Arthritis Rheum. 1995;38(1):44–8.
6. Porter D, Gadsby K, Thompson P, White J, McClinton C, Oliver S. DAS28 and rheumatoid arthritis: the need for standardization. Musculoskelet Care. 2011;9(4):222–7.
7. Scott IC, Scott DL. Joint counts in inflammatory arthritis. Clin Exp Rheumatol. 2014;32(Suppl. 85):S7–12.
8. Sokka T, Pincus T. Joint counts to assess rheumatoid arthritis for clinical research and usual clinical care: advantages and limitations. Rheum Dis Clin N Am. 2009;35(4):713–22.
9. Smolen JS, Landewé RBM, Bijlsma JWJ, et al. EULAR recommendations for the management of rheumatoid arthritis with synthetic and biological disease-modifying antirheumatic drugs: 2019 update. Ann Rheumatic Dis. 2020;79:685–99.
10. Aletaha D, Neogi T, Silman AJ, Funovits J, Felson DT, Bingham CO, et al. 2010 Rheumatoid arthritis classification criteria: an American College of Rheumatology-European League Against Rheumatism collaborative initiative. Ann Rheum Dis. 2010;69:1580–8.
11. Wakefield RJ, Balint PV, Szkudlarek M, Filippucci E, Backhaus M, D'Agostino MA, et al. OMERACT 7 special interest group. Musculoskeletal ultrasound including definitions for ultrasonography pathology. J Rheumatol. 2005;32:2485–7.
12. Szkudlarek M, Wakefield R, Backhaus M, Terslev L. The discriminatory capacity of ultrasound in rheumatoid arthritis: active vs inactive, early vs advanced, and more. Rheumatology. 2012;51(suppl 7):vii6–9.
13. Wakefield RJ, Green MJ, Marzo-Ortega H, Conaghan PG, Gibbon WW, McGonagle D, et al. Should oligoarthritis be reclassified? Ultrasound reveals a high prevalence of subclinical disease. Ann Rheum Dis. 2004;63:382–5.
14. Szkudlarek M, Court-Payen M, Jacobsen S, Klarlund M, Thomsen H, Østergaard M. Interobserver agreement in ultrasonography of the finger and toe joints in rheumatoid arthritis. Arthritis Rheum. 2003;48(4):955–62.
15. Bruyn GA, Iagnocco A, Naredo E, Balint PV, Gutierrez M, Hammer HB, et al. OMERACT definitions for ultrasonographic pathologies and elementary lesions of rheumatic disorders 15 years on. J Rheumatol. 2019;46(10):1388–93. https://doi.org/10.3899/jrheum.181095.
16. Terslev L, Naredo E, Aegerter P, et al. Scoring ultrasound synovitis in rheumatoid arthritis: a EULAR-OMERACT ultrasound taskforce-Part 2: reliability and application to multiple joints of a standardised consensus-based scoring system. RMD Open. 2017;3:e000427. https://doi.org/10.1136/rmdopen-2016-000427.
17. Schmidt WA, Schmidt H, Schicke B, Gromnica-Ihle E. Standard reference values for musculoskeletal ultrasonography. Ann Rheum Dis. 2004;63:988–94.
18. Landis JR, Koch GG. The measurement of observer agreement for categorical data. Biometrics. 1977;33:159–74.
19. Scott DL, Choy EHS, Greeves A, Isenberg DM, Kassinor D, Rankin E, et al. Standardizing joint assessment in rheumatoid arthritis. Clin Rheumatol. 1996;15(6):579–82.
20. Grunke M, Antoni C, Kavanaugh A, Hildebrand V, Dechant C, Schett G, et al. Standardization of joint examination technique leads to a significant decrease in variability among different examiners. J Rheumatol. 2010;37(4):860–4.
21. El-Hadidi K, Gamal S, Saad S. Inter-observer agreement of standard joint count examination and disease global assessment in a cohort of Egyptian Rheumatoid Arthritis patients. Reumatol Clín. 2019;15(5):258–63.

22. Hirata A, Ogura T, Hayashi N, Takenaka S, Ito H, Mizushina K, et al. Concordance of patient-reported joint symptoms, physician-examined arthritic signs, and ultrasound-detected synovitis in rheumatoid arthritis. Arthritis Care Res. 2017;69(6):801–6.
23. Salaffi F, Filippucci E, Carotti M, Naredo E, Meenagh G, Ciapetti A, et al. Inter-observer agreement of standard joint counts in early rheumatoid arthritis: a comparison with grey scale ultrasonography: a preliminary study. Rheumatology. 2008;47:54–8.

6

Cardiovascular risk assessment using ASCVD risk score in fibromyalgia: A single-centre, retrospective study using "traditional" case control methodology and "novel" machine learning

Sandeep Surendran[1], C. B. Mithun[1], Merlin Moni[2], Arun Tiwari[1] and Manu Pradeep[3*]

Abstract

Background: In autoimmune inflammatory rheumatological diseases, routine cardiovascular risk assessment is becoming more important. As an increased cardiovascular disease (CVD) risk is recognized in patients with fibromyalgia (FM), a combination of traditional CVD risk assessment tool with Machine Learning (ML) predictive model could help to identify non-traditional CVD risk factors.

Methods: This study was a retrospective case–control study conducted at a quaternary care center in India. Female patients diagnosed with FM as per 2016 modified American College of Rheumatology 2010/2011 diagnostic criteria were enrolled; healthy age and gender-matched controls were obtained from Non-communicable disease Initiatives and Research at AMrita (NIRAM) study database. Firstly, FM cases and healthy controls were age-stratified into three categories of 18–39 years, 40–59 years, and ≥ 60 years. A 10 year and lifetime CVD risk was calculated in both cases and controls using the ASCVD calculator. Pearson chi-square test and Fisher's exact were used to compare the ASCVD risk scores of FM patients and controls across the age categories. Secondly, ML predictive models of CVD risk in FM patients were developed. A random forest algorithm was used to develop the predictive models with ASCVD 10 years and lifetime risk as target measures. Model predictive accuracy of the ML models was assessed by accuracy, f1-score, and Area Under 'receiver operating Curve' (AUC). From the final predictive models, we assessed risk factors that had the highest weightage for CVD risk in FM.

Results: A total of 139 FM cases and 1820 controls were enrolled in the study. FM patients in the age group 40–59 years had increased lifetime CVD risk compared to the control group ($OR = 1.56, p = 0.043$). However, CVD risk was not associated with FM disease severity and disease duration as per the conventional statistical analysis. ML model for 10-year ASCVD risk had an accuracy of 95% with an f1-score of 0.67 and AUC of 0.825. ML model for the lifetime ASCVD risk had an accuracy of 72% with an f1-score of 0.79 and AUC of 0.713. In addition to the traditional risk factors for CVD, FM disease severity parameters were important contributors in the ML predictive models.

*Correspondence: drmanupradeep24@gmail.com
[3] Department of Pharmacology, Amrita Institute of Medical Sciences, Amrita Vishwa Vidyapeetham, Kochi, Kerala, India

Conclusion: FM patients of the 40–59 years age group had increased lifetime CVD risk in our study. Although FM disease severity was not associated with high CVD risk as per the conventional statistical analysis of the data, it was among the highest contributor to ML predictive model for CVD risk in FM patients. This also highlights that ML can potentially help to bridge the gap of non-linear risk factor identification.

Keywords: Fibromyalgia, Heart disease risk factors, Machine learning, Cardiovascular diseases

Introduction

Fibromyalgia (FM) is a debilitating condition that presents with generalized widespread pain and is often associated with sleep disturbances, fatigue, and cognitive dysfunction [1]. The prevalence rates of FM range from 1 to 3% in the general population [2].

While there is no singular pathological process that explains the development of FM; three key mechanisms include increased central nervous system response to peripheral pain stimulation via amplification of signalling, abnormal ascending pain pathways, and small fiber neuropathy [3, 4]. It is well known that other diseases with altered neuronal pathways like depression are more likely to develop cardiovascular disease (CVD). Major depression is more prevalent in people who have suffered an acute myocardial infarction, with up to 18–20% of patients meeting the criteria for depression patients using structured interviews [5]. However, this is not just a cause-effect relationship where the occurrence of a major cardiac event leads to the secondary development of depression. Patients with depression are more likely to have a cardiac event across the world. A cohort study in the South-Asian cohort population had reported that patients with depression were at an increased risk for developing CVD by 41% for men and 48% for women [6]. Western populations also showed similar results where a combination of depressive symptoms and stress in low-income persons was associated with an increased risk of incident CVD [7].

While depression and CVD are well studied, the interrelationship between FM and CVD is less described in the literature. A causal association is lent weight to by findings that FM is associated with dysfunction of the autonomic nervous system and the inflammatory system; both of which play a part in the pathophysiology of CVD [8].

A meta-analysis of the key studies on cytokines in FM has shown elevated interleukin-6 (IL-6) levels in FM patients, which is similar to a state of chronic mild inflammation [9]. IL-6 has a downstream knockdown effect on lipid metabolism and anti-inflammatory therapy with canakinumab (human anti-IL-1β monoclonal antibody) has been studied in a randomized controlled trial for CVD prevention [10, 11]. Thus, it is also possible that the neuro-immunological changes linked with FM may itself be a risk factor for CVD. CVD risk assessment in a Taiwanese cohort has shown findings that are suggestive of the same [12]. To the best of our knowledge, regional data regarding this is lacking from India.

Non-invasive CVD risk assessment tools are well described and validated in many cohorts. The most recent of these scales put forward by the American Heart Association (AHA) and American College of Cardiology is the Atherosclerotic Cardiovascular (ASCVD) risk assessment tool. Unlike the more traditionally used Framingham Risk Score, the ASCVD risk score can be applied to other races also and predicts both the 10-year and lifetime ASCVD risk of an individual [13]. This tool—ASCVD risk calculator, helps to predict future risk of CVD and is in fact, currently recommended to be used as a guide in the initiation of statin therapy [13]. As there is a paucity of studies assessing CVD risk in FM patients, this study has also adopted this tool to quantify the CVD risk.

As FM is a disease that is more common in females, an increased CVD risk in the affected females would be a relevant observation [14]. The identification of any elevated CVD risk as compared to the general population would help in stratifying such patients for interventions and primary prevention strategies.

Machine learning (ML) is the process by which the large computing capacity of modern computers is applied to analyse the varied statistical relations within a data set for an outcome prediction [15]. In the recent years, many studies have shown ability of ML to predict accurate predictions in medicine [16].

There are two main techniques of machine learning. The first is "supervised" learning when the goal is predicting a known output or target using classified/sorted data. The other type is called unsupervised learning where there are no outputs to predict; rather the aim is to find naturally occurring patterns or groupings within the unsorted data using massive statistical computing power. Both types have found applications in medicine with supervised machine learning methods being the more commonly used currently. This is largely because it is easier to create datasets that allow communication between researching physicians and data analysts. One of the best-known ML projects launched by the Microsoft

Corporation (USA) is Project Hanover which uses supervised ML and aims to help in drug research in oncology [17].

Machine learning (ML) tools are increasingly used to understand the complex interplay of the various factors associated with diseases. Recently ML tools were used to develop an algorithm to aid diagnosis of systemic lupus erythematosus by Adamichou et al. [18].

The primary objective of our study was to assess the CVD risk in female FM patients using the ASCVD risk score calculator and compare it with that of the general population.

A secondary objective of our study was to develop a supervised machine learning (ML) algorithm for studying the interactions between characteristics of the FM patients and ASCVD risk categories.

Methods

Study design (Fig. 1)

This was a retrospective case–control study done in a setting of Rheumatology outpatient department (OPD) of a quaternary care center in the southern Indian state of Kerala. Electronic medical records of FM patients were accessed after the study was approved by the institutional ethics committee.

We included the female FM patients diagnosed as per 2016 modified 2010/2011 ACR criteria, who had documented parameters needed for risk score calculation with ASCVD risk calculator (done within 6 months of diagnosis), baseline average pain score on a visual analog scale more than 5, and visited rheumatology OPD from April 2017 to April 2020 [1]. We excluded those FM patients who had any associated autoimmune disease, primary psychiatric diagnosis, breastfeeding, and patients taking any concomitant medications which could affect the fasting lipid profile.

Healthy control participants data was obtained after age and gender matching from the datasets of a population-based cross-sectional study conducted at the same quaternary center by Menon et al.- Non-communicable disease Initiatives and Research at AMrita (NIRAM) study [19].

The ASCVD risk score was calculated in both FM patients and controls, The details collected for ASCVD risk score calculation included age (in years), height (in meters), weight (in kilograms), and co-morbid conditions like hypertension, diabetes mellitus, and dyslipidemia. The FM disease severity was assessed using Fibromyalgia Impact Questionnaire-Revised (FIQR), the average pain score on the Brief Pain Inventory (BPI) form. Patients with a FIQR score of more than 60 at baseline were considered to have severe disease. The fasting lipid profile was measured using AU2700 plus Beckman Coulter (USA).

Based on the age, the study participants were categorized into three age group strata of 18–39 years, 40–59 years, and 60 years or older. The 10-year and lifetime ASCVD cardiovascular risk score was calculated for each study participant in the age group of 41–60 years. For participants less than 40 years of age, only lifetime risk could be calculated whereas for the participants of more than 60 years of age, only a 10-year risk could be calculated. The ASCVD lifetime and 10-year risk scores were further categorized into low risk and high risk based on the standard cut-off. The 10-year CVD risk of less than 7.5% was considered as low while 7.5% or more was considered high. Lifetime CVD risk less than 39% was considered low, 39% or more was considered high. The FM patients were also stratified based on disease severity and disease duration to study the association of these parameters with ASCVD risk scores.

To address the secondary objective of the study, a supervised ML algorithm was developed to study the interactions between FM disease characteristics and ASCVD risk scores. A random forest classifier ML algorithm was used for the development and training of the model to help predict the ASCVD risk category of FM patients using baseline clinical features and biochemical parameters. Baseline characteristics of higher importance for high CVD risk in FM patients were identified using this ML algorithm.

Statistical methods

We used SPSS Version 20.0 (IBM Corporation, USA) for statistical analysis. All continuous variables were summarized using mean (SD) or median (IQR). Kolmogorov–Smirnov test was used to ascertain whether the data were normally distributed. Categorical variables were expressed in counts (%). We used the Pearson Chi-Square test or Fisher's exact test for categorical variables and independent sample *t*-test or Mann–Whitney test for continuous variables. Anaconda-Python 3.0 (USA) software was used for ML analysis.

Machine learning (ML) model preparation and evaluation of the model

The 10 years and Lifetime ASCVD risk status were the target variables (high risk versus low risk) that were to be predicted in their respective models. The inputs were all other variables mentioned above and cumulatively, these included 21 parameters for each patient—age, height, weight, body mass index (BMI), presence of co-morbidities (hypothyroidism, diabetes mellitus, hypertension, and dyslipidemia), systolic- diastolic blood pressures, smoking status, BPI (total and average) score, FIQR

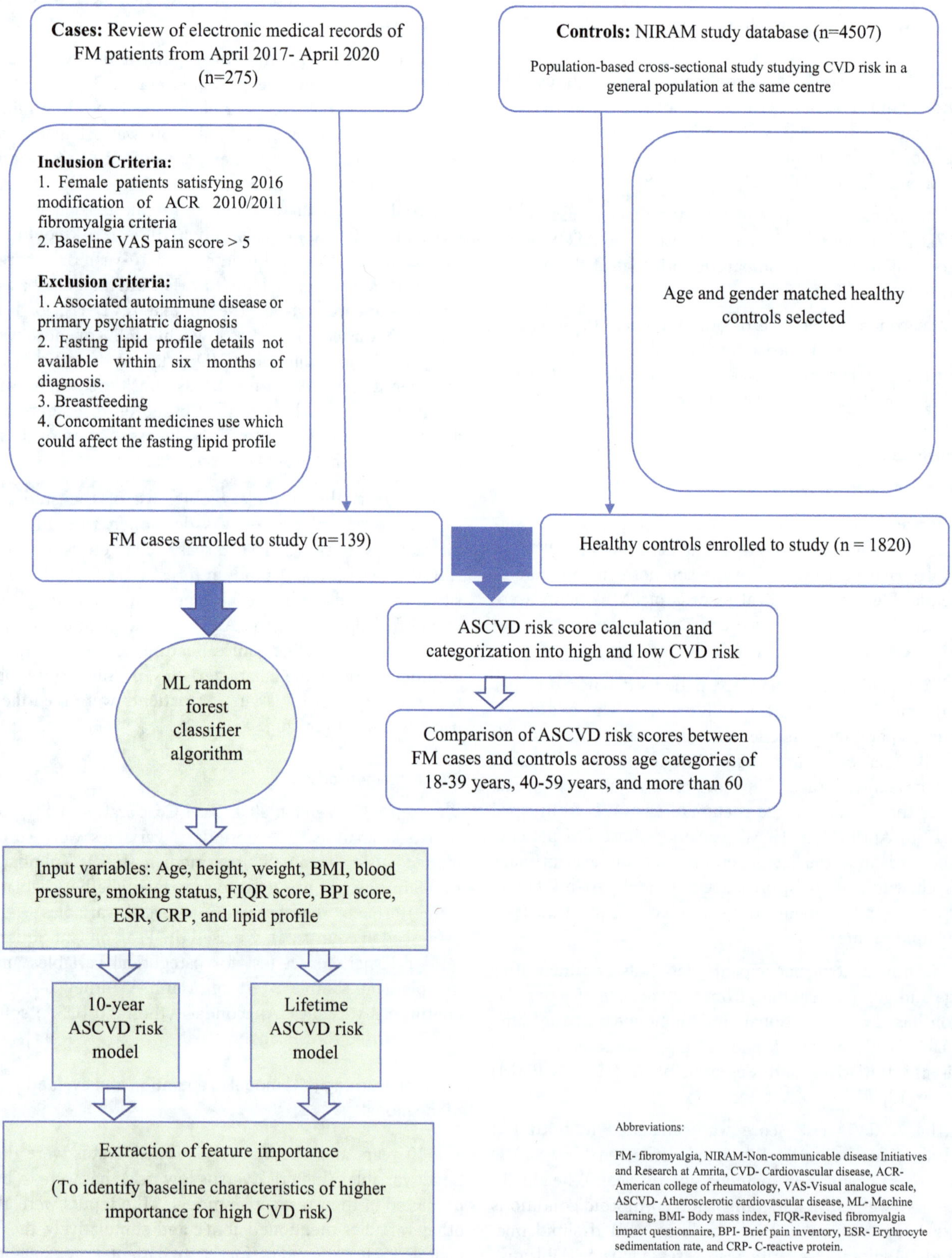

Fig. 1 Study design and methodology

score, ESR, CRP levels and lipid profile (total cholesterol, LDL, HDL levels and triglyceride). To apply the ML risk algorithms, the data was imported using Python 3.0 using JupyterLab coding environment. For the ML modeling, the Scikit-learn python library, which has been specifically developed for data science and ML, was used. The FM patients were split into the data set into training and validation subgroups. The training subgroup was derived from a random sampling of 80% of the FM patients, and the 'validation' cohort comprised the remaining 20% which was imported into a random forest classifier algorithm to help derive an ML model for the 10-year CVD risk and lifetime CVD risk, respectively. Then validation subgroup data was used by these trained algorithms to test the performance of the model. Each model's hyperparameters were determined manually with the n-estimators and using fivefold cross-validation on the training subgroup to determine the values which led to the best performance. The model with the best performance was then represented using accuracy score, f-score, area under the curve (A.U.C) for both ML models. In both the 10-year risk random classifier model and lifetime risk random classifier model in addition to model training, the feature importance and their weightage were calculated.

Table 1 Baseline characteristics of study participants

	FM cases (n = 139)	**Healthy controls (n = 1820)**
A: Baseline characteristics of FM cases and healthy control group		
Age in years (mean ± SD)	46.85 ± 10.15	48.94 ± 10.7
BMI kg/m^2 (mean ± SD)	27.34 ± 4.58	26.97 ± 3.88
Type 2 diabetes mellitus	19 (13.66%)	397 (21.81%)
Hypertension, no. (%)	30 (21.58%)	397 (21.81%)
Dyslipidaemia, no. (%)	89 (64.49%)	310 (39.40%)
B: Clinical characteristics of FM patients		
Disease duration (in years) (mean ± SD)	5.04 ± 4.51	
Baseline FIQR score (IQR)	55.33 (26.32)	
Baseline BPI average pain (IQR)	6.66 (3)	
CRP (mg/L) (mean ± SD)	4.44 ± 4.39	
ESR (mm/h) (mean ± SD)	23.31 ± 12.50	

FM, fibromyalgia; SD, standard deviation; BMI, body mass index; FIQR, revised fibromyalgia impact questionnaire; IQR, interquartile range; CRP, C-reactive protein; ESR, erythrocyte sedimentation rate

Table 2 Age stratified distribution of ASCVD risk scores in FM cases and healthy controls

Age (in years)	**ASCVD risk score†**							
	10-year risk				**Lifetime risk**			
	<7.5% (low)	**≥7.5% (high)**	**OR (CI)**	***p*-value**	**<39% (low)**	**≥39% (high)**	**OR (CI)**	***p*-value**
18–39 years								
FM cases (n = 29)	–	–	–		19	10	0.649	0.267
Healthy controls (n = 428)	–	–	–		235	193	(0.29–1.41)	
40–59 years								
FM cases (n = 97)	92	5	2.27	0.093	62	35	**1.56**	**0.044**
Healthy Control (n = 1071)	1046	25	(0.85–6.08)		787	284	**(1.01–2.42)**	
≥ 60 years								
FM cases (n = 13)	8	5	0.56	0.307	–	–	–	
Healthy control (n = 321)	151	170	(0.18–1.73)		–	–	–	

FM, fibromyalgia; ASCVD, Atherosclerotic cardiovascular disease; OR, odd's ratio; CI, 95% confidence interval; Emboldened summary estimate is statistically significant at $p < 0.05$.

† 10-year ASCVD risk calculated only for patients 40 years and more; Lifetime ASCVD risk calculated for patients who are less than 60 years of age

Results

A total of 139 FM cases and 1820 age and gender-matched healthy controls were enrolled in the study. Table 1 shows the baseline characteristics of study participants.

Table 2 shows the age-stratified distribution of ASCVD risk scores between the FM cases and healthy controls. The lifetime risk of CVD is significantly higher in the FM cases of age group 40–59 years than the age and gender-matched healthy controls ($OR = 1.56$, $95\%\ CI = 1.01$–2.42, $p = 0.043$).

Table 3 shows ASCVD risk scores of FM patients stratified for FM disease severity and disease duration. There is no difference noted in CVD risk with FM disease severity and duration ($p > 0.05$).

Machine learning (ML) analysis and features importance

Out of a total of 139 FM patients enrolled, 110 patients were of more than 40 years of age whose 10-year ASCVD risk was calculated. An ML model was derived using the SciKit Random Classifier algorithm. The best model was selected after hyperparameter tuning (manually with the n-estimators, and using fivefold cross-validation) and the precision of 96%, recall of 95% with an F1 score of 0.95 was achieved. The AUC of this 10-year ASCVD ML model was 0.825 and is shown in Fig. 2A.

Table 3 ASCVD risk scores stratified for FM disease severity and duration

	ASCVD risk score					
	10-year risk			Lifetime risk		
	Low	High	*p*-value[†]	Low	High	*p*-value[†]
FM disease severity[§]						
Severe	49	5	0.564	20	34	0.135
Mild/moderate	80	5		40	45	
FM disease duration						
2 years or more	88	7	0.914	39	56	0.546
< 2 years	41	3		21	23	

ASCVD, atherosclerotic cardiovascular disease; FM, fibromyalgia

[†] *p*-value was calculated using Pearson Chi-square and Fisher's exact test, a value of < 0.05 was considered significant

[§] FM disease severity defined by revised fibromyalgia impact questionnaire (FIQR); FIQR score > 60 was considered severe FM and FIQR score ≤ 60 considered mild-moderate FM

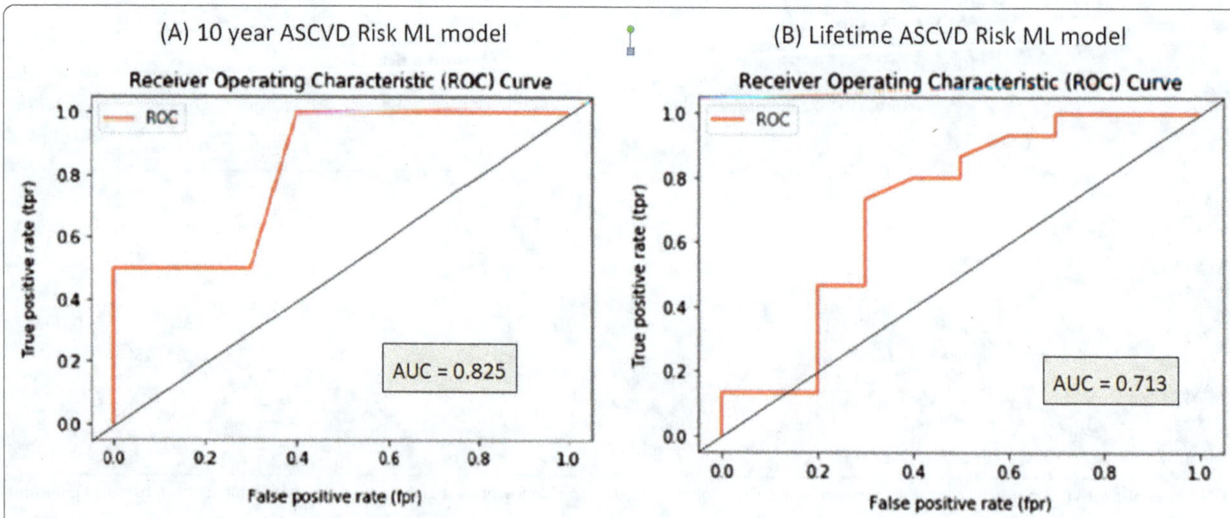

Fig. 2 R.O.C curve of the best machine learning models for ASCVD risk prediction

Table 4 Feature importance of ML predictive models of 10 years and lifetime ASCVD risk (random forest algorithm)

	Feature importance in 10-year ASCVD risk ML predictive model	Feature importance in lifetime ASCVD risk ML predictive model
Age	**0.150**	**0.074**
Height	0.063	**0.051**
Weight	**0.078**	0.035
BMI	**0.065**	0.039
Systolic blood pressure	0.043	**0.069**
Diastolic blood pressure	0.030	0.037
Diabetes mellitus	0.041	0.007
Hypertension	0.006	0.015
Dyslipidaemia	0.012	0.009
Hypothyroidism	0.023	0.013
Smoker	0.000	0.000
Disease duration	0.036	0.043
FIQR score	**0.071**	**0.062**
BPI total score	0.038	0.029
BPI average score	**0.066**	0.047
ESR	0.036	0.044
CRP	0.040	0.050
Serum total cholesterol	**0.077**	**0.179**
Serum LDL	0.041	**0.083**
Serum HDL	0.022	0.051
Serum triglycerides	**0.070**	**0.055**

Feature importance is the degree of contribution in the random forest ML predictive model. Seven parameters of high feature importance are emboldened in each ML classifier model

ML, Machine learning; ASCVD, atherosclerotic cardiovascular disease; BMI, body mass index; FIQR, revised fibromyalgia impact questionnaire; BPI, brief pain inventory; ESR, erythrocyte sedimentation rate; CRP, C-reactive protein; LDL, low-density lipoprotein; HDL, high-density lipoprotein

A lifetime ASCVD risk calculated for 126 FM patients of less than 60 years age. Using the SciKit Random Classifier algorithm again, an ML model was derived. The best model developed has a precision of 72% recall of 72% with an F1 score of 0.79 was achieved. The AUC of the lifetime ASCVD ML model was 0.713 and is shown in Fig. 2B. The feature importance in the individual models are shown in Table 4.

Discussion

In our study, the conventional case–control design showed that female FM patients of age group 40–59 years had increased lifetime ASCVD risk. Nevertheless, ASCVD risk was not increased in female FM patients of the age groups of 18–39 years and more than 60 years. Also, this conventional study design failed to show any association of ASCVD risk with FM disease severity and disease duration.

These results are in concordance with the study done in Taiwan which also shows that FM is a risk factor for CVD [12]. This finding of increased CVD risk in patients with FM is homologous to CVD risk in another related condition—major depressive disorder [20]. Depression has been demonstrated to be an independent risk factor for the onset of a wide range of cardiovascular disorders in a meta-analysis [21].

As FM pathogenesis is multifaceted and we are continuing to learn with every research, evidence to support the role of inflammation in FM etiopathogenesis is increasing. Pro-inflammatory cytokines, reactive oxygen species and inflammatory factors are considered to play a distinct role in inflammatory response in FM patients [22]. Serum CRP levels in FM patients are reported to be higher than control population which is known to improve by exercise and dietary changes [23]. This low-grade inflammation could be the common link between FM and CVD.

The CVD risk is multi-factorial but amongst the parameters used in the ASCVD risk calculator, dyslipidemia is strikingly high in fibromyalgia patients in comparison to the control population in this study (Table 1A). This is finding is consistent with various studies across the globe [24, 25]. A low-grade subclinical inflammatory process with an elevation of inflammatory cytokine (interleukin-6) is well described in fibromyalgia patients [26]. The role of IL-6 in lipid metabolism is well described and this could be the common mechanism that links the two diseases explaining our observation [10]. FM patients have lower physical fitness that could be another reason for increased CVD risk as suggested in the al-Ándalus Project [27].

Since the conventional statistical analysis showed a significantly high ASCVD risk in FM patients of age 40–59 years but failed to show any association of ASCVD risk with FM disease severity and disease duration; ML algorithms were developed and trained to understand the non-linear relationships of CVD risk in FM patients. The application of ML models showed some interesting relationships with all the possible risk factors assessed, which were overlooked by the traditional study design. Notably, the ML models, displayed the importance of FM disease severity with ASCVD risk status, in addition to other traditional CVD risk features like dyslipidemia. The high importance feature of both the 10-year ASCVD risk score and lifetime ASCVD risk ML models were age, weight, total cholesterol, FIQR score, and triglyceride level. Other features included BMI and BPI (average pain) score for the 10-year ASCVD ML model while the lifetime ASCVD risk ML model had revealed height and low-density lipoprotein levels, in addition to the aforementioned five parameters. Both models showed excellent validity after training. This demonstrates the ability of ML in identifying the non-linear relationships between the disease datasets (FM characteristics) and the target variable (ASCVD risk score) and improving prediction models.

The application of ML algorithms for the prediction of cardiovascular diseases is not novel. Data from a large cohort of 378,000 patients from a family practice database in England were analyzed using machine learning and was shown to significantly improve the accuracy of cardiovascular risk prediction when compared to 10-year ASCVD risk scores [28].

While the use of ML for data analysis from the general population for CVD risk prediction is increasingly studied; our study explores the novel application of ML in FM for studying the role of non-linear predictors of ASCVD risk (Table 4). However, in addition to the high feature importance of traditional risk factors (age, BMI, and fasting lipid profile) our ML model was able to identify that FM disease severity also had high feature importance for increasing CVD risk in female FM patients which is an interesting finding.

Given the widespread prevalence of heart disease, the importance of characterizing the "at-risk" population for CVD cannot be understated. In addition to the ASCVD risk score, carotid intimal medial thickness could be used as a surrogate marker for predicting CVD risk in future studies, as recommended by a meta-analysis report by Willeit et al. [29].

The external validity of our study could be limited as it was an observational study from a single center. Further prospective studies are required to establish causation, but as this study shows excellent internal validity, it can be used to guide future research. This study highlights a probable novel non-linear FM disease severity association with the ASCVD risk score that could help better stratify an individual FM patient for CVD risk.

Conclusion

Traditional risk factors like obesity, diabetes mellitus, hypertension, and dyslipidemia are the main pillars of CVD risk. In our study, the conventional case–control design showed that premenopausal female patients with FM could represent a new CVD risk group. The novel supervised ML study design identified FM disease severity as a high contributor feature importance for CVD risk, which was missed by the conventional study design. More definitive evidence can be gathered by future prospective studies employing non-invasive surrogate markers of CVD risk like carotid intimal medial thickness and coronary artery calcium scoring.

Acknowledgements

The authors would like to extend their note of gratitude to the clinical and administrative staff of Amrita Institute of Medical Sciences, Kochi, India for facilitating the data collection process.

Authors' contributions

SS: conceptualization, data curation, formal analysis, investigation, methodology, software, validation, visualization, writing—original draft, writing-editing. CBM: conceptualization, project administration, data curation, formal analysis, methodology, writing—review. MM: conceptualization, data curation, formal analysis, methodology, supervision, validation, visualization, writing—review. AT: conceptualization, data curation, formal analysis, methodology, validation, visualization, writing—review. MP: data curation, formal analysis, methodology, validation, visualization, writing—review. The authors read and approved the final manuscript.

Author details

[1]Department of Rheumatology, Amrita Institute of Medical Sciences, Amrita Vishwa Vidyapeetham, Kochi, Kerala, India. [2]Department of General Medicine, Amrita Institute of Medical Sciences, Amrita Vishwa Vidyapeetham, Kochi, Kerala, India. [3]Department of Pharmacology, Amrita Institute of Medical Sciences, Amrita Vishwa Vidyapeetham, Kochi, Kerala, India.

References

1. Wolfe F, et al. 2016 Revisions to the 2010/2011 fibromyalgia diagnostic criteria. Semin Arthr Rheum. 2016;46(3):319–29. https://doi.org/10.1016/j.semarthrit.2016.08.012.
2. Walitt B, Nahin RL, Katz RS, Bergman MJ, Wolfe F. The prevalence and characteristics of fibromyalgia in the 2012 National Health Interview Survey. PLoS ONE. 2015;10(9):e0138024. https://doi.org/10.1371/JOURNAL.PONE.0138024

3. Staud R, Spaeth M. Psychophysical and neurochemical abnormalities of pain processing in fibromyalgia. CNS Spectr. 2008;13(3 Suppl 5):12–7. https://doi.org/10.1017/S109285290002678X.
4. Caro XJ, Winter EF. The role and importance of small fiber neuropathy in fibromyalgia pain. Curr Pain Headache Rep. 2015;19(12):1–7. https://doi.org/10.1007/S11916-015-0527-7.
5. Thombs BD, et al. Prevalence of depression in survivors of acute myocardial infarction. J Gen Internal Med. 2006;21(1):30–8. https://doi.org/10.1111/J.1525-1497.2005.00269.X.
6. Ho Jee Y, Chang H, Ji Jung K, Ha Jee S. Cohort study on the effects of depression on atherosclerotic cardiovascular disease risk in Korea. BMJ Open. 2018. https://doi.org/10.1136/bmjopen-2018-026913.
7. Sumner JA, et al. Effects of concurrent depressive symptoms and perceived stress on cardiovascular risk in low- and high-income participants: findings from the reasons for geographical and racial differences in stroke (REGARDS) study. J Am Heart Assoc. 2016;5(10):e003930. https://doi.org/10.1161/JAHA.116.003930.
8. da Cunha Ribeiro RP, et al. Cardiac autonomic impairment and chronotropic incompetence in fibromyalgia. Arthritis Res Ther. 2011;13(6):1–5. https://doi.org/10.1186/AR3519.
9. Üçeyler N, Häuser W, Sommer C. Systematic review with meta-analysis: cytokines in fibromyalgia syndrome. BMC Musculoskelet Disord. 2011;12:1–15. https://doi.org/10.1186/1471-2474-12-245.
10. Esteve E, Ricart W, Fernández-Real JM. Dyslipidemia and inflammation: an evolutionary conserved mechanism. Clin Nutr (Edinb, Scotl). 2005;24(1):16–31. https://doi.org/10.1016/J.CLNU.2004.08.004.
11. Ridker PM, Everett BM, Thuren T, MacFadyen JG, Chang WH, Ballantyne C, Fonseca F, Nicolau J, Koenig W, Anker SD, Kastelein JJ. Antiinflammatory therapy with canakinumab for atherosclerotic disease. N Engl J Med. 2017;377(12):1119–31. https://doi.org/10.1056/NEJMOA1707914.
12. Su CH, Chen JH, Lan JL, Wang YC, Tseng CH, Hsu CY, Huang L. Increased risk of coronary heart disease in patients with primary fibromyalgia and those with concomitant comorbidity-a Taiwanese population-based cohort study. PLoS ONE. 2015;10(9):e0137137. https://doi.org/10.1371/JOURNAL.PONE.0137137.
13. Goff DC, et al. 2013 ACC/AHA guideline on the assessment of cardiovascular risk: a report of the American College of Cardiology/American Heart Association task force on practice guidelines. Circulation. 2014. https://doi.org/10.1161/01.CIR.0000437741.48606.98.
14. Wolfe F, Ross K, Anderson J, Russell IJ, Hebert L. The prevalence and characteristics of fibromyalgia in the general population. Arthritis Rheum. 1995;38(1):19–28. https://doi.org/10.1002/ART.1780380104.
15. Deo RC. Machine learning in medicine. Circulation. 2015;132(20):1920. https://doi.org/10.1161/CIRCULATIONAHA.115.001593.
16. Jordan MI, Mitchell TM. Machine learning: trends, perspectives, and prospects. Science (New York, NY). 2015;349(6245):255–60. https://doi.org/10.1126/SCIENCE.AAA8415.
17. "Project Hanover," Microsoft Research (2016). https://www.microsoft.com/en-us/research/project/project-hanover/. Accessed 24 Sept 2021.
18. Adamichou C, et al. Lupus or not? SLE Risk Probability Index (SLERPI): a simple, clinician-friendly machine learning-based model to assist the diagnosis of systemic lupus erythematosus. Ann Rheum Dis. 2021;80(6):758–66. https://doi.org/10.1136/ANNRHEUMDIS-2020-219069.
19. Menon VP, et al. Assessment of 2013 AHA/ACC ASCVD risk scores with behavioral characteristics of an urban cohort in India: preliminary analysis of noncommunicable disease Initiatives and Research at AMrita (NIRAM) study. Medicine. 2016;95(49):e5542–e5542. https://doi.org/10.1097/MD.0000000000005542.
20. Gracely RH, Ceko M, Bushnell MC. Fibromyalgia and depression. Pain Res Treat. 2012. https://doi.org/10.1155/2012/486590.
21. van der Kooy K, van Hout H, Marwijk H, Marten H, Stehouwer C, Beekman A. Depression and the risk for cardiovascular diseases: systematic review and meta analysis. Int J Geriatr Psychiatry. 2007;22(7):613–26. https://doi.org/10.1002/GPS.1723.
22. Benlidayi IC. Role of inflammation in the pathogenesis and treatment of fibromyalgia. Rheumatol Int. 2019;39(5):781–91. https://doi.org/10.1007/S00296-019-04251-6
23. Metyas S, Rezk T, Arkfeld D, Leptich T. Autoinflammation and immunomodulation in inflammatory fibromyalgia syndrome: a review. Curr Rheumatol Rev. 2017;13(2):98–102. https://doi.org/10.2174/1573397112666160919120530.
24. Sicras-Mainar A, Blanca-Tamayo M, Navarro-Artieda R, Rejas-Gutiérrez J. Use of resources and costs profile in patients with fibromyalgia or generalized anxiety disorder in primary care settings. Aten Primaria. 2009;41(2):84. https://doi.org/10.1016/J.APRIM.2008.09.008.
25. Gurer G, Sendur OF, Ay C. Serum lipid profile in fibromyalgia women. Clin Rheumatol. 2006;25(3):300–3. https://doi.org/10.1007/S10067-005-0004-5.
26. Mendieta D, et al. IL-8 and IL-6 primarily mediate the inflammatory response in fibromyalgia patients. J Neuroimmunol. 2016;290:22–5. https://doi.org/10.1016/J.JNEUROIM.2015.11.011.
27. Borges-Cosic M, et al. Sedentary time, physical activity, and sleep quality in fibromyalgia: the al-Ándalus project. Scand J Med Sci Sports. 2019;29(2):266–74. https://doi.org/10.1111/SMS.13318.
28. Weng SF, Reps J, Kai J, Garibaldi JM, Qureshi N. Can machine-learning improve cardiovascular risk prediction using routine clinical data? PLoS ONE. 2017;12(4):e0174944. https://doi.org/10.1371/JOURNAL.PONE.0174944.
29. Willeit P, et al. Carotid intima-media thickness progression as surrogate marker for cardiovascular risk. Circulation. 2020;142:621–42. https://doi.org/10.1161/CIRCULATIONAHA.120.046361.

7

Cardiac magnetic resonance imaging in patients with Behçet's disease

Ali A. Ahmed[1], Samar Tharwat[1*], Nihal M. Batouty[2], Ahmed El Bahy[3], Ahmed M. Tawfik[2] and Dina A. Shahin[1]

Abstract

Background: Behçet's disease (BD) is a multisystemic vasculitis that may affect the heart. However, the incidence and nature of cardiac involvement in BD have not been clearly documented yet. The aim of this study was to delineate the cardiac magnetic resonance imaging (MRI) appearances of cardiac involvement in BD patients.

Methods: This cross-sectional observational study was carried out 30 BD patients without known cardiac disease. Patients were subjected to history taking, physical examination, echocardiography and cardiac MRI.

Results: At least one abnormality on cardiac MRI was observed in 20/30 patients (66.67%). Myocardial oedema was observed in 3 patients (10%) and late gadolinium enhancement in 1 patient (3.3%). Pericardial effusion was found in 3 patients (10.0%), global hypokinesia in 6 patients (20.0%) and intra-cardiac thrombosis in only 1 patient (3.3%). Pulmonary artery was dilated in 4 patients (13.3%). Left ventricular (LV) and right ventricular (RV) end diastolic volume were altered in 4 patients (13.3%) and 7 patients (23.3%) respectively. LV and RV end systolic volume were abnormal in 7 patients (23.3%) and 5 patients (16.7%) respectively. There was aortic valve regurge in 2 patients (6.7%), tricuspid valve regurge in 9 patients (30%), and mitral valve regurge in 9 patients (30%). Dilated left main coronary artery was found in 2 patients (6.7%) and arrhythmogenic right ventricular dysplasia in only one patient 1 patient (3.3%). On logistic regression analysis, BD activity index score was a significant predictor of cardiac abnormalities.

Conclusion: BD may cause cardiac abnormalities without clinical manifestations and cardiac MRI may represent a tool for early detection of these subtle abnormalities. Higher BD activity index scores are strongly linked to cardiac problems.

Keywords: Behçet's disease, Heart, Cardiac MRI

Background

Behçet disease (BD) is a chronic, relapsing inflammatory disorder of unknown etiology [1]. Although BD occurs worldwide, it is most prevalent along the "Silk road" region extending from Japan to the Middle Eastern countries [2]. The exact pathogenesis is still unknown, but it is a multifactorial disease classified as vasculitis. It may be triggered by many environmental factors as infection in genetically predisposed persons [3].

BD was first described as a trisymptom complex of recurrent oral and genital ulcers and uveitis [4] and later recognized as a multisystem disease with neurological, pulmonary, gastrointestinal, musculoskeletal, vascular and cardiac involvement [5].

Venous pathology and thrombotic complications are hallmarks of BD. However, cardiac involvement is rare and underestimated [6]. All cardiac layers may be involved resulting in pericarditis, myocarditis, endocarditis, intracardiac thrombosis and valvular disease [7]. Early recognition of cardiac involvement is important being associated with poor prognosis. There are only few

*Correspondence: samartharwat2000@yahoo.com
[1] Rheumatology and Immunology Unit, Internal Medicine Department, Faculty of Medicine, Mansoura University Hospital, Mansoura University, El Gomhouria St, Mansoura, Dakahlia Governorate, Egypt

data on cardiac manifestations in BD. Additionally, routine methods assessing heart involvement in BD patients such as echocardiography are not sensitive nor specific [8].

Cardiac magnetic resonance imaging (MRI) is a noninvasive, non-radiating safe modality that can be valuable in assessing cardiac structure and function [9]. The aims of the present study were to evaluate usefulness of cardiac MRI in BD patients without known cardiac disease and to detect areas of hyperenhancement after IV administration of gadolinium. To the best of our knowledge, this is the first study to investigate silent cardiac involvement in patients with BD using Cardiac MRI.

Methods

Patients

This is an observational analytical cross-sectional study conducted on 30 patients with BD. Patients were recruited from Rheumatology and Immunology unit at Mansoura University Hospital, Egypt between May 2018 to December 2019. All patients met the following inclusion criteria: (a) age > 18 years (b) classified as having BD according to the International Criteria for Behcet's Disease (ICBD) [10] (c) BD duration more than one year (d) without known cardiac disease or manifestations. Exclusion criteria included: diabetes mellitus, hypertension, ischemic heart diseases, liver cell failure, overlap with other autoimmune diseases, and coexistent infection or malignancy. Patients with glomerular filtration rate below 30 ml/min/1.73 m^2 or had cardiac pacemaker or cochlear implants were also excluded from the start. The study protocol was approved by the Institutional Research Board of the Faculty of Medicine, Mansoura University (approval registration number: MS/18.02.44). The study was explained to all patients, and informed written consent was obtained from all of them before starting the study.

Demographic, clinical and laboratory data

For the included patients, sex, age and BD duration were recorded. BD cumulative manifestations affecting the eye, gastrointestinal tract, joints, skin, blood vessels and central nervous system were evaluated and registered by an experienced rheumatologist. BD activity within the past 4 weeks was also evaluated using Behçet's Disease Current Activity Form 2006 (BDCAF) (http://www.behcet.ws).

The following investigations were evaluated and recorded at the same day of clinical assessment: complete blood count (CBC), erythrocyte sedimentation rate (ESR), C-reactive protein (CRP) and serum creatinine (SCr).

Transthoracic echocardiographic evaluation

Transthoracic echocardiographic evaluation of each patient was done by an experienced internist who was blinded to the clinical data. All patients were scanned by the same physician using commercial imaging analysis software (Philips Affiniti 50) with high frame rates (>60 frames/s) and evaluated according to the American Society of Echocardiography [11].

Cardiac MRI protocol

Each patient was evaluated by cardiac MRI within 24 h after clinical and echocardiographic assessment. Cardiac MRI was performed on a 1.5-T scanner (Philips Ingenia, Best, Netherlands). Retrospective ECG gating was used, and sequences were obtained with breath hold. Routine cine steady-state free-precession (SSFP) sequence was used to obtain a stalk of contiguous slices in the short-axis, axial, three chamber and four chambers. Parameters were TR = 3.2 ms, TE = 1.6 ms, field of view (FOV) 350 mm^2, slice thickness = 5 mm, no slice gap. Intravenous contrast agent (DOTAREM, Magnevest) was injected at a dose of 0.2 mmol/kg. After 10–15 min of contrast injection, T1-weighted inversion recovery sequence (PSIR-TFE-BH) was acquired in the short axis and 4 chamber planes with the following parameters: FOV 350 × 350 mm^2, slice thickness 8–10 mm, acquisition matrix 220 × 176, voxel size 1.6 × 1.9 × 10, TR/TE 6.1 ms/3 ms, flip angle 25°, and inversion time (TI) 250–425 ms. T2-weighted images were acquired in the short axis plane with a triple inversion recovery fast spin echo with the following parameters: TR, 1500 ms, TE 30 ms, FA 90°, FOV 350 × 350 mm^2, matrix 196–149 and slice thickness 8 mm.

Cardiac morphology and function were evaluated by an experienced radiologist blinded to echocardiography reports, using the dedicated cardiac MR software. Left ventricle and right ventricle volume and function were assessed by manually tracing the endocontours at endsystole and end-diastole. No sedation was used, and all patients were in sinus rhythm during the examination.

Cardiac MRI Post processing and image analysis

Cardiac morphology and function were evaluated by an experienced radiologist, blinded to echocardiography reports, using extended MR 130 Workspace 2.6.3.5, Philips medical systems Netherland. Semi-automated method was used to trace the endocardial contours of both left and right ventricles and LV epicardial contours on each slice from base to apex on short axis plane for left ventricle and axial plane for right ventricle on end systole and end diastole. The end diastolic volume (EDV) and end systolic volume (ESV) were recorded. The Stroke volume (SV) was obtained as the difference between EDV and ESV. The ejection fraction (EF) is the SV/EDV. The end diastolic wall mass of left ventricle (LVM) was calculated as the total myocardial volume multiplied by specific gravity of myocardial tissue (1.05 g/mL). Both ventricular end diastolic volume indexed (EDVi) and the left ventricular mass indexed (LVMi) were measured by dividing the EDV and myocardial mass by the BSA. Late contrast enhancement and myocardial oedema were evaluated on PSIR-TFE-BH sequence and T2 with triple inversion recovery sequence.

Statistical analysis

The collected data were coded, processed, and analysed using IBM SPSS for Windows version 24 (IBM Corp., Armonk, NY). After examining the distribution of continuous variables for normality using the Shapiro–Wilk test, data were expressed as mean and standard deviation if normally distributed or as median, minimum, and maximum if not normally distributed. Qualitative data were presented as frequencies and relative percentages. The Mann–Whitney test and independent samples t-test were used to compare continuous variables. The chi-square test was used to assess the differences between qualitative variables. The Spearman's rank-order correlation was used to determine the strength and direction of a linear relationship between two non-normally distributed continuous variables and/or ordinal variables. Logistic regression analysis was carried out to identify the potential predictors for cardiac MRI abnormalities. A ROC curve was also generated and the area under the curve (AUC) was calculated for BDCAF score to identify the cut off points above which cardiac MRI abnormalities are likely. *P* values of ≤ 0.05 were considered significant.

Results

Patients' characteristics and echocardiographic findings

A total of 30 BD patients were included in the study. The patients' characteristics and transthoracic echocardiographic findings are described in Table 1. Among the studied patients, 21 (70%) were males and their mean age was 32.3 years (SD 8.9). The median duration of BD was 3 years with a range from1.5–7 years. Echocardiography detected tricuspid valve regurge in 8 patients (26.7%) and global myocardium hypokinesia in 6 patients (20%).

Cardiac MRI evaluation

Cardiac MRI showed at least one abnormality in 25 (83.33%) of the studied 30 BD patients. The main cardiac MRI findings are shown in Table 2. Increased signal

Table 1 Demographic, clinical, laboratory, echocardiographic and treatment characteristics of patients (n = 30)

Characteristic	Value
Demographic and clinical characteristics	
Age (years), M ± SD	32.3 ± 8.9
Sex	
Male, n (%)	21 (70)
Female, n (%)	9 (30)
Behçet's disease duration (years), median (min–max)	3 (1.5–7)
Height (cm), M ± SD	171.03 ± 5.49
Weight (kg), M ± SD	75.37 ± 9.22
BMI (kg/m^2), M ± SD	25.82 ± 3.37
Heart rate (bpm), M ± SD	89.50 ± 7.69
SBP (mmHg), M ± SD	127.5 ± 6.53
DBP (mmHg), M ± SD	78.33 ± 9.49
Behcet disease activity index score, M ± SD	4.60 ± 1.4
≤4, n (%)	15 (50)
>4, n (%)	15 (50)
Cumulative manifestations of Behcet disease, n (%)	
Orogenital Ulcers	30 (100)
Uveitis	23 (76.7)
Cutaneous manifestations	11 (36.7)
Musculoskeletal manifestations	10 (33.3)
Gastrointestinal tract manifestations	1 (3.3)
Deep venous thrombosis	4 (13.3)
Laboratory characteristics	
Complete blood count	
Hb (g/dL), M ± SD	11.83 ± 1.01
WBCs (10^3 /mm^3), M ± SD	4.63 ± 1.5
PLT (10^3 /mm^3), M ± SD	222.8 ± 53.6
Serum creatinine (mg/dL), M ± SD	0.91 ± 0.11
Erythrocyte sedimentation rate (mm/hr), M ± SD	35.33 ± 10.08
Positive C-reactive protein, n (%)	14 (46.7)
Echocardiographic findings	
Ejection fraction (%), M ± SD	59.73 ± 5.09
Pericardial effusion, n (%)	2 (6.7)
Global hypokinesia, n (%)	6 (20)
Aortic valve regurge, n (%)	1 (3.3)
Tricuspid valve regurge, n (%)	8 (26.7)
Intra-cardiac thrombosis, n (%)	1 (3.3)
Medications used for treatment, n (%)	
Colchicine	30 (100)
Steroids	30 (100)
Azathioprine	14 (46.7)
Cyclosporine	14 (46.7)
Anticoagulants	5 (16.7)
Biological agents	10 (33.3)
Dose of steroids (mg /day), median (min–max)	20 (0–60)

BMI, body mass index; DBP, diastolic blood pressure; SBP, systolic blood pressure

Table 2 Findings of cardiac MRI of the studied Behçet's patients (n=30)

Findings of cardiac MRI	The study patients (n=30)
End diastolic volume (ml), M±SD	
Left ventricle	79.36±19.71
Right ventricle	85.46±23.09
End systolic volume (ml), M±SD	
Left ventricle	31.59±9.59
Right ventricle	40.84±12.15
Stroke volume (ml), M±SD	
Left ventricle	46.74±12.29
Right ventricle	46.27±11.53
Ejection fraction (%), M±SD	
Left ventricle	60.20±5.81
Right ventricle	53.70±4.74
End diastolic wall mass (g/m^2), M±SD	61.46±11.2
Signs of myocarditis, n (%)	
Myocardial edema	3 (10)
Late gadolinium enhancement	1 (3.3)
Cardiac valves, n (%)	
Aortic valve regurge	2 (6.7)
Pulmonary valve regurge	0
Tricuspid valve regurge	9 (30)
Mitral valve regurge	9 (30)
Blood vessels	
Mid ascending aorta diameter (mm), M±SD	28.18±3.07
Aortic sinus root diameter (mm), M±SD	29.98±2.76
Main pulmonary artery diameter (mm), M±SD	23.74±3.45
Pulmonary /aortic ratio, M±SD	0.80±0.16
Right pulmonary artery diameter (mm), M±SD	16.09±2.24
Left pulmonary artery diameter (mm), M±SD	16.71±2.38
Increased Pulmonary /aortic ratio, n (%)	3 (10)
Dilated main pulmonary artery, n (%)	4 (13.3)
Bilateral pulmonary artery aneurysm and embolism, n (%)	1 (3.3)
Dilated left main coronary artery (coronary aneurysm), n (%)	2 (6.7)
SVC thrombosis	1 (3.3)
Other findings, n (%)	
Pericardial effusion	3 (10)
Global hypokinesia	6 (20)
Arrythmogenic right ventricular dysplasia*	1 (3.3)
Right ventricular thrombus	1 (3.3)

SVC, Superior vena cava

*Major criterion of ARVD by MRI; dyskinesia of right ventricular free wall with right ventricular end diastolic volume indexed to body surface area more than 110 ml/m^2

intensity on T2 weighted images (Fig. 1) was found in 3 patients (10%) while myocardial delayed contrast enhancement was detected in only one patient (3.3%). Tricuspid and mitral valves showed evidence of regurge in 9 patients (30%). Four of the 30 studied patients (13.3%) showed dilatation at the main pulmonary artery while only one patient (3.3%) showed aneurysmal dilatation and thrombosis of both right and left pulmonary arteries. Aneurysmal dilatation was observed at the left main coronary artery in 2 patients (6.7%). Superior vena cava (SVC) was thrombosed in only 1 patient (3.3%).

Pericardial effusion was detected in 3 patients (10%). Additionally, global myocardium hypokinesia was present in 6 patients (20%). The right ventricle showed evidence of thrombosis in 1 patient (3.3%), and arrhythmogenic ventricular dysplasia in another 1 patient (3.3%).

No significant difference between patients with and without cardiac MRI abnormalities when compared regarding demographic, clinical and therapeutic data as shown in Table 3.

For prediction of cardiac MRI abnormalities, logistic regression analysis was carried out. Diastolic blood pressure and BDCAF score were the most significant predictors for cardiac MRI abnormalities (Table 4). As shown in Fig. 2 the AUC of BDCAF score revealed that a cut off value of>6 identifying the probability of cardiac MRI abnormalities with 84% sensitivity and 60% specificity.

Echocardiography versus cardiac MRI in detecting cardiac abnormalities

When we explored the performance of echocardiography in heart evaluation compared to cardiac MRI in BD patients, the results showed sensitivity of 64%, specificity of 100%, positive predictive value (PPV) of 100%, negative predictive value of 37.5% and accuracy of 70%. Kappa agreement was 0.372 indicating slight agreement ($P=0.45$).

Discussion

BD is a rare chronic autoinflammatory disorder that is usually seen along the Silk road including the Middle East and Far-east Asia [12]. It is characterized by four main symptoms of recurrent oral aphthous ulcers, genital ulcers, cutaneous manifestations, and ocular symptoms [13]. Cardiac involvement have been reported in about 6% of BD patients and may be subclinical [14]. Cardiac MRI is a non-invasive modality that can evaluate cardiac function and structure [15]. In the present study, we used cardiac MRI to evaluate cardiac abnormalities in a group of 30 BD patients with no known cardiac disease.

To the best of our knowledge, this is the first detailed study of cardiac abnormalities encountered in patients with BD, which utilizes cardiac MRI. Previous studies in the literature used echocardiography to analyze the spectrum of cardiac involvement in BD patients [16–18].

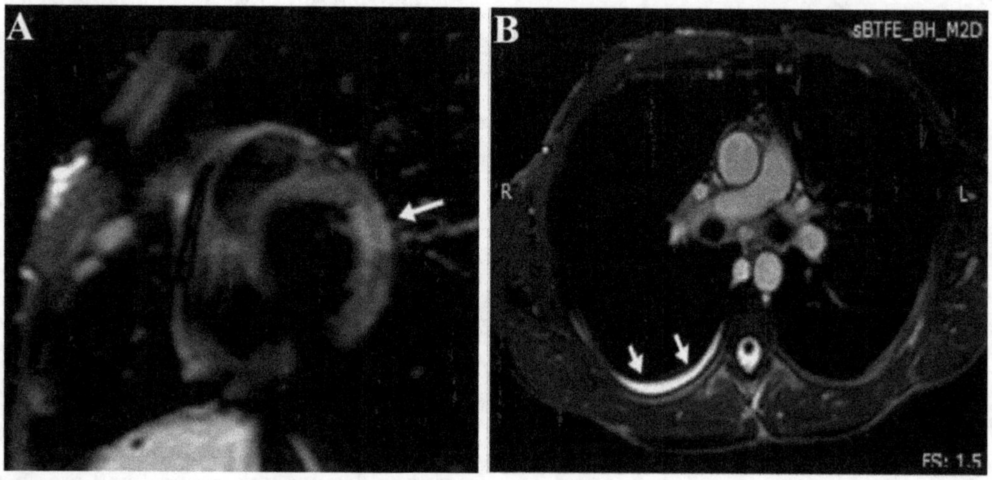

Fig. 1 Cardiac MRI of a 33-year-old male patient with Behcet's disease with **A** small patchy area of myocardial edema in lateral segment of basal myocardium of left ventricle in cardiac MRI T2 edema sequence short axis view and **B** small right sided pleural effusion in Cardiac MRI cine SSFP axial view

The main results of this study are as the following; first, the majority of BD patients (83%) had at least one abnormality on cardiac MRI. Second, cardiac MRI enabled us to evaluate the pattern of these cardiac abnormalities. Third, cardiac MRI is more sensitive than echocardiography in detecting any cardiac abnormalities in BD patients. Lastly, higher scores of BDCAF are highly suggestive of cardiac abnormalities.

One of the most striking findings to emerge from this study is the high prevalence of detected subtle cardiac abnormalities. Pathological cardiac findings were detected in 83% of our study patients. However, in the study by Geri et al.[14], cardiac lesions were found in only 6% of a cohort of 807 patients with BD. This variability may be attributed to the different tools used for assessment of the heart. These results suggest that heart affection in BD may be underestimated, and cardiac MRI is more sensitive in detecting any subtle cardiac abnormalities.

Cardiovascular involvement is a remarkable systemic affection of BD [19] and may be overlooked. Aktürk E and coworkers evaluated the left atrium using real-time three-dimensional echocardiography (RT3DE) in 30 BD patients with no cardiac symptoms and found significant impairment in left atrium volumes and mechanical functions in BD patients [17].

Myocardial edema has been detected in 10% of our patients. Additionally, one of these patients showed late gadolinium enhancement. These findings are highly suggestive of acute myocardial injury mostly myocarditis. Myocarditis is extremely rare in patients with BD [20, 21] and may contribute to cardiomegaly and cardiac fibrosis [22]. Cardiac MRI has emerged as a noninvasive diagnostic tool for early detection of myocarditis [23]. Kechida et al. have recently reported a case of BD with chest pain related to myocarditis that documented by cardiac MRI in spite of normal echocardiography [24].

Our results cast a new light on endocardial involvement in BD as valvular regurgitation was frequently observed in our cohort. The most frequently affected valves were the tricuspid and mitral valves (9/30 patients) followed by the aortic valve (2/30 patients). Endocardial involvement was also identified in previous studies [14, 25–28]. A similar pattern of results was also obtained by another study; wherein a cross-sectional study evaluated 35 BD patients using transesophageal echocardiography and revealed that mitral valve prolapse, and mitral regurgitation are the most frequent common findings of cardiac involvement in patients with BD [29].

The current study revealed dilated pulmonary artery in 4 cases and one case with bilateral pulmonary aneurysm and embolism. Pulmonary artery involvement is rare, it occurs in 1 to 7.7% of BD patients [30]. Pulmonary artery aneurysm with or without thrombosis is a typical feature of BD [31, 32].

Coronary arteries are rarely involved by aneurysms formation in vasculitis [33–35] and usually observed in Kawasaki disease [36]. In a case–control study on 476 BD patients, coronary aneurysm were present in only 9 patients [37]. Similarly, we have demonstrated coronary aneurysm in 3 patients only. Notably, they were all asymptomatic.

Our cohort revealed one case of superior vena cava (SVC) thrombosis. Involvement of great veins is a well-defined but rare complication of BD [38]. SVC thrombosis occurs in 2% of BD patients [38].

Table 3 Comparison between the studied patients with normal and abnormal cardiac MRI

Variables	With normal cardiac MRI)n = 5((% = 16.67)	With abnormal cardiac MRI (n = 25((% = 83.33)	*P* value
Demographic and clinical characteristics			
Age (years), M ± SD	26.0 ± 2.65	33.56 ± 9.22	.084
Sex			
Male, n (%)	2 (40)	19 (76)	.109
Female, n (%)	3 (60)	6 (24)	
Behçet's disease duration (years), median (min–max)	2 (2–3)	3 (1–7)	.176
Height (cm), M ± SD	171.6 ± 4.77	170.92 ± 5.71	.723
Weight (kg), M ± SD	74 ± 8.22	75.64 ± 9.54	.723
BMI (kg/m^2), M ± SD	25.08 ± 1.86	25.96 ± 3.6	.60
Heart rate (bpm), M ± SD	88 ± 4.47	89.9 ± 8.23	.641
SBP (mmHg), M ± SD	124 ± 5.47	128.2 ± 6.59	.19
DBP (mmHg), M ± SD	70 ± 7.07	80 ± 9.13	.806
Behcet disease activity index score, M ± SD			
≤4, n (%)	1(20)	14(56)	.33
>4, n (%)	4(80)	11(44)	
Cumulative manifestations of Behcet disease			
Orogenital Ulcers	5(100)	25(100)	1
Uveitis	4(80.0)	19(76.0)	1
Cutaneous manifestations	1(20.0)	10(40.0)	.63
Musculoskeletal manifestations	2 (40)	8 (32)	1
Gastrointestinal tract manifestations	1 (20)	1(4)	1
Deep venous thrombosis	1(20)	3 (12)	.53
Laboratory characteristics			
Complete blood count			
Hb (g/dL), M ± SD	11.90 ± 0.74	11.82 ± 1.07	.88
WBCs (10^3 /mm^3), M ± SD	4.26 ± 0.78	4.71 ± 0.71	.21
PLT (10^3 /mm^3), M ± SD	225.0 ± 32.02	222.36 ± 57.48	.92
Serum creatinine (mg/dL), M ± SD	0.86 ± 0.09	0.916 ± 0.11	.312
Erythrocyte sedimentation rate (mm/hr), M ± SD	33.0 ± 12.04	33.0 ± 12.04	.58
Positive C-reactive protein, n (%)	2(40)	12(48)	1
Medications used for treatment, n (%)			
Colchicine	5 (100)	25 (100)	1
Steroids	5 (100)	25 (100)	1
Azathioprine	4 (80)	10 (40)	.157
Cyclosporine	1 (20)	11 (44)	.62
Anticoagulants	1 (20)	4 (16)	1
Biological agents	1 (20)	9 (36)	.64

BMI, body mass index; DBP, diastolic blood pressure; Hb, hemoglobin; PLT, platelets; SBP, systolic blood pressure; WBCs, white blood cells

Among the studied 30 BD patients, cardiac MRI showed evidence of pericardial effusion in 3 patients. Pericarditis seemed to be the most frequently observed cardiac feature in BD patients, occurring in up to 40% of cardiac involvement [14]. However severe pericardial effusion is not commonly observed [25].

Only 22 cases of intracardiac thrombosis associated with BD were reported from 1992 to 2010, most of the cases were limited to the right ventricle and atrium [14]. In this cohort, we have detected one case with evidence of right ventricular thrombosis.

We could not present any difference in BD activity between patients with and without cardiac

Table 4 Logistic regression analysis for of independent predictors associated with abnormal cardiac MRI in the studied patients (n = 30)

Variable	Odds ratio (95% CI)	95% CI		*P* value
		LL	UL	
Age/years	1.25	0.97	1.59	.08
Sex (male)	4.75	0.64	35.48	.13
Behcet disease duration	1.88	0.72	4.96	.19
Heart rate	1.04	0.85	1.27	.74
SBP	1.32	0.98	1.79	.07
DBP	1.28	1.03	1.59	.03*
BMI	1.26	0.83	1.92	.28
Behcet's disease activity index	0.42	0.18	1.0	.05*
Azathioprine	0.17	0.007	4.03	.270
Cyclosporine	0.79	0.02	33.18	.902
Anticoagulants	0.81	0.03	23.56	.904
Biological agents	1.44	0.03	66.77	.853

BMI, body mass index; CI, confidence interval; DBP, diastolic blood pressure; LL, lower limit; SBP, systolic blood pressure; UL, upper limit

*$P \leq 0.05$

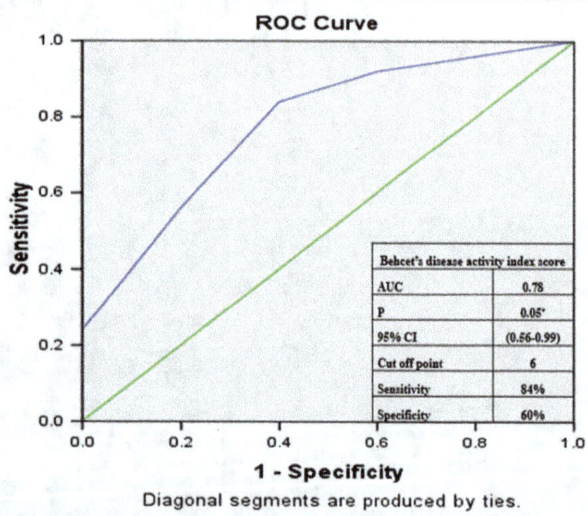

Fig. 2 Receiver operating characteristic (ROC) curve for Behcet's disease activity index score as a predictor of abnormal cardiac MRI (n = 30)

abnormalities. However, the score of BDCAF was among the most significant predictors of cardiac abnormalities in BD patients on logistic regression analysis. Others have shown that cardiac manifestations in BD patients are not proportional to systemic BD activity [39].

Finally, we admit that this study has some limitations; namely, the small sample size, the absence of a matched control group and the cross-sectional nature with only a single evaluation of the heart status in BD patients. Also, there was no information about serum level of important cardiac enzymes as troponin and CK-MB. Advanced cardiac MRI tools as T1/T2 mapping and extra-cellular volume (ECV) quantifications were not part of this study protocol. It would be highly favorable to perform future multi-parametric cardiac MRI studies on patients with BD. However, the detailed assessment of the functional and anatomical cardiac abnormalities and investigating the relation between these abnormalities and BD activity index score are strengths of this study.

Conclusion

BD may cause cardiac abnormalities without clinical manifestations and cardiac MRI may represent a tool for early detection of these subtle abnormalities. Higher BD activity index scores are strongly linked to cardiac problems. Echocardiography may be not enough for screening for cardiac involvement in BD patients and cardiac MRI is recommended especially in those with high BD activity index.

Acknowledgements

Not applicable

Authors' contributions

ST and DA conceived the hypothesis, provided clinical guidance, and interpretation of the findings, AA, NM and ST and performed data collection and drafted the manuscript. AE and AM participated in study design, conducted data analysis, and edited the final manuscript. The authors read and approved the final manuscript.

Author details

[1]Rheumatology and Immunology Unit, Internal Medicine Department, Faculty of Medicine, Mansoura University Hospital, Mansoura University, El Gomhouria St, Mansoura, Dakahlia Governorate, Egypt. [2]Diagnostic and Interventional Radiology Department, Faculty of Medicine, Mansoura University, Mansoura, Dakahlia Governorate, Egypt. [3]Mansoura University Nephrology and Dialysis Unit, Internal Medicine Department, Faculty of Medicine, Mansoura University, Mansoura, Dakahlia Governorate, Egypt.

References

1. Khairallah M, Accorinti M, Muccioli C, Kahloun R, Kempen JH. Epidemiology of Behçet disease. Ocul Immunol Inflamm. 2012;20(5):324–35. https://doi.org/10.3109/09273948.2012.723112.
2. Alpsoy EJT. Behcet's disease: a comprehensive review with a focus on epidemiology, etiology and clinical features, and management of mucocutaneous lesions. J Dermatol. 2016;43(6):620–32. https://doi.org/10.1111/1346-8138.13381.
3. Mazzoccoli G, Matarangolo A, Rubino R, Inglese M, De Cata AJC. Behçet syndrome: from pathogenesis to novel therapies. Clin Exp Med. 2016;16(1):1–12. https://doi.org/10.1007/s10238-014-0328-z.
4. Behcet HJDW. Uber rezidivierende, aphthose, durchein Virus verusachte Gaschwure am Mund, am Auge und an den Genitalien. Dermat Wochsch. 1937;105:1152–7.
5. Yurdakul S, Hamuryudan V, Yazici HJC. Behçet syndrome. Curr Opin Rheumatol. 2004;16(1):38–42. https://doi.org/10.1097/00002281-200401000-00008

6. Yahalom M, Bloch L, Suleiman K, Rosh B, Turgeman Y. Cardiovascular involvement in Behçet disease: clinical implications. Int J Angiol. 2016;25(5):e84–6. https://doi.org/10.1055/s-0035-1551796.
7. Aksu T, Tufekcioglu O. Intracardiac thrombus in Behçet's disease: four new cases and a comprehensive literature review. Rheumatol Int. 2015;35 (7):1269–79. https://doi.org/10.1007/s00296-014-3174-0.
8. Demirelli S, Degirmenci H, Inci S, Arisoy A. Cardiac manifestations in Behcet's disease. Intractable Rare Dis Res. 2015; 4(2):70–5.https://doi.org/10.5582/irdr.2015.01007.
9. Petersen SE, Aung N, Sanghvi MM, Zemrak F, Fung K, Paiva JM, et al. Reference ranges for cardiac structure and function using cardiovascular magnetic resonance (CMR) in Caucasians from the UK Biobank population cohort. J Cardiovasc Magn Reson. 2017;19(1):1–19. https://doi.org/10.1186/s12968-017-0327-9.
10. Disease ITftRotICfBs, Davatchi F, Assaad-Khalil S, Calamia K, Crook J, Sadeghi-Abdollahi B, et al. The International Criteria for Behçet's Disease (ICBD): a collaborative study of 27 countries on the sensitivity and specificity of the new criteria. J Eur Acad Dermatol Venereol. 2014; 28 (3):338–47. https://doi.org/10.1111/jdv.12107.
11. Henry WL, DeMaria A, Gramiak R, King DL, Kisslo JA, Popp RL, et al. Report of the American Society of Echocardiography Committee on nomenclature and standards in two dimensionalechocardiography. Circulation. 1980;62(2):212–7. https://doi.org/10.1161/01.CIR.62.2.212.
12. Verity D, Marr J, Ohno S, Wallace G, Stanford MJT. Behçet's disease, the Silk Road and HLA-B51: historical and geographical perspectives. Tissue Antigens 1999; 54(3):213–20. https://doi.org/10.1034/j.1399-0039.1999.540301.x.
13. Yoshimi R. The diagnosis and management of vasculo-Behçet's disease. Intern Med. 2019; 1657–18.https://doi.org/10.2169/internalmedicine.1657-18.
14. Geri G, Wechsler B, Isnard R, Piette J-C, Amoura Z, Resche-Rigon M, et al. Spectrum of cardiac lesions in Behçet disease: a series of 52 patients and review of the literature. Medicine (Baltimore). 2012;91(1):25–34. https://doi.org/10.1097/MD.0b013e3182428f49.
15. Seetharam K, Lerakis S. Cardiac magnetic resonance imaging: the future is bright. F1000Res. 2019. https://doi.org/10.12688/f1000research.19721.1.
16. Li R, Pu L, Sun Z, Wang Y, Liu G, Xie J, et al. Echocardiographic findings of cardiovascular involvement in Behçet's disease and post-operative complications after cardiac surgery. Clin Exp Rheumatol. 2018;36(6 Suppl 115):103–9.
17. Aktürk E, Yağmur J, Kurtoğlu E, Ermis N, Acikgoz N, Şener S, et al. Left atrial volume and function in patients with Behcet's disease assessed by real-time three-dimensional echocardiography. Eur Heart J Cardiovasc Imaging. 2012;13(8):650–5. https://doi.org/10.1093/ejechocard/jer301.
18. Pu L, Li R, Xie J, Yang Y, Liu G, Wang Y, et al. Characteristic echocardiographic manifestations of Behçet's disease. Ultrasound Med Biol. 2018; 44(4):825–30. https://doi.org/10.1016/j.ultrasmedbio.2017.12.010.
19. Gao N, Han W, Ci WP, Liao H, Du J .[Clinical data analysis of cardiovascular involvement in Behcet's disease]. Zhonghua Yi Xue Za Zhi.2016; 96 (19):1523–6. https://doi.org/10.3760/cma.j.issn.0376-2491.2016.19.013.
20. Higashihara M, Mori M, Takeuchi A, Ogita T, Miyamoto T, Okimoto T. Myocarditis in Behcet's disease--a case report and review of the literature. J Rheumatol. 1982; 9(4):630–3.
21. Maeda S, Tamura A, Zaizen H, Takahashi NJIM. Behçet's disease complicated by giant-cell myocarditis. Intern Med. 2014;53(15):1721. https://doi.org/10.2169/internalmedicine.53.2213.
22. Lakhanpal S, Tani K, Lie JT, Katoh K, Ishigatsubo Y, Ohokubo T. Pathologic features of Behçet's syndrome: a review of Japanese autopsy registry data. Hum Pathol. 1985;16(8):790–5. https://doi.org/10.1016/S0046-8177(85)80250-1.
23. Gannon MP, Schaub E, Grines CL, Saba SG. State of the art: evaluation and prognostication of myocarditis using cardiac MRI. J Magn Reson Imaging. 2019; 49(7):e122-e31. https://doi.org/10.1002/jmri.26611.
24. Kechida M, Jomaa W, Maatouk M. A case of behçet disease myocarditis documented using cardiac magnetic resonance imaging. Can J Cardiol. 2020;36(9):1554.e9-.e11. https://doi.org/10.1016/j.cjca.2020.05.006.
25. Pu L, Li R, Xie J, Yang Y, Liu G, Wang Y, et al. Characteristic echocardiographic manifestations of Behcet's disease. Ultrasound Med Biol. 2018;44(4):825–30. https://doi.org/10.1016/j.ultrasmedbio.2017.12.010.
26. Gao N, Han W, Ci W, Liao H, Du J. Clinical data analysis of cardiovascular involvement in Behcet's disease. Zhonghua Yi Xue Za Zhi. 2016;96(19):1523–6. https://doi.org/10.3760/cma.j.issn.0376-2491.2016.19.013.
27. Bletry O, Mohattane A, Wechsler B, Beaufils P, Valere P, Petit J, et al. Cardiac involvement in Behcet's disease. 12 cases. Presse Med. 1988;17 (45):2388–91.
28. Gürgün C, Ercan E, Ceyhan C, Yavuzgil O, Zoghi M, Aksu K, et al. [Cardiovascular involvement in Behçet's disease]. Rev Med Interne. 2014;35(2):103–11. https://doi.org/10.1016/j.revmed.2013.12.002.
29. Gürgün C, Ercan E, Ceyhan C, Yavuzgil O, Zoghi M, Aksu K, et al. Cardiovascular involvement in Behçet's disease. Jpn Heart J. 2002;43(4):389–98. https://doi.org/10.1536/jhj.43.389.
30. Erkan F. Pulmonary involvement in Behçet disease. Curr Opin Pulm Med. 1999; 5(5):314–8. https://doi.org/10.1097/00063198-199909000-00009.
31. Erkan F, Gül A, Tasali E. Pulmonary manifestations of Behçet's disease. Thorax. 2001;56(7):572–8. https://doi.org/10.1136/thx.56.7.572.
32. Hiller N, Lieberman S, Chajek-Shaul T, Bar-Ziv J, Shaham D. Thoracic manifestations of Behçet disease at CT. Radiographics. 2004; 24 (3):801–8. https://doi.org/10.1148/rg.243035091.
33. Liu H-F, Wang M, Xu Y-S, Lu X-R, Lei J-Q. Left circumflex pseudoaneurysm and left anterior descending aneurysm in coronary artery due to Behcet's disease. Chin Med J (Engl). 2018;131(21):2626. https://doi.org/10.4103/0366-6999.244119.
34. Farhat SB, Slim M. A coronary artery aneurysm revealing a Behçet's disease: a case report. Pan Afr Med J. 2020. https://doi.org/10.11604/pamj.2020.36.3.22373.
35. Maatouk M, Messaoud MB, Mnari W, Bouchahda N, Omri F, Gamra H, et al. A giant aneurysm of the left anterior descending coronary artery in the setting of Behcet's disease: case report. Cardiovasc J Afr. 2020; 31(1):e1-e3. https://doi.org/10.5830/CVJA-2019-031.
36. Abou Sherif S, Ozden Tok O, Taşköylü Ö, Goktekin O, Kilic ID. Coronary artery aneurysms: a review of the epidemiology, pathophysiology, diagnosis, and treatment. Front Cardiovasc Med. 2017; 4:24.https://doi.org/10.3389/fcvm.2017.00024.
37. Chen H, Zhang Y, Li C, Wu W, Liu J, Zhang F, et al. Coronary involvement in patients with Behçet's disease. Clin Rheumatol. 2019;38(10):2835–41. https://doi.org/10.1007/s10067-019-04640-z.
38. Uyaroglu OA, Erden A, Kilic L, Peynircioğlu B, Karadag O, Kalyoncu U. Behçet's disease; A rare refractory patient with vena cava superior syndrome treated with infliximab: a case report and review of the literature. Acta Clin Belg. 2018;74(5):364–9. https://doi.org/10.1080/17843286.2018.1522020.
39. Sun BJ, Park JH, Yoo SJ, Park Y, Kim YJ, Lee IS, et al. Intrinsic changes of left ventricular function in patients with Behçet disease and comparison according to systemic disease activity. Echocardiography. 2018;35(6):809–16. https://doi.org/10.1111/echo.13844.

8

2021 recommendations of the Brazilian Society of Rheumatology for the gynecological and obstetric care of patients with Sjogren's syndrome

Fabiola Reis Oliveira[1], Valeria Valim[2], Sandra Gofinet Pasoto[3], Marilena Leal Mesquita Silvestre Fernandes[4], Maria Lucia Lemos Lopes[5], Sonia Cristina de Magalhães Souza Fialho[6], Aysa César Pinheiro[7], Laura Caldas dos Santos[8], Simone Appenzeller[9], Tania Fidelix[8], Sandra Lucia Euzébio Ribeiro[10], Danielle Christinne Soares Egypto de Brito[11], Tatiana Libório[10], Maria Carmen Lopes Ferreira Silva Santos[12], Leandro Tanure[13], Juliana DAgostino Gennari[14], Vinicius Tassoni Civile[15], Ana Carolina Pereira Nunes Pinto[15], César Ramos Rocha-Filho[15], Samira Tatiyama Miyamoto[16], Lissiane Karine Noronha Guedes[3], Alisson Pugliesi[9*] and Virginia Fernandes Moça Trevisani[15,17]

Abstract

Sjogren's syndrome (SS) is an autoimmune disease characterized by lymphocytic infiltration of the exocrine glands and other organs. Women with SS often experience gynecological symptoms due to the disease and need extra care regarding their sexual activity, reproductive health and during pregnancy, conditions that are not properly conducted in the clinical practice. To cover this gap, a panel of experts from the Brazilian Society of Rheumatology conducted a systematic review and meta-analysis on the identification of symptoms, diagnosis, monitoring, prognosis, and treatment of these manifestations. A Focus Group meeting was held and included experts in the field and methodologists, based on a previously developed script, with themes related to the objective of the study. The most important topics were summarized and 11 recommendations were provided.

Background

Sjogren's syndrome (SS) is an autoimmune disease characterized by lymphocytic infiltration of the exocrine glands and other organs [1]. The disease may occur in isolation, when it is called primary Sjogren's syndrome (pSS), or in conjunction with rheumatoid arthritis (RA), systemic lupus erythematosus (SLE), or another rheumatic disease, when it is called secondary Sjogren's syndrome [2]. pSS is a common disease that affects 0.04–0.08% of people worldwide and has a female to male ratio of 9–14 to 1 [3]. As the process leads to progressively reduced or absent glandular secretion along with mucosal dryness, SS is characterized by symptoms ranging from xerophthalmia, xerostomia, fatigue, myalgia, and arthralgia to severe systemic symptoms with cutaneous, vascular, renal, pulmonary, or neurological involvement [2]. Besides these well-known symptoms, women with SS often experience vaginal dryness and dyspareunia, which result in a substantial disease burden as well

*Correspondence: alissonvigano@gmail.com
[9] Departamento de Ortopedia, Reumatologia e Traumatologia da Faculdade de Ciências Médicas da Universidade Estadual de Campinas (UNICAMP), R. Tessália Vieira de Camargo, 126 - Cidade Universitária, Campinas, SP CEP: 13083-887, Brazil

as reduced quality of life [4]. Despite this, little attention has been given to gynecological and obstetric variables in women with SS [5]. Knowledge of the main gynecological and obstetric characteristics is required for early diagnosis, careful monitoring, and multidisciplinary programs.

To address these gaps, the Sjögren's syndrome Committee of the Brazilian Society of Rheumatology conducted a broad systematic review of the literature on population-based studies investigating gynecological symptoms and obstetric morbidities in Sjogren's patients. The Brazilian Society of Rheumatology gathered the experts in the field and developed recommendations for the screening and management of women with these manifestations. Therefore, the current study represents an effort by this committee with the objective of retrieving the best available evidence and providing guidance for the identification of symptoms, diagnosis, monitoring, prognosis, and treatment of gynecological and obstetric manifestations in women with SS.

Methods

A systematic literature review was conducted of papers on the identification of symptoms, diagnosis, monitoring, prognosis, and treatment of gynecological and obstetric manifestations in women with Sjogren's syndrome. We searched the Cochrane Central Register of Controlled Trials, MEDLINE, Embase, LILACS, and Trip Database for studies published up to January 7th, 2021 (Fig. 1). A search strategy was designed for MEDLINE (Additional file 1: Appendix 1) and adapted for the main electronic

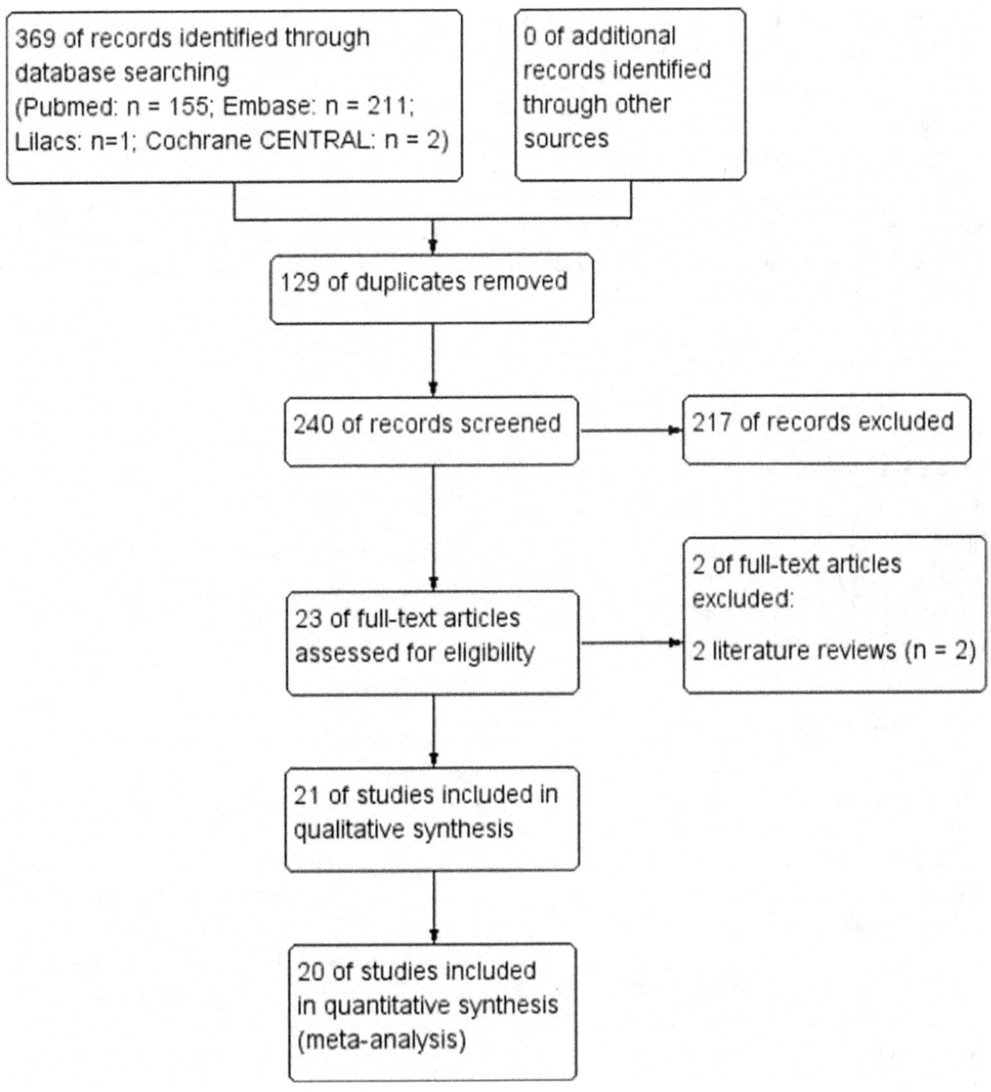

Fig. 1 Study flow diagram

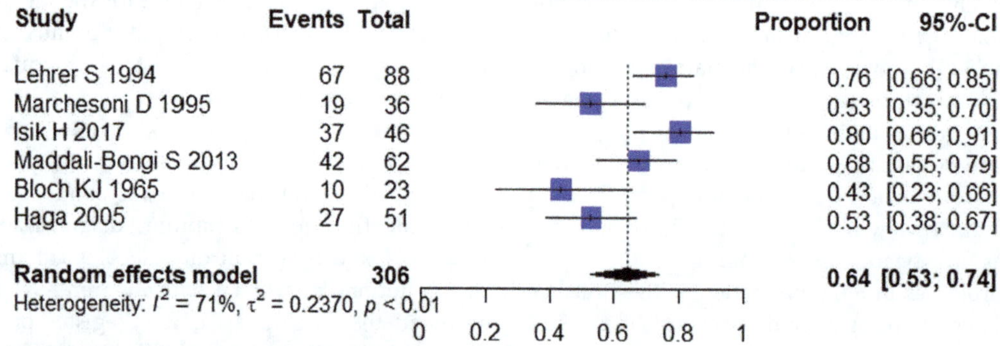

Fig. 2 Meta-analysis of the prevalence of vaginal dryness in women with Sjogren's syndrome

databases. The search was conducted without language, date, or any other type of restriction. The methodological quality of studies reporting prevalence data was evaluated using the Joanna Briggs Institute (JBI) Critical Appraisal Checklist. We pooled clinical data by extracting the number of events and total patients to perform proportion meta-analysis. For studies that presented continuous data as medians and inter-quartile ranges, or as medians and ranges, we estimated means and standard deviations following the method described by Wan et al. [6]. To present pooled results with their respective 95% confidence intervals (CI), we used the "meta" and "metafor" packages from R software (version 3.6.1). We used a generalized linear mixed model (GLMM) method with a random-effects model for pooling the results. To calculate an overall proportion, we used logit transformation. For continuous data, we pooled results of means with their respective 95% CI by the inverse variance method with a random-effects model. A panel composed by specialists in SS and members of the Sjögren's syndrome Committee of Brazilian Society of Rheumatology elaborated question and recommendations. Agreement between the recommendations was achieved in a Focus Group meeting occurred on March 10th, 2020.

Important points—gynecological care

- Women with SS experience more genital discomfort related to dryness of the mucosa, which can be the cause of dyspareunia and decreased satisfaction with sexual activity. There is a prevailing association between these complaints and indices of poor quality of life.
- The coincidence between age of onset and onset of climacteric symptoms in Sjogren's Syndrome can worsen the framework.
- These women are also more predisposed to reproductive disorders that harm fertility, although reduced gonadal reserve and premature ovarian failure are unusual.
- The impact on fertility can be evidenced by oocyte quality and quantity rates, reduced serum levels of anti-mullerian hormone, and increased Luteinizing Hormone (LH) levels. Long menstrual cycles (> 35 days) may be associated with infertility.

Gynecological recommendations

1. Active inquiry regarding genital and sexual complaints is recommended, since they are not spontaneously reported to the rheumatologist. (Hundred percent agreement).
2. Patients should be referred for follow-up with the gynecologist. (Hundred percent agreement).

Gynecological involvement

Vaginal dryness, dyspareunia, genital infections

Women with SS experience vaginal discomfort related to mucosal dryness, which can be the cause of higher rates of dyspareunia and decreased satisfaction with sexual activity in this population [7–10]. The complaints become more relevant in the climacteric period, adding vaginal atrophy related to hypoestrogenism to the preexisting dryness [11]. The most common manifestations were vaginal dryness (prevalence of 64%) and dyspareunia (62%) (Figs. 2, 3; Table 1 on Additional file 1).

Despite the changes occurring in the genital mucosa as a result of local dryness and the increased use of lubricant, there seems to be no high risk of vaginal infections in these cases [12]. Previous data show that premenopausal SS women are not more exposed to vaginal infections than healthy women of the same age, although according to some authors they exhibit more inflammation and vaginal atrophy [12, 13]. Some studies indicate that the pH and composition of the vaginal microbiota are similar between reproductive-age SS patients and

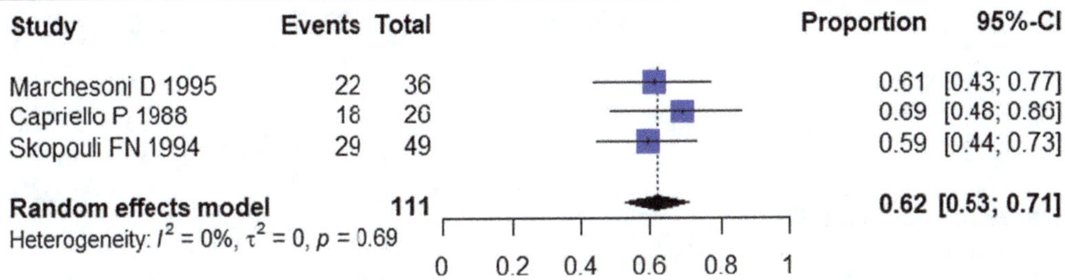

Fig. 3 Meta-analysis of the prevalence of dyspareunia in women with Sjogren's syndrome

healthy controls and the most prevalent genera in this flora (Lactobacillus, Gardnerella, and Streptococcus) are equally found in both cases [14]. In contrast, the changes in vaginal microbiota that occur postmenopause can be explained by hypoestrogenism and worsened by sicca due to SS. Lactobacilli use the breakdown products of glycogen to produce lactic acid, which contributes to low vaginal pH and thereby inhibits the growth of other bacteria. This phenomenon occurs through the influence of estrogen (premenopausal) and makes the health of this epithelium less dependent on dryness [15, 16]. Contradictorily, the oral dryness leads to proliferation of Lactobacillus in the oral mucosa, which contributes to increased dental caries and Candida infection rates [17]. Despite this, additional genital infections can be expected in SS patients considering the set of dryness, hypoestrogenism, therapeutic regimens, and degree of immunosuppression to which they are submitted.

Sexual dysfunction

Sexual dysfunction refers to a multifactorial etiology of symptoms that compromise the quality of general and sexual lives of several individuals, including rheumatic patients, proportionally related to the chronicity of the disease [18]. The evaluation of sexual dysfunction is heterogeneous in different societies, arising from cultural and religious influences. The female sexual function index (FSFI), in Rosen et al. [19], is a female inventory of symptoms that takes into account six main domains: desire, arousal, lubrication, orgasm, satisfaction, and pain. The lower the score achieved, the worse the quality of sexual life reported by the individuals [19]. Pooled results from studies evaluating sexual dysfunction in women with Sjogren's syndrome are displayed in Fig. 4.

Studies on sexual dysfunction conducted in patients with SS and controlled by healthy women in the same age group using this specific instrument demonstrate significant impairment in the sexual life of SS patients. The results show lower means of total score, a lower frequency of sexual intercourse, and a worse index in the domains of lubrication and dyspareunia [5, 20–22].

There is a clear relationship of greater sexual dysfunction with age, with the degree of vaginal dryness, and with the physical impact of the disease (intensity of pain and fatigue measured by ESSPRI) in SS patients. The use of vaginal lubricants, apparently, improves sexual satisfaction in these cases [21].

A considerable proportion of patients do not raise complaints of a gynecological or sexual nature in rheumatological appointments, since they do not associate them with the underlying disease or because of embarrassment [21, 23].

Fertility

Sjogren's syndrome preferably affects women of near-menopausal age and sometimes women of reproductive age. As in other autoimmune diseases (systemic lupus erythematosus, Hashimoto's thyroiditis, etc.), reproductive dysfunctions like reduced gonadal reserve and early ovarian failure may occur [7, 8]. Two studies assessing reproductive dysfunction in women with Sjogren's syndrome were pooled and the results are shown in Additional file 1: Appendix 2 (Fig. 5).

Nevertheless, Lehrer et al. [7], applied questionnaires on gynecological symptoms to 539 patients and the resulting data did not show statistical differences between Sjogren's syndrome females and the healthy American population with respect to fertility rate (10% vs. 10–15%), miscarriage (17% vs. 12–16%), or premature ovarian failure [7]. Skopouli et al., in a Greek cohort study from the same year, supported these findings of no impact on fertility, parity, or age at onset of menopause [8].

Currently, the reduction in fertility can be measured by several parameters. The decrease in serum anti-mullerian hormone, rise in LH serum levels, and reduced amount in quantity and quality of oocytes are some of the methods employed. However, there is no consensus that patients with SS might submit the complete investigation routinely [24]. Prolactin levels may be higher in primary SS patients but it is unclear if there is any association to clinical, hormonal or immunological outcomes [25–27].

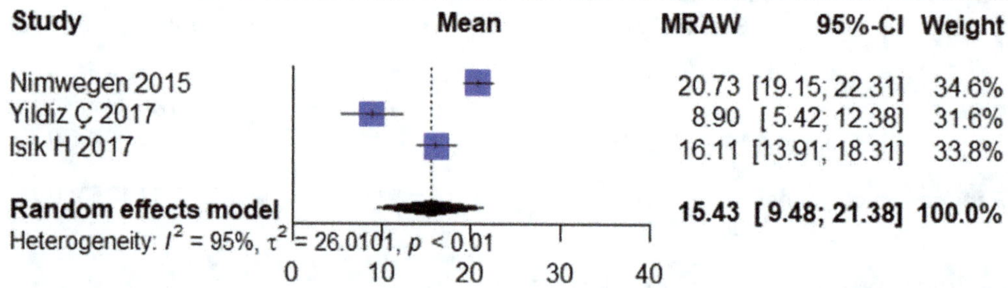

Fig. 4 Meta-analysis of the female sexual function index (FSFI) in women with Sjogren's syndrome

Long menstrual cycles lasting more than 35 days seem to have some relationship with infertility in SS [7].

Endometriosis

Endometriosis is an estrogen-dependent inflammatory disease caused by the implantation of endometrial tissue outside the uterus. It affects 2 to 10% of women of childbearing age and can cause pelvic pain, dysmenorrhea, and infertility [28, 29]. The gold standard of diagnosis is laparoscopy, only indicated in women with relevant symptoms. The phenomenon may occur through a combination of retrograde menstruation and disturbances in immune surveillance. A number of immunological changes have been described in endometriosis since the 80s, leading to the proposal of possible associations with cases of fibromyalgia, thyroiditis, multiple sclerosis, and arthritis. Apparently, SLE and SS are diseases with a higher risk ratio [30].

It remains poorly defined, however, if the immunological alterations described, such as the circulating immunoglobulin surge, detection of anti-endometrial antibodies, and changes in the chemokine profile, could be inducing endometriosis or are simply a consequence of its presence.

It is not possible to stipulate the frequency of the association of endometriosis and SS, due both to different protocols used for diagnosing the first and to the lack of data in SS cohorts.

The majority of registry studies with analysis of a large number of patients with endometriosis in Spain, Denmark, and Israel [31–33] failed to demonstrate an unequivocal association.

Contraception and hormonal replacement therapy

The use of contraceptive methods sometimes includes potential interactions among hormonal contraceptives and other medications, increase in infection risk with intrauterine devices and thrombosis [34] Menopausal hormone therapy (HT) has not been studied in SS patients. Decisions about which contraceptive methods and about the risks and benefits of HT use should be individualized and take into consideration patient´s medical status, tobacco use, family history of hormonal-dependent cancers, laboratory features such as antiphospholipid antibody, and stage of reproductive live [34].

Important points—obstetric care

- Neonatal lupus syndrome (NLS) results from the trans placental passage of maternal anti-SSA/ Ro antibodies around the eleventh week of pregnancy. The most severe manifestation is congenital heart block (CHB) which may require cardiac pacemaker implantation.
- In addition to cardiac conduction system injuries in the newborn, fetal hydrops, liver dysfunctions, cytopenias, and transient skin lesions may also occur.

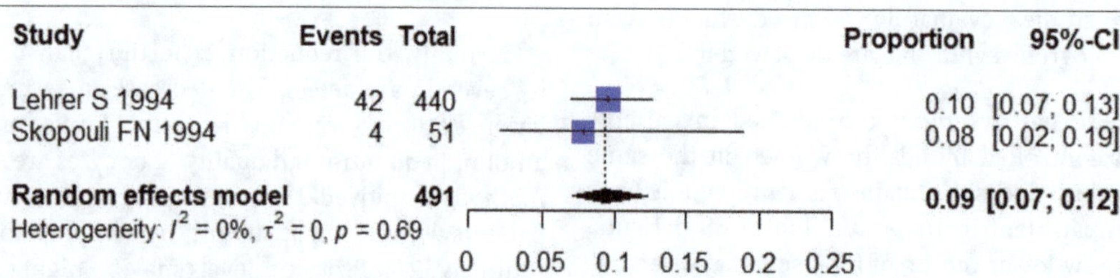

Fig. 5 Meta-analysis of the prevalence of reproductive dysfunction in women with Sjogren's syndrome

Obstetric recommendations

3. All pregnant women with SS should be assisted by a multidisciplinary team in a high-risk prenatal care center, regardless of the controversy in literature data on gestational outcomes such as spontaneous abortion rates, fetal growth restriction, or prematurity. (Hundred percent agreement).
4. It is recommended that the disease be well controlled in the 6 months before pregnancy and that the profile of antiphospholipid and anti-SSA/Ro antibodies be updated. (Hundred percent agreement).
5. Adjustment of pregnancy compatible drugs and specific vitamin supplements for pregnant women are recommended. The use of hydroxychloroquine should be encouraged in positive anti-SSA/Ro pregnant women and it is mandatory in pregnant women with a previous history of fetal heart block or other forms of neonatal lupus. (Hundred percent agreement).

Obstetric recommendations in the presence of Neonatal Lupus Syndrome risk

6. Prenatal care and delivery should be accomplished in a referral Hospital. (Hundred percent agreement).
7. Hydroxychloroquine (5 mg/kg/d) should be prescribed for all positive anti-SSA/Ro pregnant women because of its impact on reducing the recurrence of NLS (which can reach 20%) in subsequent pregnancies, compared to patients who do not use the drug. (Hundred percent agreement).
8. In these pregnant women, the effectiveness of treatment with corticosteroids, human immunoglobulin, β-sympathomimetics, or plasmapheresis is controversial. Dexamethasone may be useful in reversing carditis and incomplete blocks in addition to improving the hemodynamic conditions of the fetus. It is recommended that the decision for treatment be shared and adjusted considering each case. (Hundred percent agreement).
9. Electrocardiogram and weekly fetal echocardiography are recommended in the interval of greatest risk for the onset of heart block (16–26 weeks) and in the newborn. (Hundred percent agreement).
10. All newborns should also be evaluated with a blood count and liver assessment. The risk of these children developing an autoimmune disease in the future is not increased. (Hundred percent agreement).
11. Breastfeeding should be encouraged. (Hundred percent agreement).

Obstetric and fetal manifestations

Obstetric

Although fertility disorders are rare, the likelihood that women with autoimmune inflammatory diseases will have complicated pregnancies is much more significant. Forest plots for the incidence of obstetric and fetal outcomes in patients with Sjogren's syndrome or rheumatic diseases with reactive anti-SSA/Ro antibodies are presented in Figs. 5, 6, 7, 8 and 9. The effects of underlying disease on pregnancy and of pregnancy on maternal health differ depending on the disease, pre-existing systemic damage, profile of autoantibodies, and type of prescription regime [35]. Data on pregnancies in primary Sjogren's syndrome are scarce [5]. In preliminary studies, with retrospective data collection, anti-SSA/Ro antibodies appear as a possible factor causing pregnancy loss [36, 37]. Considering the high frequency of these antibodies in SS patients (60–90%) compared to other rheumatic diseases such as SLE (30–50%) and RA (11%), we could assume higher rates of spontaneous abortions in pSS and in pregnant women with anti-SSA/Ro [38–40]. However, the literature does not show clinical or statistical differences between the outcomes of pregnancy in seropositive or seronegative patients [38–42].

Likewise, for some authors there is a higher rate of premature births and a lower neonatal average weight, explained by pathological restriction on intrauterine growth in SSA-positive pregnant women [43, 44]. Contradictorily, other studies do not show increased rates of prematurity or fetal growth restriction [8, 42, 45]. Even if the literature data are controversial regarding gestational outcomes, all pregnant women should be assisted in a high-risk prenatal care centre [46].

Furthermore, several authors agree that there is a higher rate of cesarean sections in Sjogren's syndrome (see Additional file 1: Table 2).

For a safe pregnancy, SS patients must be well controlled for at least 6 months [46]. Adjustments for tapering and discontinuing some medications that require washout periods should be provided [47]. Mycophenolate mofetil, leflunomide, cyclophosphamide, methotrexate, and biologic disease modifying anti-rheumatic drugs like rituximab, belimumab and tocilizumab are the main drugs to be avoided [47–49]. Dietary supplementation with vitamins, minerals and folic acid should be indicated according to the specifics of each patient, by the gynecologist, in prenatal care. The use of hydroxychoroquine should be encouraged in positive anti-SSA/Ro pregnant women and it is mandatory in pregnant women with a previous history of fetal heart block or other forms of neonatal lupus [50] It´s also recommended to update the profile of antiphospholipid, anti-SSB/La and anti-SSA/Ro antibodies at this time [46, 50].

Neonatal lupus syndrome (NLS)

One of the most feared gestational complications in patients with SS is neonatal lupus syndrome, especially congenital heart block (CHB) [42].

NLS occurs as a result of passive transplacental passage of maternal anti-SSA and/or anti-SSB antibodies at the beginning of pregnancy (~ 11 weeks) [42]. It affects

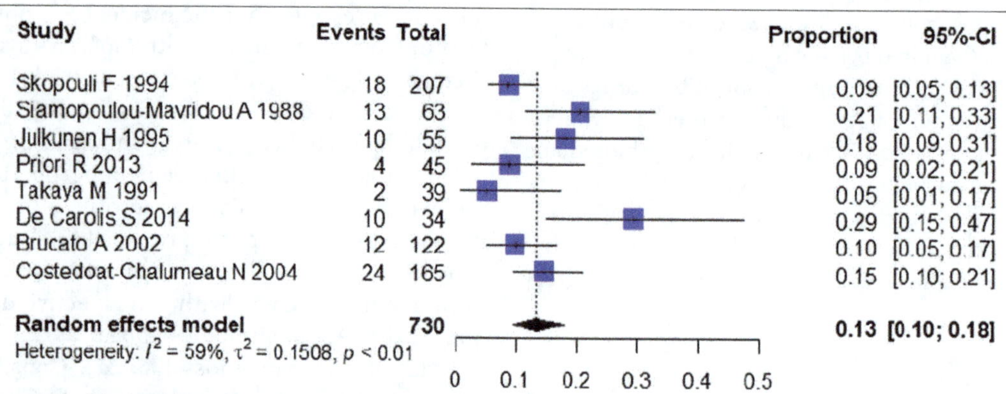

Fig. 6 Meta-analysis of the incidence of spontaneous abortion in women with Sjogren's syndrome or rheumatic diseases with reactive anti-SSA/Ro antibodies during pregnancy

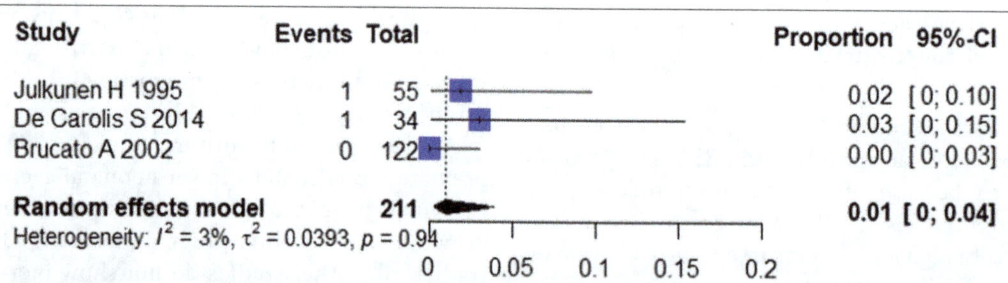

Fig. 7 Meta-analysis of the incidence of intrauterine growth retardation in fetuses of women with Sjogren's syndrome or rheumatic diseases with reactive anti-SSA/Ro antibodies

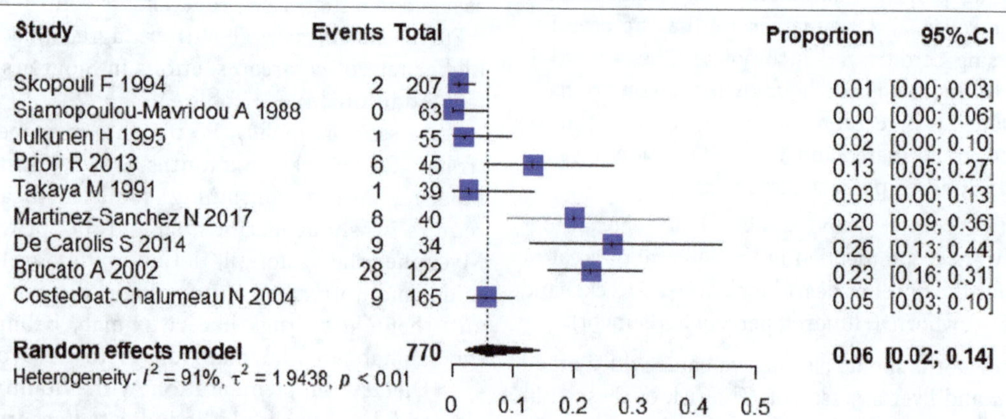

Fig. 8 Meta-analysis of the incidence of premature delivery in pregnant women with Sjogren's syndrome or rheumatic diseases with reactive anti-SSA/Ro antibodies

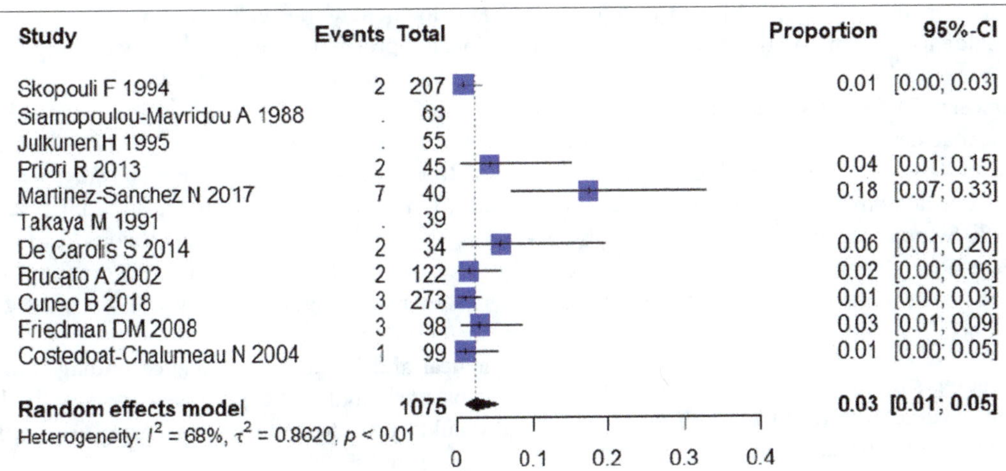

Fig. 9 Meta-analysis of the incidence of congenital autoimmune heart block in fetuses of women with Sjogren's syndrome or rheumatic diseases with reactive anti-SSA/Ro antibodies

similarly male and female fetuses and can cause cardiac disease [42–45], skin lesions, cytopenias, neurological and hepatobiliary manifestations in the newborn [51–54]. All the extracardiac injuries, usually mild and self-limited, may be present at birth or develop during the first months of life [51, 55]. Laboratory abnormalities in asymptomatic babies can be identified in up to one third of cases [51, 52, 54].

Among the most significant cardiac injuries are arrhythmogenic damage to the conduction system, such as congenital autoimmune heart block (AVBc), endocardial fibroelastosis, and myocarditis, which can progress to dilated cardiomyopathy [55–63]. The increased risk period for the development of fetal heart injury is between 16 and 26 weeks of pregnancy and it can be detected by fetal echocardiography [42, 58, 64–66]. In some studies, the prevalence of congenital autoimmune heart block (defined as atrioventricular block diagnosed in utero, at birth, or in the neonatal period) reaches 1–2% [46, 55, 56].

Irreversible third degree CBH is the most serious manifestation of NLS, requiring cardiac pacemaker implantation and beings associated with higher rates of intrauterine and perinatal mortality [57, 67]. Electric conduction blocks, regardless of degree, can be detected by prenatal ultrasound between 18 and 24 weeks of gestation [68]. Fetal bradycardia is the main finding, often the only one. Due to the existence of the gap between the transfer of maternal antibodies and development of the electric fetal conduction system (~ 12 weeks) and the late clinical observation of CHB (~ 20 weeks), without other structural fetal abnormalities, it becomes very difficult to fix any effective therapeutic intervention [68].

Sinus bradycardia, atrioventricular nodal dysfunction, and increased QT interval are also included electrocardiographic disorders [57, 58, 68].

Some fetuses (6% of all cases of AVBc) may develop dilated cardiomyopathy and die from congestive heart failure or still require a heart transplant. Valve malformations, pulmonary artery stenosis, and atrial or ventricular septal defects have been reported occasionally [59–62]. Fetal necropsy findings also reveal unsuspected fibrotic lesions of the sinoatrial node [62].

Interestingly, asymptomatic fetuses and newborn infants with incomplete AV changes can evolve with a variable spectrum of cardiac injuries, even later and in the absence of circulating maternal antibodies, suggesting that an intrinsic factor (the fetal itself or the intrauterine environment) might be relevant in the progression of lesions [63].

A cardiac pacemaker is implanted in most of these fetuses in the neonatal period. Even asymptomatic patients with AVBc have an indication for prophylactic pacemaker implantation, due to the unpredictable risk of Stokes-Adams attacks [63, 64]. Intrauterine and neonatal mortality due to AVBc affects up to 30% of cases when associated with fetal hydrops and prematurity, even with advanced intensive care support [64].

The literature is controversial regarding the effectiveness of pharmacological therapy, be it the use of fluorinated corticosteroids that are resistant to the placental enzyme action or IVIG for the prevention or treatment of CHB. The rationale for this type of management in an attempt to obtain better outcomes for the fetus would be to: 1—reduce circulating maternal antibodies and placental transfer; 2—reduce cardiac tissue inflammation before fibrosis and irreversible AVBc [69–73]. However, there is not enough evidence that this actually occurs or that the therapy can prevent AVBc, and safety of some regimes remains a concern [74–76]. In selected cases, studies support the idea that dexamethasone (but not prednisone) can reverse carditis and incomplete blocks in addition to improving the hemodynamic conditions of the fetus [71–74, 77, 78]. Sympathomimetic agent improves bradycardia but does not influence the prognosis [68, 79]. Plasmapheresis has been reported as a therapeutic option in a few case reports [80].

The multicenter study by Cuneo et al. [81], followed 315 pregnant women with anti SSA/Ro antibodies through home monitoring, using a device for measuring the fetal heart rate and rhythm twice a day, and showed that the window of opportunity for therapeutic intervention is very slight [81].

The recurrence of AVBc in a subsequent pregnancy is approximately 10 times greater [78, 82] and the rate of NLS reaches 20% [68, 83]. Hydroxychloroquine (HCQ) impacts on reducing these outcomes and it has not been related to fetal malformations or hearing and visual risks evaluated in the first year of life [74, 75, 83, 84]. Several retrospective studies suggest that women taking hydroxychloroquine are less likely to have a fetus with second- or third-degree heart block [50, 84]. Most authors recommend the administration of HCQ before conception and another part as soon as the patient with positive anti-SSA becomes pregnant [50' 83' 84].

Management of the newborn with NLS

Specific procedures are adopted according to the manifestation presented by each child [85].

Skin lesion A transient, erythematous-desquamative or erythematous-annular and photosensitive skin rash similar to that found in SLE can appear at birth (20%) and up to 2–3 months later (80%). The lesions last for the period of clearance of the circulating maternal antibodies and usually resolve spontaneously without leaving scars, and therefore do not require drug treatment [86, 87]. Histological and immunofluorescence findings are similar to subacute cutaneous lupus. Newborns with skin lesions should be protected from sun exposure until complete regression [85, 88].

Cytopenias: Thrombocytopenia, anemia, and neutropenia are described in NLS. According to Cimaz et al., [52], inconspicuous hematological variations can occur in up to 27% of those born to positive anti-SSA mothers and revert spontaneously. Cases of anemia or severe thrombocytopenia may require blood transfusions, the use of corticosteroids, and intravenous human immunoglobulin in their treatment [52, 89, 90].

Hepatic Liver disorders range from a slight increase in serum transaminases to severe cholestatic syndrome, hepatomegaly and, rarely, splenomegaly [52, 53, 91].

Neurological Non-specific CNS anomalies on cerebral image, in absent of clinical neurological findings, are

Table 1 Brazilian recommendations for the gynecological and obstetric care of women of Sjogren Syndrome

1	Active inquiry regarding genital and sexual complaints is recommended, since they are not spontaneously reported to the rheumatologist. (hundred percent agreement)
2	Patients should be referred for follow-up with the gynecologist (hundred percent agreement)
3	All pregnant women with SS should be assisted by a multidisciplinary team in a high-risk prenatal care center, regardless of the literature data on gestational outcomes such as spontaneous abortion rates, fetal growth restriction or prematurity (hundred percent agreement)
4	It is recommended that the disease be well controlled in the 6 months before pregnancy and that the profile of antiphospholipid and anti-SSA/Ro antibodies be updated. (hundred percent agreement)
5	Adjustment of pregnancy compatible drugs and specific vitamin supplements for pregnant women are recommended. The use of hydroxychloroquine should be encouraged in positive anti-SSA/Ro pregnant women and it is mandatory in pregnant women with a previous history of fetal heart block or other forms of neonatal lupus (hundred percent agreement)
6	Prenatal care and delivery should be accomplished in a referral hospital (hundred percent agreement)
7	Hydroxychloroquine (5 mg/kg/d) should be prescribed for all positive anti SSA/Ro pregnant women because of its impact on reducing the recurrence of NLS (which can reach 20%) in subsequent pregnancies, compared to patients who do not use the drug (hundred percent agreement)
8	In these pregnant women, the effectiveness of treatment with corticosteroids, human immunoglobulin, β-sympathomimetics, or plasmapheresis is controversial. Dexamethasone may be useful in reversing carditis and incomplete blocks in addition to improving the hemodynamic conditions of the fetus. It is recommended that the decision for treatment be shared and adjusted considering each case (hundred percent agreement)
9	Electrocardiogram and weekly fetal echocardiography are recommended in the interval of greatest risk for the onset of heart block (CHB) and in the newborn (12–22 weeks) (hundred percent agreement)
10	All newborns should also be evaluated with a blood count and liver assessment. The risk of these children developing an autoimmune disease in the future is not increased (hundred percent agreement)
11	Breastfeeding should be encouraged (hundred percent agreement)

reported in newborns with NLS [51, 54]. The anomalies resolve during follow-up and do not present any clinical correlate.

Cardiac The most common involvement is AVBc of the first, second, and third degrees usually without structural cardiac lesions. The treatment of intrauterine fetal atrioventricular block is often disappointing and more than 90% of affected newborns undergo definitive pacemaker implantation. Fortunately, these children can lead practically normal lives if there is no associated cardiomyopathy [92].

After birth, a progressive reduction of anti SSA/Ro blood titers occurs over 6 months.

A clinical and laboratorial follow-up should be performed in all infants, until the first year of life [51]. The risk of children with NLS developing autoimmune diseases in the future is not superior than the risk of asymptomatic children born to mothers with autoimmune diseases. There is no contraindication to breastfeeding [52, 92, 93].

The topic of neonatal lupus syndrome is vast, especially in the field of fetal heart block, and goes beyond Sjogren´s syndrome. We do not intend to exhaust all the content in this approach (Table 1).

Conclusions

Despite its importance, the gynecological and obstetric care of patients with SS are not as properly incorporated in the clinical practice, as sicca symptoms or extra glandular manifestations are. A significative prevalence of gynecological symptoms and obstetric care needs were identified in this systematic review and meta-analysis as well a high morbidity associated with them. To attend these demands and improve pSS women´s health care, our panel of specialists developed eleven recommendations, all of them with high agreement between the members. A limitation of our guideline was the absence of a patient representative or a gynecologist/obstetric in the voting panel, a strategy that will be used in future guidelines.

Supplementary Information

Additional file 1. Table 1: Gynecological symptoms in Sjogren´s syndrome patients. **Table 2**: Gestational outcomes in patients with Sjogren's syndrome or rheumatic diseases with reactive anti-SSA / Ro antibodies.

Acknowledgements

Not applicable.

Authors' contributions

All authors made contributions to the acquisition of data, have been involved in drafting the manuscript or revising it critically for important intellectual content, participated in the voting rounds, gave final approval of the version to be published and have participated sufficiently in the work to take public responsibility for appropriate portions of the content. All authors read and approved the final manuscript.

Author details

[1]Hospital das Clínicas da Faculdade de Medicina de Ribeirão Preto (HCFMRP-USP), Av. Bandeirantes, 3900, Vila Monte Alegre, Ribeirão Preto, SP CEP: 14049-900, Brazil. [2]Serviço de Reumatologia, Hospital Universitário Cassiano Antônio de Moraes, Universidade Federal do Espírito Santo, Av. Marechal Campos, 1468, Maruípe, Vitória, ES CEP: 29075-910, Brazil. [3]Disciplina de Reumatologia, Laboratório de Autoimunidade (DLC + LIM17), Hospital das Clínicas da Faculdade de Medicina da USP (HCFMUSP), R. Dr. Ovídio Pires de Campos, 225 - Cerqueira César, São Paulo, SP CEP: 05403-010, Brazil. [4]Disciplina de Reumatologia, Hospital Federal dos Servidores do Estado do Rio de Janeiro,, R. Sacadura Cabral, 178, Saúde, Rio de Janeiro, RJ CEP: 20221-903, Brazil. [5]Disciplina de Reumatologia Departamento de Clínica Médica, Universidade Federal de Ciências da Saúde de Porto Alegre (UFCSPA),, R. Sarmento Leite, 245 - Centro Histórico de Porto Alegre, Porto Alegre, RS CEP: 90050-170, Brazil. [6]Serviço de Reumatologia, Universidade Federal de Santa Catarina, R. Profa. Maria Flora Pausewang, s/n - Trindade, Florianópolis, SC CEP: 88036-800, Brazil. [7]Disciplina de Reumatologia, Departamento de Clínica Médica, Universidade Federal de Pernambuco, Av. Prof. Moraes Rego, 1235, Cidade Universitária, Recife, PE CEP: 50670-901, Brazil. [8]Departamento de Oftalmologia, Escola Paulista de Medicina-Universidade Federal de São Paulo (EPM-UNIFESP), Rua Botucatu, 820, Vila Clementino, Sao Paulo, SP CEP: 04023-062, Brazil. [9]Departamento de Ortopedia, Reumatologia e Traumatologia da Faculdade de Ciências Médicas da Universidade Estadual de Campinas (UNICAMP), R. Tessália Vieira de Camargo, 126 - Cidade Universitária, Campinas, SP CEP: 13083-887, Brazil. [10]Disciplina de Reumatologia, Universidade Federal do Amazonas, Rua Afonso Pena, 1053, Manaus, AM CEP: 69020-160, Brazil. [11]Disciplina de Reumatologia, Departamento de Medicina Interna, Centro de Ciências Médicas, Universidade Federal de Paraíba (UFPB), Campus I - Lot. Cidade Universitária, Paraíba, PB CEP: 58051-900, Brazil. [12]Departamento de Patologia, Hospital Universitário Cassiano Antônio de Moraes, Universidade Federal do Espírito Santo, Av. Marechal Campos, 1468, Maruípe, Vitória, ES CEP: 29075-910, Brazil. [13]Disciplina de Reumatologia, Universidade Federal de Minas Gerais, Av. Pres. Antônio Carlos, 6627, Pampulha, Belo Horizonte, MG CEP: 31270-901, Brazil. [14]Serviço de Reumatologia da Santa Casa de São Paulo, R. Dr. Cesário Mota Júnior, 112, Vila Buarque, São Paulo, SP CEP: 01221-020, Brazil. [15]Disciplina de Medicina de Urgência e Medicina Baseada em Evidências, Escola Paulista de Medicina-Universidade Federal de São Paulo (EPM-UNIFESP), Rua Botucatu 740 Vila Clementino, São Paulo, SP CEP: 04023-062, Brazil. [16]Departamento de Educação Integrada em Saúde, Universidade Federal do Espírito Santo (UFES), Av. Marechal Campos, 1468, Maruípe, Vitória, ES CEP: 29040-090, Brazil. [17]Disciplina de Reumatologia, Universidade de Santo Amaro, Rua Enéas Siqueira Neto, Jardim das Imbuias, São Paulo, SP CEP: 04829-300, Brazil.

References

1. Shiboski CH, Shiboski SC, Seror R, Criswell LA, Labetoulle M, Lietman TM, et al. 2016 American College of Rheumatology/European League Against Rheumatism classification criteria for primary Sjogren's syndrome: a consensus and data-driven methodology involving three international patient cohorts. Arthritis Rheumatol. 2017;69(2326–5205 (Electronic)):35–45.
2. Patel R, Shahane A. The epidemiology of Sjogren's syndrome. Clin Epidemiol. 2014;30(1179–1349 (Print)):247–55.
3. Qin B, Wang J, Yang Z, Yang M, Ma N, Huang F, et al. Epidemiology of primary Sjögren's syndrome: a systematic review and meta-analysis. Ann Rheum Dis. 2015;74(11):1983. https://doi.org/10.1136/annrheumdis-2014-205375.
4. Fox RI. Sjögren's syndrome. Lancet. 2005;366(9482):321–31. https://doi.org/10.1016/S0140-6736(05)66990-5.
5. van Nimwegen JF, Arends S, van Zuiden GS, Vissink A, Kroese FG, Bootsma H. The impact of primary Sjögren's syndrome on female sexual function.

Rheumatology (Oxford). 2015;54(7):1286–93. https://doi.org/10.1093/rheumatology/keu522.
6. Wan X, Wang W, Liu J, Tong T. Estimating the sample mean and standard deviation from the sample size, median, range and/or interquartile range. BMC Med Res Methodol. 2014;14:135. https://doi.org/10.1186/1471-2288-14-135.
7. Lehrer S, Bogursky E, Yemini M, Kase NG, Birkenfeld A. Gynecologic manifestations of Sjögren's syndrome. Am J Obstet Gynecol. 1994;170(3):835–7. https://doi.org/10.1016/s0002-9378(94)70294-2.
8. Skopouli FN, Papanikolaou S, Malamou-Mitsi V, Papanikolaou N, Moutso poulos HM. Obstetric and gynaecological profile in patients with primary Sjögren's syndrome. Ann Rheum Dis. 1994;53(9):569–73. https://doi.org/10.1136/ard.53.9.569.
9. Mulherin DM, Sheeran TP, Kumararatne DS, Speculand B, Luesley D, Situnayake RD. Sjögren's syndrome in women presenting with chronic dyspareunia. BJOG Int J Obstet Gynaecol. 1997;104(9):1019–23. https://doi.org/10.1111/j.1471-0528.1997.tb12060.x.
10. Bloch KJ, Buchanan WW, Wohl MJ, Bunim JJ. Sjogren's Syndrome. A clinical, pathological, and serological study of sixty-two cases. Medicine (Baltimore). 1965;44:187–231.
11. Marchesoni D, Mozzanega B, De Sandre P, Romagnolo C, Gambari PF, Maggino T. Gynaecological aspects of primary Sjogren's syndrome. Eur J Obstet Gynecol Reprod Biol. 1995;63(1):49–53. https://doi.org/10.1016/0301-2115(95)02224-u.
12. van der Meulen TA, van Nimwegen JF, Harmsen HJM, Liefers SC, van der Tuuk K, Kroese FGM, et al. Normal vaginal microbiome in women with primary Sjögren's syndrome-associated vaginal dryness. Ann Rheum Dis. 2019;78(5):707–9. https://doi.org/10.1136/annrheumdis-2018-214404.
13. Capriello P, Barale E, Cappelli N, Lupo S, Teti G. Sjögren's syndrome: clinical, cytological, histological and colposcopic aspects in women. Clin Exp Obstet Gynecol. 1988;15(1–2):9–12.
14. Ravel J, Gajer P, Abdo Z, Schneider GM, Koenig SSK, McCulle SL, et al. Vaginal microbiome of reproductive-age women. Proc Natl Acad Sci. 2011;108(Supplement 1):4680–7. https://doi.org/10.1073/pnas.1002611107.
15. Hummelen R, Macklaim JM, Bisanz JE, Hammond JA, McMillan A, Vongsa R, et al. Vaginal microbiome and epithelial gene array in post-menopausal women with moderate to severe dryness. PLoS ONE. 2011;6(11): e26602. https://doi.org/10.1371/journal.pone.0026602.
16. van Nimwegen JF, van der Tuuk K, Liefers SC, Verstappen GM, Visser A, Wijnsma RF, Vissink A, Hollema H, et al. Vaginal dryness in primary Sjögren's syndrome: a histopathological case–control study. Rheumatology. 2020;59(10):2806–15. https://doi.org/10.1093/rheumatology/keaa017.
17. van der Meulen TA, Harmsen HJM, Bootsma H, Liefers SC, Vich Vila A, Zhernakova A, et al. Dysbiosis of the buccal mucosa microbiome in primary Sjögren's syndrome patients. Rheumatology (Oxford). 2018;57(12):2225–34. https://doi.org/10.1093/rheumatology/key215.
18. Ferreira C, da Mota LM, Oliveira AC, de Carvalho JF, Lima RA, Simaan CK, et al. Frequency of sexual dysfunction in women with rheumatic diseases. Rev Bras Reumatol. 2013;53(1):35–46. https://doi.org/10.1016/s2255-5021(13)70004-x.
19. Rosen R, Brown C, Heiman J, Leiblum S, Meston C, Shabsigh R, et al. The Female Sexual Function Index (FSFI): a multidimensional self-report instrument for the assessment of female sexual function. J Sex Marital Ther. 2000;26(2):191–208. https://doi.org/10.1080/009262300278597.
20. Yildiz Ç, Karakuş S, Bozoklu Akkar Ö, Şahin A, Bozkurt B, Yanik A. Primary Sjögren's syndrome adversely affects the female sexual function assessed by the female sexual function index: a case–control study. Arch Rheumatol. 2017;32(2):1238. https://doi.org/10.5606/ArchRheumatol.2017.6066.
21. Isik H, Isik M, Aynioglu O, Karcaaltincaba D, Sahbaz A, Beyazcicek T, et al. Are the women with Sjögren's Syndrome satisfied with their sexual activity? Rev Bras Reumatol. 2017;57:210–6.
22. Priori R, Minniti A, Derme M, Antonazzo B, Brancatisano F, Ghirini S, et al. Quality of sexual life in women with primary Sjögren syndrome. J Rheumatol. 2015;42(8):1427–31. https://doi.org/10.3899/jrheum.141475.
23. Maddali Bongi S, Del Rosso A, Orlandi M, Matucci-Cerinic M. Gynaecological symptoms and sexual disability in women with primary Sjögren's syndrome and sicca syndrome. Clin Exp Rheumatol. 2013;31(5):683–90.
24. Karakus S, Sahin A, Durmaz Y, Aydin H, Yildiz C, Akkar O, et al. Evaluation of ovarian reserve using anti-müllerian hormone and antral follicle count in Sjögren's syndrome: preliminary study. J Obstet Gynaecol Res. 2017;43(2):303–7. https://doi.org/10.1111/jog.13216.
25. El Miedany YM, Ahmed I, Moustafa H, El Baddini M. Hyperprolactinemia in Sjogren's syndrome: a patient subset or a disease manifestation? Joint Bone Spine. 2004;71(3):203–8. https://doi.org/10.1016/S1297-319X(03)00151-9.
26. Haga HJ, Rygh T. The prevalence of hyperprolactinemia in patients with primary Sjögren's syndrome. J Rheumatol. 1999;26(6):1291–5.
27. Gutiérrez MA, Anaya JM, Scopelitis E, Citera G, Silveira L, Espinoza LR. Hyperprolactinaemia in primary Sjögren's syndrome. Ann Rheum Dis. 1994;53(6):425. https://doi.org/10.1136/ard.53.6.425-a.PMID:8037502; PMCID:PMC1005360.
28. Bulun SE. Endometriosis. N Engl J Med. 2009;360(3):268–79. https://doi.org/10.1056/NEJMra0804690.
29. Shigesi N, Kvaskoff M, Kirtley S, Feng Q, Fang H, Knight JC, et al. The association between endometriosis and autoimmune diseases: a systematic review and metaanalysis. Hum Reprod Update. 2019;25(4):486–503. https://doi.org/10.1093/humupd/dmz014.
30. Sinaii N, Cleary SD, Ballweg ML, Nieman LK, Stratton P. High rates of autoimmune and endocrine disorders, fibromyalgia, chronic fatigue syndrome and atopic diseases among women with endometriosis: a survey analysis. Hum Reprod. 2002;17(10):2715–24. https://doi.org/10.1093/humrep/17.10.2715.
31. Matorras R, Ocerin I, Unamuno M, Nieto A, Peiró E, Burgos J, et al. Prevalence of endometriosis in women with systemic lupus erythematosus and Sjögren's syndrome. Lupus. 2007;16(9):736–40. https://doi.org/10.1177/0961203307081339.
32. Nielsen NM, Jørgensen KT, Pedersen BV, Rostgaard K, Frisch M. The cooccurrence of endometriosis with multiple sclerosis, systemic lupus erythematosus and Sjogren syndrome. Hum Reprod. 2011;26(6):1555–9. https://doi.org/10.1093/humrep/der105.
33. Greenbaum H, Weil C, Chodick G, Shalev V, Eisenberg VH. Evidence for an association between endometriosis, fibromyalgia, and autoimmune diseases. Am J Reprod Immunol. 2019;81(4): e13095. https://doi.org/10.1111/aji.13095.
34. Ammaritano LR. Therapy insight: guidelines for selection of contraception in women with rheumatic diseases. Nat Clin Pract Rheumatol. 2007;3(5):273–81. https://doi.org/10.1038/ncprheum0484 (**quiz 305-6**).
35. Carvalheiras G, Faria R, Braga J, Vasconcelos C. Fetal outcome in autoimmune diseases. Autoimmun Rev. 2012;11(6–7):A520–30. https://doi.org/10.1016/j.autrev.2011.12.002.
36. Watson RM, Braunstein BL, Watson AJ, Hochberg MC, Provost TT. Fetal wastage in women with anti-Ro(SSA) antibody. J Rheumatol. 1986;13(1):90–4.
37. Hull R, Harris E, Morgan S, Hughes G. Anti-Ro antibodies and abortions in women with SLE. Lancet. 1983;2:1138.
38. Routsias JG, Tzioufas AG. Sjögren's syndrome-study of autoantigens and autoantibodies. Clin Rev Allergy Immunol. 2007;32:238–51. https://doi.org/10.1007/s12016-0078003-8.
39. Franceschini F, Cavazzana I. Anti-Ro/SSA and La/SSB antibodies. Autoimmunity. 2005;38(1):55–63. https://doi.org/10.1080/08916930400022954.
40. Satoh M, Chan EK, Ho LA, Rose KM, Parks CG, Cohn RD, et al. Prevalence and sociodemographic correlates of antinuclear antibodies in the United States. Arthritis Rheum. 2012;64(7):2319–27. https://doi.org/10.1002/art.34380.
41. Mavragani CP, Dafni UG, Tzioufas AG, Moutsopoulos HM. Pregnancy outcome and anti-Ro/SSA in autoimmune diseases: a retrospective cohort study. Br J Rheumatol. 1998;37(7):740–5. https://doi.org/10.1093/rheumatology/37.7.740.
42. Brucato A, Cimaz R, Caporali R, Ramoni V, Buyon J. Pregnancy outcomes in patients with autoimmune diseases and anti-Ro/SSA antibodies. Clin Rev Allergy Immunol. 2011;40(1):27–41. https://doi.org/10.1007/s12016-009-8190-6.
43. Priori R, Gattamelata A, Modesti M, Colafrancesco S, Frisenda S, Minniti A, et al. Outcome of pregnancy in Italian patients with primary Sjögren syndrome. J Rheumatol. 2013;40(7):1143–7. https://doi.org/10.3899/jrheum.121518
44. Hussein SZ, Jacobsson LT, Lindquist PG, Theander E. Pregnancy and fetal outcome in women with primary Sjogren's syndrome compared with women in the general population: a nested case-control study. Rheumatology (Oxford). 2011;50(9):1612–7. https://doi.org/10.1093/rheumatology/ker077.

45. Martínez-Sánchez N, Pérez-Pinto S, Robles-Marhuenda Á, Arnalich-Fernández F, Martín Cameán M, Hueso Zalvide E, et al. Obstetric and perinatal outcome in anti Ro/SSA-positive pregnant women: a prospective cohort study. Immunol Res. 2017;65(2):487–94. https://doi.org/10.1007/s12026-016-8888-5.
46. Gupta S, Gupta N. Sjögren Syndrome And Pregnancy: a literature review. Perm J. 2017;21:16–047. https://doi.org/10.7812/TPP/16-047.
47. Korpen CG, Hoeltzenbein M, Tincani A, Fischer-betz R, Elefant E, Chambers C, et al. The EULAR points to consider for use of antirheumatic drugs before pregnancy, and during pregnancy and lactation. Ann Rheumatic Dis. 2016. https://doi.org/10.1136/annrheumdis-2015-208840.
48. Flint J, Panchal S, Hurrell A, van de Venne M, Gayed M, Schreiber K, et al. BSR and BHPR guideline on prescribing drugs in pregnancy and breastfeeding-Part I: standard and biologic disease modifying anti-rheumatic drugs and corticosteroids. Rheumatology (Oxford). 2016. https://doi.org/10.1093/rheumatology/kev404.
49. Flint J, Panchal S, Hurrell A, van de Venne M, Gayed M, Schreiber K, et al. BSR and BHPR guideline on prescribing drugs in pregnancy and breastfeeding-Part II: analgesics and other drugs used in rheumatology practice. Rheumatology (Oxford). 2016. https://doi.org/10.1093/rheumatology/kev405.
50. Tunks RD, Clowse MEB, Miller SG, Brancazio LR, Barker PCA. Maternal autoantibody levels in congenital heart block and potential prophylaxis with antiinflammatory agents. Am J Obstet Gynecol. 2013;208(1):64.e1-7. https://doi.org/10.1016/j.ajog.2012.09.020.
51. Zuppa AA, Riccardi R, Frezza S, Gallini F, Luciano RM, Alighieri G, Romagnoli C, De Carolis S. Neonatal lupus: Follow-up in infants with anti-SSA/Ro antibodies and review of the literature. Autoimmun Rev. 2017;16(4):427–32. https://doi.org/10.1016/j.autrev.2017.02.010.
52. Cimaz R, Spence DL, Hornberger L, Silverman ED. Incidence and spectrum of neonatal lupus erythematosus: A prospective study of infants born to mothers with anti-Ro autoantibodies. J Pediatr. 2003;142(6):678–83. https://doi.org/10.1067/mpd.2003.233.
53. Motta M, Rodriguez-Perez C, Tincani A, Lojacono A, Chirico G. Outcome of infants from mothers with anti-SSA/Ro antibodies. J Perinatol. 2007;27(5):278–83. https://doi.org/10.1038/sj.jp.7211688.
54. Boros CA, Spence D, Blaser S, Silverman ED. Hydrocephalus and macrocephaly: new manifestations of neonatal lupus erythematosus. Arthritis Rheum. 2007;57(2):261–6. https://doi.org/10.1002/art.22543.
55. Julkunen H, Kaaja R, Kurki P, Palosuo T, Friman C. Fetal outcome in women with primary Sjögren's syndrome. A retrospective case-control study. Clin Exp Rheumatol. 1995;13(1):65–71.
56. Costedoat-Chalumeau N, Amoura Z, Lupoglazoff JM, Huong DL, Denjoy I, Vauthier D, et al. Outcome of pregnancies in patients with anti-SSA/Ro antibodies: a study of 165 pregnancies, with special focus on electrocardiographic variations in the children and comparison with a control group. Arthritis Rheum. 2004;50(10):3187–94. https://doi.org/10.1002/art.20554.
57. Gerosa M, Cimaz R, Stramba-Badiale M, Goulene K, Meregalli E, Trespidi L, et al. Electrocardiographic abnormalities in infants born from mothers with autoimmune diseases—a multicentre prospective study. Rheumatology. 2007;46(8):1285–9. https://doi.org/10.1093/rheumatology/kem073.
58. Brucato A, Frassi M, Franceschini F, Cimaz R, Faden D, Pisoni MP, et al. Risk of congenital complete heart block in newborns of mothers with anti-Ro/SSA antibodies detected by counterimmunoelectrophoresis: a prospective study of 100 women. Arthritis Rheum. 2001;44(8):1832–5. https://doi.org/10.1002/1529-0131(200108)44:8%3c1832::Aidart320%3e3.0.Co;2-c.
59. Eronen M, Sirèn MK, Ekblad H, Tikanoja T, Julkunen H, Paavilainen T. Short- and long-term outcome of children with congenital complete heart block diagnosed in utero or as a newborn. Pediatrics. 2000;106(1 Pt 1):86–91. https://doi.org/10.1542/peds.106.1.86.
60. Moak JP, Barron KS, Hougen TJ, Wiles HB, Balaji S, Sreeram N, et al. Congenital heart block: development of late-onset cardiomyopathy, a previously underappreciated sequela. J Am Coll Cardiol. 2001;37(1):238–42. https://doi.org/10.1016/s07351097(00)01048-2.
61. Udink ten Cate FE, Breur JM, Cohen MI, Boramanand N, Kapusta L, Crosson JE, et al. Dilated cardiomyopathy in isolated congenital complete atrioventricular block: early and long-term risk in children. J Am Coll Cardiol. 2001;37(4):1129–34. https://doi.org/10.1016/s0735 1097(00)01209 2
62. Ho SY, Esscher E, Anderson RH, Michaëlsson M. Anatomy of congenital complete heart block and relation to maternal anti-Ro antibodies. Am J Cardiol. 1986;58(3):291–4. https://doi.org/10.1016/0002-9149(86)90064-0.
63. Askanase AD, Friedman DM, Copel J, Dische MR, Dubin A, Starc TJ, et al. Spectrum and progression of conduction abnormalities in infants born to mothers with anti-SSA/Ro anti-SSB/La antibodies. Lupus. 2002;11(3):145–51. https://doi.org/10.1191/0961203302lu173oa.
64. Altman CA, Sheth SS. Could timing be everything for antibody-mediated congenital heart? J Am Coll Cardiol. 2018;72(16):1952–4. https://doi.org/10.1016/j.jacc.2018.08.1039.
65. Glickstein JS, Buyon JP, Friedman D. The fetal PR interval: pulsed Doppler echocardiographic assessment. Am J Cardiol. 2000;86:236–9.
66. Friedman D, Buyon J, Kim M, Glickstein JS. Fetal cardiac function assessed by Doppler myocardial performance index (Tei index). Ultrasound Obstet Gynecol. 2003;21:33–6.
67. Buyon JP, Hiebert R, Copel J, et al. Autoimmune-associated congenital heart block: mortality, morbidity, and recurrence rates obtained from a national neonatal lupus registry. J Am Coll Cardiol. 1998;31:1658–66.
68. Friedman DM, Kim MY, Copel JA, Davis C, Phoon CK, Glickstein JS, et al. Utility of cardiac monitoring in fetuses at risk for congenital heart block: the PR Interval and Dexamethasone Evaluation (PRIDE) prospective study. Circulation. 2008;117(4):485–93. https://doi.org/10.1161/circulationaha.107.707661.
69. Rosenthal D, Druzin M, Chin C, Dubin A. A new therapeutic approach to the fetus with congenital complete heart block: preemptive, targeted therapy with dexamethasone. Obstet Gynecol. 1998;92(4 Pt 2):689–91. https://doi.org/10.1016/s00297844(98)00149-5.
70. Yang CH, Chen JY, Lee SC, Luo SF. Successful preventive treatment of congenital heart block during pregnancy in a woman with systemic lupus erythematosus and anti Sjögren's syndrome A/Ro antibody. J Microbiol Immunol Infect. 2005;38(5):365–9.
71. Copel JA, Buyon JP, Kleinman CS. Successful in utero therapy of fetal heart block. Am J Obstet Gynecol. 1995;173(5):1384–90. https://doi.org/10.1016/0002-9378(95)906215.
72. Saleeb S, Copel J, Friedman D, Buyon JP. Comparison of treatment with fluorinated glucocorticoids to the natural history of autoantibody-associated congenital heart block: retrospective review of the research registry for neonatal lupus. Arthritis Rheum. 1999;42(11):2335–45. https://doi.org/10.1002/15290131(199911)42:11%3c2335.
73. Kaaja R, Julkunen H. Prevention of recurrence of congenital heart block with intravenous immunoglobulin and corticosteroid therapy. Arthritis Rheum. 2003;48(1):280–1.
74. Izmirly PM, Saxena A, Sahl SK, Shah U, Friedman DM, Kim MY, et al. Assessment of fluorinated steroids to avert progression and mortality in anti-SSA/Ro-associated cardiac injury limited to the fetal conduction system. Ann Rheum Dis. 2016;75(6):11615. https://doi.org/10.1136/annrheumdis-2015-208311.
75. Costedoat-Chalumeau N, Amoura Z, Le Thi HD, Wechsler B, Vauthier D, Ghillani P, et al. Questions about dexamethasone use for the prevention of anti-SSA related congenital heart block. Ann Rheum Dis. 2003;62(10):1010–2. https://doi.org/10.1136/ard.62.10.1010.
76. Levesque K, Morel N, Maltret A, Baron G, Masseau A, Orquevaux P, et al. Description of 214 cases of autoimmune congenital heart block: results of the French neonatal lupus syndrome. Autoimmun Rev. 2015;14(12):1154–60. https://doi.org/10.1016/j.autrev.2015.08.005.
77. Buyon JP, Clancy RM. Neonatal lupus: review of proposed pathogenesis and clinical data from the US-based Research Registry for Neonatal Lupus. Autoimmunity. 2003;36(1):41–50. https://doi.org/10.1080/0891693031000067340.
78. Buyon JP, Hiebert R, Copel J, Craft J, Friedman D, Katholi M, et al. Autoimmune associated congenital heart block: demographics, mortality, morbidity and recurrence rates obtained from a national neonatal lupus registry. J Am Coll Cardiol. 1998;31(7):1658–66. https://doi.org/10.1016/s0735-1097(98)00161-2.
79. Miyoshi T, Maeno Y, Sago H, Inamura N, Yasukohchi S, Kawataki M, et al. Evaluation of transplacental treatment for fetal congenital bradyarrhythmia: nationwide survey in Japan. Circ J. 2012;76:469–76.
80. Barclay CS, French MA, Ross LD, Sokol RJ. Successful pregnancy following steroid therapy and plasma exchange in a woman with anti-Ro (SS-A) antibodies. Case report Br J Obstet Gynaecol. 1987;94(4):369–71. https://doi.org/10.1111/j.14710528.1987.tb03107.x.

81. Cuneo BF, Sonesson SE, Levasseur S, Moon-Grady AJ, Krishnan A, Donofrio MT, et al. Home monitoring for fetal heart rhythm during anti-Ro pregnancies. J Am Coll Cardiol. 2018;72(16):1940–51. https://doi.org/10.1016/j.jacc.2018.07.076.
82. Julkunen H, Eronen M. The rate of recurrence of isolated congenital heart block: a population-based study. Arthritis Rheum. 2001;44(2):487–8. https://doi.org/10.1002/1529-0131(200102)44:2%3c487::Aid-anr70%3e3.0.Co;2-d.
83. Levy RA, Vilela VS, Cataldo MJ, Ramos RC, Duarte JL, Tura BR, et al. Hydroxychloroquine (HCQ) in lupus pregnancy: double-blind and placebo-controlled study. Lupus. 2001;10(6):401–4. https://doi.org/10.1191/096120301678646137.
84. Izmirly PM, Costedoat-Chalumeau N, Pisoni CN, Khamashta MA, Kim MY, Saxena A, et al. Maternal use of hydroxychloroquine is associated with a reduced risk of recurrent anti-SSA/Ro-antibody-associated cardiac manifestations of neonatal lupus. Circulation. 2012;126(1):76–82. https://doi.org/10.1161/circulationaha.111.089268.
85. Vanoni F, Lava SA, Fossali EF, Cavalli R, Simonetti GD, Bianchetti MG, et al. Neonatal systemic lupus erythematosus syndrome: a comprehensive review. Clin Rev Allergy Immunol. 2017;53(3):469–76. https://doi.org/10.1007/s12016-017-8653-0.
86. Lee LA, Weston WL. Cutaneous lupus erythematosus during the neonatal and childhood periods. Lupus. 1997;6(2):132–8. https://doi.org/10.1177/096120339700600208.
87. Neiman AR, Lee LA, Weston WL, Buyon JP. Cutaneous manifestations of neonatal lupus without heart block: characteristics of mothers and children enrolled in a national registry. J Pediatr. 2000;137(5):674–80. https://doi.org/10.1067/mpd.2000.109108.
88. Walling HW, Sontheimer RD. Cutaneous lupus erythematosus: issues in diagnosis and treatment. Am J Clin Dermatol. 2009;10:365–81.
89. Watson R, Kang JE, May M, Hudak M, Kickler T, Provost TT. Thrombocytopenia in the neonatal lupus syndrome. Arch Dermatol. 1988;124(4):560–3.
90. Kanagasegar S, Cimaz R, Kurien BT, Brucato A, Scofield RH. Neonatal lupus manifests as isolated neutropenia and mildly abnormal liver functions. J Rheumatol. 2002;29(1):187–91.
91. Laxer RM, Roberts EA, Gross KR, Britton JR, Cutz E, Dimmick J, et al. Liver disease in neonatal lupus erythematosus. J Pediatr. 1990;116(2):238–42. https://doi.org/10.1016/s0022-3476(05)82880-x.
92. Martin V, Lee LA, Askanase AD, Katholi M, Buyon JP. Long-term followup of children with neonatal lupus and their unaffected siblings. Arthritis Rheum. 2002;46(9):2377–83. https://doi.org/10.1002/art.10638.
93. Cimaz R. Any increased risk of autoimmune disease? Lupus. 2004;13(9):736–9. https://doi.org/10.1191/0961203303lu1093oa.
94. Haga HJ, Gjesdal CG, Irgens LM, Ostensen M. Reproduction and gynaecological manifestations in women with primary Sjögren's syndrome: a case-control study. Scand J Rheumatol. 2005;34(1):45–8. https://doi.org/10.1080/03009740510017959.
95. Siamopoulou-Mavridou A, Manoussakis MN, Mavridis AK, Moutsopoulos HM. Outcome of pregnancy in patients with autoimmune rheumatic disease before the disease onset. Ann Rheum Dis. 1988;47(12):982–7. https://doi.org/10.1136/ard.47.12.982.
96. Takaya M, Ichikawa Y, Shimizu H, Uchiyama M, Moriuchi J, Arimori S. Sjögren's syndrome and pregnancy. Tokai J Exp Clin Med. 1991;16(2):83–8.
97. De Carolis S, Salvi S, Botta A, Garofalo S, Garufi C, Ferrazzani S, et al. The impact of primary Sjogren's syndrome on pregnancy outcome: our series and review of the literature. Autoimmun Rev. 2014;13(2):103–7. https://doi.org/10.1016/j.autrev.2013.09.003.
98. Brucato A, Doria A, Frassi M, Castellino G, Franceschini F, Faden D, et al. Pregnancy outcome in 100 women with autoimmune diseases and anti-Ro/SSA antibodies: a prospective controlled study. Lupus. 2002;11(11):716–21. https://doi.org/10.1191/0961203302lu252oa.

9

Attitudes of patients with a rheumatic disease on drug use in the COVID-19 pandemic

Belkıs Nihan Coskun[1*], Burcu Yagiz[2], Yavuz Pehlivan[1] and Ediz Dalkilic[1]

Abstract

Background: Anti-rheumatic drugs can increase the predisposition to infection, and patients may be unaware of continuing their treatment during the COVID-19 pandemic.

Objective: This study aimed to assess whether patients maintain their treatment for rheumatic conditions during the pandemic period and determine the factors responsible for discontinuation.

Methods: Patients were randomly selected from the prospectively collected database of our tertiary referral center. The patients were interviewed by telephone through a standardized closed-ended questionnaire, which is targeting the continuity of the treatment plan and the considerations related to the individual choice. The patients were asked whether they hesitated to visit the hospital for follow-up or intravenous drug administration.

Results: A total of 278 patients completed the questionnaire. While 62 of the patients (22.3%) had reduced or interrupted the treatment, only 11 patients (3.9%) stopped the treatment completely. A significant difference was observed between the duration of illness and the discontinuation of treatment. ($p = 0.023$) There was a significant difference in disease activity between the group that stopped treatment and continued treatment. ($p = 0.001$) There was no statistically significant difference in other demographic characteristics. One hundred thirty-five patients (48.6%) made the treatment decision by themselves, and 80% continued the treatment. Reasons for stopping the treatment were anxiety (48.4%), not being able to go to the hospital for intravenous treatment (45.1%), and not being able to find the drug (6.5%).

Conclusion: Since patients with long-term illnesses were found to be significantly more likely to stop their treatment, this group of patients should be monitored.

Keywords: Anti-rheumatic drugs, Biological treatments, COVID-19, Discontinuation, Rheumatic patients

Introduction

In December 2019, coronavirus disease 2019 (COVID-19), caused by severe acute respiratory coronavirus 2 (SARS-CoV-2), first emerged in Wuhan, China. The virus spread quickly worldwide due to its high disease trans mission rate [1, 2]. Since the diagnosis of the first cases, nearly 120 million people were confirmed as positive, and 2.6 million died in the COVID-19 pandemic by the end of March 2021 [3].

While the disease is usually asymptomatic or with minor symptoms in many cases, 15–20% develop interstitial pneumonia and acute respiratory distress syndrome (ARDS) [4]. Several risk factors are responsible for the development of severe symptoms, including older age, comorbidities such as hypertension (HT), diabetes mellitus (DM), obesity, high-dose corticosteroid use, and immunodeficiency [5].

Patients with rheumatic diseases have an inherent risk for bacterial, viral, or opportunistic infections compared

*Correspondence: belkisnihanseniz@hotmail.com
[1] Division of Rheumatology, Uludağ University Faculty of Medicine (Uludağ Üniversitesi Tıp Fakültesi Romatoloji Bilim Dalı), Görükle, Nilüfer, Bursa 16059, Turkey

to the general population. Also, the use of immunosuppressive medications such as conventional synthetic disease-modifying anti-rheumatic drugs (csDMARDs), biological disease-modifying anti-rheumatic drugs (bDMARDs), and corticosteroids in patients with autoimmune rheumatoid disease, increase the risk of these infections [6, 7].

Uncontrolled disease activity is one of the most sensitive and specific independent infection risk predictors, especially during the pandemic. On the other hand, the immunosuppressive treatment may increase the risk of infection, and therefore, the patients may hesitate to continue their ongoing treatment plan [8, 9].

There is currently a lack of information regarding the effect of SARS-CoV-2 on patients suffering from rheumatoid diseases. However, several international associations of rheumatoid diseases such as the European League against Rheumatology (EULAR), American College of Rheumatology (ACR), British Society for Rheumatology (BSR), and Italian Society for Rheumatology (SIR) recommend continuing immunosuppressive therapies to prevent relapses [10–13]. This advice helps prevent relapses that may occur when therapy is eventually stopped [14].

There is limited data on patients' preferences on the continuation of the treatment during the pandemic phase. Patient surveys from Greece, Italy, and Latin America reported a compliance rate between 85 and 97.8% [14–16]. This study aimed to survey whether the patients diagnosed with rheumatoid arthritis (RA) and ankylosing spondylitis (AS) continue their medications during the pandemic phase and determine the factors responsible for discontinuation.

Methods

Following the approval by the institutional board review, a telephone survey was conducted between the dates 1/7/2020 and 20/7/2020. The patients were interviewed by telephone through a standardized closed-ended questionnaire.

Patients characteristics

The patients diagnosed with RA or AS receiving corticosteroids, non-steroidal anti-inflammatory drugs, csDMARDs, bDMARDs and selective targeted synthetic disease-modifying (tsDMARDs) treatments were expected to participate in the study. The 2010 EULAR/ACR guidelines were used to diagnose patients with RA [17]. In diagnosing SpA patients, the modified New York criteria and EULAR criteria for axial and peripheral SPA 2009 were used [18, 19].

Patients were randomly selected from a prospectively collected database of our tertiary referral center. The participation of a total number of 300 patients was targeted. Every 5th patient was chosen for the survey on the database as the randomization procedure. The patients with a follow-up duration longer than 6 months were included in the study. Patients under the age of 18 and who had invalid contact information were excluded.

The demographic information including age, gender, the region of residence (urban, sub-neighborhood, rural), the education level (First, second, third), employment status, smoking, rheumatological diagnosis, disease duration, current treatments, comorbidity (HT, coronary heart disease, DM, chronic obstructive pulmonary disease (COPD)) was obtained from the database.

Questionnaire features and application method

A single rheumatologist (BNC) interviewed with all of the patients. The patients were asked whether they continued their ongoing treatment plan and how they decided to continue or stop treatment after 15th March 2020 when the first COVID-19 cases were reported in Turkey. The patients were asked if they hesitated to visit the hospital for follow-up or intravenous drug administration. Also, patients were asked whether they referred to a hospital due to COVID-19 symptoms and whether they had a history of hospitalization for an infection in the past year. The perception of disease control was evaluated by using the Visual Analog Scale.

Statistical analysis

SPSS version 22.0 was used for statistical analysis. Data were presented as the mean and standard deviation or, when applicable, number and percentage. For categorical data comparisons, Fischer's Exact Test was used, and the independent t-test was used to determine parameters when applicable. A p-value of less than 0.05 was considered statistically significant.

Results

A total of 278 patients (146 RA, 132 AS) completed the survey as shown in Fig. 1. The mean age of the patients was 47.53 ± 13.02 years (19–78). One hundred seventy-nine patients (64.4%) were female. A total of 62 (%22.3) patients discontinued or interrupted their ongoing treatment plan. Only 11 patients (3.9%) completely stopped their treatment. A comparison of the demographic variables in patients according to the continuation status was reported in Table 1. While the mean disease duration in patients who continued to their treatment plan was 11.15 ± 8 years, and the mean disease duration in patients who interrupted/stop their treatment plan was 13.93 ± 9.79 years. Disease duration was significantly higher as a contributing factor ($p = 0.023$). A significant difference was observed between the duration of illness and the discontinuation of treatment. There was

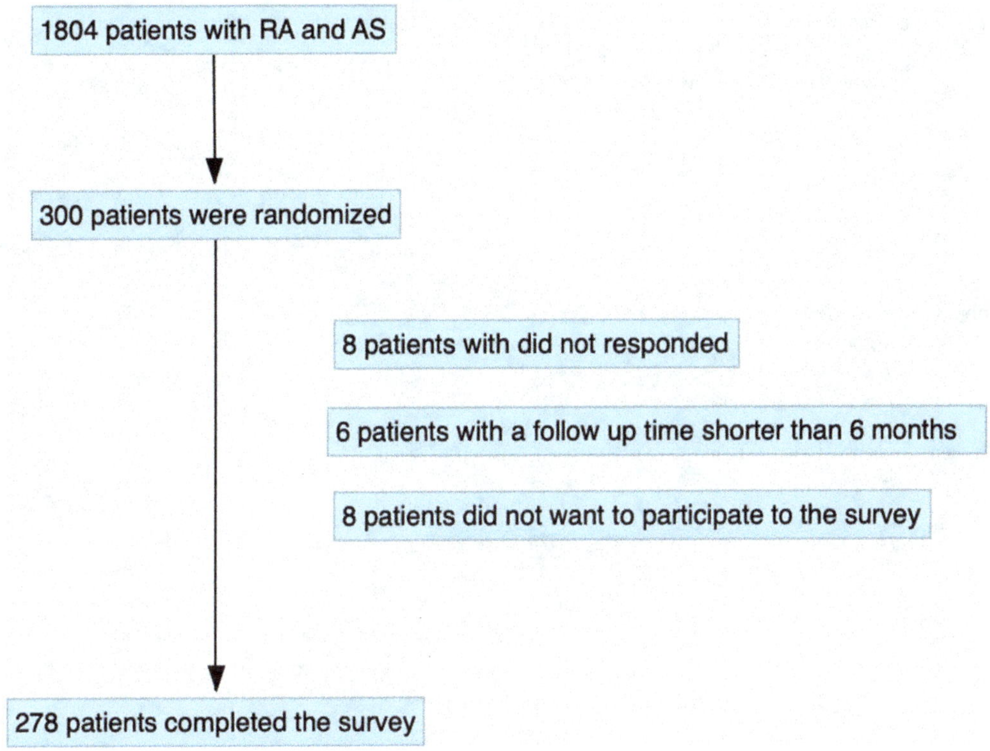

Fig. 1 Flowchart of the planning strategy of the article

a significant difference in disease activity between the group that stopped treatment and continued treatment. ($p=0.001$) There was no statistically significant difference in other demographic characteristics. Table 2 listed the rate of drugs in patients with their continuous status. The continuation rate of DMARDS, bDMARDs, tsDMARD, csDMARDs was 73.3%, 83.3%, 95.4%, respectively. Low-dose glucocorticoids and NSAIDs were maintained in 95.5% and 96.4% of the patients, respectively.

One hundred and thirty-five patients (48.6%) made the treatment decision independently, 80% continued the treatment. One hundred eleven patients (39.9%) made a co-decision with the rheumatologist, and 76.6% maintained the treatment. The other 32 patients (11.5%) decided by consultation with other healthcare professionals such as family physicians, nurses, and pharmacists. Of these cases, 71.9% continued the treatment ($p=0.571$). It was found that the decision on the medication was made mainly by contacting the rheumatologist. The reasons for stopping/interrupting medication were anxiety (48.4%), inability to visit the hospital for intravenous treatment (45.1%), and inability to obtain the drug (6.5%). 89.6% of the patients had concerns about visiting the hospital. There were only three patients (1.1%) who had an infection requiring hospitalization last year. In the past 3 months four patients with suspected COVID-19 symptoms such as cough and back pain were admitted to the emergency room. The COVID-19 tests performed on these patients have been reported to be negative.

Discussion

The inherent risk of infection in rheumatic patients, in addition to the medication's immunosuppressive effects, can lead patients to remain concerned regarding treatment continuity. Any patients who suspected the treatment's immunosuppressive effects stopped or disrupted their current treatment either in compliance with their own decisions or in line with the health authorities' recommendations. Patients may also have trouble reaching physicians for information or cannot access their intravenous treatments when ambulatory health services have been shut down. Since the pandemic has not stopped and a second wave is likely, we aim to examine the actions and behaviors of treatment for patients with rheumatological conditions and explore the factors that will help them prepare more accurately.

Our study found that a great majority of the patients have retained in their current treatment with a continuation rate of 77.6%. In the first three months since the pandemic announcement, approximately one in five patients extended the treatment dose intervals, while only 11 patients stopped their medication completely.

Table 1 Comparison of the demographic variables in patients acoording to the contiuation status

	Ongoing (n = 216)	Interrupted/ stop (n = 62)	p
Age	47.75 ± 13.09	46.8 ± 12.86	0.616
Gender			0.073
Female	133 (74.3%)	46 (25.7%)	
Male	83 (83.8%)	16 (16.2%)	
Diagnosis			0.248
Rheumatoid arthritis	109 (74.7%)	37 (25.3%)	
Spondylitis	107 (81.1%)	25 (18.9%)	
BMI	26.9 ± 5.18	28.27 ± 6.39	0.083
Smoking			0.327
Active	58 (78.4%)	16 (21.6%)	
Non-smoker	134 (75.7%)	43 (24.3%)	
Previous	24 (88.9%)	3 (11.1%)	
Disease duration	11.15 ± 8	13.93 ± 9.79	**0.023**
Disease activity (VAS)	7.76 ± 1.7	6.61 ± 2.33	**0.001**
Education			0.079
Low	98 (81%)	23 (19%)	
High school	81 (80.2%)	20 (19.8%)	
University	37 (66.1%)	19 (33.9%)	
Occupation			0.771
Occupant	89 (79.5%)	23 (20.5%)	
Non-working	106 (75.7%)	34 (24.3%)	
Retired	21 (80.8%)	5 (19.2%)	
Mariatial			0.582
Single	21 (75%)	7 (25%)	
Married	187 (78.2%)	52(21.8%)	
Divorced/widowed	6 (66.7%)	3 (33.3%)	
Comorbidity			0.326
Hypertension	34 (70.8%)	14 (29.2%)	
Coroner artery disease	5 (71.4%)	2 (28.6%)	
Diabetes mellitus	14 (82.4%)	3 (17.6%)	
Pulmonery disease	2 (50%)	2 (50%)	

Bold values refer to statistical significance values

Table 2 Distribution of ongoing and Interrupted/stop drugs

Drugs	Ongoing	Interrupted/stop
bDMARD	148 (73.3%)	55 (26.7%)
Anti-TNF		
Adalimumab	30 (90.9%)	3 (9.1%)
Certolizumab	17 (85%)	3 (15%)
Etanercept	29 (74.3%)	10 (25.7%)
Golimumab	18 (81.8%)	4 (18.2%)
Infliximab	13 (56.5%)	10 (43.5%)
Tocilizumab	11 (47.8%)	12 (52.2%)
Rituximab	19 (65.5%)	10 (34.5%)
Secukinumab	3 (60%)	2 (40%)
Abatacept	3 (100%)	0 (0%)
tDMARD		
Tofasitinib	5 (83.3%)	1 (16.7%)
csDMARD	124 (95.4%)	6 (4.6%)
Methotrexate	69 (95.8%)	3 (4.2%)
Leflunomide	40 (100%)	0 (0%)
Sulfasalazine	15 (100%)	0 (0%)
Hydroxychloroquine	70 (93.3%)	5 (6.7%)
Low-dose glucocorticoids	84 (95.4%)	3 (4.6%)
NSAIDs	134 (96.4%)	5 (3.6%)

Similarly, in a study of 500 patients, Fragoulis et al. reported that 11 patients (2.2%) stopped immunosuppressive drug therapy [15]. Another Latin American study revealed that 90% (n = 293) of patients did not modify their drug schedule [16]. In various studies conducted in Italy, America, Spain and Turkey, it was reported that approximately 75–80% of patients did not change their treatment [20–23].

Following the pandemic's announcement, EULAR, ACR, BSR, SIR, and Turkish Rheumatology Association issued recommendations in March–April that patients with rheumatic disease should not stop medication treatment since any discontinuation in treatment can lead to a relapse of rheumatological diseases and may increase the risk of infection further. Due to the positive effects of both national and international recommendations, drug treatments may have been left to a lesser extent [10–13, 24].

In our research, patients were found to postpone or delay their treatments, most notably because they were fearful of the predisposition to infection induced by their therapies (48.4%). Similarly, fear of contagion COVID-19 infection, which is the most common reason for stopping or delaying treatment, has been reported in other studies with rates as high as 80% [21, 25]. The second most common reason was the lack of service in hospitals that refer to intravenous treatment (45.1%). The discontinuation rate due to the inability to obtain the medication (6.5%) was very low.

Before the pandemic, patients evaluated by rheumatologists in routine practice in our country were able to access biological treatments only after obtaining a committee report and prescription was written. However, after the announcement of the pandemic, patients with a prior committee report had the right to obtain their biological drugs from the pharmacy without seeing the doctor and without a prescription by the permission of Ministry of Health of The Republic of Turkey [26]. This condition may be an essential factor for patients to continue drug treatment.

In the present study, the group that stopped treatment was found to have a longer disease duration than those who did not stop. Patients using long-term immunosuppressive drugs have been shown to have a predisposition to anxiety and behavioral disorders. This situation may explain why discontinuation is high in patients with a long disease duration due to anxiety [27]. No statistically significant difference between the group that stopped the treatment and the group that did not was found when comparing education level, age, profession, comorbidities, and body mass index. Although this result was not statistically significant, we found a high propensity to stop among those with high education. Fragoulis et al. found that the discontinuation rates were associated with specific clinical and social conditions such as unemployment status and COPD [15]. In this study, four patients had pulmonary disease. Two of them continued treatment while two intermittently used it.

Typically, extreme COVID-19 symptoms were associated with obesity, age, comorbidities such as lung disease, DM, history of previous serious infections, long-term corticosteroid therapy, and higher underlying rheumatic disease activity [28, 29]. We observed a trend in obese patients to avoid drug therapy while not statistically significant.

The steroid drugs are among the most essential medicines used in managing rheumatological disorders, in terms of increased risk of infection [30]. Although it is generally known as a tendency to infection, discontinuation of steroids and other immunosuppressive drug treatments has not been recommended by associations such as EULAR, ACR [10, 11]. A recent study also reported the efficacy of low-dose steroid therapy in the treatment of severe COVID-19 infections [31]. Approximately 1/3 of the present study patients were using steroids with a discontinuation rate of 3.4%. In a retrospective analysis published in China, 6 of the 21 rheumatic patients with COVID-19 infection were using glucocorticoid therapy before infection. All of these patients were found to improve. During the follow-up, four patients received steroids due to rheumatologic disease reactivation. A total of 37.5 mg glucocorticoid treatment was administered to 10 patients during the treatment [32]. Continuing the ongoing steroid treatment is necessary to stop reactivation of the condition and to prevent potential infections.

Patients with immunocompromises are at high risk of multiple infectious diseases, including infections with the viruses. TNF-α, IL-6, and IL-1 are crucial pro-inflammatory cytokines in body defense. Blocking these cytokines may cause especially infections with intracellular infectious agents; however, it creates a predisposition to all kinds of infections[33]. Due to the increased risk of infection, the use of bDMARD may be a concern in patients during the COVID-19 period. Although the increased risk of serious infections has been reported in meta-analyses to date in those receiving biological treatments, we do not have clear data on whether this risk increases COVID-19 infection [10].

In the present study, the bDMARD usage rate was 73.3%, with a discontinuation rate of 27%. Although there are no clinical studies on whether these drugs negatively affect the course of COVID-19 infection in patients using anti-TNF agents, few case reports are available in the literature. There is no proven data to show that these drugs have positive or negative effects [34–36].

Tocilizumab (TCZ), a monoclonal antibody against interleukin-6 (IL-6), has recently emerged as an alternative therapy for COVID-19 patients at risk for cytokine storms. Which inflammatory cytokine is most important in the pathogenesis of COVID-19 is currently unknown, although IL-6 appears to be crucial [37]. The cytokine storm causing ARDS because of excessive immune reaction may be fatal in COVID-19 infection. Therefore, anti-cytokine intervention may not affect the risk of viral infection and viral clearance but may inhibit the hyperinflammatory state in COVID-19, which can be beneficial [37]. No data has been shown that it is protective against COVID-19 infection in TCZ users due to rheumatic disease. 52.5% of our patients had interrupted TCZ treatment. All of those who interrupted were receiving TCZ treatment intravenously. The interruption was due to the inability to reach the hospital, but all patients continued their medication, albeit with a delay.

Hydroxychloroquine (HCQ), an anti-malarial drug, acts by increasing endosomal PH. It inhibits immune activation by preventing signaling and cytokine production through Toll-like Receptors (TLR) at the cellular level. It has an inhibitory effect on viral replication in ex vivo, but this has never been demonstrated in randomized controlled trials [38].

There is no data supporting the use of HCQ as a preservative, and it is not included in the guidelines. In Italy, 4 of 320 chronic rheumatology patients were found to be Covid-19 positive, and these four patients were infected while using HCQ. None of these patients with a mean age of 58 ± 5 years, who also used biological therapy, had a severe respiratory syndrome or death [39, 40].

Only 6.7% of our patients had interrupted the treatment due to the inability to obtain the drug. Although its effectiveness in prophylaxis has not been demonstrated, learning the use of HCQ in the treatment of COVID-19 may have aroused more interest in the drug in patients. Effective and acceptable use of HCQ in the treatment of SARS-CoV-2 may be one factor that has increased drug retention.

Vitamin D modulates the innate and adaptive immune system, and its deficiency has been understandably linked to an increase in autoimmunity and infection predisposition [41]. Grant et al. (2020) pointed to the importance of vitamin D in reducing the incidence of COVID-19 infections in the respiratory tract [42]. The rate of using vitamin D supplements in our patients 21.2%. Vitamin C is one of the critical components that makes a strong immune system of water-soluble vitamins. The specific types of products and food must be known in the current situation for combating COVID-19 to improve our immune system [43]. The rate of using vitamin C supplements in our patients was 5.4%.

At the beginning of the epidemic, tight closure policies were implemented in most countries of the world. In the first three months of the epidemic in Turkey, there was a period of strict isolation, especially for people over the age of 65 years and under the age of 18 years.

In the same period, people with chronic diseases were deemed on administrative leave, many workplaces switched to online working order and many patients were self-quarantined. In a period when such strict measures are taken, it seems possible that rheumatism patients will make changes such as the anxiety of getting COVID 19 infection and reduction in drug treatment. There may also be an increased interest in supplements to protect patients from infection.

The limited number of patients is the main limitation of the current study. In this study, although it was theoretically possible to reach a higher number by sending e-mails to all patients in the database, only telephone access was selected to analyze the data in better quality due to the consideration of the socio-cultural status and low education level of the patients.

Conclusions

The adherence of rheumatology patients to treatment was investigated in this study in the early period after the announcement of the COVID-19 pandemic, and it was found that treatment adherence was high. It was determined that the most important factor in the discontinuation of the drug was the concern of infection with COVID 19. It was observed that treatment was considerably more stopped, particularly in patients with longer illness duration. Therefore, it may be intended to provide patients with better information not to disrupt therapy.

Acknowledgements

We thank our colleagues from Uludağ University Faculty of Medicine, Division of Rheumatology who provided insight and expertise that greatly assisted the research.

Authors' contributions

BNC is the owner of the research topic and organised the research team. BNC and BY were responsible for the writing of the article. YP was responsible for the statistics. ED reviewed the literature. All authors read and approved the final manuscript.

Author details

[1]Division of Rheumatology, Uludağ University Faculty of Medicine (Uludağ Üniversitesi Tıp Fakültesi Romatoloji Bilim Dalı), Görükle, Nilüfer, Bursa 16059, Turkey. [2]Division of Rheumatology, Afyonkarahisar State Hospital, Afyon, Turkey.

References

1. Munster VJ, Koopmans M, van Doremalen N, van Riel D, de Wit E. A novel coronavirus emerging in China—key questions for impact assessment. N Engl J Med. 2020;382(8):692–4. https://doi.org/10.1056/NEJMp2000929.
2. Zhu S, Guo X, Geary K, Zhang D. Emerging therapeutic strategies for COVID-19 patients. Discoveries. 2020;8(1): e105. https://doi.org/10.15190/d.2020.2.
3. WHO Coronavirus Disease (COVID-19) Dashboard. [Internet]. (cited 2021 Mar 14). https://covid19.who.int/.
4. Favalli EG, Ingegnoli F, De Lucia O, Cincinelli G, Cimaz R, Caporali R. COVID-19 infection and rheumatoid arthritis: faraway, so close! Autoimmun Rev. 2020;19(5): 102523. https://doi.org/10.1016/j.autrev.2020.102523.
5. Li X, Xu S, Yu M, Wang K, Tao Y, Zhou Y, et al. Risk factors for severity and mortality in adult COVID-19 inpatients in Wuhan. J Allergy Clin Immunol. 2020. https://doi.org/10.1016/j.jaci.2020.04.006.
6. Sfriso P, Ghirardello A, Botsios C, Tonon M, Zen M, Bassi N, et al. Infections and autoimmunity: the multifaceted relationship. J Leukoc Biol. 2010;87(3):385–95. https://doi.org/10.1189/jlb.0709517.
7. Girschick HJ, Guilherme L, Inman RD, Latsch K, Rihl M, Sherer Y, et al. Bacterial triggers and autoimmune rheumatic diseases. Clin Exp Rheumatol. 2008;26(1 SUPPL. 48).
8. Scott DL, Wolfe F, Huizinga TWJ. Rheumatoid arthritis. Lancet. 2010;376(9746):1094–108. https://doi.org/10.1016/S0140-6736(10)60826-4.
9. Furst DE. The risk of infections with biologic therapies for rheumatoid arthritis. Semin Arthritis Rheum. 2010;39(5):327–46. https://doi.org/10.1016/j.semarthrit.2008.10.002.
10. European League Against Rheumatism (EULAR), Guidance for Patients duringCovid-19 Outbreak, (2020) Updated March 17th [Internet]. https://www.eular.org/eular_guidance_for_patients_covid19_outbreak.cfm. April 25th, 2020
11. American College of Rheumatology (Acr), Guidance for Patients during Covid-19Outbreak, (2020) Updated April 14th.
12. British Society for Rheumatology (Bsr), Guidance for Patients during Covid-19 Outbreak, (2020) Updated July 29th.
13. Italian Society for Rheumatology (SIR), Guidance during Covid-19 Outbreak,(2020) Updated March 20th.
14. Zen M, Fuzzi E, Astorri D, Saccon F, Padoan R, Ienna L, et al. SARS-CoV-2 infection in patients with autoimmune rheumatic diseases in northeast Italy: a cross-sectional study on 916 patients. J Autoimmun. 2020;112(May): 102502. https://doi.org/10.1016/j.jaut.2020.102502.
15. Fragoulis GE, Evangelatos G, Arida A, Bournia V-K, Fragiadaki K, Karamanakos A, et al. Treatment adherence of patients with systemic rheumatic diseases in COVID-19 pandemic. Ann Rheum Dis. 2020. https://doi.org/10.1136/annrheumdis-2020-217935.
16. Pineda-Sic RA, Galarza-Delgado DA, Serna-Pena G, Castillo-Torres SA, Flores-Alvarado DE, et al. Treatment adherence behaviours in rheumatic disease during pandemic COVID-19: a Latin American experience. Ann Rheum Dis. 2020. https://doi.org/10.1136/annrheumdis-2020-218198.
17. Aletaha D, Neogi T, Silman AJ, Funovits J, Felson DT, Bingham CO, et al. 2010 Rheumatoid arthritis classification criteria: an American College of Rheumatology/European League Against Rheumatism collaborative initiative. Arthritis Rheum. 2010;62(9):2569–81. https://doi.org/10.1002/art.27584.
18. Rudwaleit M, Van Der Heijde D, Landewé R, Listing J, Akkoc N, Brandt J, et al. The development of Assessment of SpondyloArthritis international Society classification criteria for axial spondyloarthritis (part II): validation and final selection. Ann Rheum Dis. 2009;68(6):777–83. https://doi.org/10.1136/ard.2009.108233.
19. Rudwaleit M, Van Der Heijde D, Landewé R, Akkoc N, Brandt J, Chou CT, et al. The Assessment of SpondyloArthritis international Society classification criteria for peripheral spondyloarthritis and for spondyloarthritis in general. Ann Rheum Dis. 2011;70(1):25–31. https://doi.org/10.1136/ard.2010.133645.

20. Favalli EG, Monti S, Ingegnoli F, Balduzzi S, Caporali R, Montecucco C. Incidence of COVID-19 in patients with rheumatic diseases treated with targeted immunosuppressive drugs: what can we learn from observational data? Arthritis Rheumatol. 2020;72(10):1600–6. https://doi.org/10.1002/art.41388.
21. Rosenbaum JT, Hamilton H, Choi D, Weisman MH, Reveille JD, Winthrop KL. Biologics, spondylitis and COVID-19. 2020;79(12): 1663–1665. doi: https://doi.org/10.1136/annrheumdis-2020-217941.
22. López-Medina C, Ladehesa-Pineda L, Gómez-García I, Puche-Larrubia MÁ, Sequí-Sabater JM, Armenteros-Ortiz P, Ortega-Castro R, Garrido-Castro JL, Escudero-Contreras AC-EE. Treatment adherence during the COVID-19 pandemic and the impact of confinement on disease activity and emotional status: a survey in 644 rheumatic patients. Jt Bone Spine. 2020;88(2): 105085. https://doi.org/10.1016/j.jbspin.2020.105085.
23. Kalyoncu U, Pehlivan Y, Akar S, Kaşifoğlu T, Kimyon G, Karada ĞÖ, Dalkiliç HE, Ertenli Aİ, Kiliç L, Ersözlü ED, Bes C, Emmungil H, Mercan R, Ediboğlu E, Alpay Kanitez N, Bilgin E, Çolak S, Koca SS, Gönüllü E, Küçükşahin O, Coşkun BN, Yağiz BK. Preferences of inflammatory arthritis patients for biological disease-modifying antirheumatic drugs in the first 100 days of covid-19 pandemic. Turk J Med Sci. 2021. https://doi.org/10.3906/sag-2012-5.
24. Turkish Rheumatology Association Coronavirus (Covid-19) Outbreak Recommendations (2020) March 27th Title.
25. Costantino F, Bahier L, Tarancón LC, Leboime A, Vidal F, Bessalah L, Breban MDM. COVID-19 in French patients with chronic inflammatory rheumatic diseases: clinical features, risk factors and treatment adherence. Jt Bone Spine. 2021;88(1): 105095. https://doi.org/10.1016/j.jbspin.2020.105095.
26. Ministry of Health of The Republic of Turkey Access [Internet]. https://www.titck.gov.tr/duyuru/eczacilara-ve-tum-ilgililere-duyurulur-16032020090441
27. Venerito V, Lopalco G, Iannone F. COVID-19, rheumatic diseases and immunosuppressive drugs: an appeal for medication adherence. Rheumatol Int. 2020;40(5):827–8. https://doi.org/10.1007/s00296-020-04566-9.
28. Santos CS, Morales CM, Álvarez ED, Castro CÁ, Robles AL, Sandoval TP. Determinants of COVID-19 disease severity in patients with underlying rheumatic disease. Clin Rheumatol. 2020;39(9):2789–96. https://doi.org/10.1007/s10067-020-05301-2.
29. Pablos JL, Galindo M, Carmona L, Lledó A, Retuerto M, Blanco R, et al. Clinical outcomes of hospitalised patients with COVID-19 and chronic inflammatory and autoimmune rheumatic diseases: a multicentric matched cohort study. Ann Rheum Dis. 2020. https://doi.org/10.1136/annrheumdis-2020-218296.
30. Johannes WGJ JW. Glucocorticoid therapy. In: Firestein GS, editor. Kelley and Firestein's Textbook of Rheumatology. 10th ed. 2017; p. 932–57.
31. Johnson RM, Vinetz JM. Dexamethasone in the management of covid -19. BMJ. 2020;370:1–2. https://doi.org/10.1136/bmj.m2648.
32. Ye C, Cai S, Shen G, Guan H, Zhou L, Hu Y, et al. Clinical features of rheumatic patients infected with COVID-19 in Wuhan. China Ann Rheum Dis. 2020;79(8):1007–13. https://doi.org/10.1136/annrheumdis-2020-217627.
33. Rothan HA, Byrareddy SN. The epidemeology and pathogensis of coronavirus (Covid-19) outbreak. J Autoimmun. 2020;109(January):1–4. https://doi.org/10.1016/j.jaut.2020.102433.
34. Coskun Benlidayi I, Kurtaran B, Tirasci E, Guzel R. Coronavirus disease 2019 (COVID-19) in a patient with ankylosing spondylitis treated with secukinumab: a case-based review. Rheumatol Int. 2020. https://doi.org/10.1007/s00296-020-04635-z.
35. Queiro Silva R, Armesto S, González Vela C, Naharro Fernández C, González-Gay MA. COVID-19 patients with psoriasis and psoriatic arthritis on biologic immunosuppressant therapy versus apremilast in North Spain. Dermatol Ther. 2020. https://doi.org/10.1111/dth.13961.
36. Duret PM, Sebbag E, Mallick A, Gravier S, Spielmann L, et al. Recovery from COVID-19 in a patient with spondyloarthritis treated with TNF-alpha inhibitor etanercept. Ann Rheum Dis. 2020;79(9):1251–2. https://doi.org/10.1136/annrheumdis-2020-217362.
37. Schett G, Manger B, Simon D, Caporali R. COVID-19 revisiting inflammatory pathways of arthritis. Nat Rev Rheumatol. 2020;16(8):465–70. https://doi.org/10.1038/s41584-020-0451-z.
38. Schrezenmeier E, Dörner T. Mechanisms of action of hydroxychloroquine and chloroquine: implications for rheumatology. Nat Rev Rheumatol. 2020;16(3):155–66. https://doi.org/10.1038/s41584-020-0372-x.
39. Spinelli FR, Ceccarelli F, Di Franco MCF. To consider or not antimalarials as a prophylactic intervention in the SARS-CoV-2 (Covid-19) pandemic. Ann Rheum Dis. 2020;79(5):666–7. https://doi.org/10.1136/annrheumdis-2020-217367.
40. McInnes I. Response to: 'Hydroxychloroquine shortages during the COVID-19 pandemic' by Mendel et al. Ann Rheum Dis. 2020. https://doi.org/10.1136/annrheumdis-2020-217954.
41. Aranow C. Vitamin D and the immune system. J Investig Med. 2011;59(6):881–6. https://doi.org/10.231/JIM.0b013e31821b8755.
42. Grant WB, Lahore H, McDonnell SL, Baggerly CA, French CB, Aliano JL, et al. Evidence that vitamin d supplementation could reduce risk of influenza and covid-19 infections and deaths. Nutrients. 2020;12(4):1–19. https://doi.org/10.3390/nu12040988.
43. Aman F, Masood S. How nutrition can help to fight against covid-19 pandemic. Pakistan J Med Sci. 2020;36(COVID19-S4):121–3. https://doi.org/10.12669/pjms.36.COVID19-S4.2776.

10

Assessment of gait in patients with fibromyalgia during motor and cognitive dual task walking

Goran Radunović[1], Zoran Veličković[1], Melanija Rašić[1], Saša Janjić[1], Vladana Marković[2] and Saša Radovanović[3*]

Abstract

Background: The aim of the study was to assess gait pattern of patients diagnosed with fibromyalgia (FM) while performing demanding motor and/or cognitive dual tasks while walking. Further, idea was to explore possible correlations of dual task gait pattern alterations to patients' functional status and presence or absence of clinical symptoms associated with FM.

Methods: Twenty-four female FM patients and 24 healthy female subjects performed a basic walking task, a dual motor, a dual mental (cognitive) and a combined, dual motor and cognitive task simultaneously. Quantitative spatial (stride length) and temporal (cycle time, swing time and double support time) gait parameters were measured using GAITRite walkway system and their variability was assessed. Patients underwent clinical examination including assessment of functional status, pain and fatigue level, psychiatric and cognitive manifestations.

Results: The motor, cognitive and combined dual tasks affect gait performance in FM patients. Difference in tasks between FM and healthy subjects was found as double support time prolongation. Comparison of tasks showing that cycle time in FM was longer than controls and stride length was shorter in patients for all conditions, while no changes were found in any of the gait parameters variability. Further, mental/cognitive dual tasks had a larger effect than motor tasks. Correlations were also found between depression and functional status of the patients and the gait parameters.

Conclusions: Gait is affected in FM patients while dual task walking. No changes in stride-to-stride variability point that patients preserve stability in complex walking situations. Analysis of gait may provide additional information for the FM identification based on presence of clinical features and cognitive status. Correlation of dual task gait alterations with occurrence of clinical symptoms and influence of cognitive changes on gait pattern could additionally define FM subgroups.

Keywords: Cycle time, Stride, Gait variability, GAITRite walkway system

Introduction

Fibromyalgia (FM) is a chronic incapacitating disease characterized by multi-focal, widespread pain. Spectrum of the disease has been broadened to include symptoms such as tenderness, fatigue, non-refreshing sleep, musculoskeletal stiffness, cognitive dysfunction, mood disorders, poor balance, muscle weakness, functional impairments and disability [1, 2]. Establishing correct diagnosis is still challenging due to the lack of objective clinical or laboratory markers, with many patients waiting up to 5 years for the diagnosis. To minimize the subjectivity of clinical judgment, several diagnostic criteria were elaborated [3–5].

*Correspondence: sasar@imi.bg.ac.rs
[3] Institute for Medical Research, University of Belgrade, Dr Subotića 4, 11129 Belgrade, Serbia

Gait is under strong input of cognitive functions, particularly attention and executive function [6, 7]. In addition to clinical features [8, 9] and biomarkers [10], gait analysis was even proposed as an objective measurement for quantifying and subgrouping FM patients [11, 12]. It was shown that gait is affected in FM patients during dual walking tasks [13–17]. In studies measuring gait while FM patients performed several motor tasks [14, 15], or during base walking [17–19] and walking with different velocities [16, 17], patients showed significant differences in spatio-temporal gait parameters [16–19] compared to healthy control subjects. Given that cognitive impairment in FM is one of the emerging key symptoms, quantitative gait analysis under motor and cognitive dual tasks could point toward influence of cognitive changes on gait pattern. Furthermore, better understanding of gait changes might lead to better characterization of FM patients, and possibly could distinguish FM subgroups [11, 12].

Our objective was to assess quantitative spatiotempo ral gait parameters in female FM patients in comparison to healthy controls during base walk and while performing motor, cognitive and combined, both motor and cognitive dual tasks. Further, aim was also to explore possible correlations of dual task gait pattern alterations to patients' functional status and presence or absence of clinical symptoms associated with FM.

Methods

Patients

Twenty-four female patients (mean age 55.08 ± 11.28 years) were consecutively recruited at the Institute of Rheumatology, Medical faculty, University of Belgrade, Serbia. Patients' diagnoses were based on revised diagnostic criteria for FM [5] and were regularly seen at the Institute for at least one year after the diagnosis was established. We recruited and examined 24 consecutive patients that fulfilled inclusion/exclusion criteria in the period of July–December 2019. Twenty-four healthy age and gender matched subjects (mean age 55.17 ± 11.18 years) served as a control group (HC). HC were recruited among healthy employees of the Medical Faculty, University of Belgrade. Subjects with conditions that could impair independent walking (neurological disorders, orthopedic diseases or other medical conditions, use of cane or walker) were not included. Additionally, patients with major psychiatric disorders, including major depression were not included in the study. All patients were on stable treatment for at least 2 months prior to inclusion in the study, both fibromyalgia treatment and use of antidepressant therapy, if any. The study was approved by Institutional Ethical Committee and written informed consent was obtained from each participant prior to the inclusion in this study. The study was performed in accordance with the ethical standards of the Declaration of Helsinki and its later amendments.

Experimental protocol

Gait parameters were measured using GAITRite electronic walkway of 5.5 m (CIR Systems, Havertown, PA) during base walk at preferred velocity and while performing dual motor, dual mental and combined tasks [20, 21]. All participants performed six passes (three times down the pathway and back) at self-paced velocity, starting and ending their walks approximately 1.5 m before and after the walkway. Then they turn around and start their next pass. The motor dual task consisted of walking with a large ("pint") glass which was filled with water, with the aim of not spilling the water. The mental/cognitive dual task was serial "7" subtraction while walking, starting from randomly chosen numbers 90, 95 or 100. The combined motor and cognitive task comprised of serial subtractions as described, while walking with glass with water. The walking distance consisted of app 50 m (six passes × 8–9 m) for each task (basic, motor, mental, and combined) which finally amounted to 200 m of walking, sufficient to assess gait variability [20, 21].

Assessment of gait data

We measured spatiotemporal parameters—cycle time (CT), stride length (SL), swing time (SWT) and double support time (DST). Variability of gait parameters was calculated through the coefficient of variation (CV)—variability normalized to mean value (CV = 100 × SD/mean) [22]. These parameters were chosen because of their association with executive functions, cognitive decline and/or gait rhythmicity in different patient and non-patient populations [6, 7]. Data from the activated sensors are collected and the GAITRite software calculated spatiotemporal parameters.

Assessment questionnaires

The following assessment questionnaires were used to estimate functional status of patients, pain and fatigue level, presence of depression, as well as cognitive functions status. The evaluator performing clinical assessments was a single, blinded, and experienced physician/rheumatologist.

Fibromyalgia Impact Questionnaire Revised (FIQR)

The FIQR is the instrument for measuring functional status in FM patients. It includes 21 items that are answered on numeric rating scale of 0-to-10, with 10 reflecting greatest impairment. The time frame is the 7 days, with the items distributed across three associated domains: "function" (9 items); "overall impact" (2 items); and "severity of symptoms" (10 items). The scoring system is as follows: the physical function domain (0-to-90) is divided by 3, the overall impact domain (0-to-20) is not transformed, and the severity of symptoms domain (0-to-100) is divided by 2 [23].

Krupp Fatigue Severity Score (FSS)

Severity and impact of fatigue was measured by FSS [24]. Patients were asked to rate their level of agreement (toward seven) or disagreement (toward zero) with nine statements. A score of 36 and above (out of a maximum of 63) indicated the presence of significant fatigue. A higher score indicates greater fatigue. FSS is most effective as a measure of disability-related fatigue arising from a chronic, debilitating illness.

Visual Analog Scale of pain intensity

The visual analog scale (VAS) is a validated, subjective measure for acute and chronic pain. Scores are recorded by making a handwritten mark on a 10-cm line that represents a continuum between "no pain" and "worst pain" (or more precisely between 0 and 100%).

The Short Form (36) Health Survey

All patients completed the SF-36 questionnaire as a measure of health related quality of life [25]. The SF-36 is a generic instrument that measures eight general health concepts: physical functioning (PF), role physical (RP), bodily pain (BP), general health (GH), vitality (VT), social functioning (SF), role emotional (RE) and mental health (MH). Two main scores are available to summarize these scales: physical composite score (PCS) and mental composite score (MCS), as well as total SF-36 score. All these scores fall within a 0–100 scale, with higher scores reflecting better health related quality of life.

Euroqol 5 dimensions (EQ 5D 3L)

All patients completed the 3-level version of EuroQol 5 dimensions (EQ-5D-3L). The EQ-5D-3L essentially consists of 2 pages: the EQ-5D descriptive system and the EQ visual analogue scale (EQ VAS). The first part records the severity of the problem in each of the five dimensions, and the second part contains a 20-cm vertical visual analogue scale ranging from 0 to 100, where 0 corresponds to the worst imaginable health states and 100 corresponds to the best health states. Its five dimensions are mobility, self-care, usual activities, pain/discomfort, and anxiety/depression, and each dimension has three levels of severity (no problems, moderate problems, and extreme problems). Health status is labeled with a five-digit number that represents the severity level in each dimension [26].

Mini Mental State Examination (MMSE)

The MMSE is an 11-question assessment tool to test domains—orientation of time and place, registration of 3 words, attention and calculation (recall of 3 words, language and visual construction). The test is scored from 0 to 30, where higher scores indicate better cognitive performance, and a score below 24 suggests dementia [27].

Hamilton Depression Rating Scale (HAM-D)

This 17-item scale questioning the depressive complaints in the past week. The maximum score is 53 points. The scoring is as follows: 0–7 points indicates "no depression", 8–15 points indicates "mild depression", 16–28 points indicates "moderate depression", 29 points and above indicates "severe depression" [28].

Beck's Depression Inventory (BDI)

Beck's Depression Inventory was used to assess the mood [29]. This index is a validated instrument which includes 21 items measuring depression. Scores above 13 are indicating the presence of depression and scores above 21 to indicate major depression.

Statistical analysis

Shapiro–Wilk test was used for data normality assessment. Friedman test was used to analyze statistical significance through motor, cognitive and combined tests input within groups (FM and HC). The independent t-test was performed for CT, SL, SWT and DST (parametric variables) while Mann–Whitney test (non-parametric) were performed for CV CT, CV SL, CV SWT and CV DST while FM and HC walking during different conditions. According to data obtained by normality tests, we used Spearman's (rho) correlation coefficient.

The analyses were performed using SPSS 17.0 (SPSS, Chicago, IL), and p-values < 0.05 were considered significant.

Results

We included 24 female FM patients (mean age 55.08 ± 11.28 years) and 24 healthy controls (mean age 55.17 ± 11.18 years). Demographic and clinical features of patients are presented in Table 1.

Patients were on average in the range of mild depression, according to HAM-D (15.63 ± 6.03) and BDI (14.63 ± 6.36). During evaluation, 11 patients (45.8%) reported use of antidepressant therapy.

Gait parameters of FM patients and healthy control subjects (cycle time, stride length, swing time and double support time, and CVs of those parameters) were presented for all experimental conditions during base walk,

Table 1 Demographic and Clinical features of fibromyalgia patients (n=24)

Value	Mean ± SD
Disease duration (years)	11.72 ± 8.59
Time from diagnosis (years)	4.75 ± 3.42
FIQR	50.68 ± 18.20
FSS	4.77 ± 1.65
VAS	66.25 ± 18.84
SF 36 PCS	35.83 ± 14.85
SF 36 MCS	46.29 ± 19.23
SF 36 total	41.12 ± 16.84
EQ 5D 3L	62.92 ± 22.55
MMSE	29.00 ± 1.35
HAM-D	15.63 ± 6.03
BDI	14.63 ± 6.36

Values present means ± SDs—FIQR: Fibromyalgia Impact Questionnaire Revised; FSS: Krupp's Fatigue Severity Scale; VAS: visual analog scale; SF 36 PCS: The Short Form (36) Health Survey: physical composite score; SF 36 MCS: The Short Form (36) Health Survey—mental composite score; SF 36 total: The Short Form (36) Health Survey total score; EQ 5D 3L: Euroqol 5 dimensions 3-level version; HAM-D: Hamilton Depression Rating Scale; MMSE: Mini Mental State Examination; BDI: Beck Depression Inventory

dual motor task, dual mental task and combined task in Fig. 1 (gait parameters on left panels, their CVs on right panels).

Assessing the impact of motor, cognitive and combined tasks in all subjects, FM patients and HC, confirmed that these tasks affect gait performance (Friedman test). There were no differences in within group comparisons of FM patients and HCs in any of the assessed parameters, except in double support time during combined task, which was significantly prolonged in FM patients compared to HC (Fig. 1—* represents significance $p=0.022$).

Between group comparisons showed that cycle time of FM patients was significantly longer than in HC while stride length was shorter in patients for all four walking conditions. Swing time was prolonged in FM patients compared to HC for base and motor tasks, while double support time was significantly different for motor, mental and combined tasks (see Table 2, all significant differences are italic values). Further, note that CV's of all gait parameters were not significantly different in FM compared to HC in any of the walking conditions.

There was no correlation of VAS, FSS, MMSE, SF 36 physical, SF 36 total and FIQR with any of the four gait parameters and their CVs, performed in any of four walking tasks for FM patients. BDI correlate to cycle time, stride length and double support time while performing combined task ($\rho=0.58$, $p<0.01$; $\rho=-0.5$, $p<0.05$ and $\rho=0.58$, $p<0.01$, respectively). In FM patients HAM-D correlate to stride length and double support time. Correlations were also found in six other CVs of gait parameters through all four tasks (see details in Table 3). Concerning EQ 5D 3L, we found correlation for SWT and CV SWT and CV DST in most of the walking tasks, respectively. Correlations of SF 36 mental are also shown in Table 3.

Discussion

Study findings indicate that gait was impaired in FM patients, and gait performance correlates to clinical symptoms associated with fibromyalgia. Compared to their matched HC, FM female patients have shown significant differences in spatio-temporal gait parameters (CT, SL, SWT and DST) while their CV's were not significantly different in any of the walking conditions. Those findings were different to earlier literature findings [16–18].

In studies measuring gait while female FM patients performed several motor tasks [14, 15], or during base walking [17] and walking with different velocities [16, 17], results did not support gender-specific differences [16]. In general, women with FM have lower pain thresholds, greater diffuse pain, a higher number of tender points, higher levels of fatigue and greater sleep disturbance compared to men with FM [30–33]. However, differences in spatio-temporal gait variables were not reported [16–19]. Therefore, our study with only female patients could give conclusions irrespective of patients' gender, while making patient group more coherent concerning gait characteristics.

Our patients were in the range of mild depression (Table 1). It was shown earlier that gait in patients with depression is affected in a certain manner [e.g., 20, 34]. In our earlier study with very similar protocol, patients with major depression demonstrated slower gait in all task conditions compared to HC, while maintaining stability. Tasks that required greater cognitive involvement increased gait variability in patients, but only up to a certain level, after which patients' gait stability appeared unaffected by the increase of cognitive demand [20]. Gait in FM patients is affected similarly, showing similar pattern of gait parameters changes as described for patients with depressive disorder [20]. That could point toward important influence of depressive symptoms in FM on gait. Further, it is interesting that HAM-D scores negatively correlated to stride length in all conditions while were positively associated to DST only where cognitive input was engaged (i.e. mental and combined tasks). BDI correlated to CT, SL and DST only during combined, more complex tasks. It could be speculated that symptoms of depression influence patients to reduce stride length and double support time in comparison to their matched control subjects, such a measures to preserve stability of gait, mostly affected while cognitive, mental

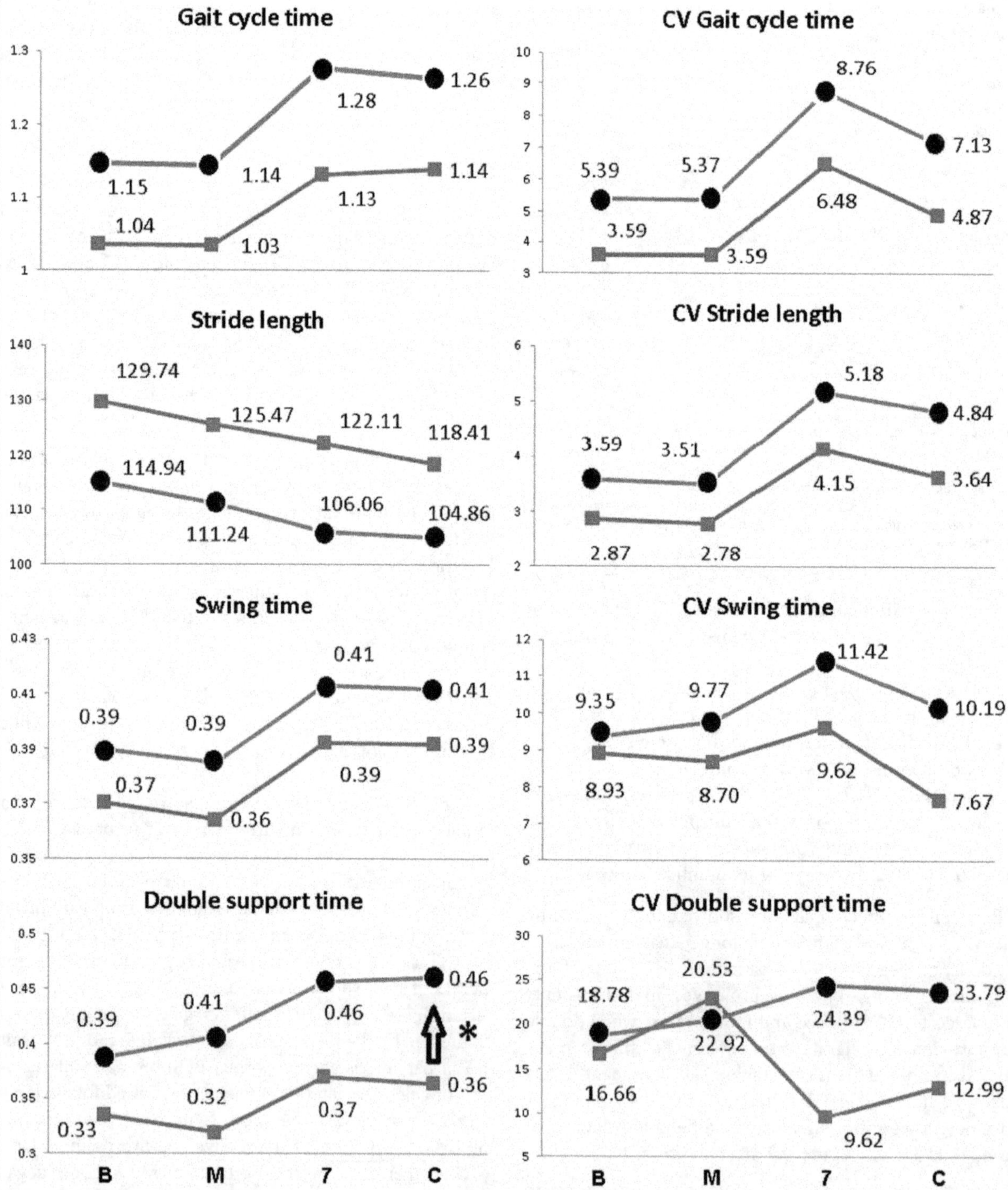

Fig. 1 Comparison between FM patients (circle) and control subjects (square). Four left panels represent FM cycle time, stride length, swing time and double support time compared to controls, while four right panels represent the CV's of cycle time, stride length, swing time and double support time. Patients and controls performing the following tasks: base walk (B), motor task (M), cognitive task (7) and combined motor and cognitive tasks (C). Each symbol represents the mean values. Note panel Double support time—*represents significance (Mann Whithey *U* test, $p=0.022$)

Table 2 Between group comparisons (FM vs HC) of gait parameters for all experimental conditions

	CT	SL	SWT	DST	CV CT	CV SL	CV SWT	CV DST
Base walk	*0.001*	*0.003*	*0.032*	0.149	0.248	0.303	0.837	0.621
Motor task	*0.001*	*0.003*	*0.041*	*0.039*	0.103	0.103	0.398	0.711
Mental task	*0.005*	*0.003*	0.125	*0.038*	0.266	0.138	0.293	0.564
Combined task	*0.006*	*0.009*	0.123	*0.014*	0.278	0.120	0.090	0.334
	t test				Mann–Whitney test			

CT Cycle Time, *SL* Stride Length, *SWT* Swing Time, *DST* Double support time, *CV* Coefficient of variation

Table 3 Correlations of HAM-D, EQ-5D-3L and SF 36m to gait parameters in all walking tasks

	CT	SL	SWT	DST	CV CT	CV SL	CV SWT	CV DST
HAM-D								
Base walk	0.13	−0.4*	−0.34	0.35	0.49*	0.46*	0.29	0.21
Motor task	0.39	−0.42*	−0.34	0.36	0.48*	0.29	0.32	0.15
Mental task	0.35	−0.5*	−0.11	0.51*	0.26	0.36	0.58**	0.42*
Combined task	0.41	−0.58**	0.20	0.69**	0.32	0.32	0.58**	0.31
EQ 5D 3L								
Base walk	0.19	0.06	0.57**	−0.20	−0.27	−0.04	0.44*	−0.59**
Motor task	0.28	0.07	0.49*	−0.15	−0.40	−0.01	−0.43*	−0.45*
Mental task	0.12	0.13	0.32	−0.11	−0.21	−0.13	−0.61**	0.5*
Combined task	−0.05	−0.27	0.49*	−0.30	−0.21	−0.13	−0.55*	−0.48*
SF 36m								
Base walk	0.05	0.35	0.28	−0.19	−0.40	−0.33	−0.25	−0.34
Motor task	−0.07	0.32	0.18	−0.14	−0.43*	−0.18	−0.23	−0.23
Mental task	−0.16	0.38	0.2	−0.25	−0.36	−0.37	−0.53**	−0.42*
Combined task	−0.41	0.55*	0.18	−0.55*	−0.35	−0.41	−0.46*	−0.31

HAM-D: Hamilton Depression Rating Scale; EQ 5D 3L: Euroqol 5 dimensions 3-level version; SF 36m: The Health Survey Mental composite score. Correlations of other used assessment questionnaires and gait parameters were described in Result section.

ρ (rho) = Spearman correlation, *$p < 0.05$, **$p < 0.01$

tasks requirements were employed. That might prevent negative cognitive input on gait stability, shortening the strides and increasing time with both feet on the ground, reducing gait variability in such complex situations. However, our patients were not suffering from major depression and were on stable antidepressant treatment, suggesting possible impact of FM per se.

Patients' gait is examined under dual task conditions, and possible impairments in dual task walking are estimated in relation to mental/cognitive and motor engagement. CT and SL were different between FM and HC for all experimental conditions (Table 2). Further, SWT was different in base and motor tasks, while it was not different during mental and combined tasks. That finding could mean that FM patients behave differently from HC, and during tasks without cognitive employment, their gait pattern is changed. The parameters affected by base walk or motor performance might be linked to clinical symptoms associated with FM, such as presence of chronic pain, bradykinesia, stiffness or fatigue [13–15, 17], and that could be responsible for gait alterations. Further, tasks with cognitive inputs (mental and combined) show no significant influence. That could be explained by importance and strong input of cognition on gait, on both groups, where HC also change their gait pattern while performing a secondary mental task [e.g., 7, 35, 36] (Table 2, Fig. 1). Additional tasks did not significantly affect described gait parameters changes, changes are already present, to preserve stability. Additionally, FM patients had considerable prolongation of DST while performing combined task (Table 2 and Fig. 1), stressing certain level of postural instability [37]. Since swing time and double support time were reported to reflect posture and balance [7, 21, 37], that could be the action to increase stability due to increased attention and awareness of patients of requirement to fulfill the complex given tasks. On the other hand, gait variability was not significantly increased as earlier described in the study where FM females were tested [17], but trend of greater CVs across all tasks was observed that did not reach statistical significance, possibly due to smaller sample in our study. Alternatively, our patients tend to preserve stability in those dual tasks, complex walking situations.

In order to assess the influence of the disease clinical characteristics, we correlated gait parameters in all experimental conditions to the questionnaires and patients' reports. There were no significant correlation of VAS, FSS, MMSE, SF 36 physical, SF 36 total and FIQR with any of the four gait parameters and their CVs, performed in any of four walking tasks for FM patients. Correlates of depression status (BDI and HAM-D) are particularly present for stride length, and that was discussed earlier. Correlations of EQ 5D 3L and SF 36m—severity of the health status and quality of life in the domain of mental health with evaluated gait parameters are shown in Table 3. Most of the correlations were with the parameters SWT, CV of SWT and DST. As it was said earlier, swing time and double support time were reported to reflect posture and balance, possibly as a function of preserved central mechanisms [7, 21, 37]. Therefore our patients preserve gait stability and adapt gait pattern for complex requirements while walking, probably because of their perceived deteriorated health status and its mental component that could change gait and evoke walking instability. Attention should be paid to depression status of FM patients in order to either improve gait pattern or to use that tests to define FM subgroup and focus on treatment of depression. Same is true for assessment of severity of the perceived health status (e.g. EQ 5D 3L) and quality of life patients' experiencing, especially in the domain of mental health (e.g. SF 36m).

Limitation of the study was the design where we performed single center, observational, cross-sectional study and we could suggest that longitudinal studies would strengthen the study findings and recommendations. Also, lower prevalence of FM in man limited us to perform study in female patients only. Finally, the number of our female patients took antidepressant medication and, therefore, the effect of this medication on gait characteristics could not be completely neglected.

Conclusions

It could be concluded that gait is affected in FM patients during dual walking tasks. Cognitive tasks, alone or combined with motor task, had a larger effect than motor tasks. However, no changes in stride-to-stride variability indicated that patients preserve stability in complex walking situations, in spite of potential clinical symptoms effect. Therefore, analysis of gait may provide additional information for the FM identification based on presence of certain clinical symptoms and cognitive status. Attention also should be paid to depression status of patients to either improve gait pattern or to use that tests to define FM subgroups. According to these results we could further support the approach that correlation of dual task gait pattern alterations to existence of FM symptoms and cognitive changes influencing gait pattern could successfully define FM subgroups.

Acknowledgements

The study has been supported by the Ministry of Education, Science and Technological Development, Republic of Serbia.

Authors' information

GR, ZV, MR and SJ are rheumatologists, experienced in fibromyalgia treatment and research. VM and SR are neurologists, experienced in gait research.

Authors' contributions

All listed authors participated significantly in this study. Study aim creation, conceptualization and design: GR and SR. Acquisition of data—recordings of patients and control subjects: SR, ZV, MR and SJ. Analysis and interpretation of data: GR, ZV, VM and SR. Drafting of the manuscript: SR, VM and GR. Critical revision of the manuscript for important intellectual content: SR. Statistical analysis: GR, VM. Study supervision and final approval: SR and GR. All authors read and approved the final manuscript.

Author details

[1]Institute of Rheumatology, Faculty of Medicine, University of Belgrade, Resavska 69, Belgrade, Serbia. [2]Neurology Clinic, Faculty of Medicine, University of Belgrade, Dr Subotića 6, Belgrade, Serbia. [3]Institute for Medical Research, University of Belgrade, Dr Subotića 4, 11129 Belgrade, Serbia.

References

1. Borchers AT, Gershwin ME. Fibromyalgia: a critical and comprehensive review. Clin Rev Allergy Immunol. 2015;49:100–51.
2. Clauw DJ. Fibromyalgia and related conditions. Mayo Clin Proc. 2015;90:680–92.
3. Wolfe F, Clauw DJ, Fitzcharles MA, Goldenberg DL, Katz RS, Mease P, et al. The American College of Rheumatology preliminary diagnostic criteria for fibromyalgia and measurement of symptom severity. Arthritis Care Res (Hoboken). 2010;62:600–10.
4. Wolfe F, Clauw DJ, Fitzcharles MA, Goldenberg DL, Häuser W, Katz RS, et al. Fibromyalgia criteria and severity scales for clinical and epidemiological studies: a modification of the ACR Preliminary Diagnostic Criteria for Fibromyalgia. J Rheumatol. 2011;38:1113–22.
5. Wolfe F, Clauw DJ, Fitzcharles MA, Goldenberg DL, Katz RS, Mease P, et al. Revisions to the 2010/2011 fibromyalgia diagnostic criteria. Semin Arthritis Rheum. 2016;46:319–29.
6. Yogev G, Giladi N, Peretz C, Springer S, Simon ES, Hausdorff JM. Dual tasking, gait rhythmicity, and Parkinson's disease: which aspects of gait are attention demanding? Eur J Neurosci. 2005;22:1248–56.
7. Yogev-Seligmann G, Hausdorff JM, Giladi N. The role of executive function and attention in gait. Mov Disord. 2008;23:329–42.
8. Giesecke T, Williams DA, Harris RE, Cupps TR, Tian X, Tian TX, et al. Subgrouping of fibromyalgia patients on the basis of pressure-pain thresholds and psychological factors. Arthritis Rheum. 2003;48:2916–22.
9. Wilson HD, Robinson JP, Turk DC. Toward the identification of symptom patterns in people with fibromyalgia. Arthritis Rheum. 2009;61:527–34.
10. Gracely RH, Ambrose KR. Neuroimaging of fibromyalgia. Best Pract Res Clin Rheumatol. 2011;25:271–84.
11. Auvinet B, Chaleil D, Cabane J, Dumolard A, Hatron P, Juvin R, et al. The interest of gait markers in the identification of subgroups among fibro myalgia patients. BMC Musculoskelet Disord. 2011;12:258.
12. Auvinet B, Chaleil D. Identification of subgroups among fibromyalgia

patients. Reumatismo. 2012;64:250–60.
13. Auvinet B, Bileckot R, Alix AS, Chaleil D, Barrey E. Gait disorders in patients with fibromyalgia. Jt Bone Spine. 2006;73:543–6.
14. Costa ID, Gamundí A, Miranda JG, França LG, De Santana CN, Montoya P. Altered functional performance in patients with fibromyalgia. Front Hum Neurosci. 2017;11:14.
15. Martín-Martínez JP, Villafaina S, Collado-Mateo D, Fuentes-García JP, Pérez-Gómez J, Gusi N. Impact of cognitive tasks on biomechanical and kinematic parameters of gait in women with fibromyalgia: a cross-sectional study. Physiol Behav. 2020;227:113171.
16. Heredia-Jimenez J, Orantes-Gonzalez E. Gender differences in patients with fibromyalgia: a gait analysis. Clin Rheumatol. 2019;38:513–22.
17. Heredia-Jimenez J, Orantes-Gonzalez E, Soto-Hermoso VM. Variability of gait, bilateral coordination, and asymmetry in women with fibromyalgia. Gait Posture. 2016;45:41–4.
18. Heredia-Jiménez JM, Aparicio García-Molina VA, Porres Foulquie JM, Delgado Fernández M, Soto-Hermoso VM. Spatial-temporal parameters of gait in women with fibromyalgia. Clin Rheumatol. 2009;28:595–8.
19. Heredia-Jimenez JM, Soto-Hermoso VM. Kinematics gait disorder in men with fibromyalgia. Rheumatol Int. 2014;34:63–5.
20. Radovanović S, Jovičić M, Marić NP, Kostić V. Gait characteristics in patients with major depression performing cognitive and motor tasks while walking. Psychiatry Res. 2014;217:39–46.
21. Radovanović S, Perić S, Savić-Pavićević D, Dobričić V, Pešović J, Kostić V, et al. Comparison of temporal and stride characteristics in myotonic dystrophies type 1 and 2 during dual-task walking. Gait Posture. 2016;44:194–9.
22. Menz HB, Latt MD, Tiedemann A, MunSanKwan M, Lord SR. Reliability of the GAITRite walkway system for the quantification of temporo-spatial parameters of gait in young and older people. Gait Posture. 2004;20:20–5.
23. Bennett RM, Friend R, Jones KD, Ward R, Han BK, Ross RL. The Revised Fibromyalgia Impact Questionnaire (FIQR): validation and psychometric properties. Arthritis Res Ther. 2009;11:415.
24. Krupp LB, LaRocca NG, Muir-Nash J, Steinberg AD. The fatigue severity scale. Application to patients with multiple sclerosis and systemic lupus erythematosus. Arch Neurol. 1989;46:1121–3.
25. Beyazal MS, Tüfekçi A, Kırbaş S, Topaloğlu MS. The impact of fibromyalgia on disability, anxiety, depression, sleep disturbance, and quality of life in patients with migraine. Noro Psikiyatr Ars. 2018;55:140–5.
26. Collado-Mateo D, Dominguez-Muñoz FJ, Adsuar JC, Garcia-Gordillo MA, Gusi N. Effects of exergames on quality of life, pain, and disease effect in women with fibromyalgia: a randomized controlled trial. Arch Phys Med Rehabil. 2017;98:1725–31.
27. Folstein MF, Folstein SE, McHugh PR. "Mini-mental state". A practical method for grading the cognitive state of patients for the clinician. J Psychiatr Res. 1975;12:189–98.
28. Hamilton M. A rating scale for depression. J Neurol Neurosurg Psychiatry. 1960;23:56–62.
29. Beck AT, Ward CH, Mendelson M, Mock J, Erbaugh J. An inventory for measuring depression. Arch Gen Psychiatry. 1961;4:561–71.
30. Wolfe F, Ross K, Anderson J, Russell IJ. Aspects of fibromyalgia in the general population: sex, pain threshold, and fibromyalgia symptoms. J Rheumatol. 1995;22:151–6.
31. Yunus MB, Celiker R, Aldag JC. Fibromyalgia in men: comparison of psychological features with women. J Rheumatol. 2004;31:2464–7.
32. Miró E, Martínez MP, Sánchez AI, Prados G, Lupiáñez J. Men and women with fibromyalgia: relation between attentional function and clinical symptoms. Br J Health Psychol. 2015;20:632–47.
33. Yunus MB, Inanici F, Aldag JC, Mangold RF. Fibromyalgia in men: comparison of clinical features with women. J Rheumatol. 2000;27:485–90.
34. Lemke MR, Wendorff T, Mieth B, Buhl K, Linnemann M. Spatiotemporal gait patterns during over ground locomotion in major depression compared with healthy controls. J Psychiatr Res. 2000;34:277–83.
35. Kressig RW, Beauchet O, European GAITRite Network Group. Guidelines for clinical applications of spatio-temporal gait analysis in older adults. Aging Clin Exp Res. 2006;18:174–6.
36. Hausdorff JM, Edelberg HK, Mitchell SL, Goldberger AL, Wei JY. Increased gait unsteadiness in community-dwelling elderly fallers. Arch Phys Med Rehabil. 1997;78:278–83.
37. Marchese R, Bove M, Abbruzzese G. Effect of cognitive and motor tasks on postural stability in Parkinson's disease: a posturographic study. Mov Disord. 2003;18:652–8.

11

Depression is associated with increased disease activity and higher disability in a large Italian cohort of patients with rheumatoid arthritis

Sara Pezzato[1], Chiara Bonetto[2], Cristian Caimmi[1], Simona Tomassi[2], Ilaria Montanari[1], Maria Giulia Gnatta[2], Elena Fracassi[1], Doriana Cristofalo[2], Maurizio Rossini[1], Antonio Carletto[1*] and Sarah Tosato[2]

Abstract

Introduction: Depression is a quite common comorbidity in patients with rheumatoid arthritis (RA) and is thought to influence its severity. This study aims to estimate, in a large cohort of Italian patients with RA, the prevalence of depression and to investigate the clinical correlates of depression in terms of disease activity and disability.

Methods: This is a cross-sectional study enrolling 490 outpatients with RA (80% female, mean age 59.5). The Hospital Anxiety and Depression Scale (HADS) was used to assess the presence of depression with a cut-off of 11. We collected data about disease activity and disability with DAS28, TJC-68, PhGA, PGA, VAS, DAS28, SDAI, CDAI and HAQ.

Results: Prevalence of depression was 14.3% (95% CI: 11-17%). Depressed patients, when compared with not depressed ones, were found to have higher scores for TJC-68 ($p=0.011$), PhGA ($p=0.001$), PGA ($p=0.001$), VAS ($p=0.001$), DAS28 ($p=0.007$), SDAI ($p=0.001$), CDAI ($p=0.001$) and HAQ ($p=0.001$). Out of the 70 depressed patients, 30 subjects, already known to be depressed in the past, were still depressed at the time of the assessment, with only 11 (15.7%) under antidepressants. A multivariate analysis showed that male sex, higher PGA score, use of antidepressants and higher HAQ score were significantly associated with an increased risk of depression.

Conclusions: Our study shows that depression is common in RA and may affect its activity mainly via an alteration in the perception of the disease. Although its important implications, depression is still under-diagnosed and its management is inadequate.

Keywords: Depression, Rheumatoid arthritis, Disease activity, Disability

Introduction

Rheumatoid arthritis (RA) is a chronic inflammatory disease with a prevalence of 0.5–1% in Europe, with the lower values in southern countries [1]. It primarily involves peripheral joints, damaging cartilages and bones, and leads progressively to disability. RA shows also systemic manifestations and it has been associated to systemic comorbidities, as depressive and anxiety disorders [2].

In patients with RA, the prevalence of depression ranges between 14.8 and 22.5%, which is two to three times higher than in the general population [3], reaching a 47% lifetime risk [4, 5]. In addition, about 39% of patients affected by RA have also sub-threshold depressive symptoms [5]. Finally, depression occurs twice as

*Correspondence: antonio.carletto@aovr.veneto.it
[1] Rheumatology Unit, University of Verona, Policlinico G.B. Rossi, Piazzale Scuro, 10, 37134 Verona, VR, Italy

often in females with RA as compared to males suffering from RA [6].

The presence of depression has been associated with increased pain perception [4], increased level of physical disability [7], enhanced health care costs [6], and greater mortality [4]. Notably, it has been demonstrated a significant association between persistent depression and high continuous disease activity, measured by the Clinical Disease Activity Index (CDAI) [8]. Notably, most of the activity scores commonly used in rheumatology are based also on subjective measures that may be affected by the psychological status [9] and may further influence the assessment of disease activity.

Finally, depression was found to be a strong negative predictor of remission [10], thus should be evaluated in every patient in order to increase the probability of a good disease control.

Since there is a possibly bidirectional relationship between the severity of both rheumatic disease and depressive disorders, it is fundamental to study the clinical correlates of depression in RA patients in order to improve the clinical outcome of RA.

The present study aims (1) to estimate, in a large sample of Italian patients affected by Rheumatoid Arthritis, the prevalence of depressive disorders; and (2) to investigate the clinical correlates of depression in terms of RA disease activity and disability. Specifically, we hypothesized that RA individuals affected by depression were characterized by higher levels of RA disease activity and disability when compared to non-depressed ones. The present study offers the opportunity to increase our knowledge on the comorbidity by investigating depression and its clinical correlates, as part of the routine clinical monitoring, in a large real life RA sample from a real-world outpatient setting. Studying the clinical correlates of depression in RA is a relevant issue in order to define appropriate screening and treatment programs to prevent worse outcome for both depression and RA.

Material and methods

This is an observational, cross-sectional study examining the clinical correlates of depressive disorders in a cohort of patients affected by Rheumatoid Arthritis on DMARDs treatment for at least one year. Individuals followed at the Unit of Rheumatology, University Hospital of Verona, Italy, in the period between March 2016 and February 2017 were enrolled during a routine outpatient visit. The inclusion criteria were: (1) age $\geq$ 18 years; (2) RA diagnosis according to the American College of Rheumatology (ACR)/ European League Against Rheumatism (EULAR) 2010 [11]. Individuals with fibromyalgia, connective tissue diseases (LES, Sjogren, sclerodermas, dermatomyositis, polymyositis), vasculitis, gout, infective arthritis, rheumatic polymyalgia or other severe systemic diseases were excluded.

A comprehensive set of standardized instruments was used to collect socio-demographic and clinical information.

Specifically, RA-related characteristics including disease duration, 28 tender/swollen joints count (TJC 28/SJC 28) [12], 68 tender/swollen joints count (TJC 68/SJC 68), Visual Analogue Scale (VAS, 0–100 mm) for joint pain, Physician Global Assessment (PhGA, 0–10) and Patient Global Assessment (PGA, 0–10), were collected. RA disease activity and disability were assessed with 28-joints Disease Activity Score (DAS28) [1], Simplified Disease Activity Index (SDAI) [1], Clinical Disease Activity Index (CDAI) [1] and Health Assessment Questionnaires (HAQ) [13]. Patients were assessed for the presence of any comorbidity and for smoking. Data about current rheumatic medications, antidepressants or benzodiazepines were recorded. Body Mass Index (BMI, kg/m^2) was calculated as following: weight was measured without shoes, and in light indoor clothes, using a balance beam scale; height was measured without shoes using a fixed stadiometer.

Blood samples were collected to detect the presence of anti-citrullinated protein antibody (ACPA) and/or rheumatoid factor (RF), erythrocyte sedimentation rate (ESR, mm/hour), C-reactive protein (CRP; mg/L), vitamin D level (25-OH-D3, nmol/L).

Depressive and anxious symptomatology was assessed using the Hospital Anxiety and Depression Scale (HADS) [8]. The HADS is a self-administered instrument validated in a hospital setting and developed for evaluating depression in somatic primary or secondary care [9]. It is composed by two subscales, one for depression (HADS-D) and one for anxiety (HADS-A), each constituted by seven items. Every item is scored from 0 to 3, and higher scores indicate more severe symptoms. Total sum score ranges from 0 to 21 for HADS-D. For the present study, we decided to use only the HADS-D with a cut-off of 11, allowing us to identify with greater specificity depressed subjects.

The investigation was carried out in accordance with the latest version of the Declaration of Helsinki [14].

Statistical analyses

Descriptives were given for all variables. Comparisons between depressed patients (HADS-D score $\geq$ 11) and not depressed patients (HADS-D score < 11) were assessed by Chi-square tests for categorical variables and t-tests (2 independent groups) for continuous variables. Each socio-demographic and clinical variable which resulted significantly different in the two groups was entered into a univariable linear regression model with HADS-D score as the dependent variable. Subsequently, only those variables associated at $p < 0.10$ entered into a series of multivariable hierarchical linear regression models (model 1: demographics; model 2: plus RA-related variables; model 3: plus RA therapy; model 4: plus psychotropic therapy; model 5: plus RA disease activity and disability indices). The R-square change at each step was used to determine the variance explained by each set of variables. Collinearity among the independent variables was explored by calculating the individual variance inflation factors. In the final model, these values ranged between 1.10 and 3.29, thus indicating the absence of multicollinearity. All tests were 2-tailed. Statistical analyses were performed using SPSS 22 for Windows.

Results

Prevalence of depression and its association with socio-demographic characteristics

We assessed 490 patients with RA (80% female, with mean age of about 60 years). We found that the prevalence of depression was 14.3% (95% CI: 11–17%). Indeed, out of the 490 participants, 70 patients scored ≥ 11 in HADS-D questionnaire (Table 1). Depression was more frequent in females and in unemployed patients ($p = 0.001$ and $p = 0.034$, respectively). No other socio-demographic characteristics were associated with depression.

The association between depression and clinical characteristics

We found that out of 70 depressed patients, 30 (42.9%) reported a personal history of depression. Moreover, patients with depression, when compared to non-depressed ones, have higher TJC68 ($p = 0.011$), PhGA ($p < 0.011$), PGA ($p < 0.011$) and VAS ($p < 0.011$) (Table 2). There were no differences between the two groups in terms of duration of illness, RF and/or ACPA seropositive form, number of erosions, family history of rheumatic disease, TJC28, SJC28, SJC66 and biological characteristics.

Most patients (90.8%) presented at least one comorbidity, with the cardiovascular the most represented one (56.1%) (Table 3). Regarding comorbidity, there were no differences between the two groups.

By considering medications (Table 4), almost half of the cohort (49.4%) used steroids, with a difference between depressed (60.0%) and not depressed (47.6%) patients ($p = 0.050$). One hundred and four patients (21.2%) used to take NSAIDs for ten or more days per month, with a significant difference between depressed (32.9%) and not depressed (19.3%) patients ($p = 0.010$).

There were no differences between the two groups in terms of cDMARDs and biologics' use. Out of the 70 depressed patients, 11 (15.7%) were under antidepressant treatment given a personal history of depression. On the other hand, a significantly lower proportion of non-depressed patients has had a previous diagnosis of depression and were taking anti-depressant drugs at the moment of assessment (4.5%, $p < 0.001$). Finally, depressed patients were found to take a higher number of drugs, i.e. anti-rheumatic drugs plus psychotropic therapy (6.4 versus 5.0, $p < 0.001$).

The association between depression and RA activity and disability

Depressed and not depressed patients were compared on RA activity and disability (Table 5) by means of

Table 1 Socio-demographic characteristics of RA patients and their association with depression (n = 490)

Socio-demographics	Total sample (n = 490)	Depression according to HADS-D (cut-off ≥ 11)		*p*-value (Chi-square or t test)
		Not depressed (n = 420)	Depressed (n = 70)	
Age (years), mean (sd)	59.5 (12.2)	59.2 (12.1)	61.5 (12.9)	0.141
Female, n (%)	392 (80.0%)	326 (77.6%)	66 (94.3%)	0.001
Marital status, n (%)				
Unmarried	57 (11.6%)	48 (11.5%)	9 (12.9%)	0.190
Married	355 (72.4%)	311 (74.0%)	44 (62.8%)	
Widowed	38 (7.8%)	30 (7.1%)	8 (11.4%)	
Divorced	40 (8.2%)	31 (7.4%)	9 (12.9%)	
With children, n (%)	395 (80.6%)	339 (80.7%)	56 (80.0%)	0.889
Low education, n (%)	299 (61.0%)	253 (60.2%)	46 (65.7%)	0.428
Occupation, n (%)				
Employed	192 (39.2%)	173 (41.2%)	19 (27.1%)	0.034
Unemployed	298 (60.8%)	247 (58.8%)	51 (72.9%)	

Low education: primary/secondary school

Table 2 Clinical characteristics and their association with depression (n = 490)

Clinical characteristics	Total sample (n = 490)	Depression according to HADS-D (cut-off ≥ 11)		*p*-value (Chi-square or t test)
		Not depressed (n = 420)	Depressed (n = 70)	
Positive personal history for depression, n (%)	106 (21.6%)	76 (18.1%)	30 (42.8%)	< 0.001
RF and/or ACPA positive, n (%)	292 (59.6%)	246 (58.6%)	46 (65.7%)	0.294
BMI (kg/m^2), mean (sd)	25.7 (4.8)	25.7 (4.8)	26.0 (5.1)	0.606
Smoker, n (%)	64 (13.1%)	57 (13.6%)	7 (10.0%)	0.565
Positive family history for rheumatologic disease, n (%)	127 (25.9%)	104 (24.8%)	23 (32.8%)	0.184
Erosions, n (%)	212 (43.3%)	179 (42.6%)	33 (47.1%)	0.516
Disease duration (years), mean (sd)	12.5 (9.6)	12.5 (9.6)	12.4 (9.5)	0.931
TJC 28, mean (sd)	2.1 (3.5)	2.0 (3.5)	2.6 (3.9)	0.197
SJC 28, mean (sd)	1.1 (2.2)	1.1 (2.3)	1.2 (2.1)	0.647
TJC 68, mean (sd)	2.6 (4.0)	2.4 (3.8)	3.7 (4.9)	0.011
SJC 66, mean (sd)	1.4 (2.7)	1.4 (2.7)	1.7 (2.4)	0.324
PhGA, mean (sd)	4.4 (2.7)	4.2 (2.7)	5.5 (2.5)	< 0.001
PGA, mean (sd)	5.3 (2.4)	5.1 (2.4)	6.6 (2.2)	< 0.001
VAS pain, mean (sd)	5.0 (2.7)	4.8 (2.7)	6.3 (2.2)	< 0.001
ESR, mean (sd)	19.9 (16.6)	19.6 (16.6)	21.9 (16.2)	0.276
CRP, mean (sd)	5.6 (8.8)	5.8 (9.3)	4.2 (4.3)	0.179
Vitamin D, mean (sd)	68.8 (28.3)	69.0 (28.1)	68.1 (30.0)	0.806
Haemoglobin, mean (sd)	13.4 (1.3)	13.4 (1.3)	13.2 (1.3)	0.105

RF rheumatoid factor; ACPA anti-citrullinated protein antibodies; BMI Body Mass Index, TJC tender joint count; SJC swollen joint count; PhGA physician global assessment; PGA patient global assessment; VAS visual analogue scale; ESR erythrocyte sedimentation rate; CRP C-reactive protein

Table 3 Presence of comorbidities and their association with depression (n = 490)

Comorbidities	Total sample (n = 490)	Depression according to HADS-D (cut-off ≥ 11)		*p*-value (Chi-square or t test)
		Not depressed(n = 420)	Depressed (n = 70)	
Comorbidities, n (%)	445 (90.8%)	379 (90.2%)	66 (94.3%)	0.373
Cardiovascular	275 (56.1%)	231 (55.0%)	44 (62.9%)	0.243
Endocrinological	127 (25.9%)	105 (25.0%)	22 (31.4%)	0.302
Neoplastic	58 (11.8%)	49 (11.7%)	9 (12.9%)	0.841
Pulmonary	43 (8.8%)	36 (8.6%)	7 (10.0%)	0.651
Neurological	9 (1.8%)	8 (1.9%)	1 (1.4%)	0.999
Gastroenterological	144 (29.4%)	117 (27.9%)	27 (38.6%)	0.088
Rheumatological	218 (44.5%)	177 (42.1%)	41 (58.6%)	0.013

DAS28-CRP, SDAI, CDAI and HAQ scores and their categories of activity/disability (remission, low, moderate, high).

Depressed patients scored significantly higher on all RA activity and disability scores. Moreover, by considering the categories of DAS28-CRP, SDAI and CDAI, the percentage of depressed patients increases from remission to moderate disease activity group, where it reaches its maximum, while decreases in high disease activity group. On the contrary, the trend between depression and disability shows that depression became more frequent in subjects with severe and very severe disability accordingly to HAQ scores ($p = 0.001$).

A series of univariable linear regression models with HADS-D score as the dependent variable and each of the variables pertaining to conceptual blocks (demographics, RA-related variables, RA therapy, psychotropic therapy, disease activity and disability indices) as the independent one was estimated. Those variables which resulted associated at $p < 0.10$ with the HADS-D score were entered into multivariable linear regression models, beginning from demographics and adding variables from the other

Table 4 Association between anti-rheumatic and psychotropic therapy and depression (n = 490)

Therapy	Total sample (n = 490)	Depression according to HADS-D (cut-off ≥ 11)		*p*-value (Chi-square or t test)
		Not depressed (n = 420)	Depressed (n = 70)	
RA therapy				
Corticosteroids, n (%)	242 (49.4%)	200 (47.6%)	42 (60.0%)	0.050
NSAIDs (> 10 per month), n (%)	104 (21.2%)	81 (19.3%)	23 (32.9%)	0.010
Vitamin D, n (%)	388 (79.2%)	328 (78.1%)	60 (85.7%)	0.146
Anti-rheumatic drugs				
Only cDMARDS, n (%)	199 (40.6%)	170 (40.5%)	29 (41.4%)	0.937
Only anti-TNFα, n (%)	67 (13.7%)	57 (13.6%)	10 (14.3%)	
cDMARDS plus anti-TNFα, n (%)	105 (21.4%)	92 (21.9%)	13 (18.6%)	
No cDMARDS, no anti-TNFα, n (%)	119 (24.3%)	101 (24.0%)	18 (25.7%)	
Psychotropic therapy				
Antidepressants, n (%)	30 (35.9%)	19 (4.5%)	11 (15.7%)	< 0.001
Total number of drugs, mean (sd)	5.2 (2.5)	5.0 (2.4)	6.4 (2.8)	< 0.001

cDMARDS: conventional disease-modifying antirheumatic drugs; anti-TNFα: anti-tumor necrosis factors drugs; Total number of drugs: anti-rheumatic drugs plus psychotropic therapy

conceptual blocks (Table 6). Males (model 1) have lower levels of depression than females (variance explained 3.3%); addition of RA-related variables (model 2) raised the variance explained up to 10.7%, with PGA score significantly associated with higher depression levels. Corticosteroids and NSAIDs (model 3) were not associated with depression score, while the use of antidepressants and the total number of assumed drugs (model 4) increased the variance by 2.2%, with both variables being significantly associated with higher depression levels. Finally, when disease activity and disability indices (SDAI and HAQ, respectively) were added (model 5), the model explained 14.5% of the variance, with higher HAQ being associated with higher depression score. At this step, however, the total number of assumed drugs was no longer statistically significant.

Discussion

This study evaluates the prevalence of depression and its clinical correlates in terms of disease activity and disability in a large sample of patients affected by RA. We found a prevalence of depression equal to 14.3% (95% CI: 11–17%), that is almost three times higher than the prevalence in the general population [15]. Depression should therefore be considered such as one of the commonest comorbidities of RA and it should always be evaluated with screening tests, and treated whether necessary, to improve clinical outcomes [16]. We also found that depressed patients had higher disease activity and increased disability indices (SDAI and HAQ, respectively). This result underlines the importance of distinguishing between an increased illness activity and an altered disease perception secondary to depression.

Previous studies showed great variability in the prevalence of depression in patients suffering from RA, reaching up to 34–48% [10, 12]. This variability may be explained by the different instruments and heterogeneity in criteria used to diagnose depression [17]. To avoid an overestimation of depression, we decided to use HADS-D with a cut-off of 11, allowing to identify with greater specificity depressed subjects, since it excludes elements that may reflect physical rather than psychological problems. Specifically, the HADS-D does not contain questions that investigate quality of sleep, fatigue and appetite, symptoms that are common in both depression and RA, as it happens in other questionnaires as Hamilton Rating Scale for Depression (HAM-D) [18]. Regarding the choice of the cut off for the HADS, a previous study [19] used a cut-off ≥ 8, thus including patients with borderline depression leading to a risk to overestimate the prevalence of depression. A systematic review [13] has identified 30 studies in RA patients in which HADS-D with a cut-off ≥ 11 was used; an average prevalence of depression of 14.8% emerged, which is very close to our result.

Regarding the socio-demographic correlates of depression, we found a significantly higher prevalence of depression among female patients (16.8%) compared to males (4.1%), in line with previous studies [14, 20, 21]. This evidence may be explained by the higher prevalence of depression in the general population among women [15]. In addition, women tend to undergo more frequently medical treatment, thus increasing the likelihood

Table 5 Association between RA activity/disability and depression (n = 490)

Disease activity and disability indices	Total sample (n = 490)	Depression according to HADS-D (cut-off ≥ 11)		*p*-value (Chi-square or t test)
		Not depressed (n = 420)	Depressed (n = 70)	
DAS28-CRP, mean (sd)	2.9 (1.1)	2.8 (1.1)	3.2 (0.9)	0.007
DAS28-CRP, n (%)				
Remission	231 (47.1%)	209 (49.7%)	22 (31.4%)	0.008
Low	82 (16.7%)	71 (16.9%)	11 (15.8%)	
Moderate	160 (32.7%)	125 (29.8%)	35 (50.0%)	
High	17 (3.5%)	15 (3.6%)	2 (2.8%)	
SDAI, mean (sd)	13.4 (8.2)	12.9 (8.2)	16.3 (7.5)	0.001
SDAI, n (%)				
Remission	34 (6.9%)	32 (7.6%)	2 (2.8%)	0.001
Low	176 (35.9%)	163 (38.8%)	13 (18.6%)	
Moderate	243 (49.6%)	193 (46.0%)	50 (71.4%)	
High	37 (7.6%)	32 (7.6%)	5 (7.1%)	
CDAI, mean (sd)	12.9 (8.0)	12.3 (8.0)	15.9 (7.4)	0.001
CDAI, n (%)				
Remission	32 (6.5%)	30 (7.1%)	2 (2.8%)	0.001
Low	184 (37.6%)	171 (40.8%)	13 (18.6%)	
Moderate	223 (45.5%)	177 (42.1%)	46 (65.7%)	
High	51 (10.4%)	42 (10.0%)	9 (12.9%)	
HAQ, mean (sd)	0.8 (0.7)	0.7 (0.7)	1.2 (0.7)	< 0.001
HAQ, n (%)				
Mild	133 (27.1%)	125 (29.8%)	8 (11.4%)	< 0.001
Moderate	220 (44.9%)	193 (46.0%)	27 (38.6%)	
Severe	109 (22.2%)	84 (20.0%)	25 (35.7%)	
Very severe	28 (5.7%)	18 (4.2%)	10 (14.3%)	

DAS28 28-joint Disease Activity Score; SDAI Simplified Disease Activity Index; CDAI Clinical Disease Activity Index; HAQ Health Assessment Questionnaires

DAS28-CRP: remission if ≤ 2.19, low if between 2.19 and 2.60, moderate if between 2.60 and 4.07, high if > 4.07

SDAI: remission if ≤ 3.3, low if between 3.3 and 11, moderate if between 11 and 26, high if > 26

CDAI: remission if ≤ 2.8, low if between 2.8 and 10, moderate if between 10 and 22, high if > 22

HAQ: mild disability if ≤ 0.1, moderate disability if between 0.1 and 1, severe disability if between 1 and 2, very severe disability if > 2

of detecting depression [22]. Furthermore, men tend not to complain about their psychological disturbances; on the contrary women express themselves more emotionally, obtaining higher scores in questionnaires [23]. In our cohort, the percentage of depressed patients is significantly higher in those without an occupation (17.1%) than in workers (9.9%). Our results are in line with previous studies [26], suggesting that the employment status is protective against the development of depression in RA. An association between lower income and depression has also been detected [26]: less economic resources may reduce attention and spending for health. On the contrary, other studies reported a positive correlation between employment and depressive symptoms [24]. We have not distinguished retired from unemployed subjects, therefore, at least half of this group is composed by old retired people (i.e. unemployed and aged ≥ 65 years), who could have negative feelings of worthlessness, fear of the future and sense of isolation, which are psychological feelings leading to the development of depressive symptoms [27]. Conversely, RA itself, causing disability, makes more difficult to find or keep a job, especially if it is a manual one.

On the other hand, 30 patients with a previous diagnosis of depression were still depressed at the time of the assessment. Out of them, 11 were depressed although under antidepressants. The remaining 19 depressed subjects were not diagnosed or treated despite a previous history of depression. A positive history for depression should be considered a risk factor for the persistence or recurrence of depression in RA. Moreover, we found that a considerable portion of patients (n = 40) with undetected depression had a negative history of depression. Thus, this under-recognized

Table 6 Multivariable hierarchical linear regression models with HADS-D score as dependent variable (n = 490)

Independent variables	Dependent variable: HADS-D score Beta coefficients (*p*-value)				
	Model 1	**Model 2**	**Model 3**	**Model 4**	**Model 5**
Socio-demographics					
Being male	− 1.85 (< 0.001)	− 1.42 (0.001)	− 1.41 (0.001)	− 1.41 (0.001)	− 1.18 (0.007)
RA-related variables					
PhGA		0.42 (< 0.001)	0.40 (< 0.001)	0.35 (< 0.001)	0.29 (0.002)
PGA		0.06 (0.387)	0.05 (0.488)	0.04 (0.582)	0.05 (0.587)
RA therapy					
Corticosteroids			0.21 (0.547)	− 0.16 (0.657)	− 0.32 (0.383)
NSAIDs (> 10 per month)			0.55 (0.196)	0.48 (0.254)	0.37 (0.382)
Antidepressants				1.96 (0.007)	2.06 (0.004)
Total number of drugs				0.16 (0.035)	0.10 (0.180)
Disease activity and disability indices					
SDAI					− 0.03 (0.422)
HAQ					0.97 (0.002)
Goodness of fit indices					
Adj R-squared %	3.3%	10.7%	10.7%	12.9%	14.5%
AIC	2723.9	2686.9	2688.9	2678.3	2671.4
BIC	2732.3	2703.7	2714.1	2711.9	2713.4
LR Chi2	–	41.0	1.9	14.6	10.9
p > Chi2	–	< 0.001	0.379	< 0.001	0.004

depression should be addressed with an appropriate screening and treatment, keeping in mind that even among patients who were under antidepressants, 34.1% were still depressed according to HADS-D, suggesting that in almost one third of cases those drugs are ineffective or maybe at inadequate dosage. These patients should be evaluated by a psychiatrist to optimize their therapy and followed up closely by the rheumatologist.

Considering the variables used to determine indices of disease activity, in our study there is a significant relationship between depression and TJC, PGA, PhGA and VAS, while no association was found between depression and disease duration, sieropositivity, erosions, markers of inflammation, or swollen joints. Our data further support the association between depression and higher pain perception that may affect mainly subjective measurements, such as tender joints count, PGA and VAS, as reported [25, 26]. Notably, it has been calculated that each extra point of depression measured with HADS results in an increase of 0.59 in TJC and 2.07 in the PGA score [28]. Even if clinical measures based on patients' reports could have important limitations, since they can reflect the subjective perception of illness, influenced by many factors (beliefs, culture, mood), some studies have suggested that those measures are better in terms of prediction of long-term outcomes, compared to objective parameters [29]. Indeed, we observed that objective measurements of disease activity (disease duration, ESR, CRP and SJC) were not associated with depressive symptoms, as reported in other studies [7, 18, 27, 30, 31], but in contrast with other ones [12, 17], in which objective scores affected mood.

Secondly, we found a significant association between RA disease activity and depression and between disability and depression, assessed through DAS28, SDAI, CDAI and HAQ, respectively. These findings were in line with previous studies [7, 12, 20]. Patients who experience a more active form of RA, with greater pain and inflammation, are at higher risk of developing depressive disorders. On the other hand, the presence of depression in individuals with a chronic disease such as RA may increase inflammation and reduce the pain threshold, making the disease more active and less prone to remission, compared to patients without mental disorders [19–21]. Our results underline that HAQ is the index that best correlates with depression, suggesting that physical disability deeply influence mental wellbeing. When we correlated depression with DAS28, CDAI and SDAI indices/scores we found, against our expectations, a greater prevalence of depressive disorders among patients with moderate disease activity compared to high disease activity. A possible explanation could be that patients with a very active disease are more frequently examined by a rheumatologist, accordingly to the treat-to-target management [32], and this carefulness may potentially reduce depression. Therefore, moderate disease activity could be the category at the highest risk of developing depression, pointing to the importance of screening and monitoring depression in these patients.

The hypothesis that depressive symptoms in patients with RA may worsen pain and lead to greater assumption of analgesics is further confirmed by our evidence that patients treated with NSAIDs had higher prevalence of depression. It is worth mentioning that NSAIDs use is usually self-prescribed, linked to the patient's perception of their health status rather than being a treatment prescribed by the physician on the basis of objective measures. In our study, we found no significant association between the use of specific anti-rheumatic drugs and depressive disorders. On the other hand, one should keep in mind that it is also possible that patients with a more active RA may have an increased risk of depression [8], so the relationship between RA and depression could be bidirectional.

Depressive symptoms are also associated with physician perception of disease severity and may influence the way patients communicate pain and affecting clinician's empathy. Depressive symptoms could also overlap with some symptoms of RA, simulating a more active and severe arthritis. Furthermore, depression may create resistance or non-adherence to treatment [33] and this may require a greater therapeutic and patient-management effort.

This paper has several strengths. To our best knowledge, this is the first large study performed in Italy analyzing data from a large sample of patients (N = 490) affected by RA. We recruited all subjects within the routine clinical practice, rather than a sample recruited with strict selection criteria, during a whole year in order to increment the generalizability of our results. We used a set of standardized questionnaires, covering a broad number of potential correlates of depression in RA, with special attention to disease activities and disability. Finally, this study arises from a strict collaboration between rheumatologist and psychiatrist leading to a multidisciplinary approach to such a relevant RA comorbidity, in both design and analysis of this paper.

The main limitation is the cross-sectional design of the study that cannot allow us to draw causal inferences on the relationship between depression and RA. Moreover, although we used the HADS, which is a well-validated and reliable screening tool, the diagnosis of depression was not confirmed by a psychiatrist.

Conclusions

In conclusion, our study shows that depression is common in RA and can lead to an alteration in the perception of the disease since the presence of depression is associated with higher disease activity, pain perception, physical disability. This suggests the importance for the rheumatologist to screen and monitor depression in patients affected by RA in order to treat them appropriately. In addition, recognizing and treating depression may increase treatment adherence, further improving disease control. Although it could sound obvious, one should not forget that treating depression has significant positive effects on patients' well-being that is one of the main target of the rheumatologist work. Finally, since depression is still under-diagnosed and almost one third of the patients treated with antidepressants does not benefit from the treatment, a close collaboration between rheumatologists and psychiatrists is desirable for an adequate diagnosis and appropriate therapy.

Abbreviations

25-OH-D3: Vitamin D; ACPA: Anti-citrullinated protein antibody; BMI: Body Mass Index; CDAI: Clinical Disease Activity Index; CRP: C-reactive protein; DAS28: 28-Joints Disease Activity Score; HADS-A: Hospital Anxiety and Depression Scale anxiety; HADS-D: Hospital Anxiety and Depression Scale depression; HAQ: Health Assessment Questionnaires Disability Index; PGA: Patient Global Assessment; RA: Rheumatoid arthritis; RF: Rheumatoid factor; SDAI: Simplified Disease Activity Index; SJC: Swollen joints count; TJC: Swollen joints count; VAS: Visual Analogue Scale.

Acknowledgements

Not applicable.

Authors' contributions

All authors read and approved the final manuscript and have had substantial contributions to the conception or design of the work or the acquisition, analysis, or interpretation of data for the work.

Author details

[1] Rheumatology Unit, University of Verona, Policlinico G.B. Rossi, Piazzale Scuro, 10, 37134 Verona, VR, Italy. [2] Department of Neuroscience, Biomedicine and Movement Sciences, Section of Psychiatry, University of Verona, Verona, Italy.

References

1. Alamanos Y, Voulgari PV, Drosos AA. Incidence and prevalence of rheumatoid arthritis, based on the 1987 American College of Rheumatology criteria: a systematic review. Semin Arthritis Rheum. 2006;36:182–8.
2. Kojima M, Kojima T, Suzuki S, Oguchi T, Oba M, Tsuchiya H, et al. Depression, inflammation, and pain in patients with rheumatoid arthritis. Arthritis Rheum. 2009;61:1018–24.
3. van den Hoek J, Roorda LD, Boshuizen HC, van Hees J, Rupp I, Tijhuis GJ, et al. Long-term physical functioning and its association with somatic comorbidity and comorbid depression in patients with established rheumatoid arthritis: a longitudinal study. Arthritis Care Res (Hoboken). 2013;65:1157–65.

4. Kotsis K, Voulgari PV, Tsifetaki N, Machado MO, Carvalho AF, Creed F, et al. Anxiety and depressive symptoms and illness perceptions in psoriatic arthritis and associations with physical health-related quality of life. Arthritis Care Res (Hoboken). 2012;64:1593–601.
5. Matcham F, Rayner L, Steer S, Hotopf M. The prevalence of depression in rheumatoid arthritis: a systematic review and meta-analysis. Rheumatology. 2013;52:2136–48.
6. Albrecht K. Gender-spezifische Unterschiede der Komorbidität bei rheumatoider Arthritis. Z Rheumatol. 2014;73:607–14.
7. Matcham F, Ali S, Irving K, Hotopf M, Chalder T. Are depression and anxiety associated with disease activity in rheumatoid arthritis? A prospective study. BMC Musculoskelet Disord. 2016;17:155.
8. Kuriya B, Joshi R, Movahedi M, Rampakakis E, Sampalis JS, Bombardier C. High disease activity is associated with self-reported depression and predicts persistent depression in early rheumatoid arthritis: results from the Ontario best practices research initiative. J Rheumatol. 2018;45:1101–8.
9. Edwards RR, Calahan C, Mensing G, Smith M, Haythornthwaite JA. Pain, catastrophizing, and depression in the rheumatic diseases. Nat Rev Rheumatol. 2011;7:216–24.
10. Michelsen B, Kristianslund EK, Sexton J, Hammer HB, Fagerli KM, Lie E, et al. Do depression and anxiety reduce the likelihood of remission in rheumatoid arthritis and psoriatic arthritis? Data from the prospective multicentre NOR-DMARD study. Ann Rheum Dis. 2017;76:1906–10.
11. Joyce AT, Smith P, Khandker R, Melin JM, Singh A. hidden cost of rheumatoid arthritis (RA): estimating cost of comorbid cardiovascular disease and depression among patients with RA. J Rheumatol. 2009;36:743–52.
12. van Gestel AM, Prevoo MLL, van't Hof MA, van Rijswijk MH, van de Putte LBA, van Riel PLCM. Development and validation of the European League against rheumatism response criteria for rheumatoid arthritis: comparison with the preliminary American College of Rheumatology and the world health organization/international league against rheumatism criteria. Arthritis Rheum. 1996;39:34–40.
13. Ranza R, Marchesoni A, Calori G, Bianchi G, Braga M, Canazza S, Canesi B, Fumagalli M, Mastaglio C, Mathieu A, et al. The Italian version of the functional disability index of the health assessment questionnaire. A reliable instrument for multicenter studies on rheumatoid arthritis. Clin Exp Rheumatol. 1993;11:123–8.
14. World Medical Association. World Medical Association Declaration of Helsinki: ethical principles for medical research involving human subjects. JAMA. 2013;310:2191–4.
15. Sjöberg L, Karlsson B, Atti AR, Skoog I, Fratiglioni L, Wang HX. Prevalence of depression: comparisons of different depression definitions in population-based samples of older adults. J Affect Disord. 2017;221:123–31.
16. Dalili Z, Bayazi MH. The effectiveness of mindfulness-based cognitive therapy on the illness perception and psychological symptoms in patients with rheumatoid arthritis. Complement Ther Clin Pract. 2019;34:139–44.
17. Smolen JS, Aletaha D, McInnes IB. Rheumatoid arthritis. Lancet. 2016;388:2023–38.
18. Hamilton M. A rating scale for depression. J Neurol Neurosurg Psychiat. 1960;23:56–62.
19. Montazeri A, Vahdaninia M, Ebrahimi M, Jarvandi S. The Hospital Anxiety and Depression Scale (HADS): translation and validation study of the Iranian version. Health Qual Life Outcomes. 2003;28:1–14.
20. Zigmond AS, Snaith RP. The hospital anxiety and depression scale (HADS). Acta Psychiatr Scand. 1983;67:361–70.
21. Bjelland I, Dahl AA, Haug TT, Neckelmann D. The validity of the Hospital Anxiety and Depression Scale. An updated literature review. J Psychosom Res. 2002;52:69–77.
22. Prothero L, Barley E, Galloway J, Georgopoulou S, Sturt J. The evidence base for psychological interventions for rheumatoid arthritis: a systematic review of reviews. Int J Nurs Stud. 2018;82:20–9.
23. Abdel-Nasser AM, Abd El-Azim S, Taal E, El-Badawy SA, Raskerd JJ, Valkenburg HA. Depression and depressive symptoms in rheumatoid arthritis patients: an analysis of their occurrence and determinants. Br J Rheumatol. 1998;37:391–7.
24. Roubille C, Richer V, Starnino T, McCourt C, McFarlane A, Fleming P, et al. Evidence-based recommendations for the management of comorbidities in rheumatoid arthritis, psoriasis, and psoriatic arthritis: expert opinion of the Canadian Dermatology-Rheumatology Comorbidity Initiative. J Rheumatol. 2015;42:1767–80.
25. Jamshidi AR, Banihashemi AT, Paragomi P, Hasanzadeh M, Barghamdi M, Ghoroghi S. Anxiety and depression in rheumatoid arthritis: an epidemio logic survey and investigation of clinical correlates in Iranian population. Rheumatol Int. 2016;36:1119–25.
26. Rathbun AM, Harrold LR, Reed GW. Temporal effect of depressive symptoms on the longitudinal evolution of rheumatoid arthritis disease activity. Arthritis Care Res (Hoboken). 2015;67:765–75.
27. Doshi JA, Cen L, Polsky D. Depression and retirement in late middle-aged U.S. workers. Health Serv Res. 2008;43:693–713.
28. Wang S-L, Chang C-H, Hu L-Y, Tsai S-J, Yang AC, You Z-H. Risk of developing depressive disorders following rheumatoid arthritis: a nationwide population-based study. PLoS ONE. 2014;9:e107791.
29. Derry HM, Padin AC, Kuo JL, Hughes S, Kiecolt-Glaser JK. Sex Differences in depression: does inflammation play a role? Curr Psychiatry Rep. 2015;17:78.
30. Lin M-C, Guo H-R, Lu M-C, Livneh H, Lai N-S, Tsai T-Y. Increased risk of depression in patients with rheumatoid arthritis: a seven-year population-based cohort study. Clinics (Sao Paulo). 2015;70:91–6.
31. Fifield J, Reisine S, Sheehan TJ, McQuillan J. Gender, paid work, and symptoms of emotional distress in rheumatoid arthritis patients. Arthritis Rheum. 1996;39:427–35.
32. Smolen JS, Aletaha D, Bijlsma JWJ, Breedveld FC, Boumpas D, Burmester G, et al. Treating rheumatoid arthritis to target: recommendations of an international task force. Ann Rheum Dis. 2010;69:631–7.
33. Bingham CO, Moni M. Periodontal disease and rheumatoid arthritis. Curr Opin Rheumatol. 2013;25:345–53.

12

Functioning in the fibromyalgia syndrome: Validity and reliability of the WHODAS 2.0

Marina Carvalho Arruda Barreto[1], Fabianna Resende Jesus Moraleida[2], Cristiane Vitaliano Graminha[3], Camila Ferreira Leite[2], Shamyr Sulyvan Castro[2] and Ana Carla Lima Nunes[2*]

Abstract

Background: Fibromyalgia syndrome (FMS) is both a challenging and disabling condition. The International Association for the Study of Pain (IASP) classifies FMS as chronic primary pain, and it can negatively impact individuals' functioning including social, psychological, physical and work-related factors. Notably, while guidelines recommend a biopsychosocial approach for managing chronic pain conditions, FMS assessment remains clinical. The WHODAS 2.0 is a unified scale to measure disability in the light of the International Classification of Functioning, Disability and Health. Thus, this study aimed to evaluate the reliability and validity of the Brazilian version of WHODAS 2.0 for use in individuals with FMS.

Methods: Methodological study of the validity and reliability of the Brazilian version of the 36-item WHODAS 2.0 with 110 individuals with FMS. The instrument gives a score from 0 to 100, the higher the value, the worse the level of functioning. We assessed participants with Medical Outcomes Study 36-Item Short-Form Health Survey (SF-36) (0–100), Fibromyalgia Impact Questionnaire (FIQ) (0–10) and Beck Depression Inventory instrument (BDI) (0–63). The construct validity, internal consistency, and test–retest stability. We used SF-36, FIQ and BDI to study construct validity analysis. For statistical analysis, we performed the intraclass correlation (ICC), Spearman correlation, and Cronbach's alpha, with a statistical level of 5%.

Results: Most participants were female (92.27%), aged 45 (± 15) years. The test–retest reliability analysis ($n = 50$) showed stability of the instrument ($ICC = 0.54$; $\rho = 0.84$, $p < 0.05$). The test–retest correlation between the domains was moderate to strong ($\rho > 0.58$ and < 0.90). Internal consistency was satisfactory for total WHODAS 2.0 (0.91) and also for domains, ranging from 0.44 to 0.81. The construct validity showed satisfactory values with all moderately correlated with WHODAS 2.0 instruments (> 0.46 and < 0.64; $p < 0.05$). WHODAS 2.0 evaluates the functioning encompassing components of health-related quality of life, functional impact, and depressive symptoms in those with FMS.

Conclusions: WHODAS 2.0 is a reliable and valid instrument to evaluate functioning of Brazilians with FMS. It provides reliable information on individuals' health through of a multidimensional perspective, that allows for individual-centered care.

Keywords: Fibromyalgia syndrome, Disability, Chronic pain, Patient reported outcome measures, WHO

Background

Fibromyalgia Syndrome (FMS) is a disabling health condition that deserves to be highlighted [1]. The International Association for the Study of Pain (IASP) classifies FMS as chronic primary pain [2], and it can negatively impact patients' functioning including social, psychological, physical and work-related factors[3]. Notably, while

*Correspondence: aclnunes@gmail.com
[2] Department of Physical Therapy, Federal University of Ceará, Major Weyne Street, 1440, Fortaleza, CE 60430-450, Brazil

guidelines recommend a biopsychosocial approach for managing chronic pain[4, 5] FMS assessment remains clinical.

FMS has an uncertain diagnosis due to reliance on patient report of subjective symptoms, absence of a universally accepted diagnostic gold standard, and lack of a specific biomarker[1]. There is a disagreement between FMS criteria and clinician-based FMS diagnoses that suggests bias in the identification of this health condition[6]. Furthermore, individuals with FMS tend to report a complex set of concerns, including fatigue, sleep dysfunction, stiffness, depression, anxiety, poor physical capacity, and cognitive disturbance in addition to musculoskeletal pain[7, 8]. These should be described as negative aspect of functioning associated with chronic pain[3].

Increased attention to the functional impact of chronic pain is an important step forward for its management. Functioning is a relevant indicator of population health[9], as it considers the dynamic interaction between a person's health status and contextual factors[10]. The analysis of the functioning covers the structures and functions of the body, activities and participation, in addition to contextual factors, which allows to understand and measure the health status through of a multidimensional perspective [9, 11]. This concept of functioning and its application as well as the term disability, were proposed by International Classification of Functioning, Disability and Health (ICF) based on the biopsychosocial model [10, 12].

Considering the fact that people with one and the same clinical condition can vary substantially in terms of disability, there is a need to expand the assessment tools [3]. The instruments commonly used to assess outcomes in FMS are not aligned with all categories of functioning as defined by the ICF[13, 14]. The World Health Organization Disability Assessment Schedule 2.0 (WHODAS 2.0) is a tool that measure functioning based on the theoretical conceptual framework of the ICF.

The WHODAS 2.0 is a generic instrument that provides the level of functioning in the following six domains: cognition, mobility, self-care, getting along, life activities, and participation, and its psychometric properties are considered satisfactory[15]. The 12-item version of WHODAS 2.0 has already been validated for the population with FMS in the United States[16]. The 36-item version of WHODAS 2.0 is the most detailed and it allows users to generate scores for the six domains of functioning and to calculate an overall functioning score[15]. This version is not validated to evaluate individuals with FMS. Knowledge of the functioning profile of individuals with FMS is needed for more appropriate and effective clinical management, especially because FMS is a multifactorial and multisystemic condition[13]. The multimodal pain management approach refers to a biopsychosocial model of pain that directs attention to suffering, Quality of Life (QoL), and participation in family and other areas of social life[3]. The WHODAS 2.0 emerges as an alternative to address this shortage. With the validation of this instrument, a tool to globally and efficiently assess individuals with FMS will be available. The aim of our study was to evaluate the validity and reliability of the WHODAS 2.0 (Brazil) for individuals with FMS.

Materials and methods

This was a methodological study that evaluated the psychometric properties of the WHODAS 2.0 (Brazil) instrument in people with FMS. The measurement properties were defined according to the recommendations of the COnsensus-based Standards for the selection of health Measurement INstruments (COSMIN)[17].

Participants

Recruitment occurred through the referral of health professionals, active searching in a health unit, and social media dissemination. Eligible participants were male or female, 18 years of age or older, who met the FM diagnostic criteria of the 1990 American College of Rheumatology[18].

Individuals who presented any disease or disorder that led to some functional impairment that was not linked to the characteristics of FMS and/or cognitive impairment that prevented them from responding to the instruments were excluded from the study. The minimum sample size to meet the necessary criteria of the validation process was 100 individuals[19].

Our study included 110 participants and was approved by the Research Ethics Committee (n.1.918.391), in accordance with the ethical standards of the institutional and/or national research committee and with the 1964 Helsinki Declaration. All participants were informed of the objectives of the study and gave written consent for their voluntary participation in the study and the anonymous use of personal data in statistical analyses.

Outcomes

Functioning—world health organization disability assessment schedule 2.0 (WHODAS 2.0)

The functioning was measured by WHODAS 2.0 in the following six domains: cognition, mobility, self-care, getting along, life activities, and participation. For the purpose of this study, we used the interview 36-item version. It allows for scoring each domain, and the general functioning score. Each domain and the total score range from 0 to 100, where a score closer to 100 indicates worse functioning of the individual. This instrument has excellent psychometric properties based on the strong test–retest reliability values found in a study conducted in 36 countries[15]. WHODAS was translated and cross-cultural adapted to the Brazilian Portuguese and the final version was approved by WHO [20].

Fibromyalgia impact—fibromyalgia impact questionnaire (FIQ)

This instrument assesses the impact of FMS on QoL. It is currently the most widely used questionnaire in clinical practice and research and is used to assess the health status of individuals with FMS. The FIQ has 19 goal character items divided into 10 questions related to function, overall impact and symptoms. The final score ranges from 0 to 10; the higher the score, the greater the impact on QoL[21].

Quality of life—medical outcomes study 36- item short-form health survey (SF-36)

The SF-36 is a generic multidimensional questionnaire that is used to assess the self-perception of QoL and health status. Its 36 items encompass eight domains, namely: physical functioning, role physical, bodily pain, general health, vitality, social functioning, role emotional, and mental health. The final score is separated by domains, where each value can be between 0 and 100; the closer the value is to 100, the better the respondent's QoL. The instrument presented significant results and satisfactory values for intra- and inter-rater correlation. The same was found in the construct validity analysis[22].

Depressive symptoms—beck depression inventory (BDI)

The instrument was used to detect depressive symptoms. The instrument has 21 items, ranging from 0 to 3 points. The higher the individual's score, the greater the likelihood of depressive symptoms, which should be confirmed with other diagnostic tests. The instrument presented high internal consistency (0.81), and significant values, and strong correlation in the construct validity[23].

Procedures

The researchers were previously trained to apply the instruments and to confirm the diagnostic criteria for FMS. Data collection occurred in a reserved room at the universities from August 2017 to July 2019.

Categorical sociodemographic variables (gender, race, marital status, profession, comorbidity, pain body places) and continuous variables (age, number of children, years of schooling, symptom evolution time, medications, numerical rating scale—NRS) were collected by means of an evaluation questionnaire prepared by the researchers. NRS is a measure of pain intensity of 11 points (0–10). Score zero means no pain and score 10 means worst pain[24]. For eligible individuals, the WHODAS 2.0, FIQ, SF-36, and BDI instruments were applied. After 7 days, participants returned to perform the retest with the same researcher, who applied the WHODAS 2.0 instrument.

Statistical analysis

The validation process was composed of the analysis of the following psychometric properties: reliability, internal consistency, and construct validity. The analysis included the subjects who answered all necessary items of the instruments. For test–retest reliability measurement, data from 50 subjects were analyzed, a number considered adequate for analysis[19]. For the analysis of the other psychometric properties, 110 individuals were included.

Test–retest reliability is obtained when the same instrument is applied twice to the same subject with an interval of seven days between applications. The instrument is considered stable when the coefficient values are greater than 0.7[25, 26].

Internal consistency evaluates the relationship between instrument sub-items within the same domain. This was evaluated using Cronbach's alpha, which analyses the degree of covariance between the sub-items. The instrument has good internal consistency when its domains present Cronbach's alpha values between 0.7 and 0.95[26].

Construct validity investigate validity of an instrument in relationships with other outcomes measures of good quality[27]. This property was measured by application of another instrument that has already been validated for the same population. Correlation values greater than 0.7 indicate strong correlation[26, 28]. For this evaluation, the correlation between the WHODAS 2.0 and the FIQ and SF-36 instruments, which are widely used for FMS and QoL impact analysis, respectively, was performed. In addition, the correlation between the WHODAS 2.0 domains and SF-36 domains, FIQ and BDI was analyzed. Table 1 shows plausible relationships between WHODAS 2.0 domains and SF36, FIQ, BDI.

To describe the clinical, sociodemographic, and functioning characteristics of the study participants, the following descriptive measures were used: measures of central tendency (mean), dispersion (standard deviation), and relative frequency (%). The collected data were analyzed using the Stata program, adopting a significance level of $\alpha = 0.05$.

Initially, the normality of the data was tested with the Kolmogorov–Smirnov test[29]. Test–retest reliability was analyzed using the intraclass correlation coefficient (ICC), followed by the Spearman correlation test between the WHODAS 2.0 domain and total values found in the test and retest. This strategy of using two

Table 1 Hypothesized correlations between the WHODAS 2.0 domains, total WHODAS 2.0 and the SF36, FIQ and BDI instruments

WHODAS 2.0	SF36	FIQ	BDI
Cognition	✓		✓
Mobility	✓	✓	
Self-Care	✓		✓
Getting along	✓		✓
Life activity	✓	✓	
Work activity			
Domestic activity	✓	✓	
Participation	✓		✓
Total	✓	✓	✓

statistical tests is due to the nature of the tests in association with the characteristics of FM. The ICC is a measure of agreement. The correlation is considered strong when the value is higher than 0.7, moderate when it is between 0.4 and 0.7, and weak when it is less than 0.4[30]. We verified the internal consistency according to Cronbach's alpha. To assess the construct validity, we use the Spearman correlation test between the domains and the total WHODAS 2.0 score, and FIQ and SF-36.

Results

We evaluated 110 people with a diagnosis of FMS. The participant data and the average value of the instruments are described in Table 2. The sample consisted primarily of women (97.27%), aged 44.66 (±14.69) years, who had paid work (21.82%) or were unemployed due to health problems (19.09%). The pain intensity level was 6.38 (±2.56).

The measures referring to the instrument's psychometric properties are described in Table 3. Results indicate satisfactory values for internal consistency. In the test–retest reliability, we found between moderate to high ICC values (except for life activities, whose work activities were not responded by 57% of the sample), and the correlation coefficient was moderate to strong.

In the construct validity analysis, the WHODAS 2.0 showed a moderate and significant correlation with the SF-36, FIQ, and BDI. The WHODAS 2.0 domains, except for the work activity domain, showed a moderate and significant correlation with SF-36. The mobility domain and domestic activity (life activities domain) of the WHODAS 2.0 showed a moderate and significant correlation with the FIQ, and the domains of cognition and getting along showed a moderate and significant correlation with the total BDI value (Table 4).

Discussion

Our study showed that the WHODAS 2.0 is a valid and reliable instrument to measure functioning in individuals with FMS, presenting adequate psychometric properties. The WHODAS 2.0 assesses functioning of individuals with FMS, incorporating aspects of health-related QoL, functional impact, and depressive symptoms. The WHODAS 2.0 offers the opportunity to evaluate the chronic patient, as in osteoarthritis[31] or rheumatoid arthritis, according to the ICF biopsychosocial model.

The WHODAS 2.0 maintains excellent internal consistency when evaluating individuals with FM. In this way, issues from the same domain and from the entire instrument are adequately related, and the interpretation of the scores reflects the level of functioning[32, 33]. Studies that evaluated the psychometric properties of the WHODAS 2.0 in musculoskeletal and rheumatic conditions found similar results[34, 35].

Additionally, our findings showed acceptable test–retest reliability but the domains of life activity and participation showed less stability in individuals with FMS after one week. These results are probably due to FMS being a health condition with a wide variety of transient symptoms[13, 36], and changes may occur between two time points. We hypothesize that the WHODAS 2.0 is capable of detecting minimal changes in these domains, however, the responsiveness of this instrument needs to be tested in a future study. The application of instruments addressing general health at the time of reapplication of the WHODAS 2.0 could confirm this hypothesis.

The WHODAS 2.0 is an instrument that includes all ICF concepts for the evaluation of functioning[15]. Our validation results reinforced the multidimensional nature of this instrument, which covers part of the domains of the three investigated instruments such as QoL, functional impact and depressive symptoms. Additionally, the WHODAS 2.0 covers other aspects not included in this questionnaires[37]. The 12-item version WHODAS 2.0 was related to fatigue, pain, sleep difficulties, cognitive impairment, depression, and social support in individuals with FMS[16].

The scores of the investigated questionnaires were related to some of the WHODAS 2.0 domains. An example is FIQ, which had a moderate correlation with two WHODAS 2.0 domains, mobility and life activities (domestic activity). These results demonstrated whereas FIQ is a specific instrument for assessing the health impact of individuals with FM[21], it fails to evaluate other functioning related domains such as cognition, self-care, and getting along. According to Prodinger et al.

Table 2 Description of the sociodemographic, clinical, and functional characteristics

Variable	n	% (100)
Sex		
Woman	107	92.27
Man	3	2.73
Marital status		
Never married	38	34.86
Currently married	42	38.53
Separated	9	8.26
Divorced	15	13.76
Widower	3	2.75
Cohabiting	2	1.83
Race[a]		
White	14	16.86
Brown	35	42.16
Negro	30	36.14
Indigenous	4	4.82
Income[a]		
Less than 1 minimum Brazilian wage	15	18.07
1–2 minimum Brazilian wage	38	45.78
3–5 minimum Brazilian wage	23	27.72
More than 5 minimum Brazilian wage	7	8.43
Work activity		
Paid work	24	21.82
Freelance	13	11.82
Non-paid work, such as volunteer or charity	2	1.82
Student	11	10
Homemaker	14	12.73
Retired	12	10.91
Unemployed (health reasons)	21	19.09
Unemployed (other reasons)	5	4.54
Other	8	7.27
	Mean	**Standard deviation**
Age	44.66	14.69
How many years spent studying	16.10	8.83
NRS[a]	6.38	2.56
FIQ	6.73	1.55
BDI[a]	22.59	10.21
WHODAS 2.0		
Cognition	43.63	20.23
Mobility	55.73	20.72
Self-care	27.18	22.67
Getting along	32.04	23.52
Life activity	46.70	21.62
Domestic activity	7.1.54	22.14
Work activity	60.10	20.56
Participation	55.00	19.92
Total	44.97	14.93
SF36		
Physical functioning	36.10	17.70
Role physical	17.65	21.04

Table 2 (continued)

	Mean	Standard deviation
Bodily pain	23.45	20.25
General health	37.97	23.13
Vitality	24.93	21.63
Social functioning	39.95	23.41
Role emotional	29.37	34.15
Mental health	49.85	22.02
Total	32.92	12.53

[a] Value referring to 83 individuals with FMS. NRS = Numeric Rating Scale; FIQ = Fibromyalgia Impact Questionnaire; WHODAS = World Health Organization Disability Assessment Schedule; SF36 = Medical Outcomes Study 36- Item Short-Form Health Survey; BDI = Beck Depression Index

Table 3 Reliability (Cronbach's α and ICC) of the WHODAS 2.0 domains

Domains WHODAS 2.0	Cronbach's α	ICC (95%)	Test–retest correlation coefficient
Cognition	0.77	0.61 (0.34–0.87)	0.83*
Mobility	0.81	0.79 (0.40- 0.95)	0.90*
Self-care	0.76	0.67 (0.40 – 0.95)	0.79*
Getting along	0.73	0.67 (0.41–0.93)	0.65*
Life activity	0.44	0.41 (0.07- 0.74)	0.62*
Domestic activity	0.62	0.31(0.00–0.67)	0.65*
Work activity	0.53	0.49 (0.06–0.92)	0.58*
Participation	0.80	0.26 (0.00–0.60)	0.59*
Total	0.91	0.54 (0.13–0.95)	0.84*

* $p<0.05$; WHODAS = World Health Organization Disability Assessment Schedule

Table 4 Correlation coefficient matrix between the domains of WHODAS 2.0, SF36, BDI and FIQ

	WHODAS 2.0 Domains								
	Cognition	Mobility	Self-care	Getting along	Life activity	Work activity	Domestic activity	Participation	Total
SF 36									
SF36 Total	−0.4055*	−0.4716*	−0.5394*	−0.5462*	−0.4436*	−0.2242	−0.5522*	−0.4819*	−0.6435*
Physical Functioning	−0.3403*	−0.5581*	−0.4397*	−0.2362	−0.4917*	−0.3756*	−0.4509*	−0.2828*	−0.4894*
Role Physical	−0.1648	−0.2165	−0.3209*	−0.2201	−0.2657	−0.0394	−0.4692*	−0.3264*	−0.3301*
Bodily Pain	−0.1658	−0.1783	−0.0933	0.0319	−0.1750	−0.0431	−0.2258	−0.0593	−0,2001*
General Health	−0.2017	−0.3715*	−0.5347*	−0.3230*	−0.4297*	−0.2075	−0.5094*	−0.3377*	−0.4483*
Vitality	−0.2821*	−0.3880*	−0.3269*	−0.1622	−0.1715	−0.0124	−0.3146*	−0.3150*	−0.4100*
Social Functioning	−0.3268*	−0.2279	−0.1436	−0.3691*	−0.2875*	−0.2328	−0.2485	−0.2066	−0.3664*
Role Emotional	−0.0244	−0.0095	−0.2995*	−0.3411*	−0.1032	−0.0236	−0.1586	−0.0353	−0.1165
Mental Health	−0.3287*	−0.2005	−0.0588	−0.3317*	−0.1434	−0.1130	−0.1517	−0.2844*	−0.2832*
FIQ	0.3419*	0.4355*	0.3105*	0.1857	0.3894*	0.1833	0.4640*	0.3615	0.4857*
BDI	0.5005*	0.3767*	0.2828	0.5276*	0.2643	0.2528	0.2387	0.2866	0.4616*

* $p<0.05$; FIQ = Fibromyalgia Impact Questionnaire; WHODAS = World Health Organization Disability Assessment Schedule; SF36 = Medical Outcomes Study 36- Item Short-Form Health Survey; BDI = Beck Depression Index

[38], a specific instrument might raise difficulties associated with the multidimensionality and functioning. This more detailed analysis according to the WHODAS 2.0 domains allows to identify typical disabilities of the FMS[3], which cannot be performed in the 12-item version of WHODAS[15].

We observed that higher scores on health-related QoL were related to a better functioning profile in WHODAS 2.0. The total score of the SF-36 showed moderate correlation in 7 of the 8 domains of the WHODAS 2.0. However, neither the mental health, role emotional nor the bodily pain SF-36 domains seem to be well explored in WHODAS 2.0. These findings support the use of the SF-36 as an outcome which complements WHODAS 2.0, as suggested Garin et al.[35], who correlated the WHODAS 2.0 with the SF-36 for individuals with different chronic diseases, and showed a moderate correlation in all analyses. Xenouli et al.[39] divided the SF-36 domains into two blocks, physical and mental health, and correlated them with the total value of the WHODAS 2.0. The correlation between the total score of the WHODAS 2.0 and the physical health SF-36 component was strong ($r = -0.76$) in Greeks with or without disabilities, while the correlation was moderate between the WHODAS 2.0 and the SF-36 mental health component (−0.50) [39]. SF-36 was chosen because it is a generic questionnaire that makes a global analysis of the QoL of the individual[22].

The moderate correlation between BDI and WHODAS 2.0 suggests that important aspects of depressive symptoms are covered in this functioning tool, especially through the domains of cognition, mobility and getting along with people. Still it SF-36 and the BDI assess different outcomes when compared to the WHODAS 2.0[22, 23]. In addition, the instruments refer to different periods of symptom presentation, which can influence the patient's report[21, 23]. Still, these instruments were included because they are the most used to assess individuals with FMS. Our study is the first to investigate the correlation of the WHODAS 2.0 with FIQ and BDI.

We had some limitations in this study. We did not reapply a concurrent instrument at the time of the second application of the WHODAS 2.0, which limits the perception of individual conditions on the day of the retest. Another limitation is the functioning in life activities because it includes the work activities that are not applied to all individuals. We highlight that the findings of the present study are unprecedented since the psychometric properties of the the 36-item version WHODAS 2.0 have not been tested for FMS individuals.

Conclusions

We propose the WHODAS 2.0 as a reliable and valid instrument for assessing functioning of individuals with FM. It provides reliable information on individuals' health based on structures and functions of the body, activities and participation, in addition to contextual factors, that allows for individual-centered care. Based on our findings we recommend using the instrument to assess health status and to monitor health interventions.

Abbreviations

FMS: Fibromyalgia syndrome; QoL: Quality of life; ICF: International classification of functioning, disability and health; WHODAS 2.0: World health organization disability assessment schedule 2.0; FIQ: Fibromyalgia Impact Questionnaire; SF-36: Medical outcomes study 36-item short-form health survey; BDI: Beck depression inventory; NRS: Numerical rating scale; ICC: Intraclass correlation coefficient.

Acknowledgements

To the Movement project of the Department of Physiotherapy, Federal University of Ceará.

Authors' contributions

MCAB collected data, contributed to the writing of the article, statistical analysis and final review; FRJM contributed to data collection, article writing and final review; CVG contributed to data collection and final review; CCL contributed to the writing of the article and final review; SSC performed the statistical analysis, contributed to the writing of the article and final review; ACLN supervised the project, contributed to data collection, statistical analysis, article writing and final review. All authors read and approved the final manuscript.

Author details

[1]Department of Public Health, Universidade Federal do Ceará, Ceará, Fortaleza, Brazil. [2]Department of Physical Therapy, Federal University of Ceará, Major Weyne Street, 1440, Fortaleza, CE 60430-450, Brazil. [3]Department of Physical Therapy, Universidade Federal do Triângulo Mineiro, Ceará, Uberaba, Brazil.

References

1. Benlidayi IC. Fibromyalgia as a challenge for patients and physicians. Rheumatol Int. 2018;38(12):2345. https://doi.org/10.1007/s00296-018-4138-6.
2. Treede R-D, Rief W, Barke A, et al. Chronic pain as a symptom or a disease: the IASP Classification of Chronic Pain for the International Classification of Diseases (ICD-11). Pain. 2019;160(1):19–27.
3. Nugraha B, Gutenbrunner C, Barke A, et al. The IASP classification of chronic pain for ICD-11: functioning properties of chronic pain. Pain. 2019;160(1):88–94.
4. Macfarlane GJ, Kronisch C, Dean LE, et al. EULAR revised recommendations for the management of fibromyalgia. Ann Rheum Dis. 2017;76(2):318–28. https://doi.org/10.1136/annrheumdis-2016-209724.
5. Clauw DJ, Essex MN, Pitman V, et al. Reframing chronic pain as a disease, not a symptom: rationale and implications for pain management. Postgrad Med. 2019;131(3):185–98. https://doi.org/10.1080/00325481.2019.1574403.
6. Marques AP, Santo ASE, Berssaneti AA, et al. A prevalência de fibromialgia: atualização da revisão de literatura. Rev Bras Reumatol. 2017;57(4):356–63. https://doi.org/10.1016/j.rbre.2017.01.005.
7. Wolfe F, Smythe HA, Yunus MB, et al. The American College of Rheumatology 1990 Criteria for the Classification of Fibromyalgia. Report of the multicenter criteria committee. Arthritis Rheum. 1990;33(2):160–72. https://doi.org/10.1002/art.1780330203.
8. Sempere-rubio N, Aguilar-rodriguez M, Ingl M, et al. Physical condition factors that predict a better quality of life in women with fibromyalgia. Int J Environ Res Public Health. 2019
9. Stucki G, Bickenbach J. Functioning: the third health indicator in the health system and the key indicator for rehabilitation. Eur J Phy Rehabil Med. 2017;53(1):134–8. https://doi.org/10.23736/s1973-9087.17.04565-8
10. World Health Organization - WHO. International Classification of Functioning, Disability and Health (ICF). Genebra; 2001.
11. Üstün TB, Chatterji S, Bickenbach J, et al. The international classification of

functioning, disability and health: a new tool for understanding disability and health. Disabil Rehabil. 2003;25(11–12):565–71. https://doi.org/10.1080/0963828031000137063.

12. Farias N, Buchalla CM. A Classificação Internacional de Funcionalidade, Incapacidade e Saúde da Organização Mundial da Saúde: Conceitos. Usos e Perspectivas Rev Bras Epidemiol. 2005;8(2):187–93. https://doi.org/10.1590/S1415-790X2005000200011.
13. Lupi JB, Abreu DCC, Ferreira MC, et al. Brazilian Portuguese version of the Revised Fibromyalgia Impact Questionnaire (FIQR-Br): cross-cultural validation, reliability, and construct and structural validation. Disabil Rehabil. 2017;39(16):1650–63. https://doi.org/10.1080/09638288.2016.1207106.
14. Costa IS, Gamundí A, Miranda JGV, et al. Altered functional performance in patients with fibromyalgia. Front Hum Neurosci. 2017;1:1–9. https://doi.org/10.3389/fnhum.2017.00014.
15. Castro SS, Leite CF, Osterbrock C, et al. Avaliação de Saúde e Deficiência: Manual do WHO Disability Assessment Schedule (WHODAS 2.0). Uberaba: Universidade Federal do Triângulo Mineiro - UFTM; 2015. 153 p.
16. Smedema SM, Yaghmaian RA, Ruiz D, et al. Psychometric validation of the world health organization disability assessment schedule 2.0–12-item Version in persons with fibromyalgia syndrome. Journal of Rehabilitation. 2016;82(2).
17. Mokkink LB, Terwee CB, Patrick DL, et al. The COSMIN checklist for assessing the methodological quality of studies on measurement properties of health status measurement instruments: an international Delphi study. Qual Life Res. 2010;19(4):539–49. https://doi.org/10.1007/s11136-010-9606-8.
18. Wolfe F, Clauw DJ, Fitzcharles MA, et al. The American College of Rheumatology preliminary diagnostic criteria for fibromyalgia and measurement of symptom severity. Arthritis Care Res. 2010;62(5):600–10. https://doi.org/10.1002/acr.20140.
19. Terwee CB, Bot SDM, de Boer MR, et al. Quality criteria were proposed for measurement properties of health status questionnaires. J Clin Epidemiol. 2007;60(1):34–42. https://doi.org/10.1016/j.jclinepi.2006.03.012.
20. Castro SS, Leite CF. Translation and cross-cultural adaptation of the World Health Organization Disability Assessment Schedule - WHODAS 2.0. Fisioter Pesqui. 2017;24(4):385–91. https://doi.org/10.1590/1809-2950/17118724042017
21. Marques AP, Barsante Santos AM, Assumpção A, et al. Validação da versão Brasileira do Fibromyalgia Impact Questionnaire (FIQ). Rev Bras Reumatol. 2006;46(1):24–31. https://doi.org/10.1590/S0482-50042006000100006.
22. Ciconelli RM, Ferraz MB, Santos W, Meinão I, Quaresma MR. Tradução para a língua portuguesa e validação do questionário genérico de avaliação de qualidade de vida SF-36 (Brasil SF-36). Revista Brasileira De Reumatologia. 1999;39:143–50. Available from: http://www.scopus.com/inward/record.url?eid=2-s2.0-0032808921&partnerID=40&md5=8e372f8e7feece5ae4fc33228a55d3a8
23. Gorestein C, Andrade LHSG. Inventário de depressão de Beck : propriedades psicométricas da versão em português. 1998;(December 2015).
24. Hjermstad MJ, Fayers PM, Haugen DF, et al. Studies comparing Numerical Rating Scales, Verbal Rating Scales, and Visual Analogue Scales for assessment of pain intensity in adults: a systematic literature review. J pain symptom manage. 2011;41(6):1073–93. https://doi.org/10.1016/j.jpainsymman.2010.08.016.
25. Roberts P. Reliability and validity in research. Nurs Stand. 2006;20(22):41–5.
26. Souza AC, Alexandre NMC, Guirardello EB, et al. Propriedades psicométricas na avaliação de instrumentos: avaliação da confiabilidade e da validade. Epidemiol Serv Saúde. 2017;26(3):649–59. https://doi.org/10.5123/S1679-49742017000300022.
27. Boateng GO, Neilands TB, Frongillo EA, et al. Best practices for developing and validating scales for heath, social and behavioral research: a primer. Front Public Health. 2018;6(June):1–18. https://doi.org/10.3389/fpubh.2018.00149.
28. Polit DF. Assessing measurement in health: Beyond reliability and validity. Internat J Nurs Stud. 2015;52(11):1746–53. https://doi.org/10.1016/j.ijnurstu.2015.07.002.
29. Koo TK, Li MY. A Guideline of Selecting and Reporting Intraclass Correlation Coefficients for Reliability Research. J Chiropractic Med. 2016;15(2):155–63. https://doi.org/10.1016/j.jcm.2016.02.012.
30. Cohen J. Statistical power analysis for the behavioral sciences [Internet]. Vol. 2nd, Statistical Power Analysis for the Behavioral Sciences. 1988. p. 567. Available from: http://books.google.com/books?id=Tl0N2lRAO9oC&pgis=1
31. Kutlay S, Küçükdeveci AA, Elhan AH, et al. Validation of the World Health Organization disability assessment schedule II (WHODAS-II) in patients with osteoarthritis. Rheumatol int. 2011;31(3):339–46. https://doi.org/10.1007/s00296-009-1306-8.
32. Streiner DL. Starting at the beginning: An introduction to coefficient alpha and internal consistency. J Pers Assess. 2003;80(1):99–103. https://doi.org/10.1207/S15327752JPA8001_18.
33. Henson RK. Understanding internal consistency reliability estimates: A conceptual primer on coefficient alpha. Meas Eval Couns Dev. 2001;34(3):177–89. https://doi.org/10.1080/07481756.2002.12069034.
34. Baron M, Schieir O, Hudson M, et al. The clinimetric properties of the World Health Organization disability assessment schedule II in early inflammatory arthritis. Arthritis Rheum. 2008;59(3):382–90. https://doi.org/10.1002/art.23314.
35. Garin O, Ayuso-Mateos JL, Almansa J, et al. Validation of the World Health Organization Disability Assessment Schedule, WHODAS-2 in patients with chronic diseases. Health qual life outcomes. 2010;8:51. https://doi.org/10.1186/1477-7525-8-51.
36. Oliveira RM, Leite ACS, da Silva LMS, et al. Comparative analysis of functional capacity among women with fibromyalgia and low back pain. Rev Dor. 2013;14(1):39–43. https://doi.org/10.1590/S1806-00132013000100010.
37. Burckhardt CS, Clark SR, Bennett RM. The Fibromyalgia Impact Questionnaire: developed and validation. J Rheumatol. 1991;18(5):728–33.
38. Prodinger B, Cieza A, Williams DA, et al. Measuring health in patients with fibromyalgia: Content comparison of questionnaires based on the international classification of functioning, disability and health. Arthritis Rheum. 2008;59(5):650–8. https://doi.org/10.1002/art.23559.
39. Xenouli G, Xenoulis K, Sarafis P, et al. Validation of the World Health Organization Disability Assessment Schedule (WHO-DAS II) in Greek and its added value to the Short Form 36 (SF-36) in a sample of people with or without disabilities. Disabil Health J. 2016;9(3):518–23. https://doi.org/10.1016/j.dhjo.2016.01.009.

13

Effects of photobiomodulation and a physical exercise program on the expression of inflammatory and cartilage degradation biomarkers and functional capacity in women with knee osteoarthritis

Patricia Gabrielli Vassão[1*], Ana Carolina Flygare de Souza[2], Raquel Munhoz da Silveira Campos[1,3], Livia Assis Garcia[4], Helga Tatiana Tucci[2] and Ana Claudia Muniz Renno[1]

Abstract

Background: The knee osteoarthritis (OA) is a joint disease characterized by degradation of articular cartilage that leads to chronic inflammation. Exercise programs and photobiomodulation (PBM) are capable of modulating the inflammatory process of minimizing functional disability related to knee OA. However, their association on the concentration of biomarkers related to OA development has not been studied yet. The aim of the present study is to investigate the effects of PBM (via cluster) with a physical exercise program in functional capacity, serum inflammatory and cartilage degradation biomarkers in patients with knee OA.

Methods: Forty-two patients were randomly allocated in 3 groups: ESP: exercise + sham PBM; EAP: exercise + PBM and CG: control group. Six patients were excluded before finished the experimental period. The analyzed outcomes in baseline and 8-week were: the Western Ontario and McMaster Universities Osteoarthritis (WOMAC) and the evaluation of serum biomarkers concentration (IL-1β, IL-6, IL-8, IL-10 e TNF-α, and CTX-II).

Results: An increase in the functional capacity was observed in the WOMAC total score for both treated groups ($p < 0.001$) and ESP presents a lower value compared to CG ($p < 0.05$) the 8-week post-treatment. In addition, there was a significant increase in IL-10 concentration of EAP ($p < 0.05$) and higher value compared to CG ($p < 0.001$) the 8-week post-treatment. Moreover, an increase in IL-1β concentration was observed for CG ($p < 0.05$). No other difference was observed comparing the other groups.

Conclusion: Our data suggest that the physical exercise therapy could be a strategy for increasing functional capacity and in association with PBM for increasing IL-10 levels in OA knee individuals.

Trial registration: ReBEC (RBR-7t6nzr).

*Correspondence: patriciavassao@gmail.com
[1] Department of Biosciences, Federal University of São Paulo, Campus Baixada Santista, Rua Silva Jardim, 136, Santos, SP 11015-020, Brazil

Keywords: Knee osteoarthritis, Inflammation, Cytokines, Biomarkers, Photobiomodulation

Introduction

Osteoarthritis (OA) leads to degradation of articular cartilage, formation of osteophytes, decrease of joint space and degeneration of subchondral bone and is characterized as a chronic joint disease [1]. These morphological alterations culminate in an increasing of the level of articular pain, loss of function, decrease in the range of motion and muscle weakness, impairing the quality of life of the patients [2].

The pathogenesis of OA has relation with the increase of expression of specific cytokines and immune system and, which contribute to cartilage degradation [3, 4]. It has been demonstrated that patients with OA showed high levels of proinflammatory cytokines, which disturb the catabolism and anabolism processes, being responsible by inflammation and consequence articular cartilage degeneration [5]. In this context, the most important cytokines involved in this process are Tumor Necrosis Factor alpha (TNF-α), interleukin-1β (IL-1β) and interleukin -6 (IL-6) [6]. As result of degradation of cartilage, a release of protein specific tissue fragments (neo-epitopes) in cleavage of type II collagen by matrix metalloproteinases (MMPs) can be observe, especially with analyze of biomarker as C-telopeptide of type II collagen (CTX-II) [7]. Based on this, the inhibition of interleukins (ILs) activity and analysis of CTX-II as a biomarker of progression of cartilage lesion are related to radiological grades of cartilage degradation and may help to improved strategies to treat OA [8].

In this context, for OA, one of the most common treatments is based on pharmacological intervention, mainly nonsteroidal and steroidal anti-inflammatory drugs (NSAIDs) [9]. However, the continuous use of NSAIDs can lead to severe adverse effects, like gastrointestinal problems, and limited efficacy [10]. In an attempt to attenuate these problems, alternative treatments have been studied including physical exercise programs, presenting positive effects on pain control, joint dysfunction and disability in patients with OA [11]. Furthermore, Castrogiovanni et al. [12] demonstrated that the moderate physical activity (MPA) significantly increased on the expression of anti-inflammatory [interleukin-4 (IL-4) and interleukin-10 (IL-10)] biomarkers in the synovium of an OA-induced rat model. The exercise protocol has been shown to have an anti-inflammatory effect, reducing levels of biomarkers like IL-6 and TNFα and suggesting that cytokine reduction can be an effective contribution for modulating pain due to OA [13].

Another promising therapeutic intervention that has been showing positive effects on degradation of cartilage tissue in the presence of OA is the low-level laser therapy (LLLT) or more recently, photobiomodulation (PBM) [14, 15]. It is well known that PBM produces stimulatory effect on healing and has the ability of modulating the inflammatory process in different tissues, including cartilage [5, 16]. Chondroprotective effects, inhibition of cartilage degradation, decreases in the expression of chemotactic factors and inflammatory cytokines and increase antioxidant enzyme levels have been observed in several experimental model of OA in rats after PBM [17, 18]. Also, clinical trials have demonstrated that PBM is able of reducing pain, articular stiffness, knee swelling, increasing the functional performance in knee OA patients [10, 19]. Alghadir, et al. [20] showed that PBM (850 nm, 50mW, 6 J/point), applied in eight points on knee during 4 weeks/ two times per week, improved the functional capacity evaluated by Western Ontario and McMaster Universities Arthritis Index (WOMAC) in patients with knee OA (grade II or III).

Furthermore, some authors have been investigating the association of physical exercise and PBM on the management of OA symptoms [21, 22]. De Paula Gomes et al. [21] observed that PBM nine diode cluster device (one 905 nm super-pulsed diode laser with, four 875 nm light-emitting diode (LED) and four 640 nm LED) associated to a physical exercise program had positive effects on reducing pain intensity in individuals with knee OA. Similar findings were observed by Alayat et al., [23] and de Matos Brunelli Braghin et al., [24].

Although all the positive effects of physical exercise programs for treatment of OA, its association with PBM via a cluster device on the expression of ILs and biomarkers related to cartilage degradation in patients with OA has not been studied yet. In this context, based on the need of determining a more appropriate therapeutic intervention to treat patients with OA, the present study aimed to investigate the effects of the incorporation of PBM (via cluster) into a physical exercise program in serum inflammatory biomarkers (IL-1β, IL-6, IL-8, IL-10 e TNF-α), cartilage degradation biomarker (CTX-II) and functional capacity (WOMAC) in patients with knee OA.

Materials and methods

Study design and setting

This is a single-blind (participants) randomized controlled trial. Ethical approval (Ethics in Human Research Committee of the Federal University of São

Paulo- approval number 1.368.478) and written informed consent (patients signed) were obtained. The study was conducted at the Laboratory of Manual and Physical Resources and Balance Space – Fitness and Health from April 2018 to February 2020 and was logged with the Brazilian Clinical Trials Registry (RBR-7t6nzr). All participants were recruited via advertisements in local newspapers and social media.

Patients

As eligibility criteria, patients had aged between 55 and 70 years, present symptomatic OA in the previous 6 months, a diagnosis of unilateral or bilateral knee OA according to the American College of Rheumatology and a radiographic confirmation of OA (grades 2 or 3 of the Kellgren-Lawrence classification) [25]. The diagnosis of knee OA was determined through an examination and the written opinion of a specialist in rheumatic diseases. Also, patients should present BMI between 22 to 35 kg/m^2, criteria established by Pan American Health Organization [26], more than 2 points on the Numeric Rating Pain Scale and should be classified as active and irregularly active (physical activity with a frequency of at least 3 times a week or a minimum of 150 min per week, according to Criteria established by American College of Sports Medicine measures by the International Physical Activity Questionnaire – Short Version (IPAQ).

Patients were excluded if they have: fibromyalgia and/or any kind of orthopedic or rheumatic diseases that may prevent the physical exercise; surgery of the knee within the past 6 months or joint replacement. Also, patients with diagnoses of lung diseases, cardiologic alterations, uncontrolled hypertension, diabetes and had any contraindications to PBM as cancer. During the study, patients who missed two consecutive training sessions or more than 3 sessions along the treatment and who discontinued the pharmacological treatment for OA started before the study were excluded.

Randomization

All patients met all inclusion criteria to participate in the study and signed a consent form. 42 patients were randomly allocated in ESP, EAP or CG groups, as observed below:

ESP: exercise + sham PBM, patients of this group performed the physical exercise program associated to PBM sham irradiation;

EAP: exercise + active PBM, patients of this group performed the physical exercise program associated to active PBM irradiation.

CG: control group, patients of this group were not submitted to any kind of therapeutical intervention.

A researcher, who was not involved in the experiment, conducted the randomization process by a simple drawing through a computer program that created a random table of numbers and put these numbers (1, 2 and 3) on opaque envelopes corresponding the group (ESP, EAP and CG), respectively.

Evaluation and reevaluation were performed by a researcher blinded to the experimental groups. Patients were also blinded to the mode of PBM application (sham or active).

Sample size

The sample size calculation was performed using the GPower 3.0.10 program with parameters: effects size of 0.25 [27], power observed of 0.75 and $\alpha = 5\%$, considering ANOVA model for three groups. The required sample would be 12 patients for each treatment group ESP, EAP or CG with a total of 36 patients. Each treatment group was started with 14 patients for possible dropout.

Experimental procedures

After the initial evaluation, the following experimental procedures were made 48 h before and 48 h after interventions: blood collection and functional capacity analysis (WOMAC). Participants of the control group were oriented to maintain the same habits and do not start any new treatment for the period of 8 weeks.

Assessments

WOMAC questionnaire

The functional capacity of lower limb and knee joint could be evaluated by using Western Ontario and McMaster Universities Osteoarthritis (WOMAC). The WOMAC is a self-administered reliable and valid questionnaire for patients with hip and knee OA and used for assessment of pain, stiffness joints, and physical activity of patients with hip and knee OA [28, 29]. The total score range of 0–96 and increased scores indicate a higher level of disability and lower level of quality of life.

Blood collection and serum biomarkers measurement

One biomedical collected 8 ml of peripheral blood samples from each patient before and after intervention period. After collected, the samples were centrifuged to prepare the plasma and stored at -80 °C in cryogenic tubes until in measurement. All the samples were sent to a certificate laboratory for analyses. The enzyme-linked immunosorbent assays (ELISA) kits were used to analyze the levels of CTX-II (MyBioSource), IL-1β and IL-10 (Enzo Life Sciences, Inc.) and IL-6, IL-8 e TNF-α (Fine Test®) following the procedures recommended by the manufacturer with automated pipetting.

Interventions

Both groups, ESP and EAP, received the intervention excepted CG (waitlist).

Physical exercise program

The physical exercise protocol used was adapted from the study by Silva et al. [30] and Foley et al., [31]. A protocol with warming (5 min on treadmill), 6 strength exercises (Hip abductors and adductors chair, SLR – *seated leg raise,* Glute Bridge (Hip lift), Knee flexors and extensors chair) and stretching of major muscle groups was used for this purpose. The patients were subjected to a physical exercise protocol twice a week (Monday and Wednesday) for 8 consecutive weeks performed individually and supervised by a physical therapist. The application of the physical exercise protocol occurred according to 1-RM (repetition maximum) was determined each 2 weeks for prescription and load progression of the exercises. The exercise consisted 3 sets of 8 repetitions each, with 60% of 1-RM and a rest interval of 2–3 min between sets based on American Geriatrics Society [32] for patients with OA.

PBM via cluster

A cluster with 7 diodes and an infrared wavelength (808 nm) was used in continuous mode, a 0.05cm^2 spot size, 100mW power output, 2 W/cm^2 power density, 91 J/cm^2 energy density, and energy of 4 J per point/56 J per knee, 40 s per application based on recommendations of the World Association of Laser Therapy [33]. The cluster dimension is 150 mm(L) × 100 mm(W) × 55 mm(H), with 1 cm of distance between infrared diodes. After each training session for ESP and EAP, respectively, sham or active PBM was applied on medial and lateral region of knee affected for unilateral OA and applied on medial and lateral region of most affected knee for bilateral OA (with knee positioned at 45 degrees of flexion) (Fig. 1). A researcher responsible to conduct the intervention turned on the device of PBM irradiation and immediately turned off the equipment to apply the sham PBM.

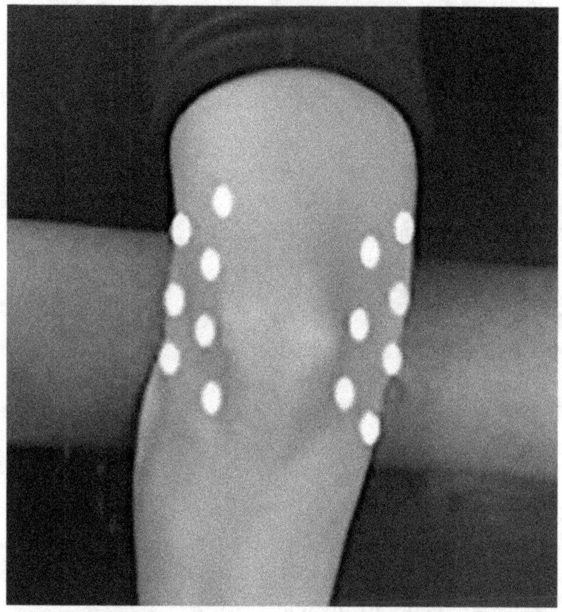

Fig. 1 PBMT irradiation points

Statistical analysis

To analyze the variables age, height, body mass, BMI, IL-1β, IL-6, IL-8, IL-10, TNF-α, CTX-II and WOMAC at groups and evaluations, were performed the analysis of variance (ANOVA *one-way* and *two-way test*) followed by Fisher's post hoc test to identify the possible differences among groups. The adopted significant value was $\alpha < 5\%$. Data were expressed as mean ± standard deviation (SD). The difference between groups was performed per-protocol analysis.

Results

Six patients (one from ESP, one from EAP and four from CG) were excluded from the study due to the absence in 2 consecutive treatment sessions. Table 1 displays the baseline values of the outcome measures, anthropometric and demographic characteristics of the participants per group. Significant difference among ESP ($p=0.024$), EAP ($p=0.009$) and CG were identified for age. The EAP group showed higher values of BMI compared to CG ($p=0.04$). The percentage of the weight range for each group was 15.4% normal weight, 69.2% overweight and 15.4% obesity for ESP; 30.8% normal weigh, 38.4% overweight and 30.8% obesity for EAP and 50% normal weigh, 40% overweight and 10% obesity for CG.

Figure 2 shows the baseline and 8-week values of WOMAC total score. The results demonstrated that there was significant difference between ESP, in the baseline compared to ESP in the 8-week ($p=0.00006$), between EAP in the baseline and EAP in the 8-week ($p=0.00002$) and between ESP and CG in the 8-week ($p=0.011$).

The results of WOMAC pain, stiffness and function subscales are demonstrated in Table 2. There was significant decrease in all domains for ESP and EAP compared baseline with 8-week evaluation ($p<0,05$) and significant decrease in WOMAC stiffness subscale for CG ($p=0.01$). Thus, in baseline values, significant difference was found

Table 1 Mean and SD of baseline values, anthropometric and demographic characteristics

Variables	ESP (n=13)			EAP (n=13)			CG (n=10)		
	Mean		SD	Mean		SD	Mean		SD
Age (years)	62.29	±	4.39 *	61.57	±	4.42 *	66.5	±	4.06
Height (m)	1.60	±	0.04	1.60	±	0.07	1.60	±	0.06
Body mass (kg)	77.06	±	10.34	78.6	±	12.67	69.9	±	7.29
BMI (kg/m²)	30.11	±	3.64	30.49	±	4.35 *	27.24	±	2.99
Unilateral and Bilateral OA (%)	23% uni 77% bi			23% uni 77% bi			50% uni 50% bi		
WOMAC pain	7.43	±	3.48	10.36	±	2.76 &	9.1	±	4.33
WOMAC stiffness	3.21	±	2.51	2.57	±	1.55	3.2	±	2.34
WOMAC function	23	±	11.36	30.5	±	7.79 &, *	21.3	±	9.25
WOMAC total	33.64	±	15.92	43.43	±	9.89	33.6	±	9.86
IL-10 (pg/ml)	8.52	±	2.09	8	±	2.48	7.21	±	1.39
IL-1β (pg/ml)	5.02	±	0.52	5.47	±	1.16	4.98	±	0.64
CTX-II (ng/ml)	4.24	±	0.78	4.10	±	1.10	4.45	±	0.48
IL-6 (pg/ml)	5.66	±	0.35	5.61	±	0.68	5.34	±	0.13
IL-8 (pg/ml)	11.28	±	2.54	11.25	±	1.77	11.26	±	1.81
TNF-α (pg/ml)	26.94	±	14.88	26.38	±	20.01	19.68	±	1.19

ESP: exercise and sham PBM group; EAP: exercise and active PBM group; CG: control group; BMI: body mass index; kg: kilograms; m: meter; uni: unilateral; bi: bilateral. IL-10: interleukin-10; IL-1β: interleukin-1β; CTX-II: C-telopeptide of type II collagen; IL-8: interleukin-8; TNF-α: Tumor Necrosis Factor alpha; WOMAC: Western Ontario and McMaster Universities Osteoarthritis

* statistical difference from CG

& statistical difference from ESP

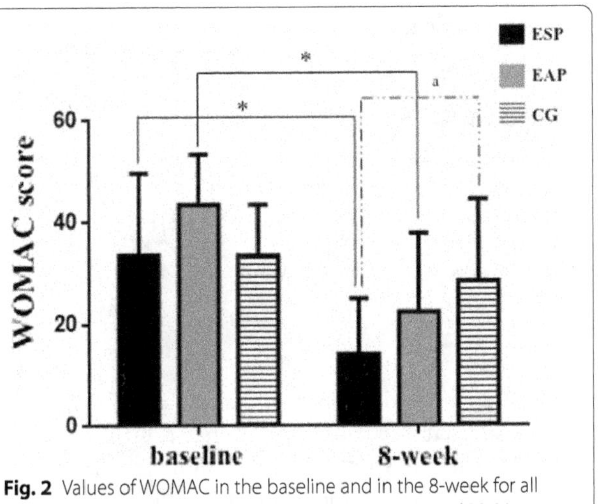

Fig. 2 Values of WOMAC in the baseline and in the 8-week for all the experimental groups. WOMAC: Western Ontario and McMaster Universities Osteoarthritis Index; ESP: exercise and sham PBM group; EAP: exercise and active PBM group; CG: control group. *statistical significance between in the baseline and in the 8-week. [a]Statistical significance from ESP group in the same condition

between the EAP and ESP in WOMAC pain (p=0.04) and function (p=0,0001) subscales, and between EAP and CG in WOMAC function subscale (p=0.02). Significant difference was found between the ESP and CG in WOMAC pain (p=0.02) and function (p=0.01) subscales 8-week.

Figure 3 shows the baseline and 8-week values of the IL-10. It is possible to observe a statistical significant difference between the values found for EAP in the baseline compared to the 8-week (p=0.047). Also, a significant difference was found between the values of EAP and CG after the experimental period (p=0.0009).

For IL-1β expression, there was a significant increase and difference between the values found in the baseline and in the 8-week for CG (p=0.016) (Fig. 4).

Table 3 shows the values found in the baseline and in the 8-week of the pro-inflammatory cytokines (IL-6, IL-8, TNF-α) and cartilage degradation biomarkers (CTX-II). For these variables, no significant difference was observed.

Discussion

The results of this study demonstrated that the physical exercise program was able of increasing the functional capacity in the patients and, the associated treatments increased IL-10 expression compared to CG after the experimental period. In addition, IL-1β expression was higher for CG comparing the values in the baseline and 8-week and no difference for the others biomarkers were observed.

Table 2 Means and SD of Western Ontario and McMaster Universities Osteoarthritis Questionnaire

Variables	ESP (n = 13)						EAP (n = 13)						CG (n = 10)					
	Baseline			8-week			Baseline			8-week			Baseline			8-week		
	Mean		SD	Mean		SD	Mean		SD	Mean		SD	Mean		SD	Mean		SD
WOMAC pain	7.43	±	3.48	3.36	±	2.87 *	10.36	±	2.76 [a]	4.79	±	4.51 *	9.1	±	4.33	7	±	4.27 [a]
WOMAC stiffness	3.21	±	2.51	1.21	±	1.48 *	2.57	±	1.55	1.43	±	1.28 *	3.2	±	2.35	1.7	±	1.7 *
WOMAC function	23	±	11.36	9.5	±	7.38 *	30.5	±	7.79 [a]	16.14	±	10.7 *	21.3	±	9.25 [b]	19.8	±	11.45 [a]
WOMAC total score	33.64	±	15.92	14.07	±	10.99*	43.43	±	9.89	22.36	±	15.49*	33.60	±	9.86	28.50	±	15.95 [a]

ESP exercise and sham PBM group, EAP exercise and active PBM group, CG control group, WOMAC: Western Ontario and McMaster Universities Osteoarthritis

* statistical significance between in the baseline and in the 8-week

[a] statistical significance from ESP group in the same condition

[b] statistical significance from EAP group in the same condition

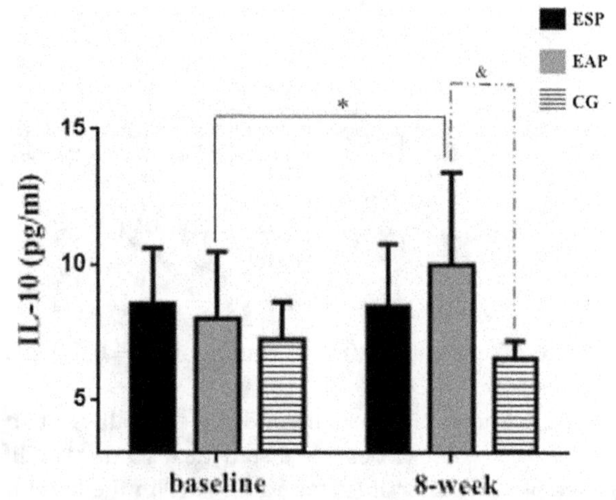

Fig. 3 Values of IL-10 concentration in the baseline and in the 8-week for all the experimental groups. IL-10: interleukin-10; ESP: exercise and sham PBM group; EAP: exercise and active PBM group; CG: control group. *statistical significance between in the baseline and 8-week values. &statistical significance between in the 8-week values

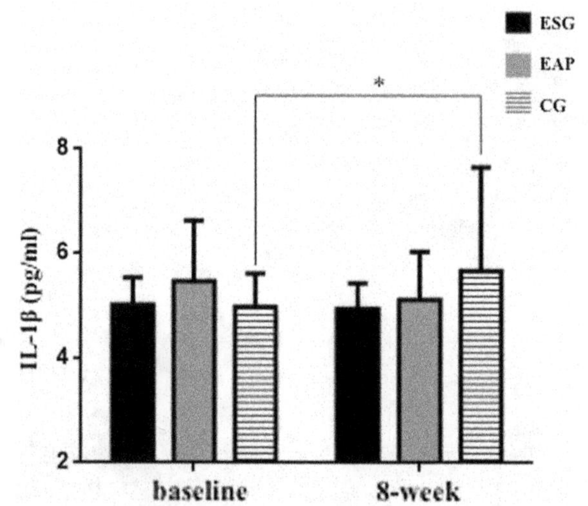

Fig. 4 Values of IL-1β concentration baseline and 8-week for all the experimental groups. IL-1ß: interleukin-1ß; ESP: exercise and sham PBM group; EAP: exercise and active PBM group; CG: control group. *Statistical significance between in the baseline and 8-week intervention values

Knee OA is clinically associated with pain and loss of functional capacity, reaching 25% of the population over the age of 60 years [34]. As described above, the lower WOMAC score demonstrated by the physical exercised patients (irradiated or not with PBM) is possibly related to the increase in muscle strength after the exercise program, improving the joint stability and the level of pain, and consequently, leading to the improvement of the functional capacity. Interestingly, PBM did not produce any extra positive effect in the exercised patients. Data from the literature do not corroborate the findings of the present study demonstrating a superior effect measured by WOMAC in exercised and irradiated patients with OA [35–37]. Kheshie et al. [36] also observed a decrease in WOMAC subscales in patients with OA treated with physical exercises and PBM. One hypothesis that can be raised is that the PBM parameters used in this study were not sufficient to produce an additional effect in the exercised patients.

Furthermore, it is well known that IL-10 has an important anti-inflammatory role in OA, presenting a chondroprotective effect and, inhibiting chondrocyte apoptosis [38]. Our results showed that the active PBM associated with physical exercises significantly increased IL-10 expression after the experimental period of treatment. Assis et al., [17] also observed an increase of IL-10 expression in an experimental study, submitting rats with OA to a program of aerobic exercises and PBM irradiation. All the positive effects may be related to the effects

Table 3 Means and SD of IL-10, IL-1b, IL-6, IL-8, TNF-α and CTX-II

Variables	ESP (n = 13)						EAP (n = 13)						CG (n = 10)					
	Baseline			8-week			Baseline			8-week			Baseline			8-week		
	Mean		SD	Mean		SD	Mean		SD	Mean		SD	Mean		SD	Mean		SD
IL-10 (pg/ml)	8.52	±	2.09	8.44	±	2.33	8.00	±	2.48	9.98	±	3.42*&	7.21	±	1.39	6.54	±	0.63
IL-1b (pg/ml)	5.02	±	0.52	4.94	±	0.49	5.47	±	1.16	5.11	±	0.92	4.98	±	0.64	5.67	±	1.99*
CTX II (ng/ml)	4.24	±	0.78	4.38	±	0.63	4.10	±	1.10	4.26	±	0.65	4.45	±	0.48	4.07	±	0.98
IL-6 (pg/ml)	5.66	±	0.35	5.57	±	0.24	5.61	±	0.68	5.65	±	0.86	5.34	±	0.13	5.37	±	0.22
IL-8 (pg/ml)	11.28	±	2.54	11.76	±	2.97	11.25	±	1.77	11.40	±	1.73	11.26	±	1.81	11.89	±	1.85
TNF-α (pg/ml)	26.94	±	14.88	26.24	±	12.11	26.38	±	20.01	23.00	±	8.59	19.68	±	1.19	19.42	±	1.09

* statistical significance between in the baseline and 8-week values

& statistical significance between in the 8-week values compare to CG group

ESP: exercise and sham PBM group; EAP: exercise and active PBM group; CG: control group

of physical exercises and PBM on inflammatory markers. Physical exercises (and the related muscle contraction) produce a mechanotransduction stimulus, which maintain homeostasis of articular cartilage and contribute to attenuate OA physiological events [39]. As a consequence, physical exercise programs have anabolic, anti-inflammatory and antioxidant effects in OA patients [40]. Moreover, many studies have demonstrated the anti-inflammatory effects of PBM [41, 42]. PBM is able to modulate mRNA gene expression of IL-10 in acute and chronic inflammatory phase and decreases the expression of this cytokine and consequently modulates the inflammatory process of OA [43]. Taking together, the combined treatments presented a positive effect on IL-10 expression, which could represent a modulation of the inflammatory process.

IL-1β is considered one of the main cytokines in OA development and the literature points out that the reduction of IL-1β production is an indication of the attenuation of cartilage degenerative process related to OA [44]. CG demonstrated a significant increase of IL-1β expression after the experimental period. Similarly, an experimental study using rats with OA also observed a higher IL-1β expression in the control animals compared to the treated ones CG [45]. In this context, it can be suggested that the treatments were able to positively kept stable the IL-1β expression.

IL-6, a pro-inflammatory cytokine has a catabolic activity in the pathogenesis of OA. In the present study, no significant difference in IL-6 expression was observed in both experimental periods for any group. Conversely, Aguiar et al., [13] found a significant reduction in IL-6 levels in patients with knee OA, after a treatment of flexibility training and muscle strengthening, 3 times a week for 12 weeks. Furthermore, a systematic review concluded that PBM has no effect on the expression of the inflammatory cytokine IL-6 in OA animals [46]. However, experimental studies indicate that PBM is capable of modulating inflammatory mediators such as IL-6 in rats using an experimental model of joint inflammation [47]. The controversial results may be related to PBM parameters or the frequency if the treatment.

Furthermore, both treatments did not have any effect on IL-8 and TNF-α cytokines concentration. IL-8 is a chemokine produced by various inflammatory cells such as neutrophils, basophils, macrophages and T cells [48]. TNF-α, a pro-inflammatory cytokine seems to be related to IL-1β (pro-inflammatory cytokine) because are secreted by the same cells of the joint, in addition the increased presence of TNF-α stimulates the synthesis of IL-6 and IL-8 [49]. These results corroborates with Helmark et al., [50] who also observed that a resistance exercise training (25 sets of 10 repetitions at 60% of 1-RM) have not decreased the levels of IL-8 and IL-6 of patients with knee OA. Aguiar et al., [13] have not observed changes in TNF-α expression after 12 weeks of physical training using 60–80% of the maximum load of individuals with knee OA. In addition, a study applied PBM immediately after total knee arthroplasty and observed a decrease of IL-8 expression [49]. Moreover, a systematic review and meta-analysis points out that the PBM is capable of reduce considerably TNF-α expression in models of joint inflammation [47]. The results of the present study for IL-8 and TNF-α cytokines can be justified by type and modality of the load used in physical exercises once it is suggested that maximum training load seems to modulate the levels of these cytokine [51].

CTX-II is a biomarker released due to the degeneration of cartilage related to catabolic activity that leads to loss of type II collagen concentration, which is the most abundant protein of the cartilage matrix and proteoglycan matrix of cartilage [52]. There was no statistically significant difference in CTX-II levels in this study. These findings do not corroborate those of with Nambi et al. [1], which demonstrated that a protocol of PBM (905 nm, super pulsed, 1.5 J per point, 12 J per knee) and exercise in patients with knee OA during 4 weeks (twice a week) were able of inhibiting CTX-II, MMP-3 (stromelysin), MMP-8 (collagenase-2), and MMP-13 (collagenase-3) expression. However, the study mentioned analyse the levels of CTX-II fragments from urinary fraction and our study evaluated from the serum fraction of peripheral blood samples and this difference in analyse can justify the results of the present study.

In addition, it may be suggested that PBM application, through a cluster device constitutes an advantage for treating patients with knee OA, allowing the irradiation of a larger area and optimizing the treatment [21]. Although some positive effects of the treatments in the patients in this study, some limitations can be raised as a minor number of patients in sample size. It would be extremely important to assess the presence of inflammatory markers in the synovial fluid, which would increase the accuracy of their analysis, as well as the possibility of correlating them with symptomatic variables. Also, there is an absence of a follow-up in order to provide information about the maintenance of results over time in these patients.

Conclusion

The results of this study demonstrated that the physical exercise program in association with PBM was capable of increasing IL-10 levels, and the physical exercise program improved the function capacity. However, PBM did not promote an additional effect to the positive effects of exercise in improving pro-inflammatory and cartilage degradation biomarkers, and functional capacity in women with knee OA. Thus, more studies need to be carried out, using other parameters, since the literature demonstrates heterogeneity in the parameters of treatment with PBM when associated with physical exercise, for the consolidation of an intervention protocol for patients with knee OA.

Clinical messages

- Patients who underwent physical exercise program in association with PBM for 8 weeks showed improvement in IL-10 levels after treatment and when compared to the control group who did not any intervention;
- The function capacity was improved in patients undergoing a physical exercise program;
- Only the control group had the pro-inflammatory marker (IL-1β) increased;
- Physical exercise program and its association with PBM had no effect on others pro-inflammatory and cartilage degradation biomarkers.

Abbreviations

OA: Osteoarthritis; TNF-α: Tumor Necrosis Factor alpha; IL-1β: Interleukin-1β; IL-6: Interleukin -6; MMPs: Matrix metalloproteinases; CTX-II: C-telopeptide of type II collagen; NSAIDs: Nonsteroidal and steroidal anti-inflammatory drugs; MPA: Moderate physical activity; ILs: Interleukins; LLLT: Low-level laser therapy; PBM: Photobiomodulation; WOMAC: Western Ontario and McMaster Universities Arthritis Index; LED: Light-emitting diode; ESP: Exercise sham photobiomodulation group; EAP: Exercise active photobiomodulation group; CG: Control group; ANOVA: Analysis of variance; ELISA: Enzyme-linked immunosorbent assays; SLR: Seated leg raise; RM: Repetition maximum.

Acknowledgements

Not applicable.

Authors' contributions

PGV, HTT and ACR–Conceptualization, methodology, data collection, writing-original draft preparation and editing; RMDSC and LAG–methodology, statistic work, writing-reviewing and editing. CFDS—biomedicine responsible for blood sample collection from volunteers. The author(s) read and approved the final manuscript.

Author details

[1]Department of Biosciences, Federal University of São Paulo, Campus Baixada Santista, Rua Silva Jardim, 136, Santos, SP 11015-020, Brazil. [2]Department of Human Movement Science, Federal University of São Paulo, Campus Baixada Santista, Rua Silva Jardim, 136, Santos, SP 11015-020, Brazil. [3]Post Graduate Program of Interdisciplinary Health Sciences, Federal University of São Paulo, Campus Baixada Santista, Rua Silva Jardim, 136, Santos, SP 11015-020, Brazil. [4]Scientific Institute and Technological Department -University Brazil, São Paulo-Itaquera, SP, Brazil.

References

1. S GN, Kamal W, George J, Manssor E. Radiological and biochemical effects (CTX-II, MMP-3, 8, and 13) of low-level laser therapy (LLLT) in chronic osteoarthritis in Al-Kharj, Saudi Arabia. Lasers Med Sci. 2017; 32(2):297–303.
2. Duan ZX, Huang P, Tu C, Liu Q, Li SQ, Long ZL, Li ZH. MicroRNA-15a-5p regulates the development of osteoarthritis by targeting PTHrP in chondrocytes. Biomed Res Int. 2019;2019(5):3904923. https://doi.org/10.1155/2019/3904923.
3. Wojdasiewicz P, Poniatowski ŁA, Szukiewicz D. The role of inflammatory and anti-inflammatory cytokines in the pathogenesis of osteoarthritis. Mediators Inflamm. 2014;2014: 561459. https://doi.org/10.1155/2014/561459.
4. Al-Khazraji BK, Appleton CT, Beier F, Birmingham TB, Shoemaker JK. Osteoarthritis, cerebrovascular dysfunction and the common denominator of inflammation: a narrative review. Osteoarthritis Cartilage. 2018;26(4):462–70. https://doi.org/10.1016/j.joca.2018.01.011.
5. Tomazoni SS, Frigo L, Dos Reis Ferreira TC, Casalechi HL, Teixeira S, de Almeida P, Muscara MN, Marcos RL, Serra AJ, de Carvalho PTC, Leal-Junior ECP. Effects of photobiomodulation therapy and topical non-steroidal anti-inflammatory drug on skeletal muscle injury induced by contusion in rats-part 1: morphological and functional aspects. Lasers Med Sci. 2017;32(9):2111–20. https://doi.org/10.1007/s10103-017-2346-z.
6. Nefla M, Holzinger D, Berenbaum F, Jacques C. The danger from within: alarmins in arthritis. Nat Rev Rheumatol. 2016;12(11):669–83. https://doi.org/10.1007/s10103-017-2346-z.
7. Severino RM, Jorge PB, Martinelli MO, deLima MV, Severino NR, Duarte Junior A. Analysis on the serum levels of the biomarker CTX-II in professional indoor soccer players over the course of one season. Rev Bras Ortop. 2015;50(3):331–5. https://doi.org/10.1016/j.rboe.2015.04.001

8. Saberi Hosnijeh F, Siebuhr AS, Uitterlinden AG, Oei EH, Hofman A, Karsdal MA, Bierma-Zeinstra SM, Bay-Jensen AC, van Meurs JB. Association between biomarkers of tissue inflammation and progression of osteoarthritis: evidence from the Rotterdam study cohort. Arthritis Res Ther. 2016;1(18):81. https://doi.org/10.1186/s13075-016-0976-3.
9. Rannou F. [Prescribe non-pharmacological treatments for lower limb osteoarthritis?]. Rev Prat 2012; 62(5):651–3. Review. French.
10. Wyszyńska J, Bal-Bocheńska M. Efficacy of high-intensity laser therapy in treating knee osteoarthritis: a first systematic review. Photomed Laser Surg. 2018;36(7):343–53. https://doi.org/10.1089/pho.2017.4425.
11. Bennell KL, Hall M, Hinman RS. Osteoarthritis year in review 2015: rehabilitation and outcomes. Osteoarthritis Cartilage. 2016;24(1):58–70. https://doi.org/10.1016/j.joca.2015.07.028.
12. Castrogiovanni P, Di Rosa M, Ravalli S, et al. Moderate physical activity as a prevention method for knee osteoarthritis and the role of synoviocytes as biological key. Int J Mol Sci. 2019;20(3):511. https://doi.org/10.3390/ijms20030511.
13. Aguiar GC, Do Nascimento MR, De Miranda AS, Rocha NP, Teixeira AL, Scalzo PL. Effects of an exercise therapy protocol on inflammatory markers, perception of pain, and physical performance in individuals with knee osteoarthritis. Rheumatol Int. 2015;35(3):525–31. https://doi.org/10.1007/s00296-014-3148-2.
14. Assis L, Milares LP, Almeida T, Tim C, Magri A, Fernandes KR, Medalha C, Muniz Renno AC. Aerobic exercise training and low-level laser therapy modulate inflammatory response and degenerative process in an experimental model of knee osteoarthritisin rats. Osteoarthr Cartil. 2016;24:169–77. https://doi.org/10.1007/s00296-014-3148-2.
15. Balbinot G, Schuch CP, Nascimento PSD, Lanferdini FJ, Casanova M, Baroni BM, Vaz MA. Photobiomodulation therapy partially restores cartilage integrity and reduces chronic pain behavior in a rat model of osteoarthritis: involvement of spinal glial modulation. Cartilage. 2019;30:1947603519876338. https://doi.org/10.1177/1947603519876338
16. Hamblin MR. Mechanisms and applications of the anti-inflammatory effects of photobiomodulation. AIMS Biophys. 2017;4(3):337–61. https://doi.org/10.3934/biophy.2017.3.337.
17. Assis L, Tim C, Magri A, Fernandes KR, Vassão PG, Renno ACM. Interleukin-10 and collagen type II immunoexpression are modulated by photobiomodulation associated to aerobic and aquatic exercises in an experimental model of osteoarthritis. Lasers Med Sci. 2018;33(9):1875–82. https://doi.org/10.1007/s10103-018-2541-6.
18. de Oliveira VL, Silva JA Jr, Serra AJ, Pallotta RC, da Silva EA, de Farias Marques AC, Feliciano RD, Marcos RL, Leal-Junior EC, de Carvalho PT. Photobiomodulation therapy in the modulation of inflammatory mediators and bradykinin receptors in an experimental model of acute osteoarthritis. Lasers Med Sci. 2017;32(1):87–94. https://doi.org/10.1007/s10103-016-2089-2.
19. Soleimanpour H, Gahramani K, Taheri R, Golzari SE, Safari S, Esfanjani RM, Iranpour A. The effect of low-level laser therapy on knee osteoarthritis: prospective, descriptive study. Lasers Med Sci. 2014;29(5):1695–700. https://doi.org/10.1007/s10103-014-1576-6.
20. Alghadir A, Omar MT, Al-Askar AB, Al-Muteri NK. Effect of low-level laser therapy in patients with chronic knee osteoarthritis: a single-blinded randomized clinical study. Lasers Med Sci. 2014;29(2):749–55. https://doi.org/10.1007/s10103-013-1393-3.
21. de Paula Gomes CAF, Leal-Junior ECP, Dibai-Filho AV, de Oliveira AR, Bley AS, Biasotto-Gonzalez DA, de Tarso Camillo de Carvalho P. Incorporation of photobiomodulation therapy into a therapeutic exercise program for knee osteoarthritis: A placebo-controlled, randomized, clinical trial. Lasers Surg Med 2018; 50(8):819–828. doi: https://doi.org/10.1002/lsm.22939.
22. Alfredo PP, Bjordal JM, Junior WS, Lopes-Martins RÁB, Stausholm MB, Casarotto RA, Marques AP, Joensen J. Long-term results of a randomized, controlled, double-blind study of low-level laser therapy before exercises in knee osteoarthritis: laser and exercises in knee osteoarthritis. Clin Rehabil. 2018;32(2):173–8. https://doi.org/10.1177/0269215517723162.
23. Alayat MSM, Atya AM, Ali MME, Shousha TM. Correction to: Long-term effect of high-intensity laser therapy in the treatment of patients with chronic low back pain: a randomized blinded placebo-controlled trial. Lasers Med Sci. 2020;35(1):297. https://doi.org/10.1007/s10103-019-02926-x.Erratumfor:LasersMedSci.201429(3):1065-73
24. de Matos Brunelli Braghin R, Libardi EC, Junqueira C, Rodrigues NC, Nogueira-Barbosa MH, Renno ACM, Carvalho de Abreu DC. The effect of low-level laser therapy and physical exercise on pain, stiffness, function, and spatiotemporal gait variables in subjects with bilateral knee osteoarthritis: a blind randomized clinical trial. Disabil Rehabil 2019; 41(26):3165–3172. doi: https://doi.org/10.1080/09638288.2018.1493160.
25. Kellgren JH, Lawrence JS. Radiological assessment of rheumatoid arthritis. Ann Rheum Dis. 1957;16:485–93.
26. Organización Panamericana de la Salud. XXXVI Reunión del Comité Asesor de Investigaciones en Salud. Encuesta Multicéntrica: Salud Bienestar y Envejecimiento (SABE) en América Latina y el Caribe [Internet]. 2011 Washington, D.C: Organización Panamericana de la Salud; Disponível em: http://envejecimiento.csic.es/documentos/documentos/paho-salud-01.pdf
27. » http://envejecimiento.csic.es/documentos/documentos/paho-salud-01.pdf
28. Abd El-Kader SM, Al-Shreef FM, Al-Jiffri OH. Impact of aerobic exercise versus resisted exercise on endothelial activation markers and inflammatory cytokines among elderly. Afr Health Sci. 2019;19(4):2874–80. https://doi.org/10.4314/ahs.v19i4.9.
29. Bellamy N, Buchanan WW, Goldsmith CH, Campbell J, Stitt LW. Validation study of WOMAC: a health status instrument for measuring clinically important patient relevant outcomes to antirheumatic drug therapy in patients with osteoarthritis of the hip or knee. J Rheumatol. 1988;15(12):1833–40.
30. Choquette D, Bellamy N, Raynauld JP. A French-Canadian version of the WOMAC osteoarthritis index. Arthritis Rheum. 1994;37:S226.
31. Silva LE, Valim V, Pessanha AP, Oliveira LM, Myamoto S, Jones A, Natour J. Hydrotherapy versus conventional land-based exercise for the management of patients with osteoarthritis of the knee: a randomized clinical trial. Phys Ther. 2008;88:12–21. https://doi.org/10.2522/ptj.20060040.
32. Foley A, Halbert J, Hewitt T, Crotty M. Does hydrotherapy improve strength and physical function in patients with osteoarthritis–a randomised controlled trial comparing a gym based and a hydrotherapy based strengthening programme. Ann Rheum Dis. 2003;62:1162–7. https://doi.org/10.1136/ard.2002.005272.
33. American Geriatrics Society Panel on Exercise and Osteoarthritis. Exercise prescription for older adults with osteoarthritis pain: consensus practice recommendations. A supplement to the AGS Clinical Practice Guidelines on the management of chronic pain in older adults. J Am Geriatr Soc 2001; 49(6):808–823 Review. Erratum in: J Am Geriatr Soc 2001 Oct;49(10):1400
34. World Association of Laser Therapy (WALT). Consensus agreement on the design and conduct of clinical studies with low- level laser therapy and light therapy for musculoskeletal pain and disorders. Photomed Laser Surg. 2006;24:761–2.
35. Alcalde GE, Fonseca AC, Bôscoa TF, et al . Effect of aquatic physical therapy on pain perception, functional capacity and quality of life in older people with knee osteoarthritis: study protocol for a randomized controlled trial. Trials 2017; 18(1):317. Published 2017 Jul 11. doi:https://doi.org/10.1186/s13063-017-2061-x.
36. Alfredo PP, Bjordal JM, Dreyer SH, Meneses SR, Zaguetti G, Ovanessian V, Fukuda TY, Junior WS, Lopes Martins RÁ, Casarotto RA, Marques AP. Efficacy of low level laser therapy associated with exercises in knee osteo arthritis: a randomized double-blind study. Clin Rehabil. 2012;26:523–33. https://doi.org/10.1016/S2255-4971(15)30407-9.
37. Kheshie AR, Alayat MS, Ali MM. High-intensity versus low-level laser ther apy in the treatment of patients with knee osteoarthritis: a randomized controlled trial. Lasers Med Sci. 2014;29(4):1371–6. https://doi.org/10.1007/s10103-014-1529-0.
38. Nazari A, Moezy A, Nejati P, Mazaherinezhad A. Efficacy of high-intensity laser therapy in comparison with conventional physiotherapy and exercise therapy on pain and function of patients with knee osteoarthritis: a randomized controlled trial with 12-week follow up. Lasers Med Sci. 2019;34(3):505–16. https://doi.org/10.1007/s10103-018-2624-4.
39. Kwon JY, Lee SH, Na HS, Jung K, Choi J, Cho KH, Lee CY, Kim SJ, Park SH, Shin DY, Cho ML. Kartogenin inhibits pain behavior, chondrocyte inflammation, and attenuates osteoarthritis progression in mice through induction of IL-10. Sci Rep. 2018; 14;8(1):13832. doi: https://doi.org/10.1038/s41598-018-32206-7.
40. Bader DL, Salter DM, Chowdhury TT. Biomechanical influence of cartilage homeostasis in health and disease. Arthritis. 2011;2011:979032. doi: https://doi.org/10.1155/2011/979032. Epub 2011 Sep 15. PMID: 22046527; PMCID: PMC3196252.
41. Cifuentes DJ, Rocha LG, Silva LA, Brito AC, Rueff-Barroso CR, Porto LC,

Pinho RA. Decrease in oxidative stress and histological changes induced by physical exercise calibrated in rats with osteoarthritis induced by monosodium iodoacetate. Osteoarthritis Cartilage. 2010;18(8):1088–95. https://doi.org/10.1016/j.joca.2010.04.004

42. Pigatto GR, Silva CS, Parizotto NA. Photobiomodulation therapy reduces acute pain and inflammation in mice. J Photochem Photobiol B. 2019;196: 111513. https://doi.org/10.1016/j.jphotobiol.2019.111513.
43. Li K, Liang Z, Zhang J, Zuo X, Sun J, Zheng Q, Song J, Ding T, Hu X, Wang Z. Attenuation of the inflammatory response and polarization of macrophages by photobiomodulation. Lasers Med Sci. 2020;35(7):1509–18. https://doi.org/10.1007/s10103-019-02941-y.
44. Casalechi HL, Leal-Junior EC, Xavier M, Silva JA Jr, de Carvalho PD, Aimbire F, Albertini R. Low-level laser therapy in experimental model of collagenase-induced tendinitis in rats: effects in acute and chronic inflammatory phases. Lasers Med Sci. 2013;28(3):989–95. https://doi.org/10.1007/s10103-012-1189-x.
45. Kapoor M, Martel-Pelletier J, Lajeunesse D, Pelletier JP, Fahmi H. Role of proinflammatory cytokines in the pathophysiology of osteoarthritis. Nat Rev Rheumatol. 2011;7(1):33–42. https://doi.org/10.1038/nrrheum.2010.196.
46. Sanches M, Assis L, Criniti C, Fernandes D, Tim C, Renno ACM. Chondroitin sulfate and glucosamine sulfate associated to photobiomodulation prevents degenerative morphological changes in an experimental model of osteoarthritis in rats. Lasers Med Sci. 2018;33(3):549–57. https://doi.org/10.1007/s10103-017-2401-9.
47. Nambi G. Does low level laser therapy has effects on inflammatory biomarkers IL-1β, IL-6, TNF-α, and MMP-13 in osteoarthritis of rat models-a systemic review and meta-analysis. Lasers Med Sci. 2021;36(3):475–84. https://doi.org/10.1007/s10103-020-03124-w.
48. Alves AC, Vieira R, Leal-Junior E, dos Santos S, Ligeiro AP, Albertini R, Junior J, de Carvalho P. Effect of low-level laser therapy on the expression of inflammatory mediators and on neutrophils and macrophages in acute joint inflammation. Arthritis Res Ther. 2013;15(5):R116. https://doi.org/10.1186/ar4296.
49. Hoff P, Buttgereit F, Burmester GR, Jakstadt M, Gaber T, Andreas K, Matziolis G, Perka C, Röhner E. Osteoarthritis synovial fluid activates pro-inflammatory cytokines in primary human chondrocytes. Int Orthop. 2013;37(1):145–51. https://doi.org/10.1007/s00264-012-1724-1.
50. Langella LG, Casalechi HL, Tomazoni SS, Johnson DS, Albertini R, Pallotta RC, Marcos RL, de Carvalho PTC, Leal-Junior ECP. Photobiomodulation therapy (PBMT) on acute pain and inflammation in patients who underwent total hip arthroplasty-a randomized, triple-blind, placebo-controlled clinical trial. Lasers Med Sci. 2018;33(9):1933–40. https://doi.org/10.1007/s10103-018-2558-x.
51. Helmark IC, Mikkelsen UR, Børglum J, Rothe A, Petersen MC, Andersen O, Langberg H, Kjaer M. Exercise increases interleukin-10 levels both intraarticularly and peri-synovially in patients with knee osteoarthritis: a randomized controlled trial. Arthritis Res Ther. 2010;12(4):R126. https://doi.org/10.1186/ar3064.
52. Greiwe JS, Cheng B, Rubin DC, Yarasheski KE, Semenkovich CF. Resistance exercise decreases skeletal muscle tumor necrosis factor alpha in frail elderly humans. FASEB J. 2001;15(2):475–82. https://doi.org/10.1096/fj.00-0274com.

14

Factors associated with anxiety and depression in rheumatoid arthritis patients

Miyabi Uda[1], Motomu Hashimoto[2,3], Ryuji Uozumi[4], Mie Torii[1], Takao Fujii[5], Masao Tanaka[2], Moritoshi Furu[2], Hiromu Ito[2], Chikashi Terao[6,7,8,9], Wataru Yamamoto[10], Genichi Sugihara[11], Yukako Nakagami[11,12], Tsuneyo Mimori[13,14] and Kazuko Nin[1*]

Abstract

Background: The management of anxiety and depression symptoms in rheumatoid arthritis (RA) patients is vital. Previous study findings on this topic are conflicting, and the topic remains to be thoroughly investigated. This study aimed to clarify the association of RA disease activity with anxiety and depression symptoms after controlling for physical disability, pain, and medication.

Methods: We conducted a cross-sectional study of RA patients from the Kyoto University Rheumatoid Arthritis Management Alliance cohort. We assessed patients using the Disease Activity Score (DAS28), Health Assessment Questionnaire Disability Index (HAQ-DI), and Hospital Anxiety and Depression Scale (HADS). Anxiety and depression symptoms were defined by a HADS score ≥ 8. We analyzed the data using multivariable logistic regression analyses.

Results: Of 517 participants, 17.6% had anxiety symptoms and 27.7% had depression symptoms. The multivariable logistic regression analysis demonstrated that DAS28 was not independently associated with anxiety symptoms (odds ratio [OR] [95% confidence interval; CI] 0.93 [0.48–1.78]; $p = 0.82$) and depression symptoms (OR [95% CI] 1.45 [0.81–2.61]; $p = 0.22$). However, DAS28 patient global assessment (PtGA) severity was associated with anxiety symptoms (OR [95% CI] 1.15 [1.02–1.29]; $p = 0.03$) and depression symptoms (OR [95% CI] 1.21 [1.09–1.35]; $p < 0.01$). Additionally, HAQ-DI scores > 0.5 were associated with anxiety symptoms (OR [95% CI] 3.51 [1.85–6.64]; $p < 0.01$) and depression symptoms (OR [95% CI] 2.65 [1.56–4.50]; $p < 0.01$). Patients using steroids were more likely to have depression than those not using steroids (OR [95% CI] 1.66 [1.03–2.67]; $p = 0.04$).

Conclusions: No association was found between RA disease activity and anxiety and depression symptoms in the multivariable logistic regression analysis. Patients with high PtGA scores or HAQ-DI-based non-remission were more likely to experience anxiety and depression symptoms, irrespective of disease activity remission status. Rather than focusing solely on controlling disease activity, treatment should focus on improving or preserving physical function and the patient's overall sense of well-being.

Keywords: Rheumatoid arthritis, Anxiety, Depression, Patient global assessment (PtGA), Quality of life

Background

Symptoms of anxiety and depression are more prevalent in rheumatoid arthritis (RA) patients than in the general population [1, 2]. Studies have shown that 26–46% of RA patients have anxiety symptoms, and 14.8–34.2% have

*Correspondence: nin@kuhp.kyoto-u.ac.jp
[1] Department of Human Health Sciences, Kyoto University Graduate School of Medicine, 53 Shogoin Kawahara-cho, Sakyo-ku, Kyoto 606-8507, Japan

depression symptoms [1]. RA patients with these conditions have worse outcomes, including poor medication adherence [3], worse response to treatment [3], higher medical costs [4–6], high mortality [7, 8], and lower quality of life (QOL) [6, 9, 10]. Therefore, it is important to examine the risk factors of anxiety and depression symptoms in RA patients and incorporate the management of psychological factors into treatment.

Research has been conducted in this area to improve RA prevention and treatment. However, it is difficult for rheumatologists to observe anxiety and depression symptoms in ambulatory care. In this study, self-report questionnaires such as the Hospital Anxiety and Depression Scale (HADS) [11] were used to assess anxiety and depression symptoms in RA patients. Because of the burden on patients and the time required, it is difficult to administer questionnaires in everyday medical settings. Therefore, we focused on disease activity evaluation during medical examinations. If disease activity and its components correlate with anxiety and depression symptoms in RA patients after excluding other factors that may affect such symptoms, then anxiety and depression could be assessed through disease activity. Thus, the results of disease activity assessment could be used in daily medical care as an index for anxiety and depression symptoms.

RA is an autoimmune inflammatory disease that causes joint deformation and physical dysfunction [12]. Physical disability [13–15] and pain [16–18] are known risk factors for anxiety and depression symptoms in RA patients. Recent studies have demonstrated that these conditions are associated with systemic inflammation caused by pro-inflammatory cytokines such as tumor necrosis factor-α, interleukin-1β, and interleukin-6 [19, 20]. Cytokines are also believed to cause depression by hyperactivation of the hypothalamic–pituitary–adrenal axis [21], and studies have reported that C-reactive protein (CRP) levels are associated with anxiety and depression symptoms in RA patients [22].

Disease activity that reflects the above factors may be associated with anxiety and depression symptoms in RA patients. However, study findings on the correlation between disease activity and anxiety and depression are inconsistent. Some studies have suggested a positive association between RA disease activity and anxiety and depression symptoms [23, 24], whereas others have not identified an association [9]. A key reason for this is that other factors associated with anxiety and depression symptoms, such as physical disability, pain, and medication, have not been investigated [9, 23].

There are few comparisons of the prevalence of anxiety and depression across diseases with similar progression patterns, and findings are inconsistent. In an early (2009) study, Arne et al. showed that patients with chronic obstructive pulmonary disease had a higher prevalence of depression than patients with RA or diabetes mellitus [25]. A comparison of patients with rheumatic diseases showed that depression was more prevalent in patients with systemic lupus erythematosus and fibromyalgia (34% and 39%, respectively) than in those with RA (15%) [26]. Similarly, a recent study of the disease impact of fibromyalgia, rheumatoid arthritis, spondyloarthritis, and Sjögren's syndrome found a higher prevalence of depression and anxiety in fibromyalgia patients than in RA patients [27]. In contrast, a case control study of depression and insomnia in patients with RA and those with osteoarthritis found that approximately 75% of RA patients reported depression compared with 50% of osteoarthritis patients, although the difference was not significant. Both groups of patients also experienced stress-related insomnia [28], suggesting that subjective experiences of stress and well-being may have a greater effect than inflammation on psychological status in RA patients.

We hypothesized that disease activity and its components are associated with anxiety and depression symptoms, even after excluding the effects of pain, disability, and medication on anxiety and depression. Using a rigorous cohort study, we aimed to identify the factors associated with anxiety and depression symptoms in RA patients by simultaneous evaluation of disease activity, pain, physical disability, and medication.

Methods

Patients and setting

We performed a cross-sectional analysis of patients who visited the outpatient RA center of Kyoto University Hospital between May 1 and December 31, 2014, and whose data were collected in the 2014 Kyoto University Rheumatoid Arthritis Management Alliance (KURAMA) cohort [29]. All patients fulfilled the 1987 or 2010 American College of Rheumatology and the European League against Rheumatism RA classification criteria [30]. We excluded patients with psychiatric disorders, such as bipolar disorder and schizophrenia. The presence of these disorders was determined by one questionnaire item, which asked patients if they were attending an outpatient appointment in the psychiatry department or in the psychosomatic medicine department; the medical records of psychiatry outpatients were then checked to verify diagnoses of psychiatric disorders. We also excluded patients who did not complete a HADS questionnaire [11]. The study protocol was approved by the Kyoto University Graduate School and Faculty of Medicine, Ethics Committee, and all procedures were performed in accordance with the 1964 Declaration of Helsinki and its later amendments or comparable ethical standards.

Clinical assessments and outcomes

RA disease activity was assessed using the Disease Activity Score-CRP (DAS28-CRP), which is based on a 28-joint assessment; 28 tender joint count (TJC), and 28 swollen joint count (SJC); CRP; and the patient global assessment (PtGA) [31, 32] to determine each patient's total RA score. DAS28-CRP-based clinical remission/non-remission and DAS4 variables (comprising TJC, SJC, CRP, and PtGA) were also used. Clinical remission of disease activity was defined as a DAS28-CRP score < 2.6 [31, 32].

The Health Assessment Questionnaire Disability Index (HAQ-DI) [33] was used to assess physical disability. This is an eight-category questionnaire with 20 subscales that measure functional disability. Each item is scored on a scale of 0–3 (0: without any difficulty; 1: with some difficulty; 2: with much difficulty; and 3: unable to do), and the average value of the eight categories was calculated. Functional remission was defined as HAQ-DI scores ≤ 0.5. Pain was evaluated using either the Visual Analogue Scale (VAS), on which items were scored from 0 (no pain) to 100 (maximum pain), or the TJC. Other data, such as age, sex, duration of disease, medication (biological disease-modifying anti-rheumatic drugs [bDMARDs], methotrexate, and steroids), were collected from the KURAMA cohort [29]. Confounding factors included age, sex, pain, HAQ-DI score, and medication use. Age and duration of disease were measured as total scores, and binary sex and medication data were used for the analysis.

The primary study outcomes were anxiety and depression symptoms. The outcomes were evaluated using the HADS [11], a 14-item questionnaire with seven subscales for anxiety and depression symptoms. Each item is scored on a scale of 0–3, the total score range for each condition is 0–21. Scores of 0–7 indicate no or few anxiety or depression symptoms, 8–10 indicate mild anxiety or depression, and ≥ 11 indicate severe anxiety or depression. The HADS has been widely used in Japan to screen patients with a variety of diseases, and has been previously validated for use with the Japanese population [34]. In this study, we defined anxiety and depression as a HADS anxiety score ≥ 8 and HADS depression score ≥ 8, respectively [11].

Statistical analysis

We followed Peduzzi [35, 36] in estimating the required sample size. The logistic model required 10 events per variables and the required sample size = (10 cases/variable) × (number of variables) ÷ probability of occurrence. The mean probability of occurrence was estimated from rates of anxiety (26–46%; mean: 36%) and depression (14.8–34.2%; mean: 24.5%) previously reported [1]. Using this method, we calculated that the estimated required sample size was 440.

Unless otherwise stated, the data are presented as the mean and 95% confidence interval (CI) for normally distributed continuous data, the median and interquartile range for non-normally distributed continuous data, or as frequencies (%). First, we examined the associations between RA patient characteristics and anxiety and depression symptoms using a univariable logistic regression and calculated the odds ratio (OR) and 95% confidence interval (CI). We then conducted a multivariable logistic regression to investigate the associations between DAS28-CRP-based remission and anxiety and depression symptoms. Based on clinician judgment and the univariable analysis results, explanatory variables were selected and adjusted for age, HAQ-DI, pain, and medication use (bDMARDs, methotrexate, and steroids). We also conducted a multivariable logistic regression using DAS4 variables scores instead of DAS28-CRP-based remission to determine which factors may separately contribute to anxiety and depression symptoms in RA patients. All analyses were performed using JMP 14.0 (SAS Institute Inc., Cary, NC, USA).

Results

Patient characteristics

We assessed 542 RA patients and excluded 25 because they had psychiatric disorders such as bipolar disorder and schizophrenia. Of the remaining 517 patients, 9 were excluded from the anxiety analyses because of incomplete HADS anxiety questionnaires. Additionally, 10 were excluded from the depression analyses because of incomplete HADS depression questionnaires. Finally, 508 patients were included in the final analyses of anxiety symptoms, and 507 patients in the analyses of depression symptoms (Fig. 1). Table 1 shows the patient characteristics. The mean DAS28-CRP score was 1.91 (95% CI 1.83–1.98), and 360 (78.9%) patients achieved DAS28-CRP-based remission. The mean HAQ-DI score was 0.75 (95% CI 0.68–0.82), and 252 (51.3%) patients achieved HAQ-DI-based remission. The mean disease duration was 160.9 (95% CI 148.8–173.1) months. Of all patients, 91 (17.6%) had anxiety symptoms, and 143 (27.7%) had depression symptoms as measured by the HADS (Table 1).

Association between clinical variables and anxiety symptoms

First, we performed a univariable logistic regression. DAS28-CRP-based non-remission, TJC, SJC, CRP, PtGA severity, HAQ-DI-based non-remission, pain severity, and steroid use were selected as possible

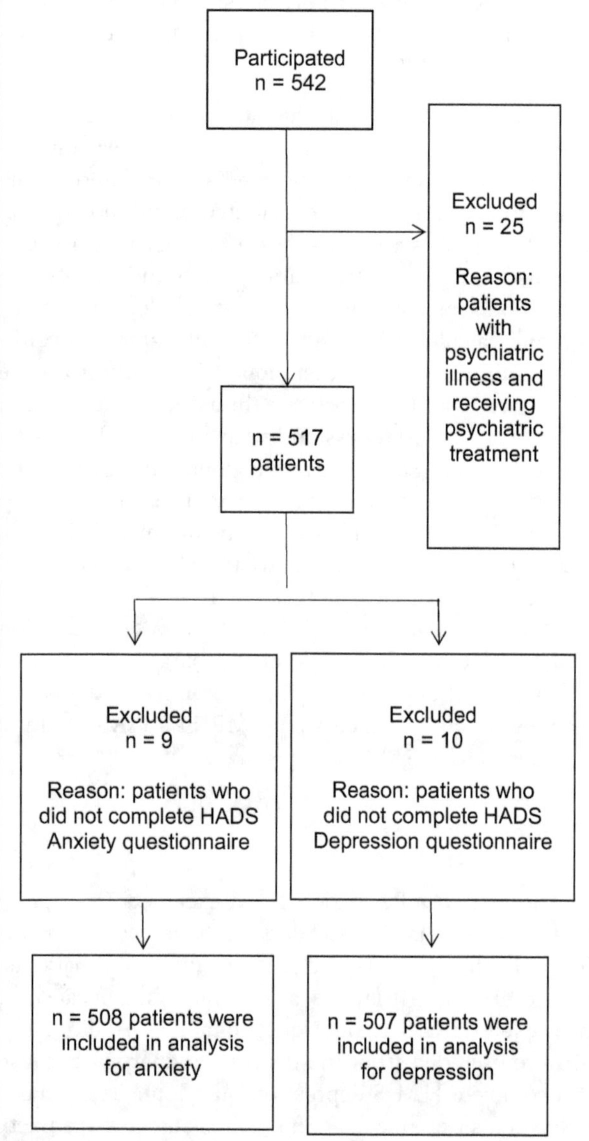

Fig. 1 Flowchart of patient selection. *HADS* Hospital Anxiety and Depression Scale

Table 1 Characteristics of patients with rheumatoid arthritis

Characteristics	**Overall N = 517**
Sex (female)	429 (83.0)
Age, years	62.5 (61.4–63.6)
Disease duration, months	160.9 (148.8–173.1)
Stage	
I	114 (22.1)
II	125 (24.2)
III	96 (18.6)
IV	180 (35.0)
Disease activity	
DAS28-CRP	1.91 (1.83–1.98)
DAS28-CRP remission†	360 (78.9)
Low disease activity†	57 (12.5)
Moderate disease activity†	37 (8.1)
High disease activity†	2 (0.5)
TJC	0.82 (0.69–0.96)
SJC	0.80 (0.67–0.93)
PtGA	29.1 (27.0–31.2)
CRP	0.40 (0.33–0.47)
HAQ-DI	0.75 (0.68–0.82)
HAQ-DI remission	252 (51.3)
Pain VAS	27.6 (25.4–29.9)
Treatment	
Biological DMARD	187 (36.2)
Methotrexate	345 (66.7)
Steroid	159 (30.8)
Anxiety and depression	
Anxiety	91 (17.6)
Depression	143 (27.7)

Data are presented as mean (95% confidence interval) or number (%). Remission: DAS28-CRP $<$ 2.6; VAS range: 0 (no pain) to 100 (maximum pain); Anxiety: HADS-A score $\geq$ 8, Depression: HADS-D score $\geq$ 8

DAS28 Disease Activity Score in 28 joints, *TJC* tender joint count, *SJC* swollen joint count, *PtGA* patient global assessment, *CRP* C-reactive protein, *HAQ-DI* Health Assessment Questionnaire Disability Index, *HADS-A* Hospital Anxiety and Depression Scale-Anxiety subscale, *HADS-D* Hospital Anxiety and Depression Scale-Depression subscale, *DMARD* disease-modifying anti-rheumatic drug, *VAS* Visual Analogue Scale

† N = 456 for DAS28-CRP remission owing to 61 missing responses

factors associated with anxiety symptoms. We then conducted a multivariable logistic regression (Table 2). In Model 1, patients with DAS28-CRP-based non-remission were no more likely to have anxiety symptoms (OR [95% CI] 0.93 [0.48–1.78]; $p = 0.82$). Patients with HAQ-DI-based non-remission were more likely to have anxiety symptoms than those in remission (OR [95% CI] 3.51 [1.85–6.64]; $p < 0.01$). Additionally, younger patients tended to have more anxiety symptoms (OR [95% CI] 0.83 [0.68–1.01]; $p = 0.07$). In Model 2, pain VAS score was excluded from the explanatory variables because of collinearity between pain VAS scores and PtGA scores (correlation coefficient, $r = 0.78$) (Table 3). Furthermore, we used the DAS4 component TJC as a pain variable instead of pain VAS score. Consequently, patients with severe PtGA scores had a notably greater likelihood of anxiety (OR [95% CI] 1.15 [1.02–1.29]; $p = 0.03$). Similar to Model 1, Model 2 showed that patients with HAQ-DI-based non-remission were more likely to have anxiety symptoms than those with HAQ-DI-based remission (OR [95% CI] 3.21 [1.69–6.08]; $p < 0.01$).

Table 2 Multivariate analyses of association between clinical factors and anxiety in patients with rheumatoid arthritis (N = 508)

	Univariable analysis		Multivariable analysis			
	Odds ratio (95% CI)	p value	Model 1		Model 2	
			Odds ratio (95% CI)	p value	Odds ratio (95% CI)	p value
Sex	0.99 (0.55, 1.89)	0.98	0.88 (0.45, 1.71)	0.71	0.83 (0.43, 1.63)	0.59
Age (10 years)	1.01 (0.84, 1.29)	0.98	0.83 (0.68, 1.01)	0.07	0.83 (0.68, 1.01)	0.06
DAS28-CRP non-remission	1.99 (1.12, 3.36)	0.01	0.93 (0.48, 1.78)	0.82		
TJC	1.18 (1.03, 1.35)	0.02			1.02 (0.85, 1.22)	0.85
SJC	1.14 (0.98, 1.34)	0.08			0.97 (0.79, 1.19)	0.76
CRP	1.23 (0.90, 1.65)	0.17			1.01 (0.70, 1.43)	0.98
PtGA (0–10)	1.29 (1.18, 1.42)	< 0.01			1.15 (1.02, 1.29)	0.03
HAQ-DI non-remission	4.32 (2.59, 7.48)	< 0.01	3.51 (1.85, 6.64)	< 0.01	3.21 (1.69, 6.08)	< 0.01
Pain VAS (0–10)	1.24 (1.14, 1.35)	< 0.01	1.10 (0.98, 1.23)	0.12		
Biological DMARD	1.12 (0.69, 1.77)	0.65	1.07 (0.63, 1.80)	0.81	1.05 (0.62, 1.77)	0.85
Methotrexate	0.64 (0.40, 1.03)	0.06	0.67 (0.40, 1.13)	0.13	0.71 (0.42, 1.20)	0.20
Steroid	1.63 (1.01, 2.60)	0.04	1.12 (0.66, 1.92)	0.67	1.14 (0.66, 1.96)	0.64

Model adjusted for age (stratified in 10 decades), pain (VAS), HAQ-DI remission, and treatment type

VAS range: 0 (no pain) to 10 (maximum). Anxiety was measured using the HADS (HADS-A score ≥ 8). DAS28 was used for clinical remission (DAS28 score of < 2.6). DAS4 variables comprise TJC, SJC, CRP, and PtGA

CI confidence interval, *DAS28* Disease Activity Score in 28 joints, *TJC* tender joint count, *SJC* swollen joint count, *PtGA* patient global assessment, *VAS* Visual Analogue Scale, *CRP* C-reactive protein, *HAQ-DI* Health Assessment Questionnaire Disability Index, *HADS* Hospital Anxiety and Depression Scale, *DMARD* disease-modifying anti-rheumatic drug

Association between clinical variables and symptoms of depression

Similar analyses were conducted for depression symptoms. First, we performed a univariable logistic regression. DAS28-CRP-based non-remission, PtGA severity, HAQ-DI-based non-remission, pain severity, and use of methotrexate and steroids were factors identified as potentially associated with depression symptoms. We then conducted a multivariable logistic regression (Table 4). In Model 1, patients with DAS28-CRP-based non-remission were no more likely to have depression symptoms (OR [95% CI] 1.45 [0.81–2.61]; $p = 0.22$). Patients with HAQ-DI-based non-remission were more likely to have depression symptoms than those with HAQ-DI-based remission (OR [95% CI] 2.65 [1.56–4.50]; $p < 0.01$). In Model 2, pain VAS score was excluded from the explanatory variables because of collinearity. Furthermore, we used the DAS4 component TJC as a pain variable instead of pain VAS score. Patients with severe PtGA scores were more likely to have depression symptoms (OR [95% CI] 1.21 [1.09–1.35]; $p < 0.01$). Similar to Model 1, Model 2 showed that patients with HAQ-DI-based non-remission were more likely to have depression than those with HAQ-DI-based remission (OR [95% CI] 1.95 [1.15–3.31]; $p = 0.01$). Patients taking steroids were more likely to have depression than those not taking steroids (OR [95% CI] 1.66 [1.03–2.67]; $p = 0.04$).

Discussion

This was a large-scale cohort study using the KURAMA cohort [29]. We investigated the association of RA disease activity with anxiety and depression symptoms after adjusting for physical disability, pain, and medication in RA patients. We used multiple models to investigate these associations and obtained several notable findings. First, the multivariable logistic regression analysis identified no association between DAS28-based-non-remission and anxiety and depression symptoms. Second, the severity of PtGA, a component of the DAS28 composite measure, was strongly associated with anxiety and depression symptoms, whereas other individual elements of DAS28-CRP (TJC, SJC, and CRP) were not. Third, HAQ-DI-based non-remission was independently and significantly associated with anxiety and depression symptoms. Fourth, patients taking steroids were more likely to have depression symptoms than those not taking steroids.

Findings of previous studies investigating the association between disease activity and anxiety and depression symptoms are inconsistent. Disease activity [23, 24], physical disability [13–15], and pain severity [16–18] are among the factors associated with anxiety and depression in RA patients. However, these studies have two key limitations: (1) DAS28 and pain scores were simultaneously analyzed, but HAQ-DI scores and drug use were not included as covariates [23] and (2) pain, HAQ-DI

Table 3 Correlations between variables

	Sex	Age	Disease duration	DAS28-CRP	TJC	SJC	CRP	PtGA (0–100)	HAQ DI	Pain VAS (0–100)	Biological DMARDs	Methotrexate	Steroid	Anxiety	Depression
Sex	1														
Age	−0.10	1													
Disease duration	0.16	0.28	1												
DAS28-CRP	−0.01	0.20	0.22	1											
TJC	0.03	0.10	0.12	0.81	1										
SJC	−0.01	0.14	0.17	0.67	0.53	1									
CRP	−0.14	0.13	0.08	0.39	0.21	0.27	1								
PtGA (0–100)	0.03	0.17	0.19	0.77	0.43	0.35	0.19	1							
HAQ-DI	0.06	0.31	0.40	0.56	0.42	0.36	0.24	0.58	1						
Pain VAS (0–100)	−0.06	0.14	0.20	0.67	0.41	0.31	0.15	0.78	0.54	1					
Biological DMARDs	0.11	−0.16	−0.09	−0.07	−0.04	−0.03	−0.06	−0.05	−0.02	−0.04	1				
Methotrexate	−0.02	−0.10	−0.09	−0.10	−0.05	−0.04	−0.19	−0.17	−0.17	−0.10	−0.01	1			
Steroids	−0.08	0.13	0.10	0.22	0.13	0.20	0.23	0.16	0.22	0.14	−0.02	−0.17	1		
Anxiety	0.03	−0.01	0.06	0.21	0.13	0.07	0.02	0.32	0.31	0.28	−0.01	−0.11	0.07	1	
Depression	−0.04	0.09	0.09	0.22	0.12	0.05	0.03	0.33	0.34	0.24	−0.01	−0.12	0.13	0.56	1

DAS28 Disease Activity Score in 28 joints, *CRP* C-reactive protein, *TJC* tender joint count; *SJC* swollen joint count; *PtGA* patient global assessment, *HAQ-DI* Health Assessment Questionnaire Disability Index, *VAS* Visual Analogue Scale, *DMARD*, disease-modifying anti-rheumatic drugs

Anxiety and depression were measured using the Hospital Anxiety and Depression Scale (HADS), Anxiety/Depression: HADS score ≥ 8. VAS range: 0 (no pain) to 100 (maximum pain)

Table 4 Multivariable analyses of association between clinical factors and depression in rheumatoid arthritis patients (N = 507)

	Univariable analysis		Multivariable analysis			
			Model 1		Model 2	
	Odds ratio (95% CI)	p value	Odds ratio (95% CI)	p value	Odds ratio (95% CI)	p value
Sex	0.80 (0.49, 1.34)	0.39	0.70 (0.40, 1.22)	0.21	0.61 (0.34, 1.07)	0.09
Age (10 years)	1.18 (1.01, 1.38)	0.04	1.03 (0.87, 1.24)	0.70	1.04 (0.87, 1.24)	0.68
DAS28-CRP-based non-remission	2.37 (1.47, 3.82)	< 0.01	1.45 (0.81, 2.61)	0.22		
TJC	1.10 (0.97, 1.25)	0.14			0.96 (0.81, 1.14)	0.63
SJC	1.06 (0.92, 1.21)	0.40			0.94 (0.78, 1.14)	0.55
CRP	1.01 (0.74, 0.99)	0.96			0.71 (0.50, 1.01)	0.06
PtGA (0–10)	1.27 (1.17, 1.38)	< 0.01			1.21 (1.09, 1.35)	< 0.01
HAQ-DI non-remission	2.96 (1.96, 4.53)	< 0.01	2.65 (1.56, 4.50)	< 0.01	1.95 (1.15, 3.31)	0.01
Pain VAS (0–10)	1.13 (1.05, 1.22)	< 0.01	0.98 (0.88, 1.09)	0.77		
Biological DMARDs	0.92 (0.61, 1.37)	0.68	0.84 (0.53, 1.33)	0.45	0.88 (0.55, 1.40)	0.58
Methotrexate	0.60 (0.40, 0.90)	0.01	0.72 (0.45, 1.14)	0.16	0.76 (0.48, 1.22)	0.26
Steroid	1.87 (1.24, 2.81)	< 0.01	1.48 (0.93, 2.34)	0.09	1.66 (1.03, 2.67)	0.04

Model adjusted for age (stratified in 10 decades), pain (VAS), HAQ-DI-based remission, and treatment type. DAS28 score was used to gauge clinical remission (score < 2.6). DAS4 variables comprise TJC, SJC, CRP, and PtGA. VAS range: 0 (no pain) to 10 (maximum pain)

CI confidence interval, *DAS28* Disease Activity Score in 28 joints, *CRP* C-reactive protein, *TJC* tender joint count, *SJC* swollen joint count, *PtGA* patient global assessment, *HAQ-DI* Health Assessment Questionnaire Disability Index, *VAS* Visual Analogue Scale, *DMARDs* biological disease-modifying anti-rheumatic drugs

scores, and drug use were not included as covariates [9, 24]. Therefore, the association between DAS28 score and anxiety and depression symptoms was mainly evaluated independently, and the effects of other factors may not have been fully evaluated. In this study, we found that when disease activity, disability, pain, and medication were adjusted for, DAS28-based non-remission was not independently associated with anxiety and depression. The average DAS28-CRP score in this study was 1.91 ± 0.82, which was lower than scores found in previous studies (DAS28-CRP scores 6.26–6.77). Additionally, almost 80% of patients achieved remission of disease activity (42.4–56.3% in previous studies), and disease severity was low and controlled. Therefore, after adjustment, the effects of other factors associated with anxiety and depression symptoms may be more robust than disease activity.

We also found that PtGA (a component of the DAS28-CRP composite measure) was notably associated with anxiety and depression symptom, which is similar to findings from a previous study [37]. Moreover, the multivariable analysis results suggested that inflammation (CRP, TJC, and SJC) was not associated with anxiety and depression. Previous studies have reported that systemic inflammation is a potential cause of depression [19–21] and that inflammatory markers correlate with depression [22], suggesting an association between inflammation and depression symptoms. In this study, we did not correlate the two variables because of low CRP. However, PtGA uses the VAS for overall patient self-assessment and is the main tool for measuring patient-reported outcomes [38]. The present results suggest that patient self-assessment, and not inflammation, is associated with anxiety and depression symptoms in RA patients.

PtGA reflects various factors; physical disability [39, 40], pain [18, 39], and catastrophizing pain [41] are among the factors that exacerbate PtGA scores. Santos et al. [42] excluded a priori testing for a direct association between DAS28-CRP3 variables and depression symptoms and instead tested the effects of disease activity and disease impact on patients. They found no direct association between DAS28-CRP3V and depression. They also confirmed an indirect relationship between disease activity and depression symptoms mediated by disease impact, such as pain, physical well-being, functional disability, and coping. Thus, functional disability, pain, recognition, and self-evaluation of disease were reflected in PtGA scores and related to anxiety and depression symptoms. This suggests that individual responses to stress caused by chronic disease, coping mechanisms, and subjective experiences of well-being are at least as important as inflammatory factors in the association between RA and psychological problems [28, 42].

In addition, there is a gap between doctor and patient PtGA assessments [43]. Therefore, to understand patients' anxiety and depression symptoms, it is necessary to pay attention to patients' subjective experience regardless of disease activity. Additionally, to reduce anxiety and depression symptoms in RA patients, it is important to improve patient self-assessment and well-being.

Cognitive behavioral therapy and mindfulness [44–46] reduce the tendency to catastrophize and subsequently reduce pain and distress; therefore, these approaches may be effective interventions for RA patients.

We found that HAQ-DI score, which identifies physical disability, was associated with anxiety and depression symptoms in a multivariable analysis. Previous studies have found that HAQ-DI score [13–15] is related to anxiety and depression. Regardless of acute disease activity score, functional disability measured by the HAQ-DI is associated with depression [22, 23, 47]. If disability persists, the possibility of concurrent symptoms of anxiety and depression increases, irrespective of disease activity remission. Physical disability reportedly leads to reduced ability to perform household chores and other activities and increased job loss/professional loss [47]. Impairment in the ability to perform daily life activities causes anxiety and depression [14, 47].

The effects of bone or joint damage were not clear because joint damage was not evaluated in this study. However, the patients were older and had a longer disease duration, low disease activity, and low inflammation. We suggest that anxiety and depression were caused by loss of activity in daily life owing to prolonged limited function rather than acute symptoms of disease activity. It is important to confirm the effects of the disease on daily life. In the "treat to target" approach, the goal of treatment is to restore physical function so that RA patients can participate in social activities again, thereby maintaining long-term QOL [48]. Improving QOL by supporting daily activities and possibly replacing or recovering lost activities to maintain and improve physical functions may relieve symptoms of anxiety and depression.

Finally, in Model 1, younger RA patients tended to experience anxiety symptoms. Younger RA patients may be more anxious about the future regarding factors such as disease-related concerns, medication, pregnancy, household chores, education, and job-related/professional work. In Model 2, patients taking steroids were more likely to have depression symptoms. Depression side effects may be caused by the pharmacological actions of steroids [49], so appropriate treatment strategies are needed that consider this risk of side effects.

One of the strengths of this study is that it used a large cohort to investigate the associations between disease activity and anxiety and depression symptoms while adjusting for factors that potentially affect these symptoms. Although a range of scales have been used to evaluate anxiety and depression in RA patients, the HADS was used in this study because scores are unaffected by the physical symptoms associated with the development of RA, such as fatigue and insomnia. Therefore, use of the HADS can help to avoid overestimating anxiety and depression symptoms. The HADS assesses the prevalence of anxiety and depression more accurately than other scales.

Despite our findings, this study had some limitations. First, instead of a formal psychiatric diagnosis, we used self-reported symptoms to determine anxiety and depression levels. Additionally, although we only considered the effects of currently used medication, we could not exclude the effects of prior treatment and drug amounts. Because this study was conducted at a single university hospital, selection bias may also have occurred; most patients had a lengthy disease duration and were in remission or had low disease activity. We also did not collect detailed demographic and socioeconomic data on participants, and therefore the analysis is unable to take such factors into account. Given these limitations, care must be taken in generalizing our findings.

Conclusions

After adjusting for physical disability, pain, and medication, there was no association between DAS28 and anxiety and depression symptoms. However, patients with high PtGA scores or HAQ-DI-based non-remission were more likely to experience anxiety and depression symptoms. Thus, functional disability, pain, recognition, and self-evaluation of disease were reflected in PtGA and indirectly related to anxiety and depression. To understand anxiety and depression symptoms, it is necessary to pay attention to improve or preserve physical function and patients' subjective experience regardless of disease activity.

Abbreviations

RA: Rheumatoid arthritis; DAS28: Disease Activity Score; HAQ-DI: Health Assessment Questionnaire Disability Index; OR: Odds ratio; CI: Confidence interval; PtGA: Patient global assessment; CRP: C-reactive protein; HADS: Hospital Anxiety and Depression Scale; TJC: Tender joint count; SJC: Swollen joint count; VAS: Visual Analogue Scale.

Acknowledgements

We would like to acknowledge the staff of the Rheumatoid Arthritis Center at the Kyoto University Hospital in Kyoto, Japan, who provided valuable assistance and support in collecting data for this study. We thank Diane Williams, PhD, from Edanz (www.edanz.com/ac) for editing a draft of this manuscript.

Authors' contributions

MU, MH, and KN were responsible for the conception and design of the study. MU, MH, MTorii, TF, MTanaka, MF, HI, CT, and WY acquired data. MU, MH, RU, and KN analyzed and interpreted the data. MU and RU contributed to the statistical analysis. GS, YN, and TM contributed to the interpretation of the data. MU, MH, and KN prepared the manuscript. All authors read and approved the final manuscript.

Competing interests

The Department of Advanced Medicine for Rheumatic Diseases is supported by two local governments in Japan (Nagahama City, Shiga, and Toyooka City, Hyogo) and five pharmaceutical companies (Mitsubishi Tanabe Pharma Corporation, Chugai Pharmaceutical Co., Ltd., AYUMI Pharmaceutical Corporation, Asahi Kasei Corporation, and UCB Japan Co., Ltd.). MH has received grants and/or speaker fees from Bristol-Myers Squibb, Eisai Co., Ltd., Eli Lilly and Company, and Mitsubishi Tanabe Pharma Corporation. RU has received consulting fees from Eisai Co. Ltd., Sawai Pharmaceutical Co. Ltd., and CAC Croit Corporation. TF has received speaking fees and/or honoraria from AbbVie Inc., Astellas Pharma Inc., Asahi Kasei Corporation, Chugai Pharmaceutical Co., Ltd., Eli Lilly and Company, Eisai Co., Ltd., Janssen, Kissei, Mitsubishi Tanabe Pharma Corporation, Ono Pharmaceutical Co., Ltd., Pfizer, Sanofi, Taisho Toyama Pharmaceutical Co., Ltd., Takeda Pharmaceutical Co., Ltd., and UCB Japan Co., Ltd., and has received research grants from AbbVie Inc., AYUMI Pharmaceutical Corporation, Asahi Kasei Corporation, Astellas Pharma Inc., Chugai Pharmaceutical Co., Ltd., Daiichi Sankyo Co., Ltd, Eli Lilly and Company, Eisai Co., Ltd., Kissei, Mitsubishi Tanabe Pharma Corporation, Pfizer, Nippon-Kayaku, Ono Pharmaceutical Co., Ltd., Takeda Pharmaceutical Co., Ltd., and UCB Japan Co., Ltd. MTanaka has received research grants and/or speaker fees from AbbVie GK, Asahi Kasei Pharma Corporation, Astellas Pharma Inc., AYUMI Pharmaceutical Corporation, Bristol-Myers Squibb, Chugai Pharmaceutical Co., Ltd., Eisai Co., Ltd., Eli Lilly Japan K.K., Pfizer Inc., UCB Japan Co., Ltd., Janssen Pharmaceutical K.K., Mitsubishi Tanabe Pharma Corporation, Novartis Pharma K.K., and Taisho Pharma Co., Ltd. HI has received a research grant and/or speaker fee from Bristol-Myers Squibb, Kyocera, and Asahi Kasei Corporation. TM has received research grants and/or speaker's fees from Asahi Kasei Corporation, Astellas Pharma Inc., AYUMI Pharmaceutical Corporation, Bristol-Myers Squibb, Chugai Pharmaceutical Co., Ltd., Daiichi Sankyo Co., Ltd., Eisai Co., Ltd., Mitsubishi Tanabe Pharma Corporation, Pfizer, and Sanofi. The above companies had no role in the study design, collection or analysis of data, writing of the manuscript, or the decision to submit the manuscript for publication.

Author details

[1]Department of Human Health Sciences, Kyoto University Graduate School of Medicine, 53 Shogoin Kawahara-cho, Sakyo-ku, Kyoto 606-8507, Japan. [2]Department of Advanced Medicine for Rheumatic Diseases, Kyoto University Graduate School of Medicine, Kyoto, Japan. [3]Department of Clinical Immunology, Graduate School of Medicine, Osaka City University, Osaka, Japan. [4]Department of Biomedical Statistics and Bioinformatics, Kyoto University Graduate School of Medicine, Kyoto, Japan. [5]Department of Rheumatology and Clinical Immunology, Wakayama Medical University, Wakayama, Japan. [6]Department of Rheumatology and Clinical Immunology, Graduate School of Medicine, Kyoto University, Kyoto, Japan. [7]Laboratory for Statistical and Translational Genetics, RIKEN Center for Integrative Medical Sciences, Yokohama, Japan. [8]Clinical Research Center, Shizuoka General Hospital, Shizuoka, Japan. [9]The Department of Applied Genetics, The School of Pharmaceutical Sciences, University of Shizuoka, Shizuoka, Japan. [10]Department of Health Information Management, Kurashiki Sweet Hospital, Okayama, Japan. [11]Department of Psychiatry, Kyoto University Graduate School of Medicine, Kyoto, Japan. [12]Kyoto University Health Service, Kyoto, Japan. [13]Department of Rheumatology and Clinical Immunology, Kyoto University Graduate School of Medicine, Kyoto, Japan. [14]Ijinkai Takeda General Hospital, Kyoto, Japan.

References

1. Matcham F, Rayner L, Steer S, Hotopf M. The prevalence of depression in rheumatoid arthritis: a systematic review and meta-analysis. Rheumatology. 2013;52:2136–48. https://doi.org/10.1093/rheumatology/ket169.
2. Marrie RA, Hitchon CA, Walld R, Patten SB, Bolton JM, Sareen J, et al. Increased burden of psychiatric disorders in rheumatoid arthritis. Arthritis Care Res. 2018;70:970–8. https://doi.org/10.1002/acr.23539.
3. Mattey DL, Dawes PT, Hassell AB, Brownfield A, Packham JC. Effect of psychological distress on continuation of anti-tumor necrosis factor therapy in patients with rheumatoid arthritis. J Rheumatol. 2010;37:2021–4. https://doi.org/10.3899/jrheum.100050.
4. Li X, Gignac MA, Anis AH. The indirect costs of arthritis resulting from unemployment, reduced performance, and occupational changes while at work. Med Care. 2006;44:304–10. https://doi.org/10.1097/01.mlr.0000204257.25875.04
5. Margaretten M, Julian L, Katz P, Yelin E. Depression in patients with rheumatoid arthritis: description, causes and mechanisms. Int J Clin Rheumatol. 2011;6:617–23. https://doi.org/10.2217/IJR.11.6.
6. Matcham F, Scott IC, Rayner L, Hotopf M, Kingsley GH, Norton S, et al. The impact of rheumatoid arthritis on quality-of-life assessed using the SF-36: a systematic review and meta-analysis. Semin Arthritis Rheum. 2014;44:123–30. https://doi.org/10.1016/j.semarthrit.2014.05.001.
7. Ang DC, Choi H, Kroenke K, Wolfe F. Comorbid depression is an independent risk factor for mortality in patients with rheumatoid arthritis. J Rheumatol. 2005;32:1013–9.
8. Timonen M, Viilo K, Hakko H, Sarkioja T, Ylikulju M, Meyer-Rochow VB, et al. Suicides in persons suffering from rheumatoid arthritis. Rheumatology. 2003;42:287–91. https://doi.org/10.1093/rheumatology/keg082.
9. Ho RC, Fu EH, Chua AN, Cheak AA, Mak A. Clinical and psychosocial factors associated with depression and anxiety in Singaporean patients with rheumatoid arthritis. Int J Rheum Dis. 2011;14:37–47. https://doi.org/10.1111/j.1756-185X.2010.01591.x.
10. Mikuls T, Saag K, Criswell L, Merlino L, Cerhan JR. Health related quality of life in women with elderly onset rheumatoid arthritis. J Rheumatol. 2003;30:952–7.
11. Zigmond AS, Snaith RP. The Hospital Anxiety and Depression Scale. Acta Psychiatr Scand. 1983;67:361–70. https://doi.org/10.1111/j.1600-0447.1983.tb09716.x.
12. Cutolo M, Kitas GD, van Riel PL. Burden of disease in treated rheumatoid arthritis patients: going beyond the joint. Semin Arthritis Rheum. 2014;43:479–88. https://doi.org/10.1016/j.semarthrit.2013.08.004.
13. Margaretten M, Yelin E, Imboden J, Graf J, Barton J, Katz P, et al. Predictors of depression in a multiethnic cohort of patients with rheumatoid arthritis. Arthritis Rheum. 2009;61:1586–91. https://doi.org/10.1002/art.24822.
14. Bacconnier L, Rincheval N, Flipo RM, Goupille P, Daures JP, Boulenger JP, et al. Psychological distress over time in early rheumatoid arthritis: results from a longitudinal study in an early arthritis cohort. Rheumatology. 2015;54:520–7. https://doi.org/10.1093/rheumatology/keu371.
15. Karpouzas GA, Dolatabadi S, Moran R, Li N, Nicassio PM, Weisman MH. Correlates and predictors of disability in vulnerable US Hispanics with rheumatoid arthritis. Arthritis Care Res. 2012;64:1274–81. https://doi.org/10.1002/acr.21689.
16. Dickens C, McGowan L, Clark-Carter D, Creed F. Depression in rheumatoid arthritis: a systematic review of the literature with meta-analysis. Psychosom Med. 2002;64:52–60. https://doi.org/10.1097/00006842-200201000-00008.
17. Walsh DA, McWilliams DF. Mechanisms, impact and management of pain in rheumatoid arthritis. Nat Rev Rheumatol. 2014;10:581–92. https://doi.org/10.1038/nrrheum.2014.64.
18. Odegård S, Finset A, Mowinckel P, Kvien TK, Uhlig T. Pain and psychological health status over a 10-year period in patients with recent onset rheumatoid arthritis. Ann Rheum Dis. 2007;66:1195–201. https://doi.org/10.1136/ard.2006.064287.
19. de Ridder D, Geenen R, Kuijer R, van Middendorp H. Psychological adjust ment to chronic disease. Lancet. 2008;372:246–55. https://doi.org/10.1016/S0140-6736(08)61078-8.
20. Liu Y, Ho RC, Mak A. Interleukin (IL)-6, tumour necrosis factor alpha (TNF-alpha) and soluble interleukin-2 receptors (sIL-2R) are elevated in patients with major depressive disorder: a meta-analysis and meta-regression. J Affect Disord. 2012;139:230–9. https://doi.org/10.1016/j.jad.2011.08.003
21. Du X, Pang TY. Is dysregulation of the HPA-Axis a core pathophysiology mediating co-morbid depression in neurodegenerative diseases? Front Psychiatry. 2015;6:32. https://doi.org/10.3389/fpsyt.2015.00032.
22. Kojima M, Kojima T, Suzuki S, Oguchi T, Oba M, Tsuchiya H, et al. Depression, inflammation, and pain in patients with rheumatoid arthritis. Arthritis Rheum. 2009;61:1018–24. https://doi.org/10.1002/art.24647.
23. Kekow J, Moots R, Khandker R, Melin J, Freundlich B, Singh A. Improvements in patient-reported outcomes, symptoms of depression and anxiety, and their association with clinical remission among patients with moderate-to-severe active early rheumatoid arthritis. Rheumatology. 2011;50:401–9. https://doi.org/10.1093/rheumatology/keq327.
24. Overman CL, Bossema ER, van Middendorp H, Wijngaards-de Meij L, Verstappen SM, Bulder M, et al. The prospective association between psychological distress and disease activity in rheumatoid arthritis: a multi level regression analysis. Ann Rheum Dis. 2012;71:192–7. https://doi.org/10.1136/annrheumdis-2011-200338

25. Arne M, Janson C, Janson S, Boman G, Lindqvist U, Berne C, et al. Physical activity and quality of life in subjects with chronic disease: chronic obstructive pulmonary disease compared with rheumatoid arthritis and diabetes mellitus. Scand J Prim Health Care. 2009;27:141–7. https://doi.org/10.1080/02813430902808643.
26. Wolfe F, Michaud K, Li T, Latz RS. Chronic conditions and health problems in rheumatic diseases: comparisons with rheumatoid arthritis, noninflammatory rheumatic disorders, systemic lupus erythematosus, and fibromyalgia. J Rheumatol. 2010;37:305–15. https://doi.org/10.3899/jrheum.090781.
27. Bucourt E, Martaillé V, Goupille P, Joncker-Vannier I, Huttenberger B, Réveillère C, et al. A comparative study of fibromyalgia, rheumatoid arthritis, spondyloarthritis, and Sjögren's syndrome; impact of the disease on quality of life, psychological adjustment, and use of coping strategies. Pain Med. 2021;22:372–81. https://doi.org/10.1093/pm/pnz255.
28. Kwiatkowska B, Kłak A, Raciborski F, Maślińska M. The prevalence of depression and insomnia symptoms among patients with rheumatoid arthritis and osteoarthritis in Poland: a case control study. Psychol Health Med. 2019;24:333–43. https://doi.org/10.1080/13548506.2018.1529325.
29. Terao C, Hashimoto M, Yamamoto K, Murakami K, Ohmura K, Nakashima R, et al. Three groups in the 28 joints for rheumatoid arthritis synovitis–analysis using more than 17,000 assessments in the KURAMA database. PLoS ONE. 2013;8:e59341. https://doi.org/10.1371/journal.pone.0059341
30. Aletaha D, Neogi T, Silman AJ, Funovits J, Felson DT, Bingham CO, et al. 2010 rheumatoid arthritis classification criteria: an American College of Rheumatology/European League Against Rheumatism collaborative initiative. Ann Rheum Dis. 2010;69:1580–8. https://doi.org/10.1136/ard.2010.138461.
31. Wells G, Becker JC, Teng J, Dougados M, Schiff M, Smolen J, et al. Validation of the 28-joint Disease Activity Score (DAS28) and European League Against Rheumatism response criteria based on C-reactive protein against disease progression in patients with rheumatoid arthritis, and comparison with the DAS28 based on erythrocyte sedimentation rate. Ann Rheum Dis. 2009;68:954–60. https://doi.org/10.1136/ard.2007.084459.
32. Fransen J, Creemers MC, Van Riel PL. Remission in rheumatoid arthritis: agreement of the disease activity score (DAS28) with the ARA preliminary remission criteria. Rheumatology. 2004;43:1252–5. https://doi.org/10.1093/rheumatology/keh297.
33. Bruce B, Fries JF. The Stanford Health Assessment Questionnaire: a review of its history, issues, progress, and documentation. J Rheumatol. 2003;30:167–78.
34. Kugaya A, Akechi T, Okuyama T, Okamura H, Uchitomi Y. Screening for psychological distress in Japanese cancer patients. Jpn J Clin Oncol. 1998;28:333–8. https://doi.org/10.1093/jjco/28.5.333.
35. Peduzzi P, Concato J, Feinstein AR, Holford TR. Importance of events per independent variable in proportional hazards regression analysis. II Accuracy and precision of regression estimates. J Clin Epidemiol. 1995;48:1503–10. https://doi.org/10.1016/0895-4356(95)00048-8.
36. Peduzzi P, Concato J, Kemper E, Holford TR, Feinstein AR. A simulation study of the number of events per variable in logistic regression analysis. J Clin Epidemiol. 1996;49:1373–9. https://doi.org/10.1016/s0895-4356(96)00236-3.
37. Katchamart W, Narongroeknawin P, Chanapai W, Thaweeratthakul P, Srisomnuek A. Prevalence of and factors associated with depression and anxiety in patients with rheumatoid arthritis: a multicenter prospective cross-sectional study. Int J Rheum Dis. 2020;23:302–8. https://doi.org/10.1111/1756-185X.13781.
38. van Tuyl LH, Boers M. Patient-reported outcomes in core domain sets for rheumatic diseases. Nat Rev Rheumatol. 2015;11:705–12. https://doi.org/10.1038/nrrheum.2015.116.
39. Khan NA, Spencer HJ, Abda EA, Alten R, Pohl C, Ancuta C, et al. Patient's global assessment of disease activity and patient's assessment of general health for rheumatoid arthritis activity assessment: are they equivalent? Ann Rheum Dis. 2012;71:1942–9. https://doi.org/10.1136/annrheumdis-2011-201142.
40. Verschueren P, Esselens G, Westhovens R. Predictors of remission, normalized physical function, and changes in the working situation during follow-up of patients with early rheumatoid arthritis: an observational study. Scand J Rheumatol. 2009;38:166–72. https://doi.org/10.1080/03009740802484846.
41. Boyden SD, Hossain IN, Wohlfahrt A, Lee YC. Non-inflammatory causes of pain in patients with rheumatoid arthritis. Curr Rheumatol Rep. 2016;18:30. https://doi.org/10.1007/s11926-016-0581-0.
42. Santos EF, Duarte CM, Ferreira RO, Pinto AM, Geenen R, da Silva JP. Multifactorial explanatory model of depression in patients with rheumatoid arthritis: a structural equation approach. Clin Exp Rheumatol. 2019;37:641–8.
43. Barton JL, Imboden J, Graf J, Glidden D, Yelin EH, Schillinger D. Patient-physician discordance in assessments of global disease severity in rheumatoid arthritis. Arthritis Care Res. 2010;62:857–64. https://doi.org/10.1002/acr.20132.
44. Beltman MW, Voshaar RC, Speckens AE. Cognitive-behavioral therapy for depression in people with a somatic disease: meta-analysis of randomized controlled trials. Br J Psychiatry. 2010;197:11–9. https://doi.org/10.1192/bjp.bp.109.064675.
45. DiRenzo D, Crespo-Bosque M, Gould N, Finan P, Nanavati J, Bingham CO. Systematic review and meta-analysis: mindfulness-based interventions for rheumatoid arthritis. Curr Rheumatol Rep. 2018;20:75. https://doi.org/10.1007/s11926-018-0787-4.
46. Hofmann SG, Gomez AF. Mindfulness-based interventions for anxiety and depression. Psychiatr Clin N Am. 2017;40:739–49. https://doi.org/10.1016/j.psc.2017.08.008.
47. Katz PP, Yelin EH. Activity loss and the onset of depressive symptoms: do some activities matter more than others? Arthritis Rheum. 2001;44:1194–202. https://doi.org/10.1002/1529-0131(200105)44:5%3c1194::AID-ANR203%3e3.0.CO;2-6.
48. Smolen JS, Aletaha D, Bijlsma JW, Breedveld FC, Boumpas D, Burmester G, et al. Treating rheumatoid arthritis to target: recommendations of an international task force. Ann Rheum Dis. 2010;69:631–7. https://doi.org/10.1136/ard.2009.123919.
49. Wolkowitz OM, Burke H, Epel ES, Reus VI. Glucocorticoids, mood, memory, and mechanisms. Ann N Y Acad Sci. 2009;179:19–40. https://doi.org/10.1111/j.1749-6632.2009.04980.x.

15

Neuropathic pain in knee osteoarthritis

Uğur Güngör Demir[1*], Ali Nail Demir[2] and Naciye Füsun Toraman[3]

Abstract

Background: This study aimed to investigate the relationship between the neuropathic pain in knee osteoarthritis with the body composition, anthropometric and postural features, physical function, and quality of life.

Methods: Patients with primary knee osteoarthritis, 50–70 years of age, were included in the study and divided into Group 1 with neuropathic pain and Group 2 with no neuropathic pain according to Douleur Neuropathique-4. The groups were compared in terms of demographic, clinical, radiological, laboratory findings and anthropometric measurements, body composition, physical function tests, osteoarthritis severity, quality of life, and posturography.

Results: 200 patients were included in the study. 98 (82.6% female) were in Group 1 and 102 (74.5% female) in Group 2. Age was higher in Group 1 compared to Group 2 [61 (50–70) and 57.5 (50–70), respectively, $p=0.03$]. Symptom duration was also longer in Group 1 (5.21 ± 4.76 and 3.38 ± 3.58, $p=0.002$). Body mass indices were 31.9 ± 5.6 and 30.1 ± 4.8 ($p=0.015$). Kellgren–Lawrence class, Western Ontario and McMaster Osteoarthritis Index and Short Form-36 scores were more unfavorable in Group 1. Although fall risk was similar, stability and Fourier harmony indices were impaired in Group 1 compared to Group 2 especially when the visual and proprioceptive input was blocked.

Conclusions: Almost half of the patients with knee osteoarthritis had neuropathic pain which was associated with longer symptom duration and higher age, lower education, higher body mass index, more severe radilogical findings, worse pain perception, lower physical function and quality of life, and lower stability.

Keywords: Knee osteoarthritis, Neuropathic pain, Posturography

Introduction

Osteoarthritis, which most commonly affects the knee, is a degenerative disease characterized by cartilage erosion, bony hypertrophy, subchondral sclerosis, and synovial and capsular changes [1]. Symptomatic knee osteoarthritis is common in the elderly with a prevalence of 13% in females and 10% in males over the age 60 [2, 3]. Pain is usually the presenting and the most common symptom and speculated to have nociceptive and neuropathic components along with sensitization that can be both mechanical (peripheral) and central (secondary hyperalgesia) [4, 7]. The prevalence of neuropathic pain was reported to be 5.4–52% in knee osteoarthritis [8, 12]. Neuropathic pain was reported to be associated with age, sex, body mass index, education and working status, radiological osteoarthritis severity, symptom duration, and presence of comorbid diseases in patients with knee osteoarthritis [8–13]. It also has impact on quality of life [12, 13]. Although the body composition, anthropometric measurements, postural stability, and physical function may have a potential relationship with the neuropathic component of the pain in knee osteoarthritis, they were not reported to be assessed together in that regard.

This study primarily aimed to investigate the relationship between the neuropathic pain in knee osteoarthritis with the body composition, anthropometric and postural features, physical function, and quality of life.

*Correspondence: ugurgungor90@gmail.com

[1] Department of Physical Therapy and Rehabilitation, University of Health Sciences, Antalya Training and Research Hospital, 07100 Muratpaşa, Antalya, Turkey

Methods

Patients and design

All patients admitted to the Physical Therapy and Rehabilitation Outpatient Clinic, Antalya Training and Research Hospital, between January 2018–January 2019, with the complaint of knee pain, were screened for the eligibility for the study. The inclusion criteria were (a) being between 50 and 70 years of age (b) knee pain in more than 25 days of during the last month (c) crepitation during movement (d) morning stiffness less than 30 min or radiographic osteophytes (e) Kellgren–Lawrence class I–IV knee osteoarthritis and (f) willingness to participate in the study. The exclusion criteria were (a) previous knee operation (b) rheumatic or metabolic disease (c) malignant disease (d) central or peripheral neurologic disease that may cause neuropathic pain (e) cardiopulmonary disease that may interfere with the functional tests (f) pregnancy (g) active infections (h) a standardized mini-mental status examination score of less than 26 (i) intra-articular steroid injection in the last 3 months (j) hip or ankle pathology (k) treatment for neuropathic pain in the last 6 months.

Age, sex, education, working, smoking, and marital status, symptom duration, number of comorbid diseases and drugs used, and painful areas other than knee were recorded for each patient along with the presence of postural deviations (thoracic hyperkyphosis, lombar hyperlordosis, scoliosis, genu varum and recurvatum, and pes planus).

Tests and measurements: anthropometric measurements and body composition

Standing height was measured using a wall-mounted stature meter. Waist and hip circumferences were measured using a tape measure. Weight, body mass index and composition were measured using a professional digital scale (Tanita®MC-180MA, Tanita Corp., Tokyo, Japan).

Western Ontario and McMaster Osteoarthritis Index (WOMAC)

It is a health status instrument with pain, stiffness and physical function domains designed for patients with osteoarthritis and validated in Turkish population [14, 15].

Short form-36 (SF-36)

It is a 36-item questionnaire for general health and quality of life and divided into eight domains: physical function, social function, physical role limitations, emotional role limitations, bodily pain, general mental health, vitality, and general health perceptions [16, 17].

Geriatric depression scale

It is a 30-item scale first created by Yesavage et al. [18] and validated in Turkish population [19]. A score of 0–10 was considered as no depression, 11–13 as possible depression, and 14 or higher as depression.

Physical function

A 30-s chair-stand, stair-climbing, and 6-min walk tests were performed for each patient as described previously [20–22].

Posturographic evaluation

Computerized tetra-ataxiometric posturography, Tetrax®(Sunlight Medical Ltd., Tel Aviv, Israel), was used for the assessment of static posturographic stability in eight positions: stable surface/eyes open/face forward, stable surface/eyes closed/face forward, unstable surface/eyes open/face forward, unstable surface/eyes closed/face forward, stable surface/eyes closed/head rotated 45° to the right, stable surface/eyes closed/head rotated 45° to the left, stable surface/eyes closed/head tilted back 30°, and stable surface/eyes closed/head tilted 30° forward. Fall risk index (low: 0–36, intermediate: 37–58, high: 59 or higher), stability index (the higher the index the lower the stability), and Fourier harmony index (< 0.9: abnormal stability; normal: 0.9–1) were calculated for each patient [23, 24].

Douleur neuropathique-4 (DN-4)

It is a scale composed of four questions. A score of 4 or higher indicates neuropathic pain [25, 26]. Additionally, a ten centimeter visual analogue scale (VAS) was used for the severity of the knee pain at rest and while walking (0 = no pain, 10 = extreme pain).

Radiological assessment

A standard standing anteroposterior knee X-ray with the knees in extension were obtained for each patient and severity of osteoarthritis was graded according to the Kellgren–Lawrence classification [27].

Laboratory analysis

Hemoglobin concentration, erythrocyte sedimentation rate and serum C-reactive protein, fasting plasma glucose and lipid profile (total cholesterol, LDL cholesterol, and triglyceride), serum uric acid, creatinine, and alanine aminotransferase, plasma 25-hydroxy-vitamin-D_3 and thyroid stimulating hormone levels of each patient were measured.

Study design

The patients were divided into two groups according to the DN-4 score: Group 1 with neuropathic pain (a DN-4 score of 4 or higher) and Group 2 with no significant neuropatic pain (a DN-4 score less than 4). The two groups were compared in terms of the demographic and clinical features and the tests and measurements. Since the sex was found to have a influencer effect, the study groups were further divided into the sex subgroups in the analyses.

Statistical analysis

SPSS Statistics v.18 (IBM Corp, Chicago, IL, USA) was used for the statistical analyses. Data were expressed as numbers with percentages for the categorical and means or medians with standard deviations or minimum and maximum values for the continuous variables. Categorical variables were compared by using chi-square of Fisher's exact tests. Distributions of the continuous data were analyzed by histograms and tested for normality by the Shapiro–Wilk test. Mann–Whitney U or a t-test was used for comparison of unrelated samples according to the distribution. Multiple logistic regression analysis was used to control for the factors associated with neuropathic pain. $p<0.05$ was considered statistically significant.

Results

A total of 200 patients were included in the study (Fig. 1). Demographic, clinical, and radiological features of the study groups according to sex were given in Table 1. There were 81 (82.6%) and 76 (74.5%) females in Group 1 and Group 2, respectively ($p=0.161$). Age was slightly higher in Group 1 and education status was worse in that group. Symptom duration was significantly longer in Group 1 compared to that of Group 2 (5.21 ± 4.76 vs. 3.38 ± 3.58 years, respectively). Kellgren–Lawrence classes were more unfavorable and genu varum was more frequent in Group 1 (Table 1). The mean DN-4 scores, according to which the patients were grouped, were 6.21 ± 1.47 and 1.16 ± 1.26 in Group 1 and Group 2, respectively. In both groups females had higher DN-4 scores compared to those of males but the differences did not reach to a level of statistical significance (6.35 ± 1.46 vs. 5.59 ± 1.42, $p=0.053$ and 1.25 ± 1.3 vs. 0.88 ± 1.11, $p=0.171$ in Group 1 and Group 2, respectively). Anthropometric measurements and body composition of the study groups were given in Table 2. Body mass index and body fat percentage were also slightly higher in Group 1 compared to those of Group 2. As shown in Table 3, physical function, general health status, pain perception, and quality of life indices were all worse in Group 1. Fall risk, stability and Fourier harmony indices obtained by the computerized posturography in eight positions were provided in Table 4. Fall risk was found to be higher in males in Group 1 compared to that of males in Group 2, although there was no difference between females. Stability indices in different positions were also more unfavorable in males in Group 1 (Table 4). The rates of abnormal Fourier harmony index (i.e. less than 0.9) in eight positions were similarly distributed between the study groups (47–69% in Group 1 and 52–65% in Group 2) and no sex difference was present (data not shown; see Table 4 for the absolute index values). Among age, education status, symptom duration, Kellgren–Lawrence class, number of comorbid diseases and drugs, body mass index, and depression scale score, which were found to be associated with neuropathic pain (Tables 1, 2 and 3), symptom duration ($p=0.01$), depression scale score ($p<0.001$), and Kellgren–Lawrence class ($p=0.02$) remained significant to predict neuropathic pain in multiple logistic regression.

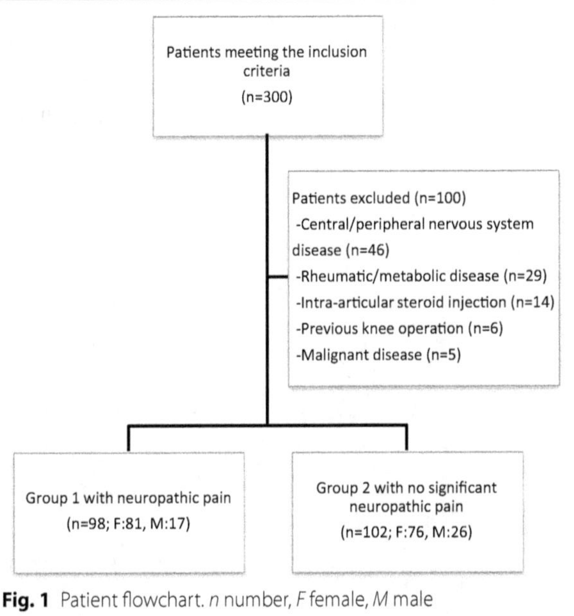

Fig. 1 Patient flowchart. *n* number, *F* female, *M* male

Hemoglobin concentration, erythrocyte sedimentation rate and serum C-reactive protein, fasting plasma glucose and lipid profile, serum uric acid, alanine aminotransferase, and plasma thyroid stimulating hormone levels were similar in Group 1 and Group 2 (data not shown). Plasma 25-hydroxy-vitamin-D_3 was slightly lower in Group 1 compared to Group 2 (median 19.6 [min:5, max:76.3] and 22.3 [min:4, max:66] ng/mL, respectively, $p=0.035$). Serum creatinine was also slightly lower in Group 1 compared to Group 2 (median 0.77 [min:0.48, max:1.41] and 0.81 [min:0.54, max:1.49] mg/dL, respectively, $p=0.034$). But in the sex-stratified comparisons plasma 25-hydroxy-vitamin-D_3 and serum creatinine

Table 1 Demographic, clinical, and radiological features of the study groups

	Group 1			Group 2			p_F	p_M	p_G
	Female (n = 81)	Male (n = 17)	Total (n = 98)	Female (n = 76)	Male (n = 26)	Total (n = 102)			
Age, years*	61 (50–70)	60.5 (51–70)	61 (50–70)	56.5 (50–70)	59 (50–69)	57.5 (50–70)	**0.010**	0.842	**0.030**
Education status, n (%)	N/P	N/P		N/P	N/P		N/P	N/P	**0.014**
Primary or lower			56 (57.1)			44 (43.1)			
Secondary or high school			32 (32.7)			32 (31.4)			
Higher education			10 (10.2)			26 (25.5)			
Working status, n (%)	N/P	N/P		N/P	N/P		N/P	N/P	0.555
Actively working			15 (15.3)			14 (13.7)			
Not working			83 (84.7)			88 (86.3)			
Marital status, n (%)	N/P	N/P		N/P	N/P		N/P	N/P	0.873
Married			77 (78.6)			89 (87.3)			
Not married			21 (21.4)			13 (12.7)			
Smoking status, n (%)	N/P	N/P		N/P	N/P		N/P	N/P	0.626
Active smoker			12 (12.2)			13 (12.7)			
Ex-smoker			32 (32.7)			27 (26.5)			
Never smoked			54 (55.1)			62 (60.8)			
Knee pain, n (%)							0.308	0.337	0.904
Unilateral	13 (16.1)	3 (17.6)	16 (16.3)	8 (10.5)	8 (30.8)	16 (15.7)			
Bilateral	68 (83.9)	14 (82.4)	82 (83.7)	68 (89.5)	18 (69.2)	86 (84.3)			
Knee crepitation, n (%)							0.234	0.136	0.059
Unilateral	6 (7.4)	1 (5.9)	7 (7.1)	10 (13.2)	6 (23.1)	16 (15.7)			
Bilateral	75 (92.6)	16 (94.1)	91 (92.9)	66 (86.8)	20 (76.9)	86 (84.3)			
Symptom duration, years	5.54 ± 4.99	3.65 ± 3.15	5.21 ± 4.76	3.8 ± 3.79	2.14 ± 2.54	3.38 ± 3.58	**0.015**	0.108	**0.002**
Kellgren–Lawrence classification, n (%)									
Right							0.133	0.170	**0.016**
Class I	7 (8.6)	1 (5.9)	8 (8.2)	13 (17.1)	9 (34.6)	22 (21.6)			
Class II	26 (32.1)	9 (52.9)	35 (35.7)	29 (38.2)	11 (42.3)	40 (39.2)			
Class III	34 (42)	6 (35.3)	40 (40.8)	28 (36.8)	5 (19.2)	33 (32.4)			
Class IV	14 (17.3)	1 (5.9)	15 (15.3)	6 (7.9)	1 (3.9)	7 (6.8)			
Left							**0.001**	0.286	**0.001**
Class I	1 (1.2)	2 (11.8)	3 (3.1)	15 (19.7)	6 (23.1)	21 (20.6)			
Class II	28 (34.7)	10 (58.8)	38 (38.7)	27 (35.6)	15 (57.7)	42 (41.2)			
Class III	34 (41.9)	5 (29.4)	39 (39.8)	25 (32.9)	3 (11.5)	28 (27.4)			
Class IV	18 (22.2)	–	18 (18.4)	9 (11.6)	2 (7.7)	11 (10.8)			
Painful areas other than knee, n (%)							**<0.001**	**0.028**	**<0.001**
Absent	11 (13.6)	6 (35.2)	17 (17.3)	36 (47.4)	18 (69.2)	54 (52.9)			
Present	70 (86.4)	11 (64.8)	81 (82.7)	40 (52.6)	8 (30.8)	48 (47.1)			
Postural deviations, n (%)									
Thoracic hyperkyphosis	28 (34.7)	8 (47.1)	36 (36.7)	25 (32.9)	8 (30.8)	33 (32.3)	0.825	0.280	0.515
Lombar hyperlordosis	44 (54.3)	10 (58.8)	54 (55.1)	39 (51.3)	13 (50)	52 (51)	0.706	0.571	0.559
Scoliosis	8 (9.8)	1 (5.9)	9 (9.2)	8 (10.5)	–	8 (7.8)	0.893	N/T	0.734
Genu varum	24 (29.6)	3 (17.6)	27 (27.5)	10 (13.2)	3 (11.5)	13 (12.7)	**0.012**	0.666	**0.009**

Table 1 (continued)

	Group 1			Group 2			p_F	p_M	p_G
	Female (n = 81)	Male (n = 17)	Total (n = 98)	Female (n = 76)	Male (n = 26)	Total (n = 102)			
Genu recurvatum	–	–	–	–	1 (3.9)	1 (1)	N/T	N/T	N/T
Pes planus	9 (11.1)	2 (11.8)	11 (11.2)	8 (10.5)	3 (11.5)	11 (10.8)	0.906	1.000	0.921
Number of comorbid diseases*	3 (0–8)	2 (0–4)	3 (0–8)	2 (0–6)	1 (0–6)	2 (0–6)	**<0.001**	0.083	**<0.001**
Number of drugs used*	2 (0–5)	2 (0–3)	2 (0–5)	1 (0–4)	1 (0–3)	1 (0–4)	**<0.001**	0.234	**<0.001**

P-value less than 0.05 ($p < 0.05$) is statistically significant

p_F; significance of difference between females in Group 1 and Group 2. p_M; significance of difference between males in Group 1 and Group 2. p_G; significance of difference between Group 1 and Group 2

n number, *N/T* not tested, *N/P* not provided

* Given as median (min–max)

Table 2 Anthropometric measurements and body composition of the study groups

	Group 1			Group 2			p_F	p_M	p_G
	Female (n = 81)	Male (n = 17)	Total (n = 98)	Female (n = 76)	Male (n = 26)	Total (n = 102)			
Weight, kg*	74.9 (52.4–118.8)	81.4 (59–102.4)	76.2 (52.4–118.8)	75.9 (53.5–110.8)	80.2 (59.6–117.4)	76.4 (53.5–117.4)	0.572	0.297	0.488
Height, cm*	155 (141–178)	170 (160–182)	157 (141–182)	157 (140–175)	167 (155–179)	159 (140–179)	**0.016**	0.432	**0.026**
Body mass index, kg/m^2	32.6 ± 5.7	28.8 ± 3.8	31.9 ± 5.6	30.8 ± 5	28.2 ± 3.8	30.1 ± 4.8	**0.037**	0.613	**0.015**
Waist circumference, cm	102.8 ± 11.7	103.5 ± 10.3	102.9 ± 11.4	99.3 ± 10.8	102.6 ± 8.4	100.1 ± 10.3	0.054	0.767	0.073
Hip circumference, cm*	114 (92–144)	107 (92–115)	112 (92–144)	113 (94–142)	104 (92–120)	109 (92–142)	0.137	0.419	0.055
Waist-to-hip ratio	0.88 ± 0.07	0.97 ± 0.06	0.9 ± 0.07	0.88 ± 0.05	0.97 ± 0.04	0.9 ± 0.06	0.672	0.958	0.691
Muscle mass, kg*	45.6 (35.6–64.9)	60.9 (51.8–73.9)	46.8 (35.6–73.9)	46 (33.3–64)	58.8 (47.5–78.5)	48.3 (33.3–78.5)	0.684	0.196	0.400
Fat mass, kg*	26.3 (13.6–58.1)	20.6 (3.4–30.6)	25.3 (3.4–58.1)	27.3 (7.8–49.8)	15.7 (6.9–34.9)	24.6 (6.9–49.8)	0.274	0.358	0.055
Body fat, %*	36.7 (24.5–48.9)	23.8 (5.7–29.9)	34 (5.7–48.9)	36.2 (10.4–45)	21.7 (11.6–29.7)	33.3 (10.4–45)	0.236	0.559	**0.039**

P-value less than 0.05 ($p < 0.05$) is statistically significant

p_F; significance of difference between females in Group 1 and Group 2. p_M; significance of difference between males in Group 1 and Group 2. p_G; significance of difference between Group 1 and Group 2

n number

* Given as median (min–max)

were similarly distributed between the groups (data not shown).

Discussion

We were able to show that almost half of the patients with knee osteoarthritis had neuropathic pain which was associated with longer symptom duration and higher age, lower education, higher body mass index, higher number of comorbid diseases and drugs used, presence of genu varum, and more severe radilogical findings. Neuropathic pain was also found to be related to the presence of painful areas other than the knee, worse pain perception, depression, lower physical function and quality of life, and lower stability when the visual and proprioceptive input was blocked.

Osteoarthritis is the most common joint disease and an important cause of mobidity [2]. The principal symptom in osteoarthritis is pain which was proposed to have nociceptive and neuropathic components [6]. Early peripheral (mechanical) and late central sensitization (secondary hyperalgesia) may augment pain perception [5–7]. The latter may predominate in some patients and the pain can not be explained entirely by nociceptive and

Table 3 Physical function tests, Western Ontario and McMaster Osteoarthritis Index (WOMAC), Short Form-36 (SF-36), geriatric depression scale (GDS), and knee pain visual analogue scale (VAS) scores of the study groups

	Group 1			Group 2			p_F	p_M	p_G
	Female (n = 81)	Male (n = 17)	Total (n = 98)	Female (n = 76)	Male (n = 26)	Total (n = 102)			
Physical function tests*									
Chair-stand /30 s	11 (2–16)	12 (6–14)	11 (2–16)	12 (5–22)	14 (8–19)	12 (5–22)	**0.002**	**0.001**	**<0.001**
Stair climbing, second									
Upwards	2.8 (1.6–21.7)	2.4 (1.4–4.7)	2.7 (1.4–21.7)	2.3 (1.2–9.4)	2 (1.4–3.8)	2.2 (1.2–9.4)	**0.003**	0.160	**<0.001**
Downwards	3 (1.5–15.2)	2.5 (1.4–5.1)	3 (1.4–12.5)	2.3 (1.3–8.5)	2 (1.4–4.3)	2.3 (1.3–8.5)	**<0.001**	0.168	**<0.001**
6-min walk, meter	360 (70–510)	425 (240–600)	360 (70–600)	420 (108–600)	420 (280–620)	430 (108–620)	**<0.001**	0.149	**<0.001**
WOMAC score*									
Pain	10 (3–19)	8 (2–16)	10 (2–19)	7 (1–15)	4 (2–12)	6 (1–15)	**<0.001**	**0.008**	**0.002**
Stiffness	2 (0–7)	0 (0–6)	2 (0–7)	0 (0–4)	0 (0–4)	0 (0–4)	**<0.001**	0.275	**<0.001**
Physical function	32 (12–59)	27 (7–55)	30 (7–59)	22.5 (1–46)	17 (5–38)	22 (1–46)	**<0.001**	**0.012**	**<0.001**
Total	12.3 (3.9–26.9)	9.2 (2–23.5)	11.5 (2–26.9)	7.4 (1.2–17.2)	5.5 (2.1–15)	6.8 (1.2–17.2)	**<0.001**	**0.012**	**<0.001**
SF-36 score*									
Physical function	35 (5–100)	40 (15–80)	35 (5–100)	45 (5–85)	67.5 (20–95)	55 (5–95)	**<0.001**	**0.033**	**<0.001**
Social function	50 (12.5–100)	75 (25–100)	50 (12.5–100)	62.5 (25–100)	81.2 (25–100)	75 (25–100)	**<0.001**	**0.036**	**<0.001**
Physical role limitation	0 (0–100)	0 (0–100)	0 (0–100)	100 (0–100)	100 (0–100)	100 (0–100)	**<0.001**	0.068	**<0.001**
Emotional role limitation	0 (0–100)	100 (0–100)	100 (0–100)	100 (0–100)	100 (0–100)	100 (0–100)	**<0.001**	0.348	**<0.001**
Bodily pain	35 (0–70)	47.5 (12.5–67)	35 (0–100)	56.2 (10–100)	57.5 (32.5–90)	57.5 (15–100)	**<0.001**	**0.010**	**<0.001**
Mental health	64 (32–88)	68 (32–72)	64 (32–88)	72 (28–92)	64 (28–84)	72 (28–92)	**<0.001**	1.000	**0.001**
Vitality	35 (10–75)	50 (30–70)	40 (10–75)	50 (15–80)	55 (5–65)	50 (5–50)	**<0.001**	0.571	**<0.001**
Health perception	35 (15–85)	50 (20–60)	40 (15–85)	50 (15–80)	55 (20–65)	55 (15–80)	**<0.001**	**0.025**	**<0.001**
GDS category, n (%)							**<0.001**	N/T	**<0.001**
No depression	31 (38.2)	14 (82.4)	45 (45.9)	58 (76.3)	25(96.2)	83 (81.4)			
Possible depression	12 (14.9)	1 (5.8)	13 (13.3)	12 (15.8)	–	12 (11.8)			
Depression	38 (46.9)	2(11.8)	40 (40.8)	6 (7.9)	1 (3.8)	7 (6.8)			
Knee pain VAS score*									
At rest	4 (0–10)	2 (0–8)	3.5 (0–10)	2 (0–6)	0 (0–6)	2 (0–6)	**<0.001**	**0.040**	**<0.001**
Walking	8 (2–10)	7 (4–10)	8 (2–10)	7 (4–10)	6 (3–10)	6.5 (3–10)	**<0.001**	**0.009**	**<0.001**

P-value less than 0.05 ($p < 0.05$) is statistically significant

p_F; significance of difference between females in Group 1 and Group 2. p_M; significance of difference between males in Group 1 and Group 2. p_G; significance of difference between Group 1 and Group 2

n number

* Given as median (min–max)

neuropathic mechanisms, with additional features such as allodynia, increased sensitivity to sound and light, sleep disturbances, fatigue, and cognitive problems. It is now called nociplastic pain [28], which probably stands as a third component of the pain in osteoarthritis. Pain, which was initially responsive to analgesics and non-steroidal anti-inflammatory drugs, may change character and gain long-lasting, more extensive and refractory features in the later course of the disease [6, 7]. At that stage, centrally acting agents, such as duloxetin and pregabalin, may work [7, 29, 30]. So characterization of the pain in osteoarthritis is of importance for proper management and patient care.

A wide range of frequency of neuropathic pain, 5.4–52%, was reported in knee osteoarthritis [8–12]. The ranges of the age (44–81 to 67–99 years) and symptom

Table 4 Fall risk, stability and Fourier harmony indices obtained by the computerized posturography in eight positions

	Group 1			Group 2			p_F	p_M	p_G
	Female (n = 81)	Male (n = 17)	Total (n = 98)	Female (n = 76)	Male (n = 26)	Total (n = 102)			
Fall risk category, n (%)							0.841	**0.029**	0.502
Low	19 (23.4)	1 (5.9)	20 (20.4)	17 (22.3)	11 (42.3)	28 (27.5)			
Intermediate	23 (28.4)	5 (29.4)	28 (28.6)	19 (25)	6 (23)	25 (24.5)			
High	39 (48.2)	11 (64.7)	50 (51)	40 (52.7)	9 (34.7)	49 (48)			
Stabililty index*									
Position 1	21.5 (9.6–90.5)	24.6 (15.5–90.6)	22 (9.6–90.6)	18.6 (8.9–114.2)	19.4 (11.3–70)	19 (8.9–114.2)	0.202	0.164	0.132
Position 2	21.2 (10.4–75.5)	29 (17.6–98.6)	22.7 (10.4–98.6)	23 (8.5–76.5)	19.4 (9–103.8)	21.7 (8.5–103.8)	0.568	**<0.001**	**0.047**
Position 3	16.2 (9.6–43.1)	19.4 (10.7–53.8)	16.5 (9.6–53.8)	15 (5.6–76.8)	14.4 (9.4–53.8)	14.7 (5.6–76.8)	**0.035**	**0.008**	**0.002**
Position 4	22 (8.7–69.1)	25.1 (15.7–75.1)	22.4 (8.7–75.1)	19.6 (6.9–59.2)	19.6 (10.6–56.9)	19.6 (6.9–59.2)	0.270	**0.021**	**0.031**
Position 5	23.1 (6.1–77)	33.9 (16.8–109.3)	24.3 (6.1–109.3)	23.1 (8.7–66.5)	21.7 (10.7–76.5)	22.5 (8.7–76.5)	0.907	**0.031**	0.312
Position 6	23 (5.5–90.3)	27.7 (19.6–73.3)	23.4 (5.5–90.3)	25.5 (9.6–60.3)	20.5 (11.8–78.9)	23.8 (9.6–78.9)	0.521	**0.003**	0.441
Position 7	23.7 (7.6–82.1)	33 (13.8–78.1)	24.4 (7.6–82.1)	24.9 (6.4–60.2)	19.9 (12.8–91.9)	23.9 (6.4–91.9)	0.769	**0.007**	0.287
Position 8	24.9 (6.1–130.2)	32 (4.7–80.2)	26.8 (4.7–130.2)	25.1 (5.9–75.5)	19.5 (12.1–92.7)	22.6 (5.9–92.7)	0.355	**0.005**	**0.013**
Fourier harmony index*									
Position 1	0.91 (0.25–1)	0.77 (0.29–0.99)	0.88 (0.25–1)	0.89 (0.33–1)	0.79 (0.39–0.99)	0.87 (0.33–1)	0.781	0.559	0.791
Position 2	0.77 (0.23–0.99)	0.76 (0.22–0.98)	0.77 (0.22–0.99)	0.85 (0.11–0.99)	0.75 (0.4–0.97)	0.84 (0.11–0.99)	**0.020**	0.551	**0.028**
Position 3	0.87 (0.22–1)	0.85 (0.34–0.97)	0.86 (0.22–1)	0.88 (0.32–0.99)	0.90 (0.6–0.99)	0.89 (0.32–0.99)	0.239	0.123	0.072
Position 4	0.85 (0.17–0.99)	0.72 (0.31–0.97)	0.84 (0.17–1)	0.86 (0.26–0.99)	0.84 (0.28–0.99)	0.85 (0.26–0.99)	0.768	0.146	0.839
Position 5	0.90 (0.42–0.99)	0.90 (0.28–0.98)	0.90 (0.28–0.99)	0.89 (0.22–0.99)	0.87 (0.45–0.98)	0.88 (0.22–0.99)	0.499	0.950	0.436
Position 6	0.88 (0.38–0.99)	0.88 (0.51–0.98)	0.88 (0.38–0.99)	0.88 (0.51–0.98)	0.93 (0.48–0.99)	0.89 (0.28–0.99)	0.545	0.164	0.172
Position 7	0.89 (0.23–0.99)	0.94 (0.48–0.98)	0.90 (0.23–0.99)	0.88 (0.28–0.99)	0.88 (0.52–0.99)	0.88 (0.5–0.99)	0.519	0.636	0.382
Position 8	0.88 (0.03–0.99)	0.86 (0.49–0.98)	0.88 (0.03–0.99)	0.86 (0.16–0.98)	0.85 (0.45–0.99)	0.86 (0.16–0.99)	0.570	0.891	0.696

P-value less than 0.05 ($p < 0.05$) is statistically significant

p_F; significance of difference between females in Group 1 and Group 2. p_M; significance of difference between males in Group 1 and Group 2. p_G; significance of difference between Group 1 and Group 2. Positions: 1, stable surface/eyes open/face forward; 2, stable surface/eyes closed/face forward; 3, unstable surface/eyes open/face forward; 4, unstable surface/eyes closed/face forward; 5, stable surface/eyes closed/head rotated 45° to the right; 6, stable surface/eyes closed/head rotated 45° to the left; 7, stable surface/eyes closed/head tilted back 30°; and 8, stable surface/eyes closed/head tilted 30° forward

n number

* Given as median (min–max)

duration (less than 1 year to 8.3 years) were quite different in these studies. Moreover, the assessment tools for neuropathic pain were different, as well. There is no gold standard tool for neuropathic pain. Three commonly used tools are painDETECT, LANSS, and DN-4 [12, 26]. The first is based on the self-reported symptoms and originally designed for patients with low back pain although modified for knee osteoarthritis [12]. DN-4 is shorter, easier to perform, and was previously reported to be more reliable than LANSS in terms of sensitivity and specificity in Turkish population [26]. Although these tools give different prevalences of neuropathic pain in knee osteoathritis, the estimate of neuropathic pain was found to be unchanged by the questionnaire type in a meta-analysis [31]. But the validity of neuropathic pain questionnaires, selection bias, methodological quality and study heterogeneity were of great concern and standardized criteria for neuropathic pain were suggested to be developed [31].

Although higher age and longer symptom duration were found to be associated with neuropathic pain in this study, these were not uniform among previous studies [8–13]. Conflicting results were possibly due to heterogeneity of the study populations. We identified a relationship between neuropathic pain and lower education in knee osteoarthritis (Table 1). Education status was not found to be associated with neuropathic pain in two previous studies, one of which was conducted in Turkish population [11, 12]. It may be an important point that both studies assessed neuropathic pain with painDETECT, a self-reported questionnaire.

As demonstrated in Table 2, and previously reported [10], knee osteoarthritis patients with neuropathic pain were slightly shorter in stature and had slightly higher body mass index and body fat percentage. These slight but significant differences are prone to type II error to be detected in smaller-scale studies [11]. Higher body mass index may be speculated to be associated with higher osteoarthritis severity, which in turn, may contribute to neuropathic pain (Table 3). Observations of beneficial effect of even slight reductions in body mass index and fat on osteoarthritis severity and symptoms may support this speculation [32].

Unfavorable osteoarthritis severity index, radiological class and postural deviation in the knee osteoarthritis patients with neuropathic pain may reflect an underlying pathophysiological relationship between osteoarthritis severity and neuropathic pain particularly if considered together with longer symtom duration and higher age in patients with neuropathic pain (Tables 1 and 3). Worse physical function tests and quality of life in those patients with neuropathic pain is possibly the result of that association but potentially has intrinsic impact on the mood, pain perception, and cognition, which may be related to central sensitization [5–7], as well. Similar results were previously reported [5, 11] along with conflicting ones [9, 11, 13, 33], again probably due to the differences in assessment tools and methodology, patient heterogeneity, and the lack of standardization.

Although fall risk was similar in knee osteoarthritis patients with or without neuropathic pain, stability and Fourier harmony indices were worse in the neuropathic pain group especially when the visual and/or proprioceptive input was blocked (Table 4). This was a novel finding and may be related to more severe osteoarthritis in the neuropathic pain group.

Increased pain perception, presence of painful areas other than the knee, and more prevalent depression in knee osteoarthritis patients with neuropathic pain indicate a more generalized psychopathological state rather than isolated neuropathic pain and may explain vulnerability to secondary hyperalgesia (Tables 1 and 3). Similar to our results, more prevalent comorbid diseases, higher number of drugs used, and a worse metabolic profile were previously reported in knee osteoarthritis patients with neuropathic pain [10]. Importantly, the sex was a significant influencer of the study results, although the frequency of female sex was similar in knee osteoarthritis patients with or without neuropathic pain.

Primary limitation of this study is the cross-sectional design that holds us to provide causal relationships regarding the study results. Type II error is also of concern in between-group male comparisons.

Conclusions

In conclusion, almost half of the patients with knee osteoarthritis had neuropathic pain which was associated with longer symptom duration and higher age, lower education, higher body mass index, more severe radilogical findings, worse pain perception, lower physical function and quality of life, and lower stability. Sex has an apparent effect on the study results. The lack of a gold standard assessment tool for neuropathic pain and a standardized methodology in knee osteoarthritis complicates comparison of the results of different studies.

Abbreviations

WOMAC: Western Ontario and McMaster Osteoarthritis Index; SF-36: Short form-36; DN-4: Douleur neuropathique-4; VAS: Visual analogue scale; LANSS: Leeds assessment of neuropathic symptoms and signs pain scale.

Acknowledgements

None.

Authors' contributions

Concept and design: UGD, AND, NFT. Data collection and processing: UGD, analysis and interpretation: UGD, literature review: UGD, NFT, writing: UGD, AND. Critical review: NFT. All authors read and approved the final manuscript.

Author details

[1]Department of Physical Therapy and Rehabilitation, University of Health Sciences, Antalya Training and Research Hospital, 07100 Muratpaşa, Antalya, Turkey. [2]Department of Physical Medicine and Rehabilitation Rheumatology Clinic, Faculty of Medicine, Akdeniz University, 07100 Antalya, Turkey. [3]Department of Physical Therapy and Rehabilitation, University of Health Sciences, Antalya Training and Research Hospital, 07100 Antalya, Turkey.

References

1. Pereira D, Peleteiro B, Araujo J, Branco J, Santos RA, Ramos E, et al. The effect of osteoarthritis definition on prevalence and incidence estimates: a systematic review. Osteoarthr Cartil. 2011;19:1270–85. https://doi.org/10.1016/j.joca.2011.08.009.
2. Corti MC, Rigon C. Epidemiology of osteoarthritis: prevalence, risk factors, and functional impact. Aging Clin Exp Res. 2003;15:359–63. https://doi.org/10.1007/BF03327356.
3. Kaçar C, Gilgil E, Urhan S, Arıkan V, Dündar Ü, Oksuz MC, et al. The prevalence of symptomatic knee and distal interphalangeal joint osteoarthritis in the urban population of Antalya, Turkey. Rheumatol Int. 2005;25:201–4. https://doi.org/10.1007/s00296-003-0415-z.
4. Ivanavicius SP, Ball AD, Heapy CG, Westwood FR, Murray F, Read SJ. Structural pathology in a rodent model of osteoarthritis is associated with neuropathic pain: increased expression of ATF-3 and pharmacological characterisation. Pain. 2007;128:272–82. https://doi.org/10.1016/j.pain.2006.12.022.
5. Hochman JR, Davis AM, Elkayam J, Gagliese L, Hawker GA. Neuropathic pain symptoms on the modified painDETECT correlate with signs of central sensitization in knee osteoarthritis. Osteoarthr Cartil. 2013;21:1236–42. https://doi.org/10.1016/j.joca.2013.06.023.
6. Schaible HG. Mechanisms of chronic pain in osteoarthritis. Curr Rheumatol Rep. 2012;14:549–56. https://doi.org/10.1007/s11926-012-0279-x.
7. Dimitroulas T, Duarte RV, Behura A, Kitas GD, Raphael JH. Neuropathic pain in osteoarthritis: a review of pathophysiological mechanisms and implications for treatment. Semin Arthritis Rheum. 2014;44:145–54. https://doi.org/10.1016/j.semarthrit.2014.05.011.
8. Oteo-Álvaro Á, Ruiz-Ibán MA, Miguens X, Stern A, Villoria J, Sánchez-Magro I, et al. High prevalence of neuropathic pain features in patients with knee osteoarthritis: a cross-sectional study. Pain Pract. 2015;15:618–26. https://doi.org/10.1111/papr.12220.
9. Ohtori S, Orita S, Yamashita M, Ishikawa T, Ito T, Shigemura T, et al. Existence of a neuropathic pain component in patients with osteoarthritis of the knee. Yonsei Med J. 2012;53:801–5. https://doi.org/10.3349/ymj.2012.53.4.801.

10. Fernandes GS, Valdes AM, Walsh DA, Zhang W, Doherty M. Neuropathic-like knee pain and associated risk factors: a cross-sectional study in a UK community sample. Arthritis Res Ther. 2018;27:215–21. https://doi.org/10.1186/s13075-018-1717-6.
11. Polat CS, Dogan A, Sezgin Ozcan D, Koseoglu BF, Kocer Akselim S. Is there a possible neuropathic pain component in knee osteoarthritis? Arch Rheumatol. 2017;32:333–8. https://doi.org/10.5606/ArchRheumatol.2017.6006.
12. Hochman JR, Gagliese L, Davis AM, Hawker GA. Neuropathic pain symptoms in a community knee OA cohort. Osteoarthr Cartil. 2011;19:647–54. https://doi.org/10.1016/j.joca.2011.03.007.
13. Hochman JR, French MR, Berminghamet SL, Hawker GA. The nerve of osteoarthritis pain. Arthrit Care Res. 2010;62:1019–23. https://doi.org/10.1002/acr.20142.
14. Bellamy N, Buchanan WW, Goldsmith CH, Campbell J, Stitt LW. Validation study of WOMAC: a health status instrument for measuring clinically important patient relevant outcomes to antirheumatic drug therapy in patients with osteoarthritis of the hip or knee. J Rheumatol. 1988;15:1833–40.
15. Tüzün E, Eker L, Aytar A, Daşkapan A, Bayramoğlu M. Acceptability, reliability, validity and responsiveness of the Turkish version of WOMAC osteoarthritis index. Osteoarthr Cartil. 2005;13:28–33. https://doi.org/10.1016/j.joca.2004.10.010.
16. Ware JE, Sherbourne CD. The Mos 36 item short-form health survey (SF-36). I. Conceptual framework and item selection. Med Care. 1992;30:473–83.
17. Koçyiğit H, Aydemir Ö, Fişek G, Ölmez N, Memiş A. Kısa Form-36 (KF36)'nın Türkçe Versiyonunun güvenilirliği ve geçerliliği. İlaç ve Tedavi Dergisi. 1999;12:102–6 (**(Turkish)**).
18. Yesavage JA, Brink TL, Rose TL, Lum O, Huang V, Adey M, et al. Development and validation of a geriatric depression screening scale: a preliminary report. Psychiatr Res. 1982;17:37–49. https://doi.org/10.1016/0022-3956(82)90033-4.
19. Ertan T, Eker E, Şar V. Geriatrik depresyon ölçeğinin Türk yaşlı nüfusunda geçerlilik ve güvenilirliği. Nöropsikiyatri Arşivi. 1997;34:62–71 (**(Turkish)**).
20. Jones CJ, Rikli RE, Beam WC. A 30-s chair-stand test as a measure of lower body strength in community-residing older adults. Res Q Exerc Sport. 1999;70:113–9. https://doi.org/10.1080/02701367.1999.10608028.
21. Bolton JWR, Weiman DS, Haynes J, Hornung CA, Olsen GN, Almond CH. Stair climbing as an indicator of pulmonary function. Chest. 1987;92:783–8. https://doi.org/10.1378/chest.92.5.783.
22. [No authors listed]. ATS statement: guidelines for the six-minute walk test. Am J Respir Crit Care Med. 2002;166:111–7. https://doi.org/10.1164/ajrccm.166.1.at1102.
23. Kohen-Raz R. Application of tetra-ataxiametric posturography in clinical and developmental diagnosis. Percept Mot Skill. 1991;73:635–56. https://doi.org/10.2466/pms.1991.73.2.635.
24. Friedrich M, Grein HJ, Wicher C, Schuetze J, Mueller A, Lauenroth A, et al. Influence of pathologic and simulated visual dysfunctions on the postural system. Exp Brain Res. 2008;186:305–14. https://doi.org/10.1007/s00221-007-1233-4.
25. Bouhassira D, Attal N, Alchaar H, Boureau F, Brochet B, Bruxelle J, et al. Comparison of pain syndromes associated with nervous or somatic lesions and development of a new neuropathic pain diagnostic questionnaire (DN-4). J Pain. 2005;114:29–36. https://doi.org/10.1016/j.pain.2004.12.010.
26. Unal-Cevik I, Sarioglu-Ay S, Evcik D. A comparison of the DN-4 and LANSS questionnaires in the assessment of neuropathic pain: validity and reliability of the Turkish version of DN-4. J Pain. 2010;11:1129–35. https://doi.org/10.1016/j.jpain.2010.02.003.
27. Kellgren JH, Lawrence JS. Radiological assessment of osteo-arthrosis. Ann Rheum Dis. 2000;16:494–502. https://doi.org/10.1136/ard.16.4.494.
28. Kosek E, Clauw D, Nijs J, Baron R, Gilron I, Harris RE, et al. Chronic nociplastic pain affecting the musculoskeletal system: clinical criteria and grading system. Pain. 2021;162:2629–34. https://doi.org/10.1097/j.pain.0000000000002324.
29. Chappell AS, Desaiah D, Seifert HL, Zhang S, Skljarevski V, Belenkov Y, et al. A double-blind, randomized, placebo-controlled study of the efficacy and safety of duloxetine for the treatment of chronic pain due to osteoarthritis of the knee. Pain Pract. 2011;11:33–41. https://doi.org/10.1111/j.1533-2500.2010.00401.x.
30. Sofat N, Harrison A, Russell MD, Ayis S, Kiely PD, Baker EH, et al. The effect of pregabalin or duloxetine on arthritis pain: a clinical and mechanistic study in people with hand osteoarthritis. J Pain Res. 2017;10:2437–49. https://doi.org/10.2147/jpr.s147640.
31. French HP, Smart KM, Doyle F. Prevalence of neuropathic pain in knee or hip osteoarthritis: a systematic review and meta-analysis. Semin Arthritis Rheum. 2017;47:1–8. https://doi.org/10.1016/j.semarthrit.2017.02.008.
32. Bliddal H, Leeds AR, Christensen R. Osteoarthritis, obesity and weight loss: evidence, hypotheses and horizons—a scoping review. Obes Rev. 2014;15:578–86. https://doi.org/10.1111/obr.12173.
33. Narayan RV, Thabah MM, Poduval M. Neuropathic pain among patients with primary knee osteoarthritis: results of a cross sectional study from a tertiary care centre in Southern India. Indian J Rheumatol. 2017;12:132–8. https://doi.org/10.4103/injr.injr_90_16.

16

Lung involvement prevalence in patients with early rheumatoid arthritis without known pulmonary disease

Francisco Paulin[1*], Anastasia Secco[2], Federico Benavidez[2], Juan José Rodríguez Moncalvo[3], Orlando Gabriel Carballo[4], Fernanda Ingenito[4], Martin Eduardo Fernández[3], Agustina Cáceres[2], Fabian Caro[3], Patricia Sasaki[2], María Laura Alberti[3], Paola Orausclio[5], Augusto Riopedre[2], Santiago Rossi[5] and María Celina de la Vega[2]

Abstract

Background: Clinically evident interstitial lung disease (ILD) affects between 10 and 42% of the patients with rheumatoid arthritis (RA). Airway involvement seems to be even more common. Most of the available evidence comes from studies performed in established RA patients. The aim of our study was to know the prevalence of non-diagnosed lung disease (airway and interstitial involvement) in patients with early RA and look for associated factors.

Methods: We designed an observational, multicenter, cross-sectional study, and included patients with RA of less than two years since diagnosis. We performed a structured questionnaire, HRCT and lung functional tests looking for lung disease, together with joint disease evaluation. We analyzed which variables were associated with the presence of lung disease on HRCT.

Results: We included 83 patients, 83% females. The median (IQR) of time since RA diagnosis was 3 (1–6) months. In the HRCT, 57 patients had airway compromisea (72%), and 6 had interstitial abnormalities (7.5%). The most common altertion found in lung functional tests was a reduced DLCO (14%). The presence of at least one abnormality in the physical exam was associated with lung involvement on HRCT [13 (21.6%) vs 0 (0%); $p = 0.026$]. Also, patients with lung involvement presented significantly lower values of FVC% and DLCO%, and higher values of RV/TLC. No variable related to joint involvement was found associated with alterations in HRCT.

Conclusion: Our study shows that a large proportion of early RA patients has abnormal findings in HRCT. Further studies are required to confirm these findings.

Keywords: Rheumatoid arthritis, Interstitial lung disease, Early rheumatoid arthritis, Airway disease

*Correspondence: francisco_paulin@yahoo.com.ar
[1] Interstitial Lung Disease Clinic, Hospital General de Agudos Juan A. Fernández, Mansilla, 2838, 1425 Buenos Aires, Argentina

Background

Rheumatoid Arthritis (RA) is the most common autoimmune disease in adults with a prevalence ranging from 0.4 to 1.3% in the general population [1]. Although joint involvement is the most prevalent and known manifestation, extra-articular manifestations represent an important issue due to the implications it may have patients´ quality-of-life and survival. In the last years, a change has been seen in the pattern of extra-articular disease occurrences because of changes in treatments and closer follow-ups [2]. Among them, the lung involvement implies one of the most relevant ones given its various manifestations and the impact it may have in the course of this disease. Lung may be affected in all its components: pleura, airway, interstitium and blood vessels, with an estimated prevalence near 30% according to different series [3]. Treatment of the articular component has experienced an important progress due to the emergence of an increasing number of agents, both biological and non-biological [4]. However, this better management of the joint disease has not been accompanied by an improvement in the course of the lung involvement, which currently represents the second cause of death after the cardiovascular disease [5]. The most severe form of lung involvement is the interstitial lung disease (ILD). The clinically evident ILD affects between 10 and 42% of the patients in different series, mainly based on the method used for its study [6, 7]. Patients with RA and ILD show a threefold higher mortality rate, and ILD is the leading cause in 7% of RA-related deaths [8, 9]. Median survival in these patients is between 3.2–6.6 years, depending on the patterns found in the High-Resolution Computerized Tomography (HRCT) or histology [10]. Airway involvement seems to be more common than ILD (up to 92% in a series), even though available evidence about it is limited [11]. Forms of airway involvement may vary, affecting the proximal as well as the small airway [3]. Patients with lung involvement seem to have elevated anti-cyclic citrullinated peptides antibodies (ACPAs) values and ACPAs have been involved not only as a marker of disease but also in the pathogenesis of severe RA [12–14]. The presence of ACPAs has been detected in patients without articular involvement. However, taking in account their pathogenicity, the organ injury could have started previously. A group of investigators showed that the active monitoring of lung disease with HRCT in RA patients may show interstitial abnormalities in 33% of the cases [15]. This scenario was defined as subclinical ILD characterized by the presence of interstitial abnormalities in HRCT in a group of asymptomatic patients or with symptoms not attributed to an ILD. 34–57% of patients with sub-clinical ILD are known to show disease progression during its course in the HRCT [15, 16]. However, this information comes from studies that included patients with established RA (with more than two years of disease duration). Therefore, we consider that the conduction of a study to evaluate the importance of an active screening of lung disease (both ILD and airway involvement) in patients with early RA is justified. Thus, the aim of our study was to know the prevalence of non-diagnosed lung disease (airway and interstitial involvement) in patients with early RA.

As a secondary objective, we propose to determine which demographic, clinical, functional and laboratory factors are associated with undiagnosed lung disease.

Materials and methods

We designed an observational, multicenter, cross-sectional study and included patients older than 18 years, with diagnosis of RA according to ACR/EULAR 2010 criteria [17]. We excluded patients with more than 2 years since the diagnosis of RA, patients previously diagnosed with RA-related lung disease, and patients that were under biologics or synthetic targeted therapies.

Patients were consecutively recruited between December 2017 and February 2020 in two rheumatology outpatient clinics and assessment of clinimetric variables related to the joint involvement was done. Patients were subsequently referred to pulmonologists for a clinical and functional respiratory evaluation. Also, a chest HRCT was performed. Data was collected in a structured form during patients' evaluation, and included: demographics (age, gender), time from diagnosis of RA (months), treatments received, erythrocyte sedimentation rate (ESR) and c reactive protein (CRP) at the time of assessment, number of tender joints, number of swollen joints, visual analog scale (VAS) for pain, VAS for activity, VAS for the rheumatologist, Disease Activity Score for 28 joints (DAS28) and CDAI (Clinical Disease Activity Index) scores, presence of extra-articular manifestations xerophthalmia, xerostomia, rheumatoid nodules), smoking history, accumulated pack/year, time and degree of dyspnea (mMRC), time of cough, presence of clubbing, presence of velcro crackles, presence of added sounds in airways (wheeze or rhonchus), saturation by pulse oximeter, lung functional parameters as FVC (liters and % theoretical value), FEV_1 (liters and % theoretical value), FEV_1/FVC (%) ratio, TLC (liters and % theoretical value), DLCO (absolute and % value). Immunology laboratory were also studied, including antinuclear antibodies (ANA) Hep2(immunofluorescence), rheumatoid factor (RF, immunoturbidimetry), and ACPAs (ELISA).

All the High Resolution Computed tomography's (HRCTs) were performed in the same center and were analyzed centrally by the same reader. The primary outcome (the presence of lung involvement) was classified into two types: interstitial abnormalities and airway disease. In the first group (interstitial abnormalities) we included the presence of honeycombing, septal thickening, reticular pattern, consolidation resembling organizing pneumonia, or ground glass opacities. In the second type (airway disease) we included the presence of centrilobular nodules, mosaic pattern or bronchiectasis.

Patients were recruited following good clinical practices (GCP) and after the signature of an ethical informed consent. The protocol was evaluated by an Ethic Committee.

Statistical analysis

Categorical variables were described based on their frequency and the continuous variables with mean and standard deviation (SD) or median and interquartile range depending on the presence of normal distribution or not. We analyzed which variables were associated with the presence of lung disease on HRCT. For comparison of categorical variables, a Chi square test or a Fisher´s test was used. For continuous variables, Student´s test or Wilcoxon´s test were used based on distribution.

Lung compromise on HRCT was divided in two different outcomes: ILD and airway involvement.

Results

We included 83 patients, 69 (83%) females, with a mean (SD) of age of 46.49 (17.09) years. Characteristics of the cohort are shown in Table 1. In the group of ever smokers (past or current smokers) the median (IQR) of pack years was 10 (5–30). The median (IQR) of time since RA diagnosis was 3 (1–6) months. Regarding symptoms referred by patients, 25 (30%) presented at least one, with cough as the most frequent (18%). Twenty patients (25%) referred a previously diagnosed respiratory disease, not related to RA. Nine patients referred a previous diagnosis of asthma, 4 referred tuberculosis, 3 recurrent pneumonia. Thirteen patients (15%) had at least one abnormal finding in the physical exam. The most common alteration found in lung functional tests was a reduced DLCO (14%). Regarding auto antibodies prevalence, 89% of patients were positive for ACPAs, 86% for RF, and 75% for ANA.

Four patients could not perform HRCT. In the HRCT, 57 patients had airway compromise (72%), and 6 had interstitial abnormalities (7.5%). In the last group, we found two patients with a pattern compatible with usual interstitial pneumonia, one with a subtle reticular pattern, one with isolated septal thickening, one with organizing pneumonia, and one with ground glass and cysts compatible with lymphoid interstitial pneumonia. From the 57 patients whose HRCT showed airway compromise, 42 showed air trapping, 18 centrilobular nodules and 6 bronchiectasis. We compared the group of patients with interstitial abnormalities with those

Table 1 General characteristics of the population of patients with early RA without known related pulmonary disease

Age, mean (SD)	46.49 (17.09)
Female gender, n (%)	69 (83.1)
Comorbidities	
Past or current somker, n (%)	42 (50.6)
Previous respiratory disease, n (%)	20 (25%)
Cariovascular disease, n (%)	4 (4.82)
Symptoms	
Dyspnea greater than I mMRC, n (%)	12 (15.6)
Months with dyspnea, median (IQR)	
Cough, n (%)	15 (18.7)
Any symptom, n (%)	25 (30.12)
Physical exam	
Ronchus, n (%)	2(2.5)
Wheezing, n (%)	2 (2.5)
Crackles, n (%)	6 (7.5)
Digital clubbing, n (%)	6 (7.5)
Abnormal physical exam, n (%)	13 (15.6)
Lung function tests	
FVC%, mean (SD)	90.4(13.9)
FVC% < 80, n (%)	7 (8.42)
FEV1/FVC < 70%, n (%)	5 (6.02)
TLC%, mean (SD)	107.6 (15.3)
TLC% < 80, n (%)	1 (1.2%)
RV/TLC% > 120, n (%)	12 (14.4)
DLCO%, mean (SD)	104.9 (24.42)
DLCO% < 80, n (%)	12 (14.4)
HRCT findings	
Airway compromise, n (%)	57/79 (72.15)
Interstitial compromise, n (%)	6/79 (7.5)
Emphysema, n (%)	10/79 (12.6)
Auto-antibodies and inflammatory parameters	
ANA, n (%)	48/64 (75)
ACPAs, n (%)	61/68 (89.7)
RF, n (%)	59/68 (86.7)
ESR, median (IQR)	28.5 (21–48)
CRP, median (IQR)	1.64 (0.74–8)
Articular evaluation	
CDAI, median (IQR)	18 (11–24)
DAS28, mean (SD)	4.53 (1.35)
HAQ, mean (SD)	1.38(0.8)
Extra articular compromise	
Sicca syndrome, n (%)	18 (21.95)
Rheumatoid nodules, n (%)	1 (1.22)
Treatment	
Methotrexate, n (%)	50 (60.9)
Leflunomide, n (%)	7 (8.5)

patients who showed airways disease in the HRCT. We did not found statistically significant differences in the median (IQR) of age [57.5 (52–61) vs 49 (42–57); $p=0.138$], proportion of female gender [6 (100%) vs 45 (83%); $p=0.278$], proportion of ever smokers [4 (66.6%) vs 33 (45%); $p=0.311$], mean (SD) of FVC% [87.3 (12.4) vs 98.4(13.1); $p=0.05$], mean (SD) of DLCO [88.1 (18.7) vs 105.1 (23.9); $p=0.095$], median (IQR) of DAS28 [4.24 (3.3–6.2) vs 4.53 (3.6–5.1); $p=0.94$], ANA positivity [6 (100%) vs 42 (72.4); $p=0.137$], ACPAs positivity [5(83.3%) vs 55(91.67%); $p=0.49$], and proportion of patients with extra articular manifestations [3 (50%) vs 57 (78%); $p=0.122$]. However, the analysis showed that patients with interstitial abnormalities tend to be older, with worse values of FVC% and DLCO%, without reaching statistical significance.

With respect to the variables associated with the presence of lung compromise on HRCT (Table 2), we found that the presence of at least one abnormality in the physical exam was associated with lung involvement [13 (21.6%) vs 0 (0%); $p=0.026$]. Also, patients with lung involvement presented significantly lower values of FVC% and DLCO%, and higher values of RV/TLC than patients without lung compromise. No variable related to joint involvement was found associated with alterations in HRCT.

Given its putative association with the presence of secondary Sjögren syndrome, which also could be associated with lung disease, we analyzed separately the presence of anti Ro antibody. The anti Ro antibody was tested in 57 patients and was positive in 11 (19.3%). Of them, 8 patients were positive for Ro60 alone, 3 were positive for both Ro60 and Ro52, and no patient was positive for Ro52 alone. The Ro antibody was more frequent in patients with interstitial abnormalities [3 (50%) vs 8 (15.6%); $p=0.044$). The association between Anti Ro and interstitial abnormalities was also observed in patients with Ro52 [2 (33%) vs 1(1.9%); $p=0.001$] and those with Ro60 [3 (50%) vs 8 (15.6%); $p=0.044$). However, we found no association between anti Ro and the presence of lung involvement, when we included airways compromise and interstitial abnormalities together (Table 2).

Table 2 Comparison of characteristics of patients with and without interstitial or airway abnormalities on HRCT

	Interstitial or airway abnormalities on HRCT (n = 60)	Absence of Interstitial or airway abnormalities on HRCT (n = 19)	P value
Age, median (IQR)	50 (42–58)	45 (33–53)	0.17
Female gender, n (%)	51 (85)	15 (78.9)	0.53
Month since RA diagnosis, median (IQR)	3 (1–7)	2 (0–5)	0.22
Smoking status (past or current), n (%)	32 (53.3)	10 (52.6)	0.95
Dyspnea and/or cough, n (%)[a]	21 (35)	4 (21)	0.25
Abnormal physical examination, n (%)[b]	13 (21.6)	0 (0)	0.026
FVC%, mean (SD)	95.6 (1.69)	103.6 (2.91)	0.022
FVC% < 80, n (%)	7 (11.6)	0 (0)	0.119
VEF1/FVC% < 70, n (%)	2 (10.53)	3 (5)	0.38
TCL%, mean (SD)	106.5 (12.05)	110.1 (23.4)	0.39
TLC < 80%, n (%)	1 (1.67)	0 (0)	0.57
RV/TLC%, mean (SD)	99.83 (31.5)	82.05 (30.08)	0.044
RV/TLC% > 120, n (%)	12 (20)	0 (0)	0.034
DLCO%, mean (SD)	91.05 (21.42)	107.6 (23.4)	0.009
DLCO < 80%, n (%)	7 (11.67)	5 (26.3)	0.121
ANA, n (%)	39 (78)	9 (64.29)	0.29
RF, n (%)	44 (86.2)	14 (93.3)	0.46
ACPA, n (%)	44 (88)	16 (100)	0.146
Anti Ro, n (%)	7/44 (15.9)	4/13 (30.7)	0.233
ESR, median (IQR)	31 (22–53)	27 (15–40)	0.113
RCP, median (IQR)	1.8 (0.7–8)	2 (1–12)	0.71
CDAI, median (IQR)	18 (11–24)	18 (12–24)	0.69
DAS28, median (IQR)	4.55 (3.81–5.4)	4.4 (3.37–4.95)	0.48
HAQ, median (IQR)	1.37 (0.7–2)	1 (0.6–1.2)	0.81
Extra articular manifestations, n (%)	12 (21.6)	6 (31.5)	0.37

[a] Dyspneagreater the I mMRC

[b] Rochus, wheezing or crackles on auscultation, or digital clubbing on examination

Discussion

In this study we found a low prevalence of interstitial compromise and high prevalence of airway involvement in a population of patients with early RA, without known related pulmonary disease. Also, we found that the presence of any type of lung involvement in the HRCT was associated with abnormalities in the physical exam, and abnormal functional tests. Also, we found that the presence of anti-Ro antibody was associated with interstitial abnormalities in the HRCT.

It has been reported that the prevalence of ILD is 10–42% among RA patients. The prevalence varies depending on detection methods and the selected patients in each publication [18]. Regarding clinically significant RA-ILD, it is identified in 2% to 10% of patients with RA, but reported estimates also vary due to the heterogeneity of RA, genetic susceptibility, and differences in disease definition and diagnostic methods [19]. Although our results showed a low interstitial lung disease prevalence compared with other studies, a possible explanation for this finding is that our studied population was compound only by early RA patients. This is an interesting point to highlight from the study. Wilsher et al. published an article which included 60 patients with early RA. Compared with our results, they found a higher prevalence of lung involvement, with ground glass opacities in HRTC in 18% of patients and reticular changes in 12%. Bronchiectasis were observed in 35% and bronchial wall thickening in 50% of the cases [20].

When we analyzed the presence of all types of lung compromise, this cohort of early RA patients showed a great proportion of airway involvement. This fact cannot be dissociated from the high prevalence of smoking found in our sample (past or current smoking near 50%), that may explain itself the airways compromise. However, this finding is consistent with studies showing the presence of RA associated antibodies evidencing an underlying autoimmune phenomenon before the appearance of clinical manifestations, in some cases several years (10 or 15) before [21]. In opposition to what we supposed, we did not find association between the smoking status and the presence of lung compromise in the HRCT. This fact may be related to the high prevalence of smoking in both groups (with and without lung disease), which can be expected in patients with RA, given the role of smoking in this disease pathogenesis. Demoruelle et al. evaluated the presence of lung abnormalities in 42 seropositive patients (RF or ACPA positive) without inflammatory arthritis (IA) [11]. They found airway compromise in 76% of the patients (thickening of bronchial wall, bronchiectasis, centrilobular opacities and air trapping) using HRCT as screening method. These findings suggest that the airway mucosa could be the place where the autoimmune response begins and highlights the importance of the lung in the development of autoantibodies and clinical RA.

The relationship between lung disease and high levels of ACPAs has been proposed by many authors, but the results are still inconclusive. Rocha-Muñoz et al. compared titers of ACPAs in 39 patients with RA-ILD vs 42 patients without RA-ILD [22]. They found a significative relationship between high ACPAs titers and interstitial compromise but the relation with prognosis couldn´t be established. A meta-analysis was conducted regarding this topic by Zhu et al. [23]. They analyzed seven observational studies (243 patients with lung disease and 1442 RA controls) and showed that the ACPA positivity was associated with RA-pulmonary related disease with a pooled OR of 2.6 (95% CI 1.561–4.403; $p<0{,}001$). In our study this relationship hasn´t been demonstrated probably because, as near 90% of our patients were seropositive, this high prevalence likely precludes detection of an association.

Functional tests in our study showed that patients with lung involvement presented significantly lower values of FVC% and DLCO%, and higher values of RV/TLC than patients without lung compromise. Also, we found that patients with interstitial abnormalities tend to be older, with worse values of FVC% and DLCO% than those with airways disease, but without reaching statistical significance. This fact may be explained by a low power of detection due to small number of included patients. Chung et al. found that certain tomographic patterns (mosaic attenuation) were significatively related with lower values of FEF 25–75% [24]. Salaffi et al. conducted a trial that showed DLCO as the most sensitive parameter to predict ILD on HRCT [25]. They performed HRCT in 151 RA patients with established disease, and a mean of seven years of disease duration. The prevalence of ILD was 19.2% in that population. Values of DLCO and FVC in the group with ILD were statistically lower, with a mean of DLCO% of 74.8 and a mean of FVC% of 86.77. Despite the difference with our results regarding ILDs prevalence, these results are consistent with our findings.

The main feature related with lung disease in our study was the presence of at least one abnormality in the physical exam. This finding was statistically associated with any type of lung involvement. In a trial published by the British Rheumatoid Interstitial Lung (BRILL) Network that analyzed ILD-RA proved by HRCT in 25 medical centers over a 25-year period, they found that seropositivity was related with ILD, as well as male gender, age of onset, and smoking [26]. The association that we found between the presence of lung involvement in the HRCT and an abnormal physical examination has been recently reported in a retrospective study that included patients with stablished RA, conducted by Kawano Dourado and coworkers, and has important implications in clinical practice [27, 28].

The association of anti-Ro antibody (in particular Ro52) with the presence of ILD has been reported in other diseases (i.e., inflammatory myopathies) [27, 28]. Our results suggests that this antibody could be a marker of interstitial involvement in RA, a fact that may have important clinical implications. However, the anti-Ro antibody could just be a marker of Sjogren Syndrome that could itself be associated with ILD, and thus, this finding needs to be confirmed by new studies, powered to detect this association.

We consider as strengths of our study that it included patients with early AR, from two rheumatology reference centers, that both HRCT and the lung functional tests together with the immunological laboratory were performed centrally with expert evaluators blind to other data. Our suggests that early lung screening with HRCT and lung functional tests can detect incipient alterations in a large number of patients. This represents an opportunity to start early treatment when indicated.

However, this study has limitations. First: the number of patients included was relatively small to estimate a real prevalence. Second: although we have considered in the analyses and reported the smoking status and the antecedent of a previous pulmonary diseases, an ideal cohort should consist of nonsmokers and patients without that conditions. Finally, the study has a cross-sectional design that does not allow us to arrive conclusions regarding causality. The longitudinal follow up of this cohort, with a larger number of patients, will allow us to elucidate this question, and to know if the prevalence of pulmonary involvement increases over time, which patients with lung disease experience a deterioration of functional parameters in the follow up, and how the different treatments influences lung disease evolution.

Conclusion

In conclusion, our study shows that a large proportion of newly diagnosed RA patients has abnormal findings in HRCT with or without clinical symptoms, and suggests that early screening for lung disease could be useful in patients with RA. Most of them are airway patterns, probably related with the pathophysiology of RA, but a significant number has interstitial pattern on HRCT. As expected, an abnormal clinical examination is associated with the presence of HRCT abnormalities, a fact with important implications in clinical practice. Further studies are needed to confirm these conclusions.

Acknowledgements

Not applicable.

Authors' contributions

FP designed the study, made the statistical analysis, and wrote the first draft of the manuscript together with AS. MF, FC and LA made the pulmonary evaluation. JJRM made the lung function tests. FB, AC, PS made the rheumatologic evaluation. SR and PO analyzed the HRCTs. GC and FI made the immunologic laboratory. MCV edited the manuscript and contributed to define the design of the study. All authors read and approved the final manuscript.

Author details

[1]Interstitial Lung Disease Clinic, Hospital General de Agudos Juan A. Fernández, Mansilla, 2838, 1425 Buenos Aires, Argentina. [2]CEIM Investigaciones Médicas, Buenos Aires, Argentina. [3]Hospital María Ferrer, Buenos Aires, Argentina. [4]Hospital General de Agudos Carlos G. Durand, Buenos Aires, Argentina. [5]Centro Diagnostico Rossi, Buenos Aires, Argentina.

References

1. Rooney BK, Silman AJ. Epidemiology of the rheumatic diseases. Curr Opin Rheumatol. 1999;11(2):91–7.
2. Myasoedova E, Crowson CS, Turesson C, et al. Incidence of extraarticular rheumatoid arthritis in Olmsted County, Minnesota, in 1995–2007 versus 1985–1994: a population-based study. J Rheumatol. 2011;38(6):983–9.
3. Antin-Ozerkis D, Evans J, Rubinowitz A, et al. Pulmonary manifestations of rheumatoid arthritis. Clin Chest Med. 2010;31(3):451–78.
4. Singh JA, Furst DE, Bharat A, et al. 2012 update of the 2008 American College of Rheumatology recommendations for the use of disease-modifying antirheumatic drugs and biologic agents in the treatment of rheumatoid arthritis. Arthritis Care Res (Hoboken). 2012;64(5):625–39.
5. Young A, Koduri G, Batley M, et al. Mortality in rheumatoid arthritis. Increased in the early course of disease, in ischaemic heart disease and in pulmonary fibrosis. Rheumatology (Oxford). 2007;46(2):350–7.
6. Zou Y-Q, Li Y-S, Ding X-N, et al. The clinical significance of HRCT in evaluation of patients with rheumatoid arthritis-associated interstitial lung disease: a report from China. Rheumatol Int. 2012;32(3):669–73.
7. Richman NC, Yazdany J, Graf J, et al. Extraarticular manifestations of rheumatoid arthritis in a multiethnic cohort of predominantly Hispanic and Asian patients. Medicine (Baltimore). 2013;92(2):92–7.
8. Olson AL, Swigris JJ, Sprunger DB, et al. Rheumatoid arthritis—interstitial lung disease—associated mortality. Am J Respir Crit Care Med. 2011;183:372–8.
9. Bongartz T, Nannini C, Medina-velasquez YF, et al. Incidence and mortality of interstitial lung disease in rheumatoid arthritis: a population based study. Arthritis Rheum. 2010;62(6):1583–91.
10. Kim EJ, Elicker BM, Maldonado F, Webb WR, Ryu JH, Van Uden JH, et al. Usual interstitial pneumonia in rheumatoid arthritis-associated interstitial lung disease. Eur Respir J. 2010;35(6):1322–8.
11. Demoruelle MK, Weisman MH, Simonian PL, et al. Airways abnormalities and rheumatoid arthritis-related autoantibodies in subjects without arthritis: early injury or initiating site of autoimmunity? Arthritis Rheum. 2012;64(6):1756–61.
12. Yin Y, Liang D, Zhao L, et al. Anti-cyclic citrullinated peptide antibody is associated with interstitial lung disease in patients with rheumatoid arthritis. PLoS ONE. 2014;9(4):1–6.
13. Rocha-Muñoz AD, Ponce-Guarneros M, Gamez-Nava JI, et al. Anti-cyclic citrullinated peptide antibodies and severity of interstitial lung disease in women with rheumatoid arthritis. J Immunol Res. 2015;2015:1–10.
14. Young A. Rheumatoid arthritis-related interstitial lung disease: associations, prognostic factors and physiological and radiological characteristics—a large multicentre UK study. Rheumatology (Oxford). 2014;53(9):1676–82.
15. Gochuico BR, Avila NA, Chow CK, et al. Progressive preclinical interstitial lung disease in rheumatoid arthritis. Arch Intern Med. 2008;168(2):159–66.
16. Dawson JK, Fewins HE, Desmond J, et al. Predictors of progression of HRCT diagnosed fibrosing alveolitis in patients with rheumatoid arthritis. Ann Rheum Dis. 2002;61(6):517–21.
17. Aletaha D, Neogi T, Silman AJ, Funovits J, Felson DT, Bingham CO, et al. 2010 Rheumatoid arthritis classification criteria: an American College of Rheumatology/European League Against Rheumatism collaborative initiative. Arthritis Rheum. 2010;62:2569–81. https://doi.org/10.1002/art.27584.

18. Dai Y, Wang W, Yu Y, et al. Rheumatoid arthritis–associated interstitial lung disease an overview of epidemiology, pathogenesis and management. Clin Rheumatol. 2021. https://doi.org/10.1007/s10067-020-05320-z.
19. Bendstrup E, Møller J, Kronborg-White S, et al. Interstitial lung disease in rheumatoid arthritis remains a challenge for clinicians. J Clin Med. 2019;2038:1–21. https://doi.org/10.3390/jcm8122038.
20. Wilsher M, Voight L, Milne D, et al. Prevalence of airway and parenchymal abnormalities in newly diagnosed rheumatoid arthritis. Respiratory Med. 2012;106(10):1441–6.
21. Nielen MM, van Schaardenburg D, Reesink HW, et al. Specific autoantibodies precede the symptoms of rheumatoid arthritis: a study of serial measurements in blood donors. Arthritis Rheum. 2004;50(2):380–6. https://doi.org/10.1002/art.20018.
22. Rocha-Muñoz AD, Ponce-Guarneros M, Gamez-Nava JI, et al. Anti-cyclic citrullinated peptide antibodies and severity of interstitial lung disease in women with rheumatoid arthritis. J Immunol Res. 2015. https://doi.org/10.1155/2015/151626.
23. Zhu J, Zhou Y, Chen X, et al. A meta analysis of the increased risk of rheumatoid arthritis-related pulmonary disease as a result of serum anticitrullinated protein antibody positivity. J Rheumatol. 2014;41:1282–9.
24. Chung MH, Lee HL, Kwon SS, et al. Air obstruction in rheumatoid arthritis: CT manifestations correlated with pulmonar function testing. Yonsei Medi J. 2004;45(3):443–52.
25. Salaffi F, Carotti M, Di Carlo M, et al. High-resolution computed tomography of the lung in patients with rheumatoid arthritis. Medicine. 2019;98:38.
26. Kelly CA, Saravanan V, Nisar M, et al. Rheumatoid arthritis-related interstitial lung disease: associations, prognostic factors and physiological and radiological characteristics—a large multicentre UK study. Rheumatology. 2014;53:1676–82.
27. Kawano-Dourado L, Doyle TJ, Bonfiglioli K, et al. Baseline characteristics and progression of a spectrum of interstitial lung abnormalities and disease in rheumatoid arthritis. Chest. 2020;158(4):1546–54. https://doi.org/10.1016/j.chest.2020.04.061.
28. Schulte-Pelkum J, Fritzler M, Mahler M. Latest update on the Ro/SS-a autoantibody system. Autoimmunity Rev. 2009;8(7):632–7. https://doi.org/10.1016/j.autrev.2009.02.010.

17

Predictors of response to etanercept-methotrexate treatment: A post hoc logistic regression analysis of a randomized, open-label study in Latin American patients with rheumatoid arthritis

Maria de la Vega[1*], Generoso Guerra Bautista[2], Ricardo Machado Xavier[3], César Pacheco-Tena[4], Gastón Solano[5], Ronald D. Pedersen[6], Annette Eva Szumski[7], Cecilia Borlenghi[8], Karina Santana[9] and Bonnie Vlahos[6]

Abstract

Background: Determining potential predictors of clinical response would allow a more personalized rheumatoid arthritis (RA) treatment approach in heterogeneous populations such as Latin American (LA) patients.

Methods: Post hoc analysis to identify baseline characteristics predictive of clinical remission in response to treatment with etanercept (ETN) plus methotrexate (MTX) in LA patients with moderate to severe MTX-resistant RA. We report data from the group of patients who received ETN 50 mg/week plus MTX (ETN + MTX, $n = 281$) in a clinical trial consisting of an initial 24-week open-label phase, followed by a 104-week extension. Remission was defined as 28-joint Disease Activity Score with erythrocyte sedimentation rate (DAS28-ESR) score < 2.6. Cutoff values to dichotomize baseline variables maximizing the detection of remission were obtained from Receiver Operator Curve analyses. Baseline dichotomized and categorical variables were analyzed altogether in a stepwise logistic regression model. Odds of attaining response at Weeks 24 and 128 were estimated for each significant predictor.

Results: At Week 24 and Week 128, 27% (66/241) and 42% (91/219) of patients in the ETN + MTX group achieved remission. On average, patients achieving remission were younger and had lower baseline ESR, lower Physician Global Assessment (PGA) scores, lower total Health Assessment Questionnaire (HAQ) scores, and lower visual analog scale (VAS) Pain scores compared with patients who did not achieve remission. The best subset of baseline variables predicting Week 24 remission in the stepwise regression model were age ≤ 49 years (odds ratio [OR] 2.93), body mass index (BMI) > 28.5 kg/m^2 (OR 3.24), disease duration > 3.7 years (OR 2.22), ESR ≤ 42 mm/h (OR 2.72), PGA ≤ 6 (OR 3.21), tender joint count ≤ 14 (OR 2.25), and total HAQ score ≤ 1.6 (OR 2.86). At Week 128, age ≤ 42 years (OR 2.21), SF-36 Mental Health Scale score > 39.6 (OR 2.16), White race (OR 4.07), > 18 swollen joints (OR 2.11), and VAS Pain ≤ 41 (OR 6.05) at baseline were the best subset of significant predictors of remission.

*Correspondence: mainadelavega.mdlv@gmail.com
[1] CEIM Investigaciones Médicas, Laprida 1307, Ciudad De Buenos Aires, 1425 Buenos Aires, Argentina

Conclusions: In LA patients with RA, younger age, higher BMI, longer disease duration, higher SF-36 Mental Health Scale score, higher swollen joint count, and overall lower disease activity predicted clinical response to ETN + MTX therapy.

Background

Rheumatoid arthritis (RA) is characterized by chronic inflammation and joint erosion, often leading to inability to work and poor quality of life [1]. The prevalence of RA in Latin America is estimated to be around 0.4% [2], compared with 0.24–1.0% worldwide [3, 4]. A majority of clinical trials investigating treatments for RA, including those of the tumor necrosis factor (TNF) inhibitor etanercept (ETN), have been conducted in patients from North America and Europe. However, the population of Latin America is highly diverse and differs from Western populations in its racial, ethnic, and socio-economic make-up [5], factors that have been associated with the treatment outcomes of RA [6, 7].

In a 24-week, randomized open-label study of methotrexate (MTX)-resistant patients with moderate or severe RA, conducted in Latin America (NCT00848354), ETN plus MTX was shown to be superior to MTX plus another conventional disease-modifying antirheumatic drug (DMARD) [8]. During the open-label, 104-week extension phase, benefits of ETN plus MTX treatment were maintained for up to 2 years [9], and a post hoc analysis demonstrated that clinical outcomes at Week 12 could be used as predictors of patient-reported outcomes at Week 24 [10].

However, as in most RA trials, treatment benefits were not distributed uniformly among the participants [8, 9]. Determining potential baseline predictors of clinical remission would allow a more personalized approach to the treatment of RA in this heterogeneous patient population. The aim of this post hoc analysis of the trial was to identify potential baseline characteristics that predict which participants were more likely to respond to treatment with ETN plus MTX at Weeks 24 and 128.

Methods

Study design and patient selection

The study design and primary outcomes have been described in detail previously [8]. Briefly, patients from Argentina, Chile, Colombia, Mexico, and Panama with moderate to severe active RA and inadequate response to MTX were included in the study. In the initial phase, participants were randomized 2:1 to receive open-label treatment with ETN 50 mg weekly plus MTX (ETN + MTX, $n = 281$) or an additional conventional DMARD (hydroxychloroquine or sulfasalazine) plus MTX ($n = 142$) for 24 weeks. The second phase (104 weeks) was an optional extension period allowing investigators to select a treatment regimen (ETN, MTX, hydroxychloroquine, or sulfasalazine, in any combination at the desired dosage) based on the participants' previous response to randomized treatment, their preference, and local product labeling [9]. Clinical efficacy endpoints at Weeks 24 and 128 included the proportion of participants who achieved response based on the 28-joint Disease Activity Score with erythrocyte sedimentation rate (DAS28-ESR) consistent with disease remission (<2.6). We report data from a post hoc analysis of predictors of response to treatment in only the group of participants randomized to receive ETN + MTX.

Statistical analysis

This observed-cases analysis included participants who were initially randomized to receive ETN + MTX (Week 24 assessment) and their subset who enrolled in the extension phase (Week 128 assessment). Clinical response at both Weeks 24 and 128 was defined as DAS28-ESR remission. Differences between Week 24 (and Week 128) remitters for demographic and baseline disease characteristics were analyzed in one-way analysis of variance (ANOVA) models (for continuous characteristics) and in chi-square tests (for categorical characteristics). Each continuous baseline variable was dichotomized twice using the Receiver Operator Curve approach from logistic regression model of Week 24 remission (or Week 128 remission). Variables were dichotomized by determining the cutoff values that maximized the sensitivity (true positive rate) plus specificity (true negative rate) of detecting Week 24 (and Week 128) remission. These dichotomized variables along with other categorical baseline variables were then analyzed altogether in a stepwise logistic regression model, and the odds of attaining response in the ETN + MTX group at Weeks 24 and 128 (observed cases) were estimated for each significant predictor, with the cutoff p-value to enter of 0.15 and stay in the model set at 0.05. Baseline characteristics used in the stepwise model as dichotomized/categorical variables included: age; body mass index (BMI); C-reactive protein (CRP); cyclic citrullinated peptide antibody positive; DAS28; disease duration; ESR; modified total Sharp score; morning stiffness; prior use of MTX, non-steroidal anti-inflammatory drugs and corticosteroids; Physician Global Assessment (PGA); race; rheumatoid factor (RF); sex; Short Form 36 (SF-36) physical component summary; SF-36 mental component summary; SF-36 vitality domain score; subject global assessment; swollen joint count; tender joint count; total Health Assessment Questionnaire (HAQ) score; visual analog scale (VAS) General Health; VAS Fatigue; and VAS Pain.

Results

Baseline characteristics

Most of the 281 patients assigned to ETN+MTX treatment were women (248; 88%); the average disease duration was 7.9 years (Table 1). A total of 269 participants from the ETN+MTX group completed the initial phase. Of those, 260 participants enrolled in the ETN+MTX group in the extension phase [9]. DAS28 remission data were available for 241 and 219 patients at Weeks 24 and 128, respectively.

At Week 24, 27% (66/241) of participants in the ETN+MTX group achieved DAS28-ESR remission. This increased to 42% (91/219) of participants at Week 128 (Table 2). On average, responders were significantly younger than non-responders ($p<0.05$ at Weeks 24 and 128). Responders also had, on average, a lower baseline ESR, lower PGA scores, lower total HAQ scores, lower VAS Pain scores (all $p<0.05$ at Week 24), and a lower rate of RF positivity ($p<0.05$ at Week 128) compared with non-responders. There were no significant differences in terms of baseline CRP (Table 2).

Table 1 Select Baseline Demographic and Clinical Characteristics of the ETN+MTX Group*. Adapted From [8]

	ETN+MTX (*n*=281)
Age, years	48.4±12.0
Women, *n* (%)	248 (88.3)
Race, *n* (%)	
White	134 (47.7)
Mestizo	60 (21.4)
African-Latin American	39 (13.9)
Other	48 (17.1)
BMI, kg/m^2	26.4±5.1
CRP, mg/L	20.7±25.4
ESR, mm/h	43.2±16.6
Disease duration, years	7.9±7.0
RF positive, *n* (%)	242 (86.1)
DAS28-ESR	6.6±0.7
HAQ total score	1.6±0.7
PGA	6.7±1.6
VAS Pain, mm (0–100 scale)	65.6±21.3

* Data are mean±SD unless stated otherwise

BMI body mass index, *CRP* C-reactive protein, *DAS28-ESR* 28-joint Disease Activity Score with erythrocyte sedimentation rate, *ETN* etanercept, *HAQ* Health Assessment Questionnaire, *MTX* methotrexate, *PGA* Physician Global Assessment, *RF* rheumatoid factor, *SD* standard deviation, *VAS* visual analog scale

Predictors of response at weeks 24 and 128

Baseline factors found to be associated with response to ETN+MTX at Weeks 24 and 128 in the one-way ANOVA models and in chi-square tests are shown in Fig. 1. The subsets of baseline factors that predicted response to ETN+MTX therapy at Weeks 24 and 128 in the stepwise regression analysis are shown in Fig. 2. Significantly higher odds of attaining remission at Week 24 were associated with a younger age (≤49 years vs>49 years; odds ratio [OR] 2.93 [95% CI 5.91–1.45]), higher BMI (>28.5 kg/m^2 vs≤28.5 kg/m^2; OR 3.24 [95% CI 1.54–6.83]), longer disease duration (>3.7 years vs≤3.7 years; OR 2.22 [95% CI 1.09–4.52]), lower ESR (≤42.0 mm/h vs>42.0 mm/h; OR 2.72 [95% CI 1.28–5.80]), lower PGA score (≤6.0 vs>6.0; OR 3.21 [95% CI 1.62–6.35]), lower prorated number of tender joints (≤14 vs>14; OR 2.25 [95% CI 1.01–5.01]), and lower total HAQ score (≤1.6 vs>1.6; OR 2.86 [95% CI 1.40–5.88]) (all $p<0.05$). Significantly higher odds of attaining remission at Week 128 were associated with a younger age (≤42 years vs>42 years; OR 2.21 [95% CI 1.16–4.21]), higher SF-36 Mental Health Scale score (>39.6 vs≤39.6; OR 2.16 [95% CI 1.15–4.05]), White versus other race (OR 4.07 [95% CI 1.48–11.11]), higher number of swollen joints (>18 vs≤18; OR 2.11 [95% CI 1.12–3.97]), and a lower VAS Pain score (≤41 mm vs>41 mm; OR 6.05 [95% CI 2.37–15.48]) (all $p<0.05$).

Discussion and conclusions

To the best of our knowledge, this is the first analysis of baseline predictors of clinical response to treatment with ETN in Latin American patients with RA. The best subset of factors that predicted clinical response to ETN+MTX therapy for 24 weeks were younger age, higher BMI, longer disease duration, and an overall lower disease activity (lower ESR, PGA, and total HAQ scores). At 128 weeks, the best subset of factors that predicted clinical response to ETN+MTX therapy were younger age, higher SF-36 score, White race, higher number of swollen joints, and lower pain.

In line with our findings, younger age of patients with RA predicted a stronger clinical response in a study of the TNF inhibitor adalimumab [11, 12] and in a study of the IL6 inhibitor tocilizumab [13]. However, age did not predict clinical response in a British registry study of the TNF inhibitor infliximab [14].

Although it could be argued that younger age may be a surrogate marker for shorter disease duration—which has

Table 2 Select Baseline Demographic and Baseline Disease Characteristics of Responders and Non-Responders (Observed Cases)

Baseline Characteristic*	Week 24			Week 128		
	Responders ($n=66$)	Non-responders ($n=175$)	*p* value**	Responders ($n=91$)	Non-responders ($n=128$)	*p* value**
Age, years	**45.4 ± 11.8**	**49.2 ± 11.7**	**0.024**	**45.7 ± 11.8**	**50.1 ± 11.8**	**0.008**
Men, *n* (%)	13 (20)	16 (9)		15 (17)	13 (10)	
Women, *n* (%)	**53 (80)**	**159 (91)**	**0.025**	76 (84)	115 (90)	0.167
Race, *n* (%)						
White	34 (52)	77 (44)	0.622	46 (51)	57 (45)	**0.015**
Mestizo	15 (23)	38 (22)		25 (28)	23 (18)	
African-Latin American	7 (11)	27 (15)		13 (14)	18 (14)	
Other	10 (15)	33 (19)		7 (8)	30 (23)	
BMI, kg/m^2	26.6 ± 5.3	26.3 ± 4.8	0.669	26.3 ± 4.4	26.4 ± 5.2	0.860
CRP, mg/L	19.5 ± 25.9	21.8 ± 25.4	0.521	22.5 ± 26.8	21.1 ± 26.1	0.707
ESR, mm/h	**37.3 ± 11.2**	**44.3 ± 17.4**	**0.003**	39.6 ± 13.8	43.1 ± 16.5	0.104
Disease duration, years	8.2 ± 7.1	7.4 ± 6.5	0.428	7.4 ± 6.4	8.0 ± 7.0	0.534
RF positive, *n* (%)	55 (83)	155 (89)	0.279	**73 (80)**	**117 (91)**	**0.016**
HAQ total score	**1.3 ± 0.7**	**1.7 ± 0.7**	**0.001**	1.5 ± 0.7	1.6 ± 0.7	0.376
VAS Pain, mm	**60.0 ± 23.6**	**66.1 ± 20.3**	**0.047**	61.6 ± 25.7	66.0 ± 18.2	0.141
PGA	**6.5 ± 1.9**	**7.2 ± 1.9**	**0.013**	6.7 ± 2.2	7.1 ± 1.8	0.122
SF-36 Mental Health Scale	41.0 ± 11.3	40.3 ± 11.0	0.665	41.5 ± 10.8	39.6 ± 11.3	0.223
Prorated number of tender joints	**22.2 ± 10.9**	**26.0 ± 11.9**	**0.024**	24.6 ± 11.1	25.5 ± 12.4	0.600
Prorated number of swollen joints	17.6 ± 7.9	18.4 ± 8.6	0.504	**19.9 ± 8.9**	**17.3 ± 8.2**	**0.029**

*Data are mean ± SD unless stated otherwise

***p* value from either a one-way ANOVA model to analyze continuous characteristics or a chis-square test to analyze categorical characteristics; baseline characteristics with *p* values < 0.05 are highlighted in bold

BMI body mass index, *CRP* C-reactive protein, *ESR* erythrocyte sedimentation rate, *HAQ* Health Assessment Questionnaire, *PGA* Physician Global Assessment, *RF* rheumatoid factor, *SD* standard deviation, *SF-36* 36-Item Short Form Survey, *VAS* visual analog scale

been shown to predict higher responses to ETN + MTX [15] and other biologics [16–18]—our analysis, surprisingly, found a marginally significant association of longer disease duration (> 3.7 years) with clinical response at Week 24 when analyzed in combination with other significant predictors in a stepwise analyses, but it was not significant on its own. However, other confounding factors may influence the relationship between disease duration and DAS28 remission. Overall, the role of disease duration as a predictor of clinical response to treatment of RA with biologic agents appears to be unclear, with the data from the British Society for Rheumatology Biologics registry [14] and a study in Japanese patients treated with infliximab, ETN, adalimumab, or tocilizumab [19] failing to establish a link between disease duration and response to treatment.

In our analysis, parameters indicating lower disease activity at baseline (ESR ≤ 42 mm/h, PGA score ≤ 6.0, tender joint count ≤ 14, and total HAQ score ≤ 1.6) were also associated with a stronger response to ETN + MTX treatment at Week 24 on their own and in combination with other significant predictors from a stepwise model. These observations are in line with a number of studies. For example, in a cohort of Chinese patients treated with a TNF inhibitor, ESR ≤ 60 mm/h and total HAQ sore ≤ 1.31 were identified as predictors of clinical response [20]. Data from the British Society for Rheumatology Biologics registry [14], as well as a study in Swedish patients [21], showed that lower baseline HAQ scores were correlated with higher response rates. Similarly, Japanese patients with higher baseline PGA scores were less likely to achieve response to biologic agents [19]. The same study identified low levels of CRP as a predictor of response, which was not the case in our analysis. In the GO-MORE study, lower tender joint count score was associated with a greater likelihood of achieving DAS28-ESR ≤ 3.2 and DAS28-ESR < 2.6 at 1 and 6 months after treatment with the anti-TNF golimumab in biologic-naïve patients with active RA despite treatment with DMARD [22]. However, in a systematic review that included 4 studies of patients with RA treated with anti-TNF therapy + MTX, tender joint count at baseline was not associated with sustained remission [23].

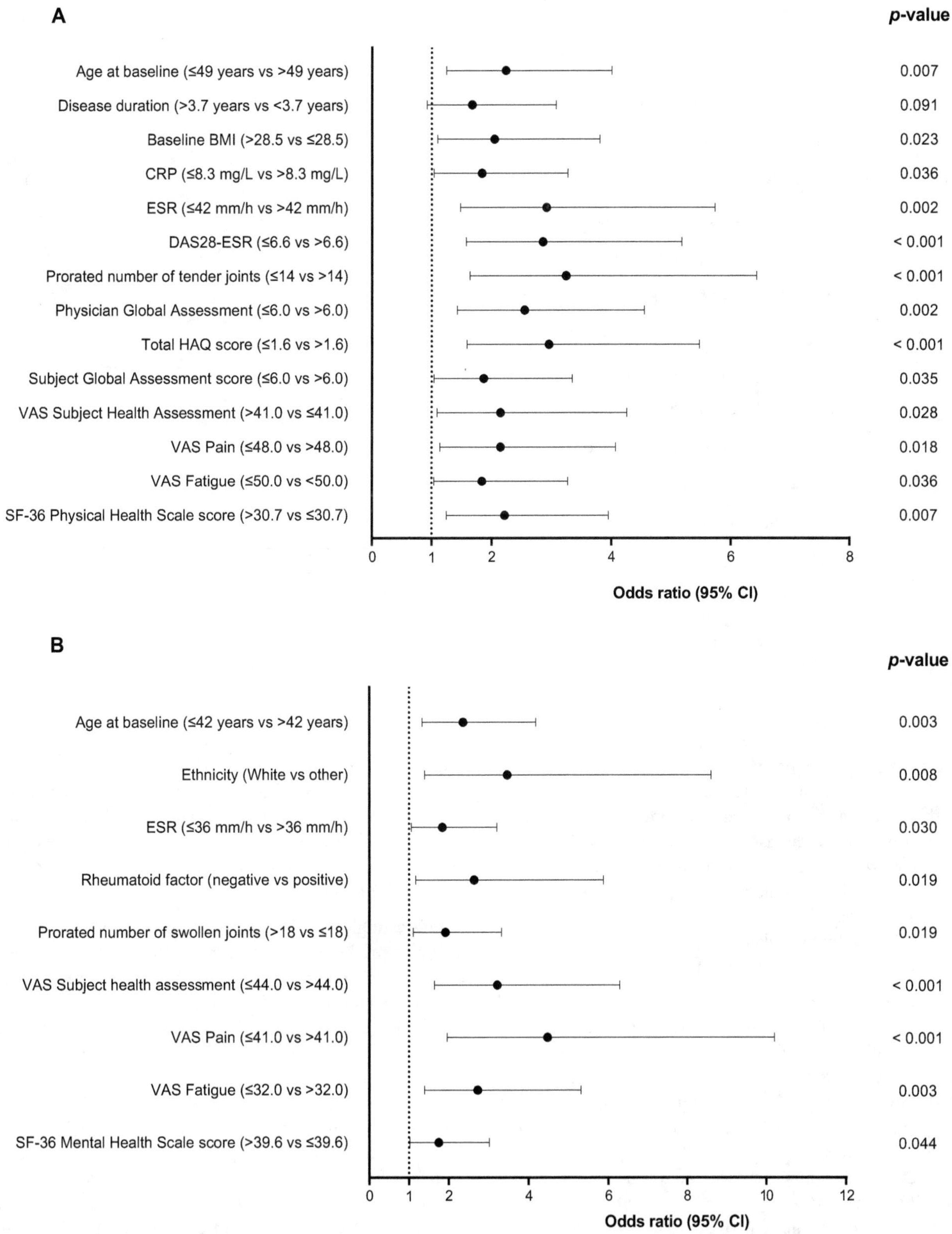

Fig. 1 Baseline Factors Associated with Response to ETN + MTX at Weeks 24 (**A**) and 128* (**B**). **Results from one-way ANOVA models and in chi-square tests. ANOVA* analysis of variance, *BMI* body mass index, *CRP* C-reactive protein, *DAS28* Disease Activity Score in 28 joints, *ESR* erythrocyte sedimentation rate, *ETN* etanercept, *SF-36* 36-Item Short Form Survey, *HAQ* Health Assessment Questionnaire, *MTX* methotrexate, *VAS* visual analog scale

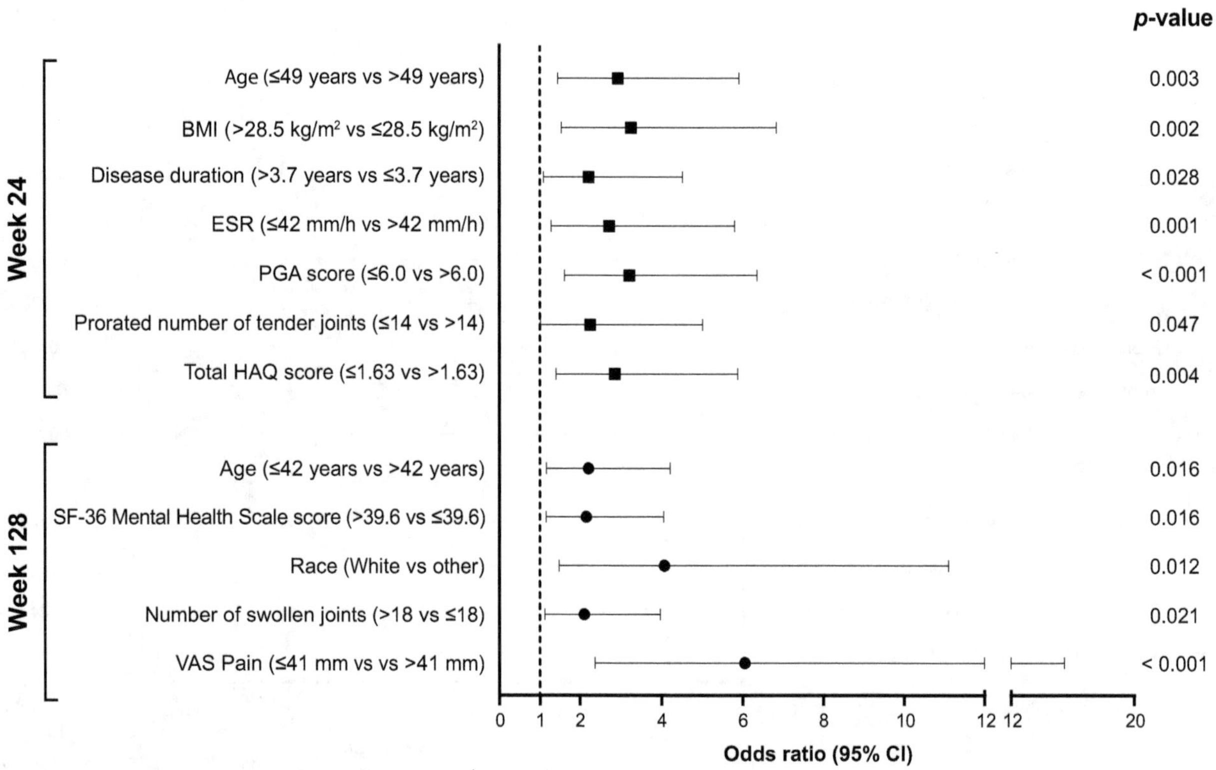

Fig. 2 Odds Ratios for Predictors of Response at Weeks 24 and 128*. *Results from a stepwise regression model of Week 24 and Week 128 DAS28-ESR remission, with list of baseline variables in the model given in the Statistical Analysis section. *BMI* body mass index, *CI* confidence interval, *ESR* erythrocyte sedimentation rate, *HAQ* Health Assessment Questionnaire, *PGA* Physician Global Assessment, *SF-36* 36-Item Short Form Survey, *VAS* visual analog scale

Conversely, a higher number of swollen joints (>18) on its own (from univariate analysis) and in combination with other significant predictors from a stepwise model, indicating higher disease activity at baseline, was associated with a stronger response at Week 128. Although synovitis can be a predictor for radiographic progression [24], an increased number of swollen joints was associated with a higher likelihood of achieving sustained remission in a UK observational study [25].

Lower pain (VAS ≤ 41 mm) and SF-36 Mental Health Scale score > 39.6 at baseline were identified as predictors of clinical response at Week 128 only in combination with other significant predictors from a stepwise model, with lower pain being only marginally significant on its own for Week 24 response. Although we could not identify any studies investigating either of these potential predictors, they may be associated with lower disease activity at baseline.

In our study, White patients (on its own and in combination with other significant predictors) were more likely to achieve clinical remission at Week 128 compared with patients of other races. This is in line with a study from the United States in which African-American and Hispanic patients with RA showed higher disease activity and worse clinical outcomes compared with White patients [26]. The role of race as a predictor is likely to be complex and include both genetic as well as socio-cultural and socio-economic factors.

Interestingly, we also identified higher BMI (>28.5 kg/m^2) as a predictor of clinical response at Week 24 when analyzed in combination with other significant predictors in a stepwise model but not on its own in a univariate model. This is in contrast with a study showing higher BMI (>30 kg/m^2) to be associated with lower response rates to infliximab [27]. In an Italian study, patients with higher BMI (>30 kg/m^2) were less likely to achieve response to infliximab, but no correlation was found for ETN and adalimumab [28]. In another study of adalimumab, BMI (>30 kg/m^2) had no impact on response rates [29]; this was also apparent in studies of rituximab [30] and tocilizumab [31]. Overall, the role of BMI as predictor of response seems to be unclear. Although higher BMI is generally associated with lower socio-economic status, 1 Brazilian study found a positive correlation between BMI and higher socio-economic status [32], which may facilitate access to health care and could therefore explain the favorable outcomes observed here.

In this stepwise regression analysis, RF positivity had no impact on clinical response. This is in line with observations from studies of ETN and infliximab [14] and of tocilizumab [13]. Based on the currently available evidence, no clear conclusion can be drawn on the role of RF positivity as predictor of response, with some studies finding a positive association although others have identified it as a negative predictor [12].

Although Week 24 and Week 128 responders to ETN+MTX were more likely to be male, sex was not a significant predictor of clinical response in our study. An earlier study in a Swedish cohort also found no significant predictive value of sex on clinical response after 3 or 6 months of therapy with ETN, infliximab, or adalimumab [21]; although males had lower DAS28 scores. This is somewhat in contrast to the findings of other studies where males were more likely to achieve clinical remission following treatment with ETN or infliximab [14], and adalimumab [11]. Within the patient population with RA, differences in severity of disease between sexes and differences in other factors, such as biological, physical, or social, may underlie any observed differences by sex.

Limitations of this study included the post hoc nature of this analysis and the absence of an adequate control group. The lack of a control group limits the ability to make conclusions about the specificity of the identified subset of predictive characteristics to the ETN+MTX treatment regimen. The low proportion of male participants makes it difficult to ascertain the impact of sex. It is not possible to generalize the results from this study, which was conducted in selected clinical trial participants, to other populations that were not sufficiently represented in the clinical trial population (e.g., men and individuals of different ages and with different disease durations).

In conclusion, this post hoc logistic regression analysis of a trial of Latin American patients with RA yielded several baseline predictors of clinical response to treatment with ETN+MTX, which may be useful for future clinical decision-making. These baseline predictors of clinical response included younger age, higher BMI, longer disease duration, higher SF-36 Mental Health Scale score, higher swollen joint count, and overall lower disease activity. Discrepancies between our findings and those from studies conducted in other geographic areas of the world, however, underline the need for further prospective studies, adequately powered to detect predictors of response.

Acknowledgements

Medical writing support was provided by Andrea Schauenburg, PhD, of Engage Scientific Solutions and was funded by Pfizer Inc.

Authors' contributions

MdlV, GGB, RMX, CP-T, AES, GS, RDP, CB, KS, BV, Conceptualization, Data curation, Writing – review and editing. All authors read and approved the final manuscript.

speaker); AES, AES is an employee of Syneos Health and was contracted by Pfizer to provide statistical support for the development of this paper; RDP, RDP was an employee of Pfizer at the time of data generation and manuscript development and own stock in Pfizer; GS, CB, KS, BV, Pfizer (stock options, employment).

Author details

[1]CEIM Investigaciones Médicas, Laprida 1307, Ciudad De Buenos Aires, 1425 Buenos Aires, Argentina. [2]Centro de Investigación Marbella, Paitilla Panamá, Panamá. [3]Hospital de Clínicas de Porto Alegre, Porto Alegre, Brazil. [4]Universidad Autónoma de Chihuahua, Chihuahua, Mexico. [5]Pfizer, San José, Costa Rica. [6]Pfizer, Collegeville, PA, USA. [7]Syneos Health, Princeton, NJ, USA. [8]Pfizer, Buenos Aires, Argentina. [9]Pfizer, Ciudad de México, Mexico.

References

1. Almoallim H, Kamil A. Rheumatoid arthritis: should we shift the focus from "Treat to Target" to "Treat to Work?" Clin Rheumatol. 2013;32:285–7.
2. Cardiel MH, Latin American Rheumatology Associations of the Pan-American League of Associations for R, Grupo Latinoamericano de Estudio de Artritis R. First Latin American position paper on the pharmacological treatment of rheumatoid arthritis. Rheumatology (Oxford). 2006;45(2):17–22.
3. Cross M, Smith E, Hoy D, et al. The global burden of rheumatoid arthritis: estimates from the global burden of disease 2010 study. Ann Rheum Dis. 2014;73:1316–22.
4. Rudan I, Sidhu S, Papana A, et al. Prevalence of rheumatoid arthritis in low- and middle-income countries: a systematic review and analysis. J Glob Health. 2015;5:010409.
5. Salzano FM, Sans M. Interethnic admixture and the evolution of Latin American populations. Genet Mol Biol. 2014;37:151–70.
6. Barton JL, Trupin L, Schillinger D, et al. Racial and ethnic disparities in disease activity and function among persons with rheumatoid arthritis from university-affiliated clinics. Arthr Care Res (Hoboken). 2011;63:1238–46.
7. Canhao H, Rodrigues AM, Mourao AF, et al. Comparative effectiveness and predictors of response to tumour necrosis factor inhibitor therapies in rheumatoid arthritis. Rheumatology (Oxford). 2012;51:2020–6.
8. Machado DA, Guzman RM, Xavier RM, et al. Open-label observation of addition of etanercept versus a conventional disease-modifying antirheumatic drug in subjects with active rheumatoid arthritis despite methotrexate therapy in the Latin American region. J Clin Rheumatol. 2014;20:25–33.
9. Machado DA, Guzman R, Xavier RM, et al. Two-year safety and efficacy experience in patients with methotrexate-resistant active rheumatoid arthritis treated with etanercept and conventional disease-modifying anti-rheumatic drugs in the Latin American region. Open Rheumatol J. 2016;10:13–25.
10. Guerra Bautista GXR, de la Vega M, Simon-Campos JA, Solano G, Pedersen RD, Vlahos B, Borlenghi C. Clinical improvements as predictors of improvements in patient-reported outcomes: post hoc analysis of a randomized, open-label study of etancerpt in Latin American patients with rheumatoid arthritis. Open Access Rheumatol Res Rev. 2019;11:275–81.
11. Burmester GR, Ferraccioli G, Flipo RM, et al. Clinical remission and/or minimal disease activity in patients receiving adalimumab treatment in a multinational, open-label, twelve-week study. Arthr Rheum. 2008;59:32–41.
12. Wijbrandts CA, Tak PP. Prediction of response to targeted treatment in rheumatoid arthritis. Mayo Clin Proc. 2017;92:1129–43.
13. Pers YM, Fortunet C, Constant E, et al. Predictors of response and remission in a large cohort of rheumatoid arthritis patients treated with

14. tocilizumab in clinical practice. Rheumatology (Oxford). 2014;53:76–84. Hyrich KL, Watson KD, Silman AJ, Symmons DP, British Society for Rheumatology Biologics R. Predictors of response to anti-TNF-alpha therapy among patients with rheumatoid arthritis: results from the British Society for Rheumatology Biologics Register. Rheumatology (Oxford). 2006;45:1558–65.
15. Emery P, Kvien TK, Combe B, et al. Combination etanercept and methotrexate provides better disease control in very early (<=4 months) versus early rheumatoid arthritis (>4 months and <2 years): post hoc analyses from the COMET study. Ann Rheum Dis. 2012;71:989–92.
16. Agarwal SK, Glass RJ, Shadick NA, et al. Predictors of discontinuation of tumor necrosis factor inhibitors in patients with rheumatoid arthritis. J Rheumatol. 2008;35:1737–44.
17. Finckh A, Liang MH, van Herckenrode CM, de Pablo P. Long-term impact of early treatment on radiographic progression in rheumatoid arthritis: a meta-analysis. Arthritis Rheum. 2006;55:864–72.
18. van der Kooij SM, le Cessie S, Goekoop-Ruiterman YP, et al. Clinical and radiological efficacy of initial vs delayed treatment with infliximab plus methotrexate in patients with early rheumatoid arthritis. Ann Rheum Dis. 2009;68:1153–8.
19. Yuasa S, Yamaguchi H, Nakanishi Y, et al. Treatment responses and their predictors in patients with rheumatoid arthritis treated with biological agents. J Med Investig. 2013;60:77–90.
20. Ding R, Li P, Song D, Zhang X, Bi L. Predictors of response to TNF-alpha antagonist therapy in Chinese rheumatoid arthritis. Clin Rheumatol. 2015;34:1203–10.
21. Kristensen LE, Kapetanovic MC, Gulfe A, Soderlin M, Saxne T, Geborek P. Predictors of response to anti-TNF therapy according to ACR and EULAR criteria in patients with established RA: results from the South Swedish Arthritis Treatment Group Register. Rheumatology (Oxford). 2008;47:495–9.
22. Vastesaeger N, Kutzbach AG, Amital H, et al. Prediction of remission and low disease activity in disease-modifying anti-rheumatic drug-refractory patients with rheumatoid arthritis treated with golimumab. Rheumatology (Oxford). 2016;55:1466–76.
23. Yun H, Xie F, Beyl RN, et al. Risk of hypersensitivity to biologic agents among medicare patients with rheumatoid arthritis. Arthritis Care Res (Hoboken). 2017;69:1526–34.
24. Cheung PP, Mari K, Devauchelle-Pensec V, et al. Predictive value of tender joints compared to synovitis for structural damage in rheumatoid arthritis. RMD Open. 2016;2:e000205.
25. Hamann PDH, Pauling JD, McHugh N, Shaddick G, Hyrich K, Group B-RC. Predictors, demographics and frequency of sustained remission and low disease activity in anti-tumour necrosis factor-treated rheumatoid arthritis patients. Rheumatology (Oxford). 2019;58:2162–9.
26. Greenberg JD, Spruill TM, Shan Y, et al. Racial and ethnic disparities in disease activity in patients with rheumatoid arthritis. Am J Med. 2013;126:1089–98.
27. Klaasen R, Wijbrandts CA, Gerlag DM, Tak PP. Body mass index and clinical response to infliximab in rheumatoid arthritis. Arthr Rheum. 2011;63:359–64.
28. Gremese E, Carletto A, Padovan M, et al. Obesity and reduction of the response rate to anti-tumor necrosis factor alpha in rheumatoid arthritis: an approach to a personalized medicine. Arthr Care Res (Hoboken). 2013;65:94–100.
29. Lafuente-Urrez RF, Perez-Pelegay J. Impact of obesity on the effectiveness of adalimumab for the treatment of psoriasis: a retrospective study of 30 patients in daily practice. Eur J Dermatol. 2014;24:217–23.
30. Ottaviani S, Gardette A, Roy C, et al. Body Mass Index and response to rituximab in rheumatoid arthritis. Joint Bone Spine. 2015;82:432–6.
31. Gardette A, Ottaviani S, Sellam J, et al. Body mass index and response to tocilizumab in rheumatoid arthritis: a real life study. Clin Rheumatol. 2016;35:857–61.
32. Silva APD, Feilbelmann TCM, Silva DC, et al. Prevalence of overweight and obesity and associated factors in school children and adolescents in a medium-sized Brazilian city. Clinics (Sao Paulo). 2018;73:e438.

18

Association of TNFSF4 polymorphisms with systemic lupus erythematosus

Yu Fu[1,2], Qing Lin[2] and Zhi-rong Zhang[2*]

Abstract

Objective: To more precisely estimate the association between the tumor necrosis factor ligand superfamily member 4 (TNFSF4) gene polymorphisms and systemic lupus erythematosus (SLE) susceptibility, we performed a meta-analysis on the association of the following single nucleotide polymorphisms (SNPs) of TNFSF4 with SLE: rs1234315, rs844648, rs2205960, rs704840, rs844644, rs10489265.

Methods: A literature-based search was conducted using PubMed, MEDLINE, Embase, Web of Science databases, and Cochrane Library databases to identify all relevant studies. And the association of TNFSF4 gene polymorphisms and SLE susceptibility was evaluated by pooled odds ratio (OR) with 95% confidence interval (CI).

Results: The meta-analysis produced overall OR of 1.42 (95% CI 1.36–1.49, $P<0.00001$), 1.41 (95% CI 1.36–1.46, $P<0.00001$) and 1.34 (95% CI 1.26–1.42, $P<0.00001$) for the rs2205960, rs1234315 and rs704840 polymorphisms respectively, confirming these three SNPs confer a significant risk for the development of SLE. On the other hand, the meta-analysis produced overall OR of 0.92 (95% CI 0.70–1.21, $P=0.54$) for the rs844644 polymorphism, suggesting no significant association. And no association was also found between either rs844648 1.11 (OR 1.11, 95% CI 0.86–1.43, $P=0.41$) or rs10489265 (OR 1.17, 95% CI 0.94–1.47, $P=0.17$) polymorphism with SLE susceptibility, respectively.

Conclusions: Our meta-analysis demonstrated that the TNFSF4 rs2205960, rs1234315 and rs844840 SNPs was significantly associated with an increased risk of SLE.

Keywords: Systemic lupus erythematosus, TNFSF4, OX40L, Genetic polymorphisms

Introduction

SLE is a chronic multisystem complex autoimmune disorder, which is characterized by pathogenic humoral and cellular immunity to self-antigen [1]. There are a series of SLE manifestations in clinic, such as a vast array of autoantibodies productions, arthritis, mucocutaneous manifestations, hematological disorders and so on [2, 3]. It is reported that the frequency of SLE occurrence is nine times higher in female than in male [4]. Although the etiology of SLE is still incompletely understood, the pathogenesis of SLE is partially owing to the loss of immune tolerance and the deposition of immune complexes. Additionally, the defective B cell suppression and excess T cell help are definitely involved in these process [5]. To our knowledge, the pathogenesis of SLE may largely be triggered by both genetic susceptibility and environmental predisposing factors [3]. And a great contribution of genetic factors to SLE susceptibility was confirmed in comparative studies between the concordance rate of monozygotic twins and dizygotic pairs [6].

*Correspondence: zrzzl@vip.sina.com
[2] Key Laboratory of Drug Targeting and Drug Delivery System of the Education Ministry, Sichuan Engineering Laboratory for Plant-Sourced Drug and Sichuan Research Center for Drug Precision Industrial Technology, West China School of Pharmacy, Sichuan University, Chengdu 610064, China

Over the last decades, great efforts have been made to identify the genes and genomic regions of SLE susceptibility through genetic association studies, especially genome-wide association studies (GWAS). And numerous susceptibility genes of SLE have been widely addressed, including HLA class II haplotypes, STAT4, MHC-I, NCF2, FCGR2B, BLK, IRF5/TNPO3, TNFAIP3, and TNFSF4 [3]. As one of susceptibility genes for SLE involved in NF-κB signaling pathway, many studies have examined the association between TNFSF4 gene polymorphisms and the risk of SLE [7–10]. The tumor necrosis factor ligand superfamily member 4 (TNFSF4, also known as OX40 ligand, OX40L, and CD252) encodes the ligand for OX40 (TNFRSF4; also known as OX40 and CD134) [11]. And OX40L is mainly expressed on activated antigen-presenting cells (APCs), such as activated B cells, dendritic cells (DCs), macrophages. OX40 transiently expresses on both activated CD4 + T cells and CD8 + T cells. The engagement of OX40 with its ligand has a dual effect on T cell responses: it can enhance Th1-mediated immune response and promote generation and maintenance of Th2, but concomitantly antagonizes Treg generation and Treg-mediated suppression [11]. OX40-OX40L interaction also promotes the survive and expansion of CD8 + T cells and the recall response of CD8 + memory T cell in vivo [12]. Furthermore, OX40-OX40L may also augment B cell differentiation and proliferation. Therefore, OX40-OX40L blockade in vivo may ameliorate autoimmunity by preventing migration and proliferation of T cells, affecting T cell polarization, altering cytokine production [9, 12].

The human TNFSF4 gene is located at 1q25. A number of studies have examined the association between TNFSF4 gene polymorphisms and the risk of SLE. For example, Zhou et al. found TNFSF4 rs2205960 with SLE susceptibility in Chinese ($P = 2.82 \times 10^{-5}$) [13]. And Zhang confirmed the association between the TNFSF4 rs1234315 SNPs and the SLE (ORs of 1.45 and P values of 1.5×10^{-16}) [14]. And a recent study also confirms TNFSF4 rsl234315 as a SLE susceptibility locus in a Chinese Guangxi population [1]. There once was a published meta-analysis about the association of TNFSF4 polymorphisms with SLE in 2012, which only focused on four common SNPs, rs2205960, rs1234315, rs844644, and rs844648 [6]. With rapid progress of SLE genetics study and massive new research data available during recent seven years, it's extremely essential to make a meta-analysis update. Thus, in the present study, we performed a meta-analysis to investigate whether six identified TNFSF4 SNPs, rs1234315, rs844648, rs2205960, rs704840, rs844644 and rs10489265 polymorphisms confer susceptibility to SLE in different ethnic groups.

Materials and methods

Identification of eligible studies and data extraction

An exhaustive literature search was conducted using PubMed, MEDLINE, Embase, Web of Science databases, and Cochrane Library databases to examine the TNFSF4 polymorphisms in SLE patients and controls (until February 2021). The following keywords and subject terms were searched in different combinations: "TNFSF4" or "tumor necrosis factor ligand superfamily member 4" or "CD252" or "OX40L" or "OX40 ligand" and "systemic lupus erythematosus" or "SLE". Additionally, potentially relevant studies were also traced from the reference lists of the identified articles. The eligible studies were included according to the following criteria: (1) it contained original data (independence among studies), (2) it used an unrelated case–control design, and (3) it provided sufficient data to calculate the odds ratio (OR). All patients included in these studies fulfilled the American College of Rheumatology criteria [15] or the ACR 1997 revised criteria [16]. When a study reported results on different subpopulations, we treated each subpopulation as a separate study in the meta-analysis. Exclusion criteria were as follows: (1) abstracts, reviews, and meta-analyses; (2) studies without patient samples; (3) studies without usable data; and for duplicate publications, only the most recent or most informative single article was included. Among these articles, the following data was extracted: (1) publication details, including first author's name and publication year; (2) TNFSF4 polymorphisms details, including single-nucleotide polymorphisms (SNPs) and minor allele (MA); (3) characteristics of studied subjects, such as the country and ethnicity of study population, numbers of SLE cases and controls, and TNFSF4 polymorphisms minor allele frequencies(MAF); (4) ORs of associations between different SNPs and SLE susceptibility, as well as their 95% CIs and P value. And original data were requested from study authors if necessary.

Evaluation of statistical associations

Allele frequencies of the TNFSF4 rs1234315, rs844648, rs2205960, rs704840, rs844644 and rs10489265 polymorphisms from each respective study were determined using the allele-counting method. And ORs with 95% CIs were determined in each study to evaluate the correlation of SNPs polymorphisms and SLE susceptibility. The data heterogeneity was examined by Cochran's Q test. When the studies contained no or moderate heterogeneity on the basis of Q test ($P > 0.10$), the fixed-effect model was adopted using the Mantel–Haenszel method, which assumes that genetic factors have similar effects on SLE susceptibility across all studies, and that observed variations between studies are caused by chance alone. By contrast, when a significant Q-statistic ($P < 0.10$) indicated heterogeneity across studies, the random effects model was applied, using the Der Simonian and Laird method, which assumes that different studies show substantial diversity, and assesses both within-study sampling errors and between-study variances. The random effects model is used in the presence of significant between-study heterogeneity. We also quantified the effect of heterogeneity using $I^2 = 100\% \times (Q - df)/Q$. The I^2-statistic measures the degree of inconsistency in the studies, and represents the proportion of inter-study variability attributable to heterogeneity rather than chance. Statistical analysis was performed by utilizing RevMan 5.3 software and STATA package version 12.0 (Stata Corporation, College Station, Texas, USA). The significance of pooled ORs was tested using the Z test ($P < 0.05$ was considered significant).

Evaluation of publication bias

Potential publication bias was assessed by the funnel plot and Begg's and Egger's test in which an asymmetric plot suggests a possible publication bias. Egger's linear regression test was used to measure the funnel plot asymmetry on the natural logarithm scale of the OR. The significance of the intercept was determined by the t test, and a $P < 0.05$ was considered to indicate significant statistical publication bias.

Results

Characteristics of the included studies

As showed in Fig. 1, 92 articles were retrieved at the beginning. Based on the described search criteria, 72 articles were collected for the initial screening after excluding the duplicate articles. Next, 24 records were excluded because they failed to provide patient samples or usable data, since they were abstracts, reviews, meta-analyses or others. And a total of 34 articles were identified as original research. Full-text articles were downloaded and carefully read for eligibility. Among them, 22 studies were excluded because of non-eligible patient samples, non-eligible experimental validations, or non-eligible outcomes. Ultimately, the searches retrieved a total of 12 studies which met the inclusion criteria to be included in the meta-analysis. All SLE patients met the diagnostic criteria of the American College of Rheumatology and Newcastle–Ottawa Quality Assessment Scale (NOS) Scores were 6–8. The characteristics of the included studies are summarized in Table 1.

Subjects were stratified in independent subgroups, and the data of each subgroup were treated as an independent study in the meta-analysis. Therefore, five relevant studies including five separate comparisons on the TNFSF4 rs1234315 polymorphism; two relevant studies including five separate comparisons on the TNFSF4 rs844648 polymorphism; eight relevant studies including ten separate comparisons on the TNFSF4 Rs2205960 polymorphism;

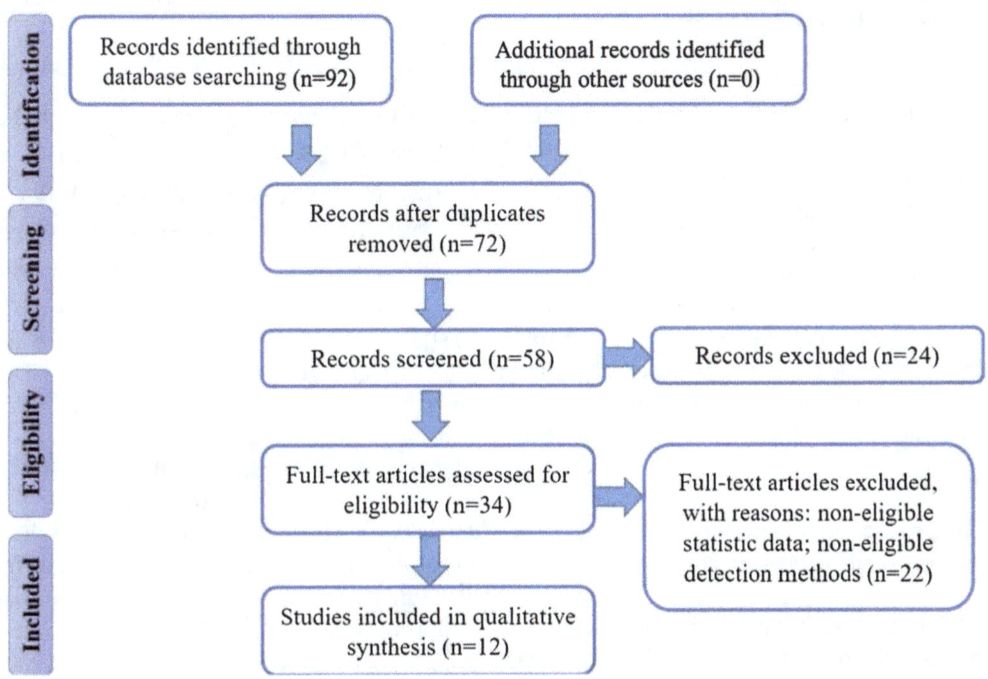

Fig. 1 Flow chart of the study search and selection

Table1 Characteristics of eligible studies in meta-analysis

Reference	Study design	Country	Population(n)		Detection method	TNFSF4 SNPs	NOS
			Case	Control			
Han et al. [17]	Case–control cohort 1	China	1047	1205	GWAS	rs1234315;	8
	Case–control cohort 2		1643	5930		Rs2205960;	
	Case–control cohort 3		1509	1120			
Zhang et al. [14]	Case–control cohort	China	1,344	4,315	RT-PCR	rs1234315	7
Yang et al. [18]	Case–control cohort 1	China;	320	1500	GWAS	rs1234315	8
	Case–control cohort 2	Thailand	2880	2700		rs704840	
Xu et al. [1]	Case–control cohort 1	China	294	282	PCR–RFLP	rs1234315,	5
Chang et al. [19]	Case–control cohort 1	China	314	920	GWAS	rs2205960,	7
	Case–control cohort 2		635	122		rs844644	
						rs844648	
Delgado Vega et al. [20]	Case–control cohort 1	Germany	259	322	GWAS	rs1234314	7
	Case–control cohort 2	Italy	258	223		rs1234317	
	Case–control cohort 3	Spain	517	901		rs844644	
	Case–control cohort 4	Argentina	278	355		rs12039904	
						rs844648	
Gupta et al. [21]	Case–control cohort 1	North Indian	394	583	RT-PCR	rs2205960	5
Zhou et al. [13]	Case–control cohort 1	China	722	804	GWAS	rs2205960	
Sanchez et al. [22]	Case–control cohort	Mestizo	794	649	GWAS	rs2205960	5
Sanchez et al. [23]	Case–control cohort 1	African American	1569	3462	GWAS	rs2205960	6
	Case–control cohort 2		155	132			
Chua et al. [8]	Case–control cohort	Malaysian	476	509	RT-PCR	rs2205960	5
						rs1234315	
						rs8446748	
						rs704840	
Orozco et al. [24]	Case–control cohort	UK	1047	9275	RT-PCR	rs10489265	6

GWAS Genome-wide association study, *NOS* Newcastle–Ottawa scale, *PCR–RFLP* polymerase chain reaction–restriction fragment length polymorphism, *RT-PCR* reverse transcription polymerase chain reaction

three relevant studies including five separate comparisons on the TNFSF4 rs704840 polymorphism; two relevant studies including five separate comparisons on the TNFSF4 rs844644 polymorphism; and two relevant studies including five separate comparisons on the TNFSF4 rs10489265 polymorphism and SLE were identified, respectively. Additionally, a total of 20 separate comparisons, involving 20,114 patients and 35,136 controls (4 European, 13 Asian, 2 African American, and 1 Latin-American populations) were included in our meta-analysis. The main characteristics of each study are described in Table 2.

Meta-analysis of the association between the TNFSF4 rs2205960, rs1234315 and rs704840 polymorphisms and SLE

Firstly, Table 3 showed a summary of the meta-analysis findings on the association between TNFSF4 polymorphisms and SLE. When the allelic effect was examined, the meta-analysis revealed an association between the TNFSF4 rs2205960 T allele and SLE in all subjects (OR 1.42, 95% CI 1.36–1.49, $P < 0.00001$) (Fig. 2a). And the analysis by ethnicity stratification detected a significant association with the rs2205960 polymorphism in both the Asian-derived samples (OR 1.42, 95%CI 1.35–1.49), and the African-derived samples (OR 1.45, 95% CI 1.30–1.62). The consistency of these findings may suggest some genetic homogeneity of SLE rs2205960 SNPs among the populations. For the rs1234315 SNP, an association was also found between SLE and the T allele in the meta-analysis (OR 1.41, 95% CI 1.36–1.46, $P < 0.00001$) (Fig. 2b). However, owing to the limited data available in the literature, those results are all from Asian-derived samples. Similarly, as for the rs704840 SNP, an association was also found in Asian-derived samples between SLE and the G allele in the meta-analysis (OR 1.34, 95% CI 1.26–1.42, $P < 0.00001$) (Fig. 2c). To sum up, overall OR for the three SNPs confer a significant risk for the development of SLE.

Table 2 Characteristics of the individual studies included in meta-analysis

Reference	Country	Ethnicity	Numbers	MAF		OR (95%)		*P* value
				Case	Control	Case	Control	
rs1234315 (T allele)								
Han et al. [17]	China	Asian	4,199	8,255	0.503	0.421	1.37 (1.29–1.45)	2.3×10^{-26}
Zhang et al. [14]	China	Asian	1,344	4,315	0.512	0.395	1.45 (1.34–1.60)	1.5×10^{-16}
Yang et al. [18]	China	Asian	3,300	4,200	0.539	0.468	1.33	1.0×10^{-3}
Xu et al. [1]	China	Asian	294	282	0.531	0.434	1.47 (1.17–1.86)	0.001
Chang et al. [19]	China	Asian	314	920	0.538	0.445	1.46 (1.21–1.75)	4.9×10^{-5}
rs844648 (A allele)								
Delgado Vega et al. [20]	Germany	European	259	322	0.470	0.400	1.29 (1.02–1.63)	3.3×10^{-2}
Delgado Vega et al. [20]	Italy	European	258	223	0.430	0.350	1.40 (1.08–1.82)	1.1×10^{-2}
Delgado Vega et al. [20]	Spain,	European	517	901	0.420	0.440	0.94 (0.80–1.10)	0.407
Delgado Vega et al. [20]	Argentina	Latin American	278	355	0.440	0.520	0.73 (0.58–0.91)	3.9×10^{-3}
Chang et al. [19]	Chinese	Asian	314	920	0.546	0.465	1.39 (1.16–1.66)	4.2×10^{-4}
rs2205960 (T allele)								
V Gupta et al. [21]	India	Asian	394	583	0.277	0.225	1.32 (1.07–1.63)	< 0.01
Zhou et al. [13]	China	Asian	722	804	0.345	0.274	1.39 (1.19–1.62)	2.8×10^{-5}
Sanchez et al. [22]	USA	African-American	767	640	0.370	0.289	1.49 (1.27–1.75)	1.7×10^{-6}
Sanchez et al. [23]	USA	African-American	2839	3441	0.070	0.049	1.44 (1.17–1.76)	5.6×10^{-4}
Han et al. [17]	China	Asian	4,199	8,255	0.347	0.268	1.46 (1.37–1.56)	2.5×10^{-32}
Gupta et al. [21]	Indian	Asian	394	583	0.225	0.277	1.32 (1.07–1.63)	< 0.01
Chua et al. [8]	Chinese	Asian	198	178	0.298	0.248	1.27 (1.00–1.61)	0.05
Chua et al. [8]	Malay	Asian	42	43	0.193	0.189	1.03 (0.64–1.65)	0.91
Chua et al. [8]	Indian	Asian	24	12	0.387	0.167	3.16 (1.41–7.05)	0.004
Chang et al. [19]	Chinese	Asian	314	920	0.331	0.227	1.69 (1.39–2.06)	1.95×10^{-7}
rs704840 (G allele)								
Chua et al. [8]	Chinese	Asian	303	283	0.451	0.394	12.6 (1.02–1.56)	0.03
Chua et al. [8]	Malay	Asian	77	82	0.353	0.360	0.97 (0.67–1.44)	0.89
Chua et al. [8]	Indian	Asian	23	22	0.371	0.306	1.34 (0.65–2.75)	0.42
Chang et al. [19]	Chinese	Asian	314	920	0.490	0.390	1.51 (1.25–1.81)	1.06×10^{-5}
Yang et al. [18]	China	Asian	3,300	4,200	0.491	0.420	1.33	1.21×10^{-3}
rs844644 (A allele)								
Chang et al. [19]	Chinese	Asian	314	920	0.545	0.458	1.41 (1.18–1.70)	1.82×10^{-4}
Delgado Vega et al. [20]	Germany	European	259	322	0.440	0.450	0.97 (0.76–1.22)	0.7691
Delgado Vega et al. [20]	Italy	European	258	223	0.390	0.500	0.64 (0.49–0.82)	5.68×10^{-4}
Delgado Vega et al. [20]	Spain,	European	517	901	0.460	0.450	1.04 (0.89–1.21)	0.6064
Delgado Vega et al. [20]	Argentina	Latin American	278	355	0.350	0.440	0.69 (0.55–0.87)	1.59×10^{-3}
rs10489265 (G allele)								
Zhou et al. [13]	China	Asian	722	804	0.348	0.287	1.33 (1.14–1.55)	3.10×10^{-4}
Orozco et al. [24]	UK	European	3962	9275	0.250	0.240	1.05 (0.99–1.12)	0.11

Meta-analysis of the association between the TNFSF4 rs844644, rs844648 and rs10489265 polymorphisms and SLE

When the allelic effect was examined, the meta-analysis produced overall ORs of 0.92 (95% CI 0.70–1.21, $P=0.54$) for the rs844644 polymorphism based on Asian-derived samples, European-derived samples, and Latin American-derived samples, which suggested that rs844644 SNP did not confer a significant risk for the development of SLE in those three ethnicities (Fig. 3a). The meta-analysis of rs844648 polymorphism also contained the samples from Asian, European, and Latin American. And the overall OR of rs844648 polymorphism was 1.11 (95% CI 0.86–1.43, $P=0.41$) (Fig. 3b), suggesting no significant association at all. As for the rs10489265 SNP, no association was also found in Asian-derived samples between

Table 3 Meta-analysis of the association between the TNFSF4 polymorphisms and SLE

Population	No. of studies	Test of association			Test of heterogeneity		
		OR	95% CI	P	I^2	P	model
rs844648 (A allele)							
Overall	5	1.11	[0.86, 1.43]	0.41	0.87	< 0.00001	Random
European	3	1.18	[0.88, 1.57]	0.26	0.82	0.004	Random
Latin American	1	0.73	[0.58, 0.91]	0.005	-	-	-
Asian	1	1.38	[1.15, 1.66]	< 0.001	–	–	–
rs2205960 (T allele)							
Overall	10	1.42	[1.36, 1.49]	< 0.00001	0	0.79	Fixed
African-American	2	1.45	[1.30, 1.62]	< 0.001	0	0.93	Fixed
Asian	8	1.42	[1.35, 1.49]	< 0.001	0	0.57	Fixed
rs844644 (A allele)							
Overall	5	0.92	[0.70, 1.21]	0.54	0.89	< 0.00001	Random
Asian	1	1.41	[1.18, 1.70]	< 0.001	–	–	–
European	3	0.87	[0.66, 1.15]	0.34	0.81	0.005	Random
Latin American	1	0.69	[0.55, 0.87]	0.001	–	–	–
rs10489265 (G allele)							
Overall	2	1.17	[0.94, 1.47]	0.17	0.87	0.006	Random
Asian	1	1.33	[1.14, 1.55]	< 0.001	–	–	–
European	1	1.06	[0.99, 1.12]	0.11	–	–	–
rs1234315 (T allele)							
Overall	5	1.41	[1.36, 1.46]	< 0.00001	0.68	0.01	Random
Asian	5	1.41	[1.36, 1.46]	< 0.00001	0.68	0.01	Random
rs704840 (G allele)							
Overall	5	1.34	[1.26, 1.42]	< 0.00001	0	0.43	Fixed
Asian	5	1.34	[1.26, 1.42]	< 0.00001	0	0.43	Fixed

SLE and the G allele in the meta-analysis (OR 1.17, 95% CI 0.94–1.47, $P=0.17$) (Fig. 3c). And the analysis by ethnicity stratification detected a significant association with the rs10489265 SNP in Asian-derived samples (OR 1.33, 95%CI 1.14–1.55, $P<0.001$), but not in European-derived samples (OR 1.06, 95%CI 0.99–1.12, $P=0.11$), which might suggest genetic heterogeneity of rs10489265 SNP among the populations. Due to the small number of studies available to date, it is difficult to assess this SNP in other populations. In conclusion, no statistically significant findings were observed on the association of rs844644, rs844648 and rs10489265 polymorphisms and SLE in our analysis.

Heterogeneity and publication bias

The P value of the Q test showed between-study heterogeneity in the overall analysis (Table 2). We conducted analyses using the random-effects models. In the analysis for the rs2205960 and rs704840 polymorphisms, no between-study heterogeneity was found. Therefore, the fixed-effects models were performed. Egger's linear regression test was used to assess the publication bias. Based on our results, there was no publication bias in all comparisons.

Discussion

In the current study, we investigated whether the major confirmed genetic risk loci of TNFSF4 gene were associated with SLE susceptibility. To our knowledge, the rs1234315 and rs2205960 in the TNFSF4 gene were both identified as a genetic risk factor for SLE, which is also consist with previous reported [6]. Since the genetic determinants often show discrepancies in different ethnic populations, overall OR for the rest four SNPs: the rs844648, rs704840, rs844644 and rs10489265 polymorphisms in the TNFSF4 gene did not confer a significant risk for the development of SLE. The replication study of different populations to clarify the genetic basis of SLE is still urgently need.

The importance of TNFSF4 as a SLE susceptibility gene was firstly underlined using both a family-based and a case–control study design [25]. It revealed that there was a single risk haplotype for SLE in the upstream region of TNFSF4, which is related to the up-expression of both cell-surface TNFSF4 and the TNFSF4 transcript,

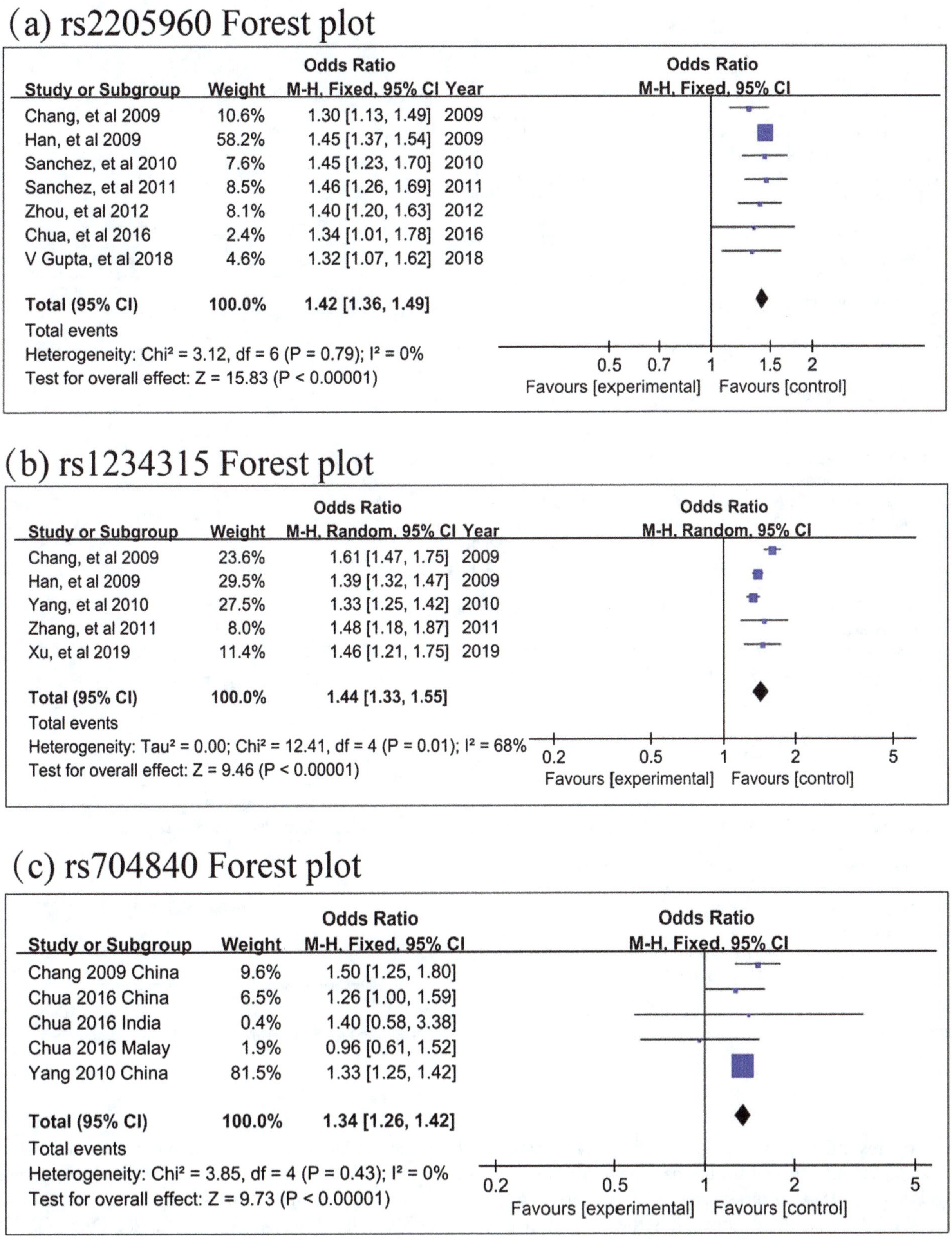

Fig.2 Forest plot for the meta-analysis of the association between the tumor necrosis factor ligand superfamily member 4 (TNFSF4) rs2205960 polymorphism (Tvs.G) (**a**), rs1234315 polymorphism (Tvs.C) (**b**), rs704840 polymorphism (**c**) and SLE

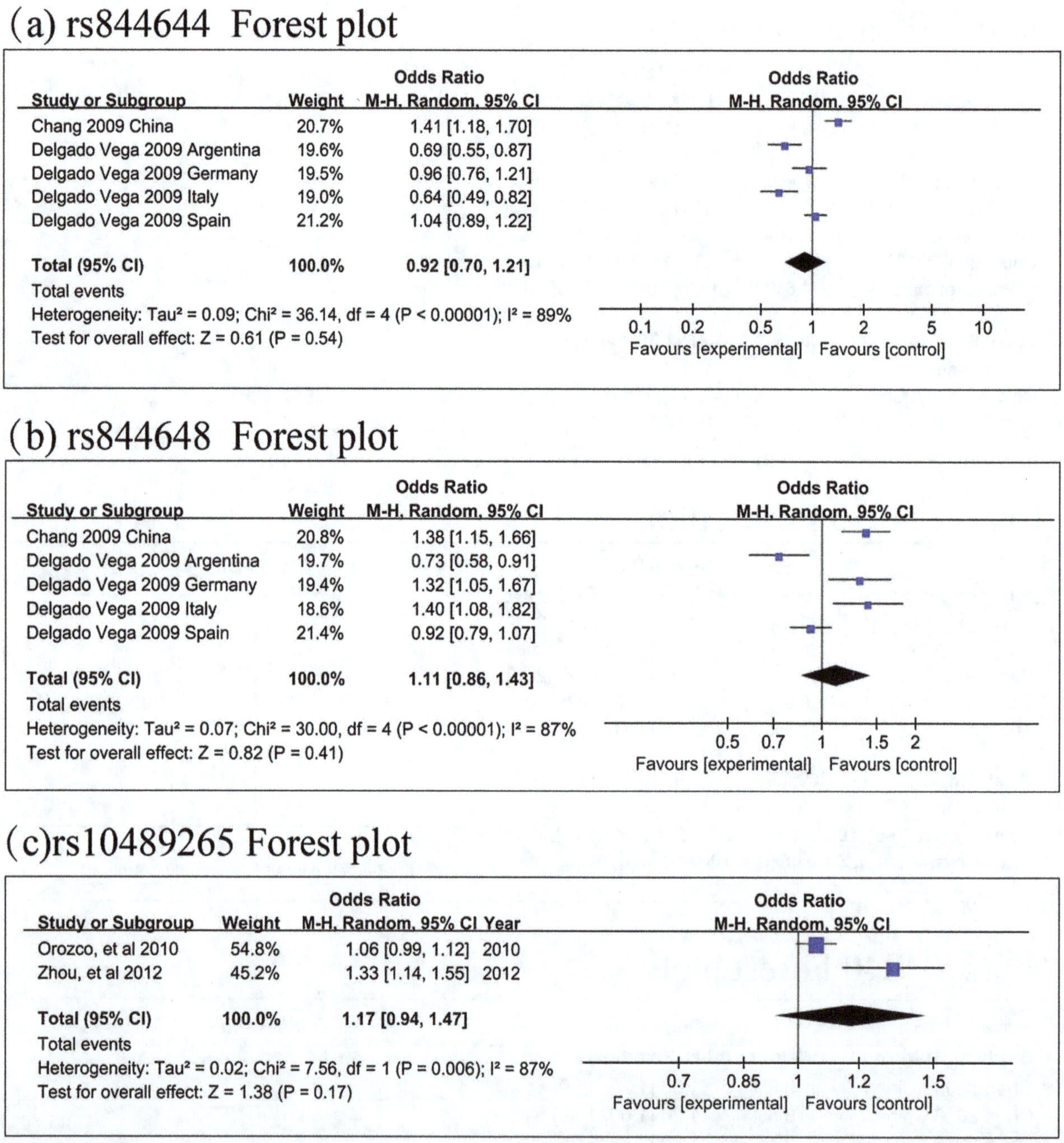

Fig.3 Forest plot for the meta-analysis of the association between TNFSF4 rs844644 polymorphism (Cvs.A) (**a**), TNFSF4 rs844648 polymorphism (Avs.G) (**b**), rs10489265 polymorphism (**c**) and SLE

probably resulting in augmenting T cell-APC interaction [25]. Consistently, several studies have demonstrated up-regulation of OX40L expression in SLE patients or SLE animal models [10, 26]. In one study the serum level of OX40L, and the percentages of OX40+CD4+T cells were suggested as indicators of lupus nephritis, and SLE, respectively [10]. Clement et al. reported that the frequency of blood active phenotype T follicular helper cells is increased in active SLE patients [27]. Several genes recently identified in WGA studies are components of B cell pathways, like OX4OL [28]. OX40-OX40L interaction may quantitatively enhance B cell proliferation, and augment the B cell hyperactivity, contributing to excess autoantibodies generation through promoting aberrant Tfh cells immunity response. Therefore, targeting OX40-OX40L interaction by blockade either OX40 or OX40L have the potential therapy for SLE [27]. Zhou et al. reported the therapeutic effect of anti-OX40L mAb in lupus-prone BXSB mice, with attenuation of concanavalin A (ConA)-induced proliferation, decrease of T helper cell cytokine secretion like IFN-γ and IL-6, and down-regulation of anti-dsDNA antibody production, by blocking the OX40-OX40L co-stimulatory pathway [29]. Collectively, those results confirmed a vital role of OX40L in the pathogenesis of SLE.

Polymorphisms in the TNFSF4 gene have been widely studied to assess the association with an increased risk for autoimmune diseases (ADs) susceptibility. A recent study confirmed the significant association between TNFSF4 rs1234315 polymorphisms and SLE and rheumatoid arthritis (RA) susceptibility both in allelic and genotypic levels in a Chinese Guangxi population [1]. Similarly, Zhang et al. also confirmed the association between the SNP and the SLE susceptibility [ORs $=1.45$ and $P=1.5\times10^{-16}$] by genotyping the SNPs rs1234315 near the TNFSF4 gene in 1,344 SLE patients and 4,315 controls of Chinese population [14]. Furthermore, the association was also confirmed in populations from East Asians, and Europeans [1]. However, some controversial results were also existed. Chua et al. did not find any significant correlation between alleles of TNFSF4 rs1234315 with SLE, and the OR values of the minor T allele in Indian, Chinese, and Malay populations were 1.45 (95% CI: 0.73–2.87), 1.20 (95% CI: 0.97–1.48), and 1.02 (95% CI: 0.70–1.49), respectively [8]. Besides the controversial results about rs1234315 polymorphisms, other TNFSF4 SNPs rs2205960, rs844644 or rs844648 polymorphisms also have the same situation. For example, Delgado-Vega et al. conducted replicated study in four countries including Germany, Italy, Spain and Argentina, and they found that rs844648 polymorphisms were strongly associated with SLE in the Argentineans and Italians, and displayed only weak association in the Germans, however, there was no statistical significance in the Spanish set, which was quite different from the first study they reported [20]. As SLE is distributed worldwide, some candidate gene and GWAS conducted in European- and Asian-derived SLE patients have identified several TNFSF4 SNPs conferring susceptibility to SLE [30–33], however, one study among those GWAS did not replicate this conclusion in African- and Hispanic-derived SLE patients [30]. Additionally, another GWAS carried out in Latin Americans failed to identify the association between TNFSF4 SNPs and SLE susceptibility [34]. Moreover, although two candidate gene studies which identified the association between TNFSF4 SNPs (rs2205960 and rs1234315) and SLE susceptibility included Mexican patients, the number of Mexican SLE patients was not well defined [22, 35]. To our knowledge, the disparity of those findings may be partially attributable to the existence of genetic heterogeneity of SLE among the populations. To validate the association, it is necessary to put the emphasis on replication in a larger scale of populations with different genetic backgrounds, especially the Latin Americans owing to limited data available currently. Besides, meta-analysis is recommended to augment sample size by the pooling of data from individual association studies, so that the statistical power to analyze genetic effects will be enhanced.

Accordingly, we summarized previously published related studies and performed a meta-analysis on the association of the TNFSF4 rs1234315, rs844648, rs2205960, rs704840, rs844644, rs10489265 polymorphisms and SLE susceptibility. Although detailed mechanisms of TNFSF4 SNPs in pathogenesis of SLE still need further explored, our study provided further potential evidence for TNFSF4 as a risk factor of SLE, which might possess some potential diagnostic and therapeutic implications and help to give some reference for SLE patients therapy.

Conclusions

Our meta-analysis demonstrated that the TNFSF4 rs2205960, rs1234315 and rs704840 SNPs was significantly associated with an increased risk of SLE in the overall population samples. It provides further evidence that the TNFSF4 gene plays a significant role in the etiology of SLE. However, despite those advantages, certain limitations were also existed in our meta-analysis. For instance, the number of included studies, and the investigative genotypes of the included studies were limited, so our attempt to conduct a more detailed subgroup analysis may also be limited. Therefore, further large-scale studies are needed to promote our understanding of the association between TNFSF4 polymorphisms and SLE susceptibility.

Abbreviations

TNFSF4: Tumor necrosis factor ligand superfamily member 4; SLE: Systemic lupus erythematosus; SNPs: Single nucleotide polymorphisms; ORs: Odds ratios; CIs: Confidence intervals; GWAS: Genome-wide association studies; APCs: Antigen-presenting cells; DCs: Dendritic cells; MA: Minor allele; MAF: Minor allele frequencies; LN: Lupus nephritis; ConA: Concanavalin A; ADs: Autoimmune diseases; RA: Rheumatoid arthritis.

Acknowledgements

Not applicable.

Authors' contributions

Conceived and designed the experiments: Yu Fu; Managed the database: Yu Fu; Contributed materials/analysis tools: Qing Lin and Zhi-rong Zhang;

Analyzed the data and wrote the paper: Yu Fu. All authors read and approved the final manuscript.

Author details

[1]College of Pharmaceutical Sciences, Southwest University, Chongqing 400715, China. [2]Key Laboratory of Drug Targeting and Drug Delivery System of the Education Ministry, Sichuan Engineering Laboratory for Plant-Sourced Drug and Sichuan Research Center for Drug Precision Industrial Technology, West China School of Pharmacy, Sichuan University, Chengdu 610064, China.

References

1. Xu J, He Y, Wang J, Li X, Huang L, Li S, et al. Influence of the TNFSF4 rs1234315 polymorphism in the susceptibility to systemic lupus erythematosus and rheumatoid arthritis. Hum Immunol. 2019;80(4):270–5. https://doi.org/10.1016/j.humimm.2018.11.006.
2. Luan H, Li P, Cao C, Li C, Hu C, Zhang S, et al. A single-nucleotide polymorphism of the STAT4 gene is associated with systemic lupus erythematosus (SLE) in female Chinese population. Rheumatol Int. 2012;32(5):1251–5.
3. Teruel M, Alarcon-Riquelme ME. Genetics of systemic lupus erythematosus and Sjogren's syndrome: an update. Curr Opin Rheumatol. 2016;28(5):506–14.
4. Zuo XB, Sheng YJ, Hu SJ, Gao JP, Li Y, Tang HY, et al. Variants in TNFSF4, TNFAIP3, TNIP1, BLK, SLC15A4 and UBE2L3 interact to confer risk of systemic lupus erythematosus in Chinese population. Rheumatol Int. 2014;34(4):459–64.
5. Mok CC, Lau CS. Pathogenesis of systemic lupus erythematosus. J Clin Pathol. 2003;56(7):481.
6. Lu MM, Xu WD, Yang J, Ye QL, Feng CC, Li J, et al. Association of TNFSF4 polymorphisms with systemic lupus erythematosus: a meta-analysis. Mod Rheumatol. 2013;23(4):686–93.
7. Lee YH, Song GG. Associations between TNFSF4 and TRAF1-C5 gene polymorphisms and systemic lupus erythematosus: a meta-analysis. Hum Immunol. 2012;73(10):1050–4.
8. Chua KH, Ooh YY, Chai HC. TNFSF4 polymorphisms are associated with systemic lupus erythematosus in the Malaysian population. Int J Immunogenet. 2016;43(5):303–9.
9. Webb GJ, Hirschfield GM, Lane PJ. OX40, OX40L and Autoimmunity: a Comprehensive Review. Clin Rev Allergy Immunol. 2016;50(3):312–32.
10. Farres MN, Al-Zifzaf DS, Aly AA, Abd Raboh NM. OX40/OX40L in systemic lupus erythematosus: association with disease activity and lupus nephritis. Ann Saudi Med. 2011;31(1):29–34.
11. Ishii N, Takahashi T, Soroosh P, Sugamura K. OX40–OX40 ligand interaction in t-cell-mediated immunity and immunopathology. 2010;105:63–98.
12. Sugamura K, Ishii N, Weinberg AD. Therapeutic targeting of the effector T-cell co-stimulatory molecule OX40. Nat Rev Immunol. 2004;4(6):420–31.
13. Zhou XJ, Lu XL, Nath SK, Lv JC, Zhu SN, Yang HZ, et al. Gene-gene interaction of BLK, TNFSF4, TRAF1, TNFAIP3, and REL in systemic lupus erythematosus. Arthritis Rheum. 2012;64(1):222–31.
14. Zhang SQ, Han JW, Sun LD, Lu WS, Yin XY, Zhang XJ, et al. A single-nucleotide polymorphism of the TNFSF4 gene is associated with systemic lupus erythematosus in Chinese Han population. Rheumatol Int. 2011;31(2):227–31.
15. Tan EM, Cohen AS, Fries JF, Masi AT, McShane DJ, Rothfield NF, et al. The 1982 revised criteria for the classification of systemic lupus erythematosus. Arthritis Rheum. 1982;25(11):1271–7.
16. Hochberg MC. Updating the American college of rheumatology revised criteria for the classification of systemic lupus erythematosus. Arthritis Rheum. 1997;40(9):1725–1725.
17. Han JW, Zheng HF, Cui Y, Sun LD, Ye DQ, Hu Z, et al. Genome-wide association study in a Chinese Han population identifies nine new susceptibility loci for systemic lupus erythematosus. Nat Genet. 2009;41(11):1234–7.
18. Yang W, Shen N, Ye DQ, Liu Q, Zhang Y, Qian XX, et al. Genome-wide association study in Asian populations identifies variants in ETS1 and WDFY4 associated with systemic lupus erythematosus. PLoS Genet. 2010;6(2):e1000841.
19. Chang YK, Yang W, Zhao M, Mok CC, Chan TM, Wong RW, et al. Association of BANK1 and TNFSF4 with systemic lupus erythematosus in Hong Kong Chinese. Genes Immun. 2009;10(5):414–20.
20. Delgado-Vega AM, Abelson AK, Sanchez E, Witte T, D'Alfonso S, Galeazzi M, et al. Replication of the TNFSF4 (OX40L) promoter region association with systemic lupus erythematosus. Genes Immun. 2009;10(3):248–53.
21. Gupta V, Kumar S, Pratap A, Singh R, Kumari R, Kumar S, et al. Association of ITGAM, TNFSF4, TNFAIP3 and STAT4 gene polymorphisms with risk of systemic lupus erythematosus in a North Indian population. Lupus. 2018;27(12):1973–9.
22. Sanchez E, Webb RD, Rasmussen A, Kelly JA, Riba L, Kaufman KM, et al. Genetically determined Amerindian ancestry correlates with increased frequency of risk alleles for systemic lupus erythematosus. Arthritis Rheum. 2010;62(12):3722–9.
23. Sanchez E, Comeau ME, Freedman BI, Kelly JA, Kaufman KM, Langefeld CD, et al. Identification of novel genetic susceptibility loci in African American lupus patients in a candidate gene association study. Arthritis Rheum. 2011;63(11):3493–501.
24. Orozco G, Eyre S, Hinks A, Bowes J, Morgan AW, Wilson AG, et al. Study of the common genetic background for rheumatoid arthritis and systemic lupus erythematosus. Ann Rheum Dis. 2011;70(3):463–8.
25. Cunninghame Graham DS, Graham RR, Manku H, Wong AK, Whittaker JC, Gaffney PM, et al. Polymorphism at the TNF superfamily gene TNFSF4 confers susceptibility to systemic lupus erythematosus. Nat Genet. 2008;40(1):83–9.
26. Yoshioka T, Nakajima A, Akiba H, Ishiwata T, Asano G, Yoshino SI et al. Contribution of ligand interaction to the pathogenesis of rheumatoid arthritis. Eur J Immunol 2000; 30(10):2815–2823
27. Jacquemin C, Schmitt N, Contin-Bordes C, Liu Y, Narayanan P, Seneschal J, et al. OX40 ligand contributes to human lupus pathogenesis by promoting T follicular helper response. Immunity. 2015;42(6):1159–70.
28. Manku H, Graham DSC, Vyse TJ. Association of the co-stimulator OX40L with systemic lupus erythematosus. J Mol Med. 2009;87(3):229–34.
29. Zhou Y-B, Ye R-G, Li Y-J, Xie C-M, Wu Y-H. Effect of anti-CD134L mAb and CTLA4Ig on ConA-induced proliferation, Th cytokine secretion, and anti-dsDNA antibody production in spleen cells from lupus-prone BXSB mice. Autoimmunity. 2008;41(5):395–404.
30. Langefeld CD, Ainsworth HC, Graham DSC, Kelly JA, Comeau ME, Marion MC, et al. Transancestral mapping and genetic load in systemic lupus erythematosus. Nat Commun. 2017;8:16021.
31. Graham DSC, Graham RR, Manku H, Wong AK, Whittaker JC, Gaffney PM, et al. Polymorphism at the TNF superfamily gene TNFSF4 confers susceptibility to systemic lupus erythematosus. Nat Genet. 2008;40:83–9.
32. Lee H-S, Kim T, Bang SY, Na YJ, Kim I, Kim K, et al. Ethnic specificity of lupus-associated loci identified in a genome-wide association study in Korean women. Ann Rheum Dis. 2014;73:1240.
33. Yang W, Shen N, Ye DQ, Liu Q, Zhang Y, Qian XX, et al. Asian Lupus Genetics, Genome-wide association study in Asian populations identifies variants in ETS1 and WDFY4 associated with systemic lupus erythematosus. PLoS Genet. 2010;6:e1000841.
34. Alarcón-Riquelme ME, Ziegler JT, Molineros J, Howard TD, Moreno-Estrada A, Sánchez-Rodríguez E, et al. Genome-wide association study in an amerindian ancestry population reveals novel systemic lupus erythematosus risk loci and the role of european admixture. Arthrit Rheumatol. 2016;68:932–43.
35. Manku H, Langefeld CD, Guerra SG, Malik TH, Alarcon-Riquelme M, Anaya JM, et al. Trans-ancestral studies fine map the SLE-susceptibility locus TNFSF4. PLoS Genet. 2013;9:e1003554.

19

Social media use in patients with fibromyalgia and its effect on symptom severity and sleep quality

Sevinç Külekçioğlu[1*] and Alp Çetin[2]

Abstract

Background: The aim of this study was to evaluate social media use in patients with fibromyalgia syndrome (FMS) and determine the effect of social media use on disease severity and sleep quality.

Materials and methods: In total, 205 social media using patients with similar characteristics were included in the study. The study group consisted of 103 patients with FMS, and the control group consisted of 102 patients without FMS. The FMS symptom severity scale and diffuse pain index were used to determine the disease severity in FMS patients, the sleep disorder short form questionnaire (PROMIS) was used to evaluate sleep quality, and the Social Media Addiction Scale-Adult Form was used to evaluate social media addiction. A visual analog scale was applied to evaluate pain in both the patient and control groups, and social media usage times were recorded.

Results: We found that pain severity, sleep disturbance and social media addiction were higher in patients with FMS than in the control group, and there was no relationship between the rates of social media use in patients with FMS and the severity and prevalence of the disease.

Conclusion: The use of social media is more frequent in patients with FMS, which can motivate healthcare professionals to evaluate social media habits in individuals with FMS.

Keywords: Fibromyalgia, Social media, Addiction, Sleep disorders, Pain, Problematic social media use

Introduction

Fibromyalgia syndrome (FMS) is a chronic disease characterized by widespread, permanent musculoskeletal system pain accompanied by symptoms such as fatigue, sleep disorders, depression, anxiety, and cognitive disorders [1]. In a recent study, the prevalence of FMS was found to be 0.2–6.6% in the general population and 2.4–6.8% in females [2]. Because of its symptoms, FMS has been found to affect daily functions both physically and psychologically [3, 4]. FMS may be seen together with various psychiatric disorders. The prevalence of emotional problems is high, and anxiety disorders, depression, and sleep disorders often accompany FMS [5–9]. Poor sleep has been reported by approximately 80% of FMS patients [10]. Epidemiological studies have shown that poor sleep quality is a risk factor for fibromyalgia, and poor sleep has been associated with the severity of symptoms in the fibromyalgia population [11, 12].

Information technology in the form of computers and the internet has entered every area of life and is increasingly spreading throughout the world [13, 14]. The implementation of the internet and internet-linked applications on mobile devices and communication systems, not just computers, has transformed people of all ages from passive users into individuals producing active content [14]. According to Internet World Statistics (2017) research, the number of internet users has reached approximately

*Correspondence: sevinckulek@gmail.com

[1] Physical Medicine and Rehabilitation, City Hospital, Bursa, Turkey

3 billion, 732 million (49.6%) worldwide [14]. Social media applications have been highlighted as the most commonly used feature of the internet [15]. According to Turkish Statistics Institution data (TUIK, 2016), the rate of internet users in Turkey is 61.2% of the population; of these, 82.4% use social media [13, 14]. There are various reasons for the high use of social media, such as establishing communication with people, publishing personal posts, following local and international news, learning, researching, and enjoyment [15–17]. It is also thought that people use social media to increase their self-confidence and to be able to share their thoughts and feelings [16, 18]. However, it has been emphasized that, as social media use increases, there is an increased risk of social media addiction and psychopathological symptoms [19–21]. Social media addiction is seen as a behavioral addiction that includes active interaction [22]. While there is an association between routine social media use and positive health outcomes, excessive use of social media has been found to be associated with depressive symptoms, anxiety, and sleep disorders [19–21, 23]. The frequent observation of anxiety, sleep disorders and depressive symptoms in FMS patients suggests that social media use may be different in FMS patients. To the best of our knowledge, there has been no previous study in the literature on the social media use of FMS patients. Against this background, the aim of the present study is not to discuss the true nature of excessive social media use but rather to address the widespread social media agenda in terms of pain and sleep disturbance. Here we emphasize the need to seek a new perspective to keep in mind when examining harmful aspects.

In this study, we aimed to evaluate the use of social media by FMS patients and determine its effect on disease severity and sleep disorders.

Patients and methods

This prospective, cross-sectional study was conducted in the Physical Medicine and Rehabilitation (PMR) Clinic of Bursa City Hospital. Overall, 205 social media user patients were included in the study. The study group included 103 patients aged > 18 years who presented at the PMR clinic and were diagnosed with FMS according to the 2016 ACR revised diagnostic criteria [24]. These patients diagnosed with FMS were treated for anxiety, sleep disturbance or depression for at least 3 months. The control group consisted of 102 patients who presented to the PMR outpatient clinic with a complaint of pain for at least 3 months, had not received any psychiatric treatment in the last 3 months, had no history of anxiety or depression, and had not been diagnosed with FMS. Patients were excluded from the study if they had a malignant disease, any central or peripheral neurological disease, cognitive problems, severe systemic disease, severe degenerative changes, or an educational level that would prevent them from completing the questionnaire. All patients' data, such as sex, educational status, marital status, occupation, age, height, weight, and body mass index (BMI), were recorded. The length of stay on social media (SSM) was recorded in minutes/day (min/d). The visual analog scale (VAS) was used to assess pain severity. The VAS is a common, simple method with robust validity and reliability. The physician explained the meaning of each number to the patients on a scale of 10 cm (cm) and asked them to mark the severity of pain. For the evaluation of sleep in all the study participants, the Patient Reported Outcomes Measurement Information System (PROMIS) 8-item sleep disorder short form questionnaire was used [25]. This self-reported form evaluates, and scores sleep quality, sleep depth, adequacy, and satisfaction with sleep in the last 7 days. To evaluate social media addiction, the Social Media Addiction Scale-Adult Form (SMAS-AF) was used, which was developed by Şahin and Yağci [14]. Before completing the form, all patients with and without FMS were informed about which applications were included in social media use (Facebook, Instagram, Twitter, and YouTube). The SMAS-AF comprises 20 items in 2 subdimensions (virtual tolerance and virtual communication), which are answered with 5-point Likert-type responses. The virtual tolerance subdimension comprises items 1–11, and the virtual communication subdimension comprises items 12–20. Item number 5 and 11 are scored in reverse. The 5-point scoring is applied as "(1) Definitely not appropriate," "(2) Not appropriate," "(3) Undecided," "(4) Appropriate" and "(5) Quite appropriate." Negative statements are reverse-scored. The maximum points obtained from the scale range from 20 to 100, with high points indicating that the individual perceives themselves to have social media addiction. To determine the disease severity in FMS patients, the FMS symptom severity scale and the widespread pain index were used [24]. The total score was recorded by adding the scores obtained from this scale and index. Recording the general characteristics of the patients, age, height, weight, BMI, and SSM time measurements were made and recorded by a specialist doctor. Questionnaires were filled out by the patients.

Statistical analysis

In the study, the descriptive statistics of the patients were given as the means and standard deviations, and the Shapiro Wilk test was used to examine the assumption of normality of the measurements. According to the results, nonparametric methods were used because the number of groups was small, and the test results were appropriate. The Mann–Whitney U test and Kruskal–Wallis test were performed to examine the measurements in groups. The chi-square test was used to examine the differences in patient characteristics according to study groups, and the Spearman correlation test was used to examine the relationships between patient measurements and disease scores. In the study, p values less than 0.05 were considered statistically significant ($\alpha = 0.05$). Analyses were finalized with the help of the SPSS 25.0 package program.

Results

The general characteristics of 205 patients participating in the study are shown in Table 1, and the measurement results are shown in Table 2. The time spent on social media was longer in patients in the FMS group; the measured VAS score, PROMIS Sleep score and SMAF score values were higher than those in the control group (Table 3) (Fig. 1); and there was no difference in the distribution of general characteristics and measurements between the FMS and control groups (Table 4). The analysis of the relationship between FMS disease severity and patient characteristics in the FMS group is shown in Table 5. Table 6 shows the analysis of the relationship between SSM duration, PROMIS sleep score, SMAE score and patient characteristics in the FMS group. Students were found to spend more time on social media than other professions. The evaluation of the relationship between patient characteristics and scores is shown in Table 7. In both groups, the relationship between the age of the patients and SSM duration was weak and inversely proportional, whereas the time spent on social media decreased as age increased. The relationship between the scores according to patient group is shown in Table 8.

Table 1 Examination of general characteristics of patients

Patient characteristics	Category	n	n %
Group	FMS	103	50.2
	Control	102	49.8
Gender	Male	182	88.8
	Female	23	11.2
Education	Primary	97	47.3
	High school	64	31.2
	University	44	21.5
Marital Status	Married	176	85.9
	Single	29	14.1
Occupation	Housewife	93	45.4
	Worker	56	27.3
	Desk job	34	16.6
	Student	8	3.9
	Retired	14	6.8

Table 2 Analysis of patient measurements

Measurement	Mean ± SD
Age	44.75 ± 11.19
Height	162.9 ± 7.56
Weight	72.02 ± 13.02
BMI	27.15 ± 4.75
SSM duration (min/day)	103.83 ± 86.51
VAS score	4.61 ± 2.02
PROMIS sleep score	21.18 ± 11.04
SMAF score	39.11 ± 11.23
FMS score	16.08 ± 3.86

SD standard deviation

Discussion

In this study, we evaluated the social media usage of FMS patients and investigated the effect of this on disease severity and sleep quality. The detected VAS score, PROMIS sleep score and SMAS score were higher in patients with FMS than in the control group, and pain severity, sleep disturbance and social media addiction were higher in patients with FMS. Although studies in the literature have shown a relationship between intense social media use and depression, anxiety, and sleep disorders, to the best of our knowledge [21, 23, 26], no study has investigated social media use in FMS patients. Depression, anxiety, and sleep problems are often seen in FMS patients, and this may be associated with more intense social media use. In this study, significantly more social media use was found in FMS patients, but interestingly, no relationship was found between the rates of social media use in patients with FMS and the severity or prevalence of the disease. These data suggest that social media use is more associated with the abovementioned symptoms accompanying FMS rather than the symptom severity and extent of FMS. Social media use may be

Table 3 Analysis of patient measurements according to groups

Measurement	Group		p
	FMS	Control	
	Mean ± SD	Mean ± SD	
Age	44.37 ± 9.63	45.13 ± 12.61	0.62
Height	162.29 ± 6.79	163.51 ± 8.24	0.25
Weight	71.5 ± 1.3	72.55 ± 12.77	0.56
BMI	27.16 ± 4.98	27.15 ± 4.53	0.98
SSM duration	153.2 ± 93.95	53.97 ± 34.73	0.01*
VAS score	5.16 ± 2.03	4.06 ± 1.85	0.01*
PROMIS sleep score	27.31 ± 8.61	14.98 ± 9.71	0.01*
SMAF score	44.56 ± 11.23	33.6 ± 8.14	0.01*

*$p < 0.05$ significant difference

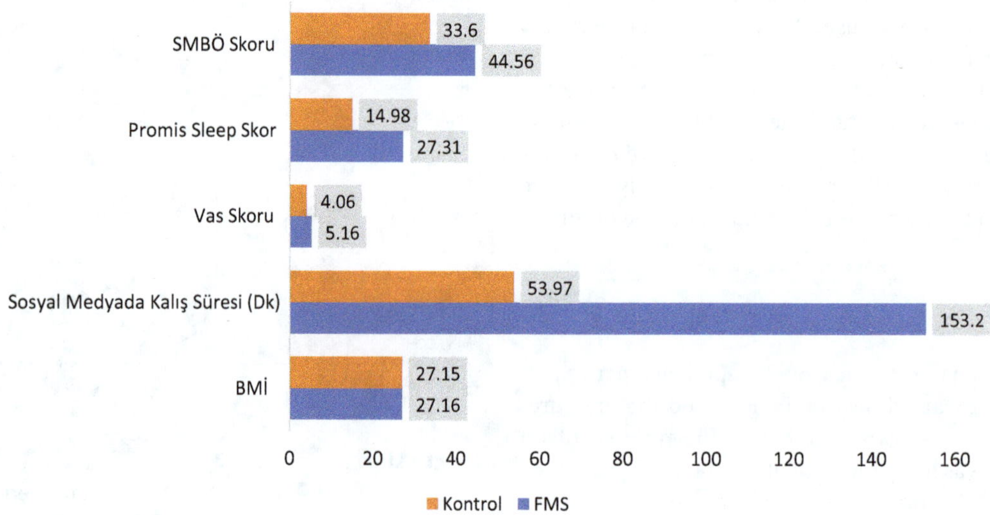

Fig. 1 Analysis of patient measurements according to groups

Table 4 Analysis of general characteristics of patients according to groups

General characteristics of patients	Group				*p*
	FMS		Control		
	n	n %	n	n %	
Gender					
Male	93	90.3	89	87.3	0.49
Female	10	9.7	13	12.7	
Education					
Primary	55	53.4	42	41.2	0.21
High school	28	27.2	36	35.3	
University	20	19.4	24	23.5	
Marital status					
Married	89	86.4	87	85.3	0.89
Single	14	13.6	15	14.7	
Occupation					
Housewife	49	47.6	44	43.1	0.82
Worker	30	29.1	26	25.5	
Desk job	14	13.6	20	19.6	
Student	4	3.9	4	3.9	
Retired	6	5.8	8	7.8	

Table 5 Analysis of the relationship between FMS disease severity and patient characteristics in the FMS group

Patient characteristics	FMS disease severity Mean ± SD	*p*
Gender		
Male	16.11 ± 3.7	0.36
Female	15.9 ± 5.4	
Education		
Primary	15.49 ± 3.43	0.19
High school	17.68 ± 4.94	
University	15.5 ± 2.59	
Marital status		
Married	15.93 ± 4.02	0.15
Single	17.07 ± 2.56	
Occupation		
Housewife	16.35 ± 3.64	0.07
Worker	15.27 ± 4.23	
Desk job	15.86 ± 2.44	
Student	16.00 ± 2.45	
Retired	18.67 ± 6.38	

affected by several factors like as age, gender, marital status, occupation, and educational level. Previous studies have shown that young people are also more likely to use social media due to their easier adaptation to technology and their desire to use technology intensively [27, 28]. Similarly, in this study, a negative relationship was found between age and duration of social media use. When the FMS group was evaluated in terms of occupations, although there was no difference in the SMAF scores of the students, the SSM duration was found to be significantly longer, and this was attributed to the fact that young people and students stay on social media more for entertainment purposes. The fact that the students in the control group had a longer SSM period supports this view. Sleep disorders are commonly seen in FMS. Previous studies have shown that 80% of FMS patients have sleep disorders [26, 29]. In accordance with the literature, in this study, there was also an association between

Table 6 Analysis of the relationship between SSM duration, PROMIS sleep score, SMAF score and patient characteristics in the FMS group

	SSM duration Mean ± SD	PROMIS sleep score Mean ± SD	SMAF score Mean ± SD	*p* ssm	*p* promis	*p* smaf
Gender						
Male	104.01 ± 85.04	21.32 ± 11.1	38.94 ± 11.27	0.26	0.31	0.35
Female	102.39 ± 99.51	20 ± 10.72	40.43 ± 11.04			
Education						
Primary	91.24 ± 67.59	21.68 ± 11.04	37.62 ± 11.3	0.09	0.23	0.41
High school	118.98 ± 107.99	21.27 ± 11.77	40.39 ± 11.77			
University	109.55 ± 86.53	19.93 ± 10.04	40.52 ± 10.02			
Marital status						
Married	98.66 ± 80.14	21.03 ± 10.87	38.88 ± 11.39	0.0	0.42	0.38
Single	135.17 ± 114.9	22.03 ± 12.18	40.52 ± 10.27			
Occupation						
Housewife	89.19 ± 73	21.1 ± 11.03	37.52 ± 11.02	0.01*	0.12	0.22
Worker	106.7 ± 90.53	22.32 ± 11.34	40.57 ± 11.39			
Desk job	113.24 ± 77.79	21.32 ± 10.24	40.5 ± 10.22			
Student	215.63 ± 142.06	17.38 ± 11.6	46.13 ± 9.93			
Retired	102.86 ± 96.65	18.93 ± 12.21	36.43 ± 13.46			

**p* value ranges from 0.01 to 0.05; there is a statistically significant difference

Table 7 Determination of the relationship between patient characteristics and scores

Group	Measurement		SSM duration	VAS score	PROMIS sleep score	SMAF score	FMS disease score
FMS	Age	r	− 0.296**	0.014	0.133	− 0.015	− 0.162
		p	0.012	0.972	0.182	0.884	0.102
	Height	r	0.145	− 0.032	− 0.012	0.157	0.015
		p	0.145	0.751	0.983	0.112	0.957
	Weight	r	− 0.017	− 0.055	0.044	0.081	0.015
		p	0.868	0.581	0.662	0.414	0.881
	BMI	r	− 0.080	− 0.054	0.058	0.016	− 0.018
		p	0.423	0.586	0.558	0.871	0.936
Control	Age	r	− 0.246**	0.066	− 0.132	− 0.120	
		p	0.013	0.511	0.187	0.231	
	Height	r	− 0.043	− 0.047	0.045	0.106	
		p	0.670	0.650	0.657	0.290	
	Weight	r	− 0.142	− 0.053	− 0.045	− 0.093	
		p	0.155	0.597	0.653	0.353	
	BMI	r	− 0.135	0.104	− 0.087	− 0.163	
		p	0.176	0.297	0.382	0.102	

**The r correlation coefficient is significant

symptom severity and sleep disorders in FMS patients [30–32]. The relationship between sleep and pain is two-way; patients may sleep badly because of pain, or pain may increase because of poor sleep [33]. In the current study, consistent with these data, sleep disorders were found at a higher rate in FMS patients than in the control group. Furthermore, in the FMS patients with greater sleep disorders, the FMS disease severity and pain scores were determined to be higher. Interestingly, contrary to previous studies, this study did not find a significant relationship between sleep disorders and social media addiction [34–36]. This may be because previous studies

Table 8 Determination of the relationship between scores according to patient groups

Group			SSM duration	VAS score	PROMIS sleep score	SMAF score	FMS disease score
FMS	SSM duration	r	1				
		p					
	VAS score	r	0.10	1			
		p	0.34				
	PROMIS sleep score	r	0.07	0.196*	1		
		p	0.49	0.05			
	SMAF score	r	0.537**	0.03	−0.03	1	
		p	0.01	0.78	0.74		
	FMS disease score	r	−0.03	0.277**	0.278**	0.01	
		p	0.74	0.01	0.01	0.99	
Control	SSM duration	r	1				
		p					
	VAS score	r	0.05	1			
		p	0.65				
	PROMIS sleep score	r	0.07	−0.03	1		
		p	0.51	0.73			
	SMAF score	r	0.414**	−0.18	−0.02	1	
		p	0.01	0.07	0.87		

**The r correlation coefficient is significant

included people who did not have FMS or any disease and found that excessive social media use causes sleep disturbance. In addition, it is thought that the sleep disorder seen in FMS is not the result of social media use but is related to the natural course of the disease. There were some limitations to this study. For example, it was cross-sectional, and the scales were completed by the patients. Although it is easy to obtain descriptive data in a cross-sectional study, it is difficult to determine cause and effect relationships. FMS patients with anxiety, depression or sleep disturbances were investigated and not compared with FMS patients without these complaints. The time period in which the networks were most used was not analyzed. In addition, the social media addiction scale used in this study is not a questionnaire of international use that has been tried and used previously in these types of studies. Nevertheless, this questionnaire was used, as it was developed for the Turkish population, was in the Turkish language, and had been subjected to validity and reliability studies.

Conclusions

Social media use was found to be higher in patients with FMS. As a result, although there was significantly more social media use in FMS, no relationship was found between the rates of social media use and the severity or prevalence of the disease in patients with FMS. These data suggest that social media use is more associated with symptoms accompanying FMS than with symptom severity and prevalence of FMS. As causality factors continue to be explored, these insights can motivate healthcare professionals to evaluate social media habits in individuals with FMS. As the first study to investigate the relationship between social media use and FMS, it can be considered that the study will serve as a guide for future more detailed studies.

Acknowledgements

Not applicable.

Authors' contributions

KS conceived the study, performed data collection, analysis, review, and interpretation, and drafted the manuscript. CA analysis, review and interpretation and contributed to the writing of the manuscript. The authors read and approved the final manuscript.

Author details

[1]Physical Medicine and Rehabilitation, City Hospital, Bursa, Turkey. [2]Faculty of Medicine, Physical Medicine and Rehabilitation, Hacettepe University, Ankara, Turkey.

References

1. Wolfe F, Smythe HA, Yunus MB, Bennett RM, Bombardier C, et al. The American College of Rheumatology 1990 criteria for the classification of fibromyalgia. Report of the multicenter criteria committee. Arthritis Rheum. 1990;33:160–72. https://doi.org/10.1002/art.1780330203.

2. Marques AP, Santo ASE, Berssaneti AA, Matsutani LA, Yuan SLK. Prevalence of fibromyalgia: literature review update. Revista Brasileira de Reumatologia (English Edition). 2017;57:356–63. https://doi.org/10.1016/j.rbre.2017.01.005.
3. Romano GF, Tomassi S, Russell A, Mondelli V, Pariante CM. Clinical challenges in the biopsychosocial interface. Adv Psychosom Med. 2015;34:61–77. https://doi.org/10.1159/000369085.
4. Dailey DL, Keffala VJ, Sluka KA. Do cognitive and physical fatigue tasks enhance pain, cognitive fatigue, and physical fatigue in people with fibromy algia? Arthritis Care Res. 2015;67:288–96. https://doi.org/10.1002/acr.22417.
5. Berkol TD, Balcioglu YH, Kirlioglu SS, Erensoy H, Vural M. Dissociative features of fibromyalgia syndrome. Neurosciences (Riyadh). 2017;22:198–204. https://doi.org/10.17712/nsj.2017.3.20160538.
6. Sluka KA, Clauw DJ. Neurobiology of fibromyalgia and chronic widespread pain. Neuroscience. 2016;338:114–29. https://doi.org/10.1016/j.neuroscience.2016.06.
7. Santos Dde M, Lage LV, Jabur EK, Kaziyama HHS, Iosifescu DV, et al. The association of major depressive episode and personality traits in patients with fibromyalgia. Clinics (Sao Paulo). 2011;66:973–8. https://doi.org/10.1590/S1807-59322011000600009.
8. Salazar A, Dueñas M, Mico JA, Ojeda B, Agüera-Ortiz L, et al. Undiagnosed mood disorders and sleep disturbances in primary care patients with chronic musculoskeletal pain. Pain Med. 2013;14(9):1416–25. https://doi.org/10.1111/pme.12165.
9. Aguglia A, Salvi V, Maina G, Rossetto I, Aguglia E. Fibromyalgia syndrome and depressive symptoms: comorbidity and clinical correlates. J Affect Disord. 2011;128:262–6. https://doi.org/10.1016/j.jad.2010.07.004.
10. Wu YL, Chang LY, Lee HC, Fang SC, Tsai PS. Sleep disturbances in fibromyalgia. A meta-analysis of case-control studies. J Psychosom Res. 2017;96:89–97. https://doi.org/10.1016/j.jpsychores.2017.03.011.
11. Écija C, Luque-Reca O, Suso-Ribera C, Catala P, Peñacoba C. Associations of cognitive fusion and pain catastrophizing with fibromyalgia impact through fatigue, pain severity, and depression: an exploratory study using structural - equation modeling. J Clin Med. 2020;9:1763. https://doi.org/10.3390/jcm9061763.
12. Choy EHS. The role of sleep in pain and fibromyalgia. Nat Rev Rheumatol. 2015;11(9):513–20. https://doi.org/10.1038/nrrheum.2015.56.
13. Duggan M, Ellison NB, Lampe C, Lenhart A, Madden M. Social media update 2014: while Facebook remains the most popular site, other platforms see higher rates of growth. Washington: Pew Research Center; 2015.
14. Şahin C, Yağcı M. Social media addiction scale-adult form: the reliability and validity study. J Ahi Evran Univ Kırşehir Fac Educ. 2017;18(1):523–38.
15. Demirci I. The adaptation of the Bergen Social Media Addiction Scale to Turk ish and its evaluation of relationship with depression and anxiety symptoms. Anatol J Psychiatry. 2019;20:15–22.
16. Fox S, Rainie H. The web at 25 in the US. [Internet & American Life Project]. Washington: Pew Research Center; 2014.
17. Subrahmanyam K, Reich SM, Waechter N, Espinoza G. Online and offline social networks: use of social networking sites by emerging adults. J Appl Dev Psychol. 2008;29:420–33. https://doi.org/10.1016/j.appdev.2008.07.003.
18. Lim MS, Choi SB. Stress caused by social media network applications and user's responses. Multimed Tools Appl. 2017;76:17685–98. https://doi.org/10.1007/s11042-015-2891-z.
19. van den Eijnden RJJM, Lemmens JS, Valkenburg PM. The social media disorder scale: validity and psychometric properties. Comput Human Behav. 2016;61:478–87. https://doi.org/10.1016/j.chb.2016.03.038.
20. Lee-Won RJ, Herzog L, Park SG. Hooked on Facebook: the role of social anxiety and need for social assurance in problematic use of Facebook. Cyberpsychol Behav Soc Netw. 2015;18:567–74. https://doi.org/10.1089/cyber.2015.0002.
21. Mohammadbeigi A, Absari R, Valizadeh F, Saadati M, Sharifimoghadam S, et al. Sleep quality in medical students; the impact of over- use of mobile cellphone and social networks. J Res Health Sci. 2016;16:46–50.
22. Griffiths M. Behavioral addiction: an issue for everybody? Empl Couns Today. 1996;3:19–25.
23. Pantic I, Damjanovic A, Todorovic J, Topalovic D, Bojovic-Jovic D, et al. Association between online social networking and depression in high school students: behavioral physiology viewpoint. Psychiatr Danub. 2012;24:90–3.
24. Yanmaz MN, Atar S, Biçer M. The reliability and validity of the Turkish version of fibromyalgia survey diagnostic criteria and symptom severity scale. J Back Musculoskelet Rehabil. 2016;29:287–93. https://doi.org/10.1136/annrheumdis-2015-eular.2026.
25. Yu L, Buysse DJ, Germain A, Moul DE, Stover A, et al. Development of short forms from the PROMIS™ sleep disturbance and Sleep-Related Impairment item banks. Behav Sleep Med. 2011;10:6–24. https://doi.org/10.1080/15402002.2012.636266.
26. Sharma MK, John N, Sahu M. Influence of social media on mental health: a systematic review. Curr Opin Psychiatry. 2020;33:467–75. https://doi.org/10.1097/YCO.0000000000000631.
27. Lenhart A, Ling R, Campell S, Purcell K. Teens, and mobile phones. Washington: Pew Internet and American Life Project; 2010.
28. Turel O, Alexander S. The benefits and dangers of enjoyment with social networking websites. Eur J Inf Syst. 2012;21:512–28. https://doi.org/10.1057/ejis.2012.1.
29. Bennett RM, Jones J, Turk DC, Russell IJ, Matallana L. An internet survey of 2596 people with fibromyalgia. BMC Musculoskelet Disord. 2007;8:27.
30. Mork PJ, Nilsen TI. Sleep problems and risk of fibromyalgia: longitudinal data on an adult female population in Norway. Arthritis Rheum. 2012;64:281–4. https://doi.org/10.1002/art.33346.
31. Andrade A, Vilarino GT, Sieczkowska SM, Coimbra DR, Bevilacqua GG, et al. The relationship between sleep quality and fibromyalgia symptoms. J Health Psychol. 2020;25:1176–86. https://doi.org/10.1177/1359105317751615.
32. Jacobson SA, Simpson RG, Lubahn C, Hu C, Belden CM, et al. Characterization of fibromyalgia symptoms in patients 55–95 years old: a longitudinal study showing symptom persistence with suboptimal treatment. Aging Clin Exp Res. 2015;27(1):75–82. https://doi.org/10.1007/s40520-014-0238-7.
33. Podsakoff PM, MacKenzie SB, Lee JY, Podsakoff NP. Common method biases in behavioral research: a critical review of the literature and recommended remedies. J Appl Psychol. 2003;88:879–903.
34. Malaeb D, Salameh P, Barbar S, Awad E, Haddad C, et al. Problematic social media use and mental health (depression, anxiety, and insomnia) among Lebanese adults: any mediating effect of stress? Perspect Psychiatr Care. 2021;57(2):539–49. https://doi.org/10.1111/ppc.12576.
35. Lin CY, Imani V, Griffiths MD, Broström A, Nygårdh A, et al. Temporal associations between morningness/eveningness, problematic social media use, psychological distress, and daytime sleepiness: mediated roles of sleep quality and insomnia among young adults. J Sleep Res. 2021;30(1):13076. https://doi.org/10.1111/jsr.13076.
36. Montag C, Hegelich S. Understanding detrimental aspects of social media use: will the real culprits please stand up? Front Sociol. 2020;5:599270. https://doi.org/10.3389/fsoc.2020.599270.

20

Chronic use of hydroxychloroquine did not protect against COVID-19 in a large cohort of patients with rheumatic diseases in Brazil

Gecilmara Salviato Pileggi[1], Gilda Aparecida Ferreira[2*], Ana Paula Monteiro Gomides Reis[3], Edgard Torres Reis-Neto[4], Mirhelen Mendes Abreu[5], Cleandro Pires Albuquerque[3], Nafice Costa Araújo[6], Ana Beatriz Bacchiega[1], Dante Valdetaro Bianchi[7], Blanca Bica[5], Eloisa Duarte Bonfa[8], Eduardo Ferreira Borba[8], Danielle Christinne Soares Egypto Brito[9], Ângela Luzia Branco Pinto Duarte[10], Rafaela Cavalheiro Espírito Santo[11], Paula Reale Fernandes[12], Mariana Peixoto Guimarães[13], Kirla Wagner Poti Gomes[14], Adriana Maria Kakehasi[2], Evandro Mendes Klumb[15], Cristina Costa Duarte Lanna[2], Claudia Diniz Lopes Marques[10], Odirlei André Monticielo[11], Licia Maria Henrique Mota[3], Gabriela Araújo Munhoz[16], Eduardo Santos Paiva[17], Helena Lucia Alves Pereira[18], José Roberto Provenza[19], Sandra Lucia Euzébio Ribeiro[18], Laurindo Ferreira Rocha Junior[20], Camila Santana Justo Cintra Sampaio[21], Vanderson Souza Sampaio[22,23,24], Emília Inoue Sato[4], Thelma Skare[25], Viviane Angelina de Souza[12], Valeria Valim[26], Marcus Vinícius Guimarães Lacerda[22,23,24], Ricardo Machado Xavier[11] and Marcelo Medeiros Pinheiro[4]

Abstract

Background: There is a lack of information on the role of chronic use of hydroxychloroquine during the SARS-CoV-2 outbreak. Our aim was to compare the occurrence of COVID-19 between rheumatic disease patients on hydroxychloroquine with individuals from the same household not taking the drug during the first 8 weeks of community viral transmission in Brazil.

Methods: This baseline cross-sectional analysis is part of a 24-week observational multi-center study involving 22 Brazilian academic outpatient centers. All information regarding COVID-19 symptoms, epidemiological, clinical, and demographic data were recorded on a specific web-based platform using telephone calls from physicians and medical students. COVID-19 was defined according to the Brazilian Ministry of Health (BMH) criteria. Mann–Whitney, Chi-square and Exact Fisher tests were used for statistical analysis and two binary Final Logistic Regression Model by Wald test were developed using a backward-stepwise method for the presence of COVID-19.

Results: From March 29th to May 17st, 2020, a total of 10,443 participants were enrolled, including 5166 (53.9%) rheumatic disease patients, of whom 82.5% had systemic erythematosus lupus, 7.8% rheumatoid arthritis, 3.7% Sjögren's syndrome and 0.8% systemic sclerosis. In total, 1822 (19.1%) participants reported flu symptoms within the 30 days prior to enrollment, of which 3.1% fulfilled the BMH criteria, but with no significant difference between

*Correspondence: gildaferreira9@gmail.com
[2] Hospital das Clínicas, Universidade Federal de Minas Gerais (UFMG), Belo Horizonte, MG, Brazil

rheumatic disease patients (4.03%) and controls (3.25%). After adjustments for multiple confounders, the main risk factor significantly associated with a COVID-19 diagnosis was lung disease (OR 1.63; 95% CI 1.03–2.58); and for rheumatic disease patients were diagnosis of systemic sclerosis (OR 2.8; 95% CI 1.19–6.63) and glucocorticoids above 10 mg/day (OR 2.05; 95% CI 1.31–3.19). In addition, a recent influenza vaccination had a protective effect (OR 0.674; 95% CI 0.46–0.98).

Conclusion: Patients with rheumatic disease on hydroxychloroquine presented a similar occurrence of COVID-19 to household cohabitants, suggesting a lack of any protective role against SARS-CoV-2 infection.

Trial registration Brazilian Registry of Clinical Trials (ReBEC; RBR – 9KTWX6).

Keywords: COVID-19, Hydroxycloroquine, Rheumatic diseases

Background

Severe Acute Respiratory Syndrome Coronavirus (SARS-CoV-2) is the etiological agent of COVID-19, a public health emergency with relevant challenges worldwide and different epidemic curves and mortality rates between countries [1, 2]. The disease has a heterogeneous clinical spectrum, from asymptomatic forms to severe systemic involvement, including pneumonia, cytokine storm syndrome, endotheliocyte damage, and thrombotic events [3–8].

Initial data have suggested that SARS-CoV-2 does not appear to cause more serious disease in immunosuppressed patients [9–11] and this clinical observation has drawn attention to a potential beneficial or 'protective' effect of medications used to control rheumatic diseases (RD) [12–15].

Chloroquine (CQ) and hydroxychloroquine (HCQ), immunomodulator drugs traditionally used to treat malaria and rheumatic diseases (RD), such as rheumatoid arthritis (RA), systemic lupus erythematosus (SLE), and primary Sjögren syndrome (pSS) [16–18], were pointed out as effective pharmacological strategies against COVID-19 in vitro and in anecdotal reports [19–21]. In addition, it could attenuate the cytokine storm observed in moderate or severe COVID-19 forms mitigating unfavorable outcomes. However, there are controversial data regarding their efficacy and safety to treat COVID-19 patients and a recent randomized controlled trial did not show any beneficial effect in patients hospitalized with mild-to-moderate disease when compared to standard care [22–27]. Gentry et al. did not found any significant difference regarding the incidence of active SARS-CoV-2 infection between patients with rheumatic diseases receiving hydroxychloroquine and patients without it [28].

Methods

Study design and participants

This study aimed to evaluate the frequency of COVID-19 in patients with RD in HCQ, in comparison with their cohabitants during the SARS-CoV-2 pandemic in Brazil. This is a cross-sectional, observational, paired study, including adult volunteers (≥18 years of age), with a known previous diagnosis of RD, using HCQ for at least 30 days before the initial consultation. According to the previously defined classification criteria, the cohort included patients with SLE [29]; RA [30]; pSS [31]; systemic sclerosis [32]; inflammatory myopathies [33]; mixed connective tissue disease [34]; hand osteoarthritis [35, 36], and chikungunya-related arthropathy [37].

Household cohabitants aged over 18, without RD and not using antimalarials for any purpose, were chosen as the control group to ensure more homogeneous environmental exposure to the SARS-CoV-2 infection among participants during the community viral transmission, instead of including rheumatic disease patients not using antimalarials, who would probably present a different set of diseases and different epidemiological exposure.

All participants with a history of solid organ or bone marrow transplantation, neoplasm in the previous 12 months, immunoglobulin use in the previous 30 days, current kidney replacement therapy, thymus disease, other immunodeficiencies, or positive HIV status were excluded.

Twenty-two tertiary rheumatology centers, representing the five geographic regions of Brazil and thus encompassing most of the population variability, joined the task-force study. The inclusion period was the first 8 weeks of community transmission in Brazil. This manuscript is part of a larger prospective study with 24-week follow-up.

Procedures

Participants were enrolled in this multi-center study and included through phone calls performed by previously trained medical students and physicians. Details were obtained of epidemiological and demographic data, as well as RD status and current treatment data. In addition, specific information about the COVID-19 symptoms, hospitalization, need for intensive care, and death was recorded in both groups and represents the main endpoints of this cohort. All the data are stored and managed using an electronic on-line platform (REDCap).

Patients taking other dosages of HCQ than 5 mg/kg/day (maximum 400 mg/ day) or using CQ were not included in the final analysis.

Outcomes

The results presented in this manuscript are from a cross-sectional database analysis at baseline (first telephone interview-inclusion visit) with the main outcome being the occurrence of COVID-19, according to the Brazilian Ministry of Health (BMH), within 30 days prior to enrollment [38]. Confirmatory tests have not been routinely performed in Brazil for patients with mild symptoms of SARS-CoV-2 infection, only for moderate-severe cases.

Outcome definitions

Participants in this study were defined with COVID-19, according to the most recent criteria established by the Brazilian Ministry of Health (BMH) during the pandemic period. The BMH criteria was applied to symptomatic patients based on the clinical, epidemiological and laboratory criteria, were considered as COVID-19 (Fig. 1).

Statistical analyses

Descriptive statistics were expressed as mean, standard deviation, as well as frequency (%) and difference 95% confidence intervals (95% CI). The Kolmogorov–Smirnov test was used to verify a normal data distribution. Two binary Final Logistic Regression Model by Wald test were developed using a backward-stepwise method for the presence of COVID-19, including Odds Ratio (OR) and their respective 95% CI. The first model considered both groups (cases and controls) and was adjusted for age, sex, lung and kidney disease, hypertension, diabetes, and influenza vaccine within the previous 30 days. The second one included only RD patients, adjusted for lung disease, corticosteroids, systemic sclerosis, and influenza vaccine within the previous 30 days. Only variables with p value below 0.2 found in the first model was added to the second model. A *P*-value under 0.05 was considered significant. The statistical analysis was performed using IBM-SPSS v.20.0 software.

Results

From March 29th to May 17th, 2020 (8-week period), a total of 9589 participants from 97 Brazilian cities were enrolled at baseline, including 5166 (53.9%) patients with RD on HCQ (5 mg/kg/day, maximum dosage of 400 mg),

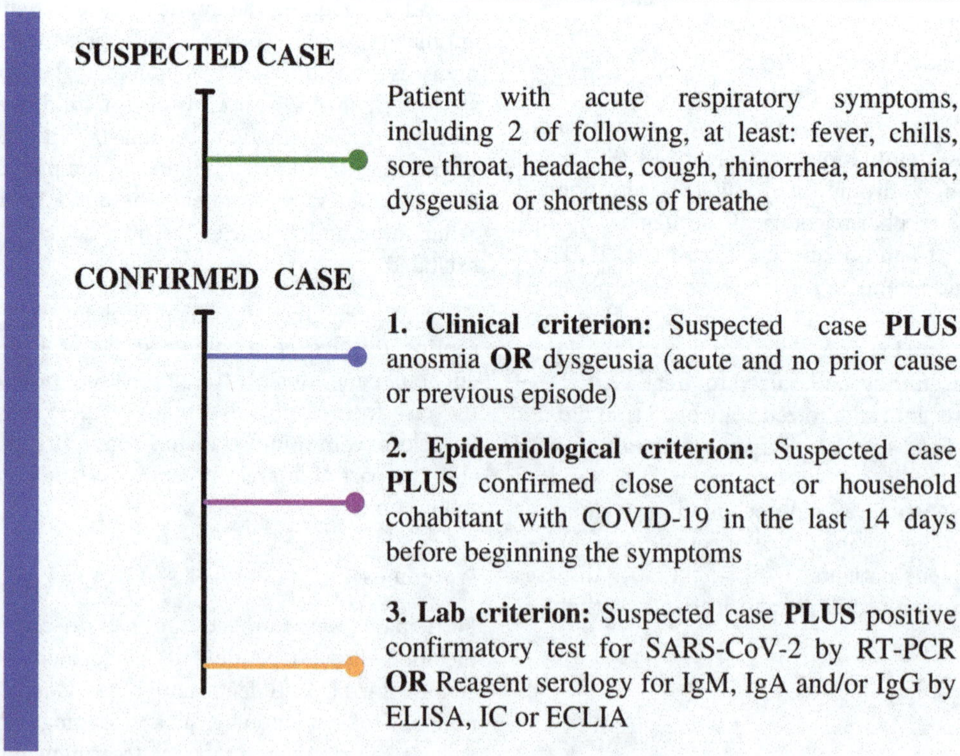

Fig. 1 Outcome definition: participants were classified according to the Brazilian Ministry of Health (BMH) criteria using the definition for COVID-19. Individuals with more than 3 days of influenza-like illness symptoms were considered for this analysis

and 4423 (46.1%) cohabitants living in the same household. Of these, 854 (8.1%) individuals were excluded according to the eligibility criteria (Fig. 2).

Although statistically different, the difference between the mean age and frequency of contact with a confirmed case of COVID-19 were not clinically relevant. There was a higher frequency of females in the patients' group and a higher frequency of males in the household cohabitants. All concomitant diseases evaluated were significantly more common in RD patients than the control group, except for diabetes. On the other hand, social distancing and influenza vaccination were reported more frequently by RD patients (Table 1).

Most of the RD patients had SLE (N=4243; 82.5%), followed by RA (N=402; 7.8%), and pSS (N=192; 3.7%). Among the 5166 RD patients, 97.5% are using HCQ, of whom 522 (10.1%) take it as monotherapy and 4644 (89.9%) combined with other therapies, such as

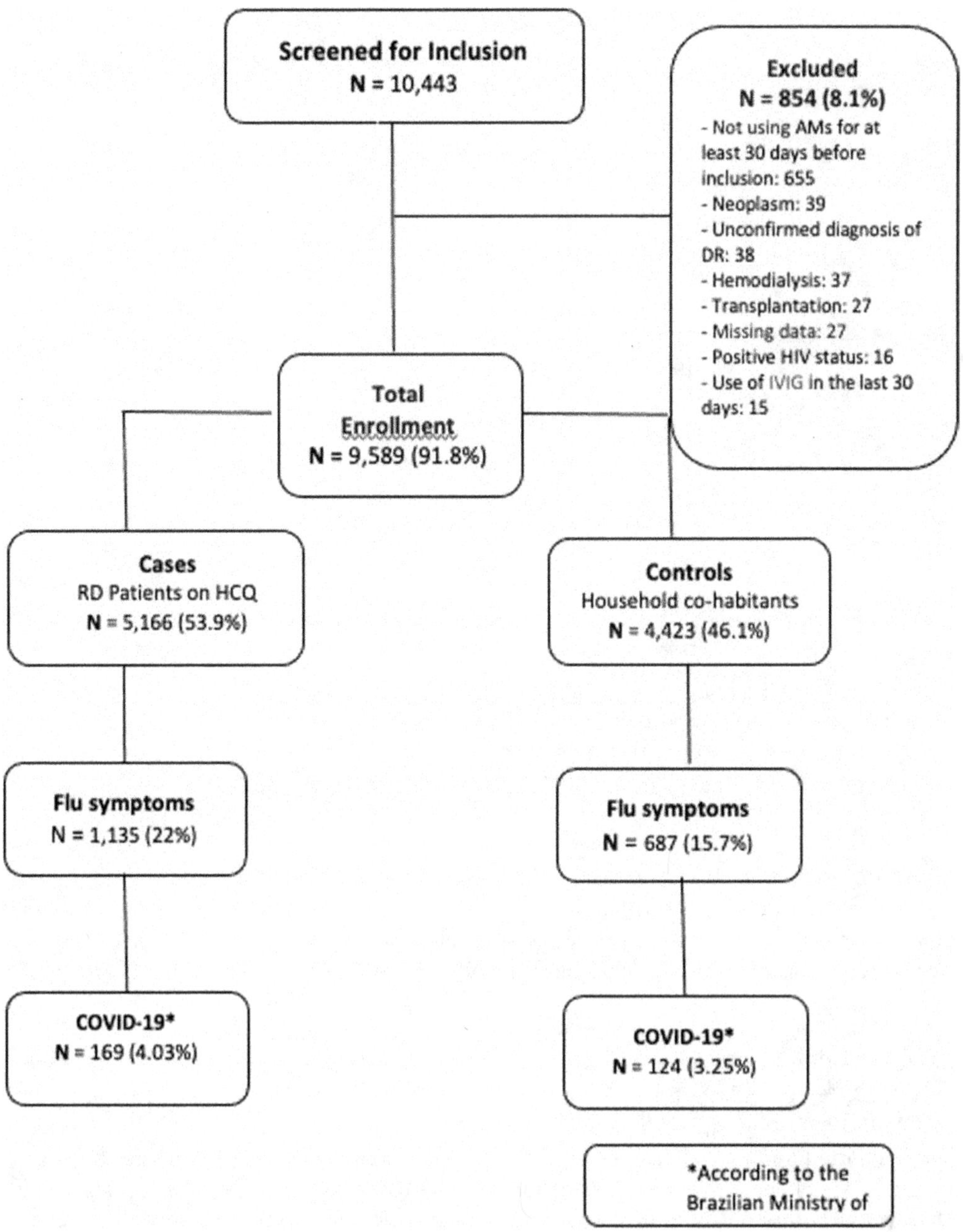

Fig. 2 Flowchart of participants enrolled in this study, considering influenza-like illness symptoms and a diagnosis of COVID-19, according to the Brazilian Ministry of Health criteria

Table 1 Epidemiological and clinical data between patients with rheumatic diseases and household contacts at baseline

Variables	All N = 9589 n (%)	RD patients N = 5166 n (%)	Household co-habitants N = 4423 n (%)	Difference (CI 95%)	p*
Age, years (SD)	43.5 (14.9)	43.1 (13.9)	44.0 (16.1)	0.90 (0.29; 1.50)	**0.039**
Sex					
Women	6617 (69.4)	4772 (92.6)	1845 (42.2)	50.4 (48.8; 52.0)	**<0.001**
Men	2912 (30.6)	382 (7.4)	2530 (57.8)		
Schooling					
Basic or illiterate	2522 (26.5)	1296 (25.1)	1226 (28)	2.9 (1.1; 4.7)	**<0.001**
High school	4027 (42.2)	2166 (42)	1861 (42.6)	0.6 (− 1.39; 2.6)	
College	2983 (31.3)	1697 (32.9)	1286 (29.4)	3.5 (1.6; 5.4)	
Profession					
Customer assistance	1911 (20.2)	946 (18.5)	965 (22.2)	3.7 (2.1; 5.3)	**<0.001**
Healthcare	683 (7.2)	443 (8.7)	240 (5.5)	3.2 (2.2; 4.2)	
Safety professionals	182 (1.9)	43 (0.8)	139 (3.2)	2.4 (1.8; 3.0)	
Education	636 (6.7)	438 (8.6)	198 (4.6)	4.0 (3.0; 4.9)	
Housewife	1662 (17.6)	1236 (24.2)	426 (9.8)	14.4 (12.9; 15.9)	
Others	4382 (46.3)	2011 (39.3)	2371 (54.6)	15.3 (13.3; 17.3)	
Contact with confirmed case of COVID-19					
No	8136 (85.3)	4484 (86.9)	3652 (83.4)	3.5 (2.1; 4.9)	**<0.001**
Yes	727 (7.6)	380 (7.4)	347 (7.9)	0.5 (− 0.6; 1.6)	
Unknown	673 (7.1)	294 (5.7)	379 (8.7)	3.0 (1.9; 4.1)	
Family unit in social distancing	5787 (60.7)	3235 (62.7)	2552 (58.4)	4.3 (2.3; 6.3)	**<0.001**
Heart disease	496 (5.3)	314 (6.2)	182 (4.3)	1.9 (1.0; 2.8)	**<0.001**
Diabetes	703 (7.5)	339 (6.7)	364 (8.5)	1.8 (0.7; 2.9)	**<0.001**
Lung disease	497 (5.3)	357 (7)	140 (3.3)	3.7 (2.8; 4;6)	**<0.001**
Kidney disease	602 (6.4)	565 (11.1)	37 (0.9)	10.2 (9.3; 11.1)	**<0.001**
Hypertension	2673 (28.6)	1692 (33.3)	981 (23)	10.3 (8.5; 12.1)	**<0.001**
Influenza vaccine within last 30 days	2584 (27.2)	1527 (29.6)	1057 (24.2)	5.4 (3.6; 7.2)	**<0.001**

Bold values indicate statistical significance ($p < 0.05$)

The results are expressed as means, standard deviation and percentages

CI, confidence interval; RD, rheumatic diseases; COVID-19, Coronavirus disease 2019

* Chi-square test

corticosteroids (37.0%) and immunosuppressant drugs (48.9%). The remaining 2.5% from antimalarials users were taking other chloroquine salts, particularly diphosphate, and they were excluded from this final analysis (Table 2).

In total, 1822 (19.1%) participants reported influenza-like illness symptoms within the 30 days prior to enrollment, of whom 293 (3.1%) individuals fulfilled the BMH criteria for a COVID-19 diagnosis [38]. In general, the frequency of self-reported influenza-like illness symptoms was significantly higher in RD patients, including those with severe symptoms (such as shortness of breath), except fever and anosmia (Table 3).

Considering a COVID-19 diagnosis, there was no significant difference in the number of cases between RD patients (4.03%) and the control group (3.25%) (OR 0.78, − 0.05; 1.60). Men (OR 0.71; 95% CI 0.52–0.98, p = 0.043) participants had lower likely of having the disease. On the other hand, individuals with previous lung disease (OR 1.63; 95% CI 1.03–2.58, p = 0.038) were more likely to present clinically confirmed COVID-19 in the final logistic regression model, after adjustments for multiple confounders, using the variables with p < 0.2 in the first (Table 4).

Considering only RD patients, having systemic sclerosis and current use of glucocorticoids (daily dosage above 10 mg) had a harmful effect for a COVID-19 diagnosis while a recent influenza vaccination had a protective role (OR 0.674; 95% CI 0.46–0.98), after multiple adjustments for sex, age, concomitant medication,

Table 2 Main rheumatic diseases and concomitant medication at baseline

	N (%)
Rheumatic disease	
Systemic lupus erythematous	4243 (82.5)
Rheumatoid arthritis	402 (7.8)
Primary Sjögren syndrome	192 (3.7)
Mixed connective tissue disease	75 (1.5)
Osteoarthritis	66 (1.3)
Systemic sclerosis	43 (0.8)
Inflammatory myopathies	34 (0.7)
Chikungunya	18 (0.4)
Other	69 (1.3)
Antimalarials	
Hydroxychloroquine (HCQ)	5035 (97.5)
HCQ use time (years), mean (SD)	7.2 (6.2)
Chloroquine diphosphate (CD)	131 (2.5)
CD use time (years), mean (SD)	10.6 (7.4)
Concomitant medication related to RD	
Glucocorticoids	1895 (36.7)
< 10 mg/day	1394 (73.6)
≥ 10 mg/day	462 (24.4)
Ibuprofen	35 (0.7)
IV Methylprednisolone (pulse)	30 (0.6)
Cyclophosphamide (oral and pulse)	73 (1.4)
Synthetic conventional DMARDs	2444 (47.3)
Methotrexate	631 (12.2)
Sulfasalazine	16 (0.3)
Azathioprine	983 (19.0)
Leflunomide	96 (1.9)
Cyclosporine	80 (1.5)
Mycophenolate mofetil	657 (12.7)
Biological or target-specific DMARDs	181 (3.5)
TNF inhibitors	17 (0.3)
Belimumab	52 (1.0)
Rituximab	81 (1.6)
Abatacept	17 (0.3)
Tocilizumab	7 (0.1)
Tofacitinib	7 (0.1)

The results are expressed as means, standard deviation and percentages; DMARDs, disease activity-modifying drugs; some individuals are taking more than one synthetic DMARD

immunosuppressant drugs, and comorbidities, regardless of chronic HCQ use, (Table 5).

Discussion

Our results showed patients with RD on HCQ had a similar likelihood of presenting a COVID-19 diagnosis, according to the BMH criteria, when compared to cohabitants living in the same household during the first 8 weeks of community transmission in Brazil. Considering that according to recent studies [12, 39], patients with RD present a similar incidence of COVID-19 to the general population but with a potentially more unfavorable outcome [40, 41] and higher mortality rate [42, 43], we were not able to confirm our preliminary hypothesis in demonstrating a potential beneficial effect of chronic HCQ use against SARS-CoV-2 [44] in a population that traditionally has a higher prevalence of respiratory diseases.

Moreover, our data showed a higher frequency of influenza-like illness symptoms, including those with greater severity, especially shortness of breath, in patients with RD when compared with controls, suggesting these individuals should maintain social distancing, especially those that work with customer assistance, such as healthcare, teaching, and safety professionals [12, 45–50]. However, it is worth highlighting that patients with RD may report more symptoms than controls due to different behavior in relation to the perception of signs and symptoms because of the information they receive about their underlying disease from healthcare professionals and the combination of disease activity, as well as that the immunosuppression may predispose them to more infectious diseases that cause influenza-like illness symptoms such as influenza, adenovirus, and others [51].

Although CQ has in vitro activity against influenza, HCQ use did not prevent infection or decrease the risk of influenza infection [52–57]. Thus, our data are supported by current evidence demonstrating a lack of association between HCQ and COVID-19 considering pre-exposure (PrEP) and post-exposure prophylaxis especially in individuals at risk, such as healthcare professionals, as well as more recent randomized clinical trials, including mild-moderate and severe forms of SARS-CoV-2 infection [22, 24, 26, 27, 58–62].

In our total sample, men had a lower risk of COVID-19 than women (OR 0.71; 95% CI 0.52–0.98). This aspect could be related to higher frequency of female in patients group than in the control group because of inclusion approach that prioritized household contact paired for age (husband and wife more frequently). Also, men participants had less comorbidities and used less glucocorticosteroids. The current literature has shown a similar incidence between men and women, but with a poorer outcome in the former [1, 63–65].

Patients with RD using a daily GC dosage above 10 mg/day (prednisone equivalent), particularly above 20 mg/day, presented a two times higher risk of COVID-19 in our cohort. These data confirm previous findings showing a harmful effect of GC on the infection rate in immune-mediated RD patients, especially lupus [66], hampering the immune response against several infectious agents,

Table 3 Self-reported influenza-like illness symptoms and a COVID-19 diagnosis in patients with rheumatic diseases and household contacts at baseline

Symptoms	All N=9589 n (%)	RD Patients N=5164 n (%)**	Household co-habitants N=4378 n (%) *	Difference (95% CI)	p*
Any	1822 (19.1)	1135 (22)	687 (15.7)	6.3 (4.7; 7.9)	**<0.001**
Fatigue	531 (5.6)	328 (6.4)	203 (4.6)	1.8 (0.9; 2.7)	**<0.001**
Headache	734 (7.7)	453 (8.8)	281 (6.4)	2.4 (1.3; 3.5)	**<0.001**
Rhinorrhea	976 (10.2)	601 (11.6)	375 (8.6)	3.0 (1.8; 4.2)	**<0.001**
Dysgeusia	242 (2.5)	146 (2.8)	96 (2.2)	0.6 (0; 1.2)	**0.049**
Shortness of breath	266 (2.8)	188 (3.6)	78 (1.8)	1.8 (1.2; 2.4)	**<0.001**
Sore throat	704 (7.4)	455 (8.8)	249 (5.7)	3.1 (2.1; 4.1)	**<0.001**
Fever	486 (5.1)	276 (5.3)	210 (4.8)	0.5 (−0.4; 1.4)	0.225
Anosmia	209 (2.2)	120 (2.3)	89 (2)	0.3 (−0.3; 0.9)	0.333
Cough	910 (9.5)	579 (11.2)	331 (7.6)	3.6 (2.4; 4.8)	**<0.001**
Fever AND Shortness of breath	123 (1.3)	80 (1.9)	43 (1.2)	0.7 (0.2; 1,2)	**0.005**
Fever AND Cough AND Shortness of breath	83 (0.9)	53 (1.3)	30 (0.8)	0.5 (0.1; 0.9)	**0.034**
BMH COVID-19 criteria	293 (3.1)	169 (4.03%)	124 (3.25%)	0.78 (−0.05; 1.60)	**0.065**

Bold values indicate statistical significance (p < 0.05)

The results are expressed as means, standard deviation and percentages

BMH, Brazilian Ministry of Health

* There are 45 missing data; **There are 2 missing

Table 4 Final logistic regression model considering all individuals enrolled at baseline

Variables	Binary analysis			Multivariate analysis	
	No symptoms N=7720 n (%)	Clinically Confirmed COVID-19 N=293 n (%)	p	OR (95% CI)	P***
Age (y), mean (SD); med. (min–max.)	43.9 (15.2); 42 (18–98)	41.6 (13.0); 41 (18–90)	**0.028***	0.989 (0.981; 0.997)	**0.008**
Group					
Household cohabitants	3691 (47.8)	124 (42.3)	0.065**	1	-
RD patients	4029 (52.2)	169 (57.7)		1.10 (0.83; 1.46)	0.526
Sex					
Women	5259 (68.2)	218 (75.4)	**0.01****	1	-
Men	2450 (31.8)	71 (24.6)		0.71 (0.52; 0.98)	**0.043**
Schooling					
Basic or illiterate	2110 (27.4)	64 (21.8)	0.091**		
High school	3280 (42.6)	139 (47.4)			
College	2317 (30.1)	90 (30.7)			
Family in social distancing	4728 (61.3)	172 (58.9)	0.402**		
Heart disease	398 (5.3)	17 (6)	0.570**		
Diabetes	585 (7.7)	17 (6)	0.292**		
Lung disease	367 (4.8)	21 (7.4)	**0.048****	1.63 (1.03; 2.58)	**0.038**
Kidney disease	465 (6.1)	23 (8.2)	0.169**		
Hypertension	2165 (28.6)	78 (27.7)	0.730**		
Influenza vaccine within 30 last days	2138 (27.8)	63 (21.6)	**0.022****		

Bold values indicate statistical significance (p < 0.05)

Outcome is clinically confirmed COVID-19 diagnosis

Y, years; SD, standard deviation; med., median; min., minimum; max., maximum

* Mann–Whitney test; **Chi-square test; ***Wald test by final logistic regression model

Table 5 Final logistic regression model regarding rheumatic disease patients enrolled at baseline

Variables	Binary analyses			Multivariate analyses	
	No symptoms N=4029 n (%)	Clinical Covid-19 N=169 n (%)	p	OR (95% CI)	P****
Influenza vaccine within last 30 days	1235 (30.7)	39 (23.1)	**0.034****	0.676 (0.465; 0.984)	**0.041**
IV Methylprednisolone (pulse)	21 (0.5)	2 (1.2)	0.236***		
Glucocorticoids					
No	2555 (63.9)	97 (58.1)	**0.004****	1	-
< 10 mg/day	1099 (27.5)	43 (25.7)		0.965 (0.662; 1.41)	0.854
> = 10 mg/day	343 (8.6)	27 (16.2)		2.07 (1.33; 3.22)	**0.001**
scDMARDs	1875 (46.5)	84 (49.7)	0.419**		
Biological or tsDMARDs	120 (3)	7 (4.1)	0.387**		
RA	317 (7.9)	16 (9.5)	0.466**		
MCTD	56 (1.4)	2 (1.2)	> 0.99***		
SS	39 (0.9)	4 (2.4)	0.042***	3.81 (1.31; 11.05)	**0.014**
SLE	3304 (82)	134 (79.3)	0.414**		
IM	26 (0.6)	1 (0.6)	0.703***		
OA	60 (1.5)	1 (0.6)	0.518***		
pSjS	150 (3.79)	6 (3.6)	0.560***		
Another RD	55 (1.4)	4 (2.4)	0.299***		

Bold values indicate statistical significance (p < 0.05)

RA, Rheumatoid arthritis; SLE, Systemic lupus erythematous; RD, Rheumatic diseases; MCTD, Mixed connective tissue disease; SS, Systemic sclerosis; IM, Inflammatory myopathies; OA, Osteoarthritis; pSjS, Primary Sjögren syndrome; sc, synthetic conventional; ts, target-specific; DMARDs, Disease Activity-Modifying Drugs; Model 3, Outcome is COVID-19 diagnosis, according to the Brazilian Ministry of Health criteria; y, years; SD, standard deviation; med., median; min., minimum; max., maximum

* Mann–Whitney test; **Chi-square test; ***Fischer's exact test; ****Wald test by final logistic regression model

including SARS-CoV-2 [67–70]. More recently, Gianfrancesco et al. also reported a higher risk of hospitalization in individuals using more than 10 mg/day (OR 2.05; 95% CI 1.06–3.96) and no significant association with HCQ, in agreement with our findings [41]. On the other hand, performing a sensitivity analysis excluding patients that received more than 10 mg/day of glucocorticoids from the RD group, and we observed quite similar findings (data not shown), suggesting that the risk for COVID-19 did not change when adjusted for corticosteroids (high vs. low dosage). It is important taking into consideration the low daily GC dosage (< 10 mg in almost 75% of them) and low proportion of current pulse therapy (around 2% of cyclophosphamide or methylprednisolone).

In the final multivariate model, systemic sclerosis was the only RD related to COVID-19, regardless of interstitial lung disease or the use of HCQ, as pointed out by some authors [71–73]. Nonetheless, an Italian phone interview study did not find any association regarding a higher risk in SS patients [39].

Interestingly, some of the main comorbidities associated with an unfavorable outcome and increased risk of death, such as diabetes, and heart and kidney diseases [1, 39, 64] were not significantly associated with COVID-19 in our patients with RD. In addition, the self-reporting of fever and/or anosmia, more specific symptoms of COVID-19, was also not different between RD patients and controls [74].

Although post influenza vaccine side effects could also have been a potential confounding factor, we found the influenza vaccine had an independent protective role in RD patients (OR 0.674; 95% CI 0.463–0.979), reducing the diagnosis of COVID-19 during the beginning of national vaccination campaign. Our data reinforce the effectiveness and safety of this approach in RD patients [75]. In addition, it is noteworthy pointing out this potential protective effect could be related to some bias, especially some behavioral attitudes (social distancing, strict masking and other self-care measurements) that are more observed in immunosuppressed patients.

To the best of our knowledge, this is the largest epidemiological study designed to evaluate the preventive role of HCQ to development of COVID-19 in patients with RD using HCQ. Some strengths should be considered, such as sampling size, the control group with the same epidemiological setting, weekly data quality monitoring, specific platform to collect all the information using serial, with national representation in pandemic times.

On the other hand, it is worth emphasizing some limitations of the study that are inherent to the COVID-19 pandemic, including the need for social distancing and specific guidance for the patients to avoid seeking medical care unless absolutely necessary. Therefore, in such a large population, we have only self-reported data, and a small number of confirmatory lab tests (RT-PCR and serology) and information on disease activity. The BMH criteria for COVID-19 have several similarities with the US criteria to define COVID-19 [76].

Another limitation was the lack of patients with RD not using HCQ as another control group. However, this approach could present other prescription biases, as SLE patients without antimalarial treatment are quite uncommon, except in those with previous toxicity (maculopathy, allergy, long-term remission, among others). The strategy of prioritizing and enrolling the household cohabitants was chosen because of the relevant epidemiological impact of COVID-19. A relevant clinical consideration is related to the severity of RD in the patients included in this cohort, since there were few patients taking biological DMARDs and cyclophosphamide. However, more recently, Zhong et al., in a Chinese retrospective study involving 6228 patients with autoimmune diseases that were enrolled in just 10 days and during sharp decline of COVID-19 outbreak in Hubei found lower risk of infection than patients taking other DMARDs (OR 0.09 [95% CI 0.01–0.94]; $p=0.044$) [77].

As future perspectives, the shortage of HCQ with potential effects after withdrawal [78–81] will be further explored during the 24-week follow-up, as well as hospitalization and mortality rate [82].

Conclusion

This study provides evidence of a non-protective role of chronic HCQ use (5 mg of the sulfate/kg/day) concerning uncomplicated COVID-19 in RD patients, regardless of comorbidities, immunosuppression therapy, and social distancing.

Abbreviations

BMH: Brazilian Ministry of Health; CI: Confidence intervals; CQ: Chloroquine; HCQ: Hydroxychloroquine; OR: Odds ratio; pSS: Primary Sjögren syndrome; RA: Rheumatic arthritis; RD: Rheumatic diseases; SLE: Systemic lupus erythematosus.

Acknowledgements

To the *Brazilian Society of Rheumatology* for technical support and rapid nationwide mobilization. To all the 395 interviewers (medical students and physicians) who collaborated in the study and the participants.

Authors' contributions

MMP, GSP, LHMH, GAF, CDLM, AMK, RMX, APMGR, ESP, ETRN, defined as Steering Committee, and MVGL conceived the study, developed the protocol and wrote the manuscript with input from all other authors. In addition, all authors are responsible for collecting data and processing, management them and statistical analysis. All authors read and approved the final manuscript.

Author details

[1]Rheumatology Unit of Escola Paulista de Medicina (Unifesp/ EPM), São Paulo, SP, Brazil. [2]Hospital das Clínicas, Universidade Federal de Minas Gerais (UFMG), Belo Horizonte, MG, Brazil. [3]Hospital Universitário de Brasília da Universidade de Brasília, EBSERH (HUB-UnB), Brasília, DF, Brazil. [4]Hospital São Paulo da Universidade Federal de São Paulo, Escola Paulista de Medicina (Unifesp/ EPM), São Paulo, SP, Brazil. [5]Hospital Universitário Clementino Fraga Filho, Universidade Federal Do Rio de Janeiro (UFRJ), Rio de Janeiro, RJ, Brazil. [6]Hospital Do Servidor Público Estadual, Instituto de Assistência Médica Ao Servidor Público Estadual (IAMSPE), São Paulo, SP, Brazil. [7]Santa Casa de Misericórdia Do Rio de Janeiro (HGSCMRJ), Rio de Janeiro, RJ, Brazil. [8]Rheumatology Division, Hospital das Clínicas HCFMUSP, Faculdade de Medicina, Universidade de São Paulo, São Paulo, SP, Brazil. [9]Hospital Universitário Lauro Wanderley, Universidade Federal da Paraíba (UFPB), João Pessoa, PB, Brazil. [10]Hospital das Clínicas da Universidade Federal de Pernambuco (UFPE), Recife, PE, Brazil. [11]Hospital de Clínicas de Porto Alegre, Universidade Federal Do Rio Grande Do Sul (UFRGS), Porto Alegre, RS, Brazil. [12]Hospital Universitário da Universidade Federal de Juiz de Fora (UFJF), Juiz de Fora, MG, Brazil. [13]Santa Casa de Misericórdia de Belo Horizonte, Belo Horizonte, MG, Brazil. [14]Hospital Geral de Fortaleza (HGF), Fortaleza, CE, Brazil. [15]Hospital Universitário Pedro Ernesto, Universidade Do Estado Do Rio de Janeiro (UERJ), Rio de Janeiro, RJ, Brazil. [16]Irmandade da Santa Casa de Misericórdia de São Paulo (ISCMSP), São Paulo, SP, Brazil. [17]Universidade Federal Do Paraná (UFPR), Curitiba, PR, Brazil. [18]Hospital Universitário Getúlio Vargas Universidade Federal Do Amazonas, Manaus, AM, Brazil. [19]Pontifícia Universidade Católica de Campinas (PUC-CAMP), Campinas, SP, Brazil. [20]Instituto de Medicina Integral Professor Fernando Figueira (IMIP/ PE), Recife, PE, Brazil. [21]Instituto de Ensino E Pesquisa No Sírio Libanês, São Paulo, SP, Brazil. [22]Fundação de Vigilância Em Saúde Do Amazonas, Manaus, AM, Brazil. [23]Instituto Leônidas and Maria Deane, Fiocruz, Manaus, AM, Brazil. [24]Fundação de Medicina Tropical Dr. Heitor Vieira Dourado, Manaus, AM, Brazil. [25]Hospital Universitário Evangélico Mackenzie (HUEM), Curitiba, PR, Brazil. [26]Hospital Universitário Cassiano Antonio de Moraes, Universidade Federal Do Espírito Santo, Vitória, ES, Brazil.

References

1. Zhou F, Yu T, Du R, Fan G, Liu Y, Liu Z, et al. Clinical course and risk factors for mortality of adult inpatients with COVID-19 in Wuhan, China: a retrospective cohort study. Lancet. 2020;395(10229):1054–62.
2. Peeri NC, Shrestha N, Rahman MS, Zaki R, Tan Z, Bibi S, et al. The SARS, MERS and novel coronavirus (COVID-19) epidemics, the newest and biggest global health threats: what lessons have we learned? Int J Epidemiol. 2020;49(3):717–26.
3. Gupta A, Madhavan MV, Sehgal K, Nair N, Mahajan S, Sehrawat TS, et al. Extrapulmonary manifestations of COVID-19. Nat Med. 2020;26(7):1017–32.
4. Zheng KI, Feng G, Liu WY, Targher G, Byrne CD, Zheng MH. Extrapulmonary complications of COVID-19: a multisystem disease? J Med Virol. 2020;93:323–35.
5. Yang W, Sirajuddin A, Zhang X, Liu G, Teng Z, Zhao S, et al. The role of imaging in 2019 novel coronavirus pneumonia (COVID-19). Eur Radiol. 2020;30:4874–82.
6. Vabret N, Britton GJ, Gruber C, Hegde S, Kim J, Kuksin M, et al. Immunology of COVID-19: current state of the science. Immunity. 2020;52(6):910–41.
7. McGonagle D, Sharif K, O'Regan A, Bridgewood C. The role of cytokines including interleukin-6 in COVID-19 induced pneumonia and macrophage activation syndrome-like disease. Autoimmun Rev. 2020;19(6):102537.
8. McGonagle D, O'Donnell JS, Sharif K, Emery P, Bridgewood C. Immune mechanisms of pulmonary intravascular coagulopathy in COVID-19 pneumonia. Lancet Rheumatol. 2020;2:e437–45.
9. Liang W, Guan W, Chen R, Wang W, Li J, Xu K, et al. Cancer patients in SARS-CoV-2 infection: a nationwide analysis in China. Lancet Oncol. 2020;21(3):335–7.
10. Al-Quteimat OM, Amer AM. The impact of the COVID-19 pandemic on cancer patients. Am J Clin Oncol. 2020;43(6):452–5.
11. Johnson KM, Belfer JJ, Peterson GR, Boelkins MR, Dumkow LE. Managing COVID-19 in renal transplant recipients: a review of recent literature and case supporting corticosteroid-sparing immunosuppression. Pharmacotherapy. 2020;40(6):517–24.

12. Favalli EG, Agape E, Caporali R. Incidence and clinical course of COVID-19 in patients with connective tissue diseases: a descriptive observational analysis. J Rheumatol. 2020;47(8):1296.
13. Mathian A, Mahevas M, Rohmer J, Roumier M, Cohen-Aubart F, Amador-Borrero B, et al. Clinical course of coronavirus disease 2019 (COVID-19) in a series of 17 patients with systemic lupus erythematosus under long-term treatment with hydroxychloroquine. Ann Rheum Dis. 2020;79(6):837–9.
14. Ouedraogo DD, Tiendrebeogo WJS, Kabore F, Ntsiba H. COVID-19, chronic inflammatory rheumatic disease and anti-rheumatic treatments. Clin Rheumatol. 2020;39(7):2069–75.
15. Sanders JM, Monogue ML, Jodlowski TZ, Cutrell JB. Pharmacologic treatments for coronavirus disease 2019 (COVID-19): a review. JAMA. 2020. https://doi.org/10.1001/jama.2020.6019.
16. Dos Reis Neto ET, Kakehasi AM, de Medeiros PM, Ferreira GA, Marques CDL, da Mota LMH, et al. Revisiting hydroxychloroquine and chloroquine for patients with chronic immunity-mediated inflammatory rheumatic diseases. Adv Rheumatol. 2020;60(1):32.
17. Fanouriakis A, Bertsias G, Boumpas DT. Hydroxychloroquine dosing in systemic lupus erythematosus: response to 'Comment on the 2019 update of the EULAR recommendations for the management of systemic lupus erythematosus by Fanouriakis et al' by Costedoat-Chalumeau et al. Ann Rheum Dis. 2020;79(8):e91.
18. Fanouriakis A, Kostopoulou M, Cheema K, Anders HJ, Aringer M, Bajema I, et al. 2019 Update of the Joint European League Against Rheumatism and European Renal Association-European Dialysis and Transplant Association (EULAR/ERA-EDTA) recommendations for the management of lupus nephritis. Ann Rheum Dis. 2020;79(6):713–23.
19. Wang M, Cao R, Zhang L, Yang X, Liu J, Xu M, et al. Remdesivir and chloroquine effectively inhibit the recently emerged novel coronavirus (2019-nCoV) in vitro. Cell Res. 2020;30(3):269–71.
20. Gautret P, Lagier JC, Parola P, Hoang VT, Meddeb L, Mailhe M, et al. Hydroxychloroquine and azithromycin as a treatment of COVID-19: results of an open-label non-randomized clinical trial. Int J Antimicrob Agents. 2020;56(1):105949.
21. Lagier JC, Million M, Gautret P, Colson P, Cortaredona S, Giraud-Gatineau A, et al. Outcomes of 3,737 COVID-19 patients treated with hydroxychloroquine/azithromycin and other regimens in Marseille, France: a retrospective analysis. Travel Med Infect Dis. 2020;36:101791.
22. Borba MGS, Val FFA, Sampaio VS, Alexandre MAA, Melo GC, Brito M, et al. Effect of high vs low doses of chloroquine diphosphate as adjunctive therapy for patients hospitalized with severe acute respiratory syndrome Coronavirus 2 (SARS-CoV-2) infection: a randomized clinical trial. JAMA Netw Open. 2020;3(4):e208857.
23. Monteiro WM, Brito-Sousa JD, Baia-da-Silva D, Melo GC, Siqueira AM, Val F, et al. Driving forces for COVID-19 clinical trials using chloroquine: the need to choose the right research questions and outcomes. Rev Soc Bras Med Trop. 2020;53:e20200155.
24. Cortegiani A, Ippolito M, Ingoglia G, Iozzo P, Giarratano A, Einav S. Update I. A systematic review on the efficacy and safety of chloroquine/hydroxychloroquine for COVID-19. J Crit Care. 2020;59:176–90.
25. Cortegiani A, Ippolito M, Ingoglia G, Einav S. Chloroquine for COVID-19: rationale, facts, hopes. Crit Care. 2020;24(1):210.
26. Cortegiani A, Ingoglia G, Ippolito M, Giarratano A, Einav S. A systematic review on the efficacy and safety of chloroquine for the treatment of COVID-19. J Crit Care. 2020;57:279–83.
27. Cavalcanti AB, Zampieri FG, Rosa RG, Azevedo LCP, Veiga VC, Avezum A, et al. Hydroxychloroquine with or without azithromycin in mild-to-moderate Covid-19. N Engl J Med. 2020;383:2041–52.
28. Gentry CA, Humphrey MB, Thind SK, Hendrickson SC, Kurdgelashvili G, Williams RJ 2nd. Long-term hydroxychloroquine use in patients with rheumatic conditions and development of SARS-CoV-2 infection: a retrospective cohort study. Lancet Rheumatol. 2020;2(11):e689–97.
29. Aringer M, Costenbader K, Dorner T, Johnson SR. SLE classification criteria items are not dependent on current activity but may accumulate over time. Response to: 'Do 2019 European League against rheumatism/American College of Rheumatology classification criteria for systemic lupus erythematosus also indicate the disease activity?' by Teng et al. Ann Rheum Dis. 2020.https://doi.org/10.1136/annrheumdis-2020-217105.
30. Aletaha D, Neogi T, Silman AJ, Funovits J, Felson DT, Bingham CO 3rd, et al. 2010 rheumatoid arthritis classification criteria: an American College of Rheumatology/European League Against Rheumatism collaborative initiative. Ann Rheum Dis. 2010;69(9):1580–8.
31. Shiboski CH, Shiboski SC, Seror R, Criswell LA, Labetoulle M, Lietman TM, et al. 2016 American College of Rheumatology/European League Against Rheumatism classification criteria for primary Sjogren's syndrome: a consensus and data-driven methodology involving three international patient cohorts. Ann Rheum Dis. 2017;76(1):9–16.
32. van den Hoogen F, Khanna D, Fransen J, Johnson SR, Baron M, Tyndall A, et al. 2013 classification criteria for systemic sclerosis: an American College of Rheumatology/European League against Rheumatism collaborative initiative. Arthritis Rheum. 2013;65(11):2737–47.
33. Lundberg IE, Tjarnlund A, Bottai M, Werth VP, Pilkington C, de Visser M, et al. 2017 European League Against Rheumatism/American College of Rheumatology classification criteria for adult and juvenile idiopathic inflammatory myopathies and their major subgroups. Arthritis Rheumatol. 2017;69(12):2271–82.
34. Sharp GC, Irvin WS, Tan EM, Gould RG, Holman HR. Mixed connective tissue disease–an apparently distinct rheumatic disease syndrome associated with a specific antibody to an extractable nuclear antigen (ENA). Am J Med. 1972;52(2):148–59.
35. Altman R, Alarcon G, Appelrouth D, Bloch D, Borenstein D, Brandt K, et al. The American College of Rheumatology criteria for the classification and reporting of osteoarthritis of the hand. Arthritis Rheum. 1990;33(11):1601–10.
36. Altman RD, Block DA, Brandt KD, Cooke DV, Greenwald RA, Hochberg MC, et al. Osteoarthritis: definitions and criteria. Ann Rheum Dis. 1990;49(3):201.
37. Javelle E, Gautret P, Simon F. Chikungunya, the emerging migratory rheumatism. Lancet Infect Dis. 2015;15(5):509–10.
38. MdSB. Boletim Epidemiológico—Doença pelo Coronavírus 2019. Ampliação da Vigilância, Medidas não Farmacológicas e Descentralização do Diagnóstico Laboratorial. In: Saúde Md, editor Brasil 2020. 2020.
39. Zen M, Fuzzi E, Astorri D, Saccon F, Padoan R, Ienna L, et al. SARS-CoV-2 infection in patients with autoimmune rheumatic diseases in northeast Italy: a cross-sectional study on 916 patients. J Autoimmun. 2020;112:102502.
40. Figueroa-Parra G, Aguirre-Garcia GM, Gamboa-Alonso CM, Camacho-Ortiz A, Galarza-Delgado DA. Are my patients with rheumatic diseases at higher risk of COVID-19? Ann Rheum Dis. 2020;79(6):839–40.
41. Gianfrancesco M, Hyrich KL, Al-Adely S, Carmona L, Danila MI, Gossec L, et al. Characteristics associated with hospitalisation for COVID-19 in people with rheumatic disease: data from the COVID-19 Global Rheumatology Alliance physician-reported registry. Ann Rheum Dis. 2020;79(7):859–66.
42. D'Silva KM, Serling-Boyd N, Wallwork R, Hsu T, Fu X, Gravallese EM, et al. Clinical characteristics and outcomes of patients with coronavirus disease 2019 (COVID-19) and rheumatic disease: a comparative cohort study from a US "hot spot." Ann Rheum Dis. 2020;80:e64.
43. Marques C, Pinheiro MM, Reis Neto ET, Dantas AT, Ribeiro FM, Melo AKG. COVID-19 in patients with rheumatic diseases: what is the real mortality risk? Ann Rheum Dis. 2020. https://doi.org/10.1136/annrheumdis-2020-218431.
44. Schrezenmeier E, Dorner T. Mechanisms of action of hydroxychloroquine and chloroquine: implications for rheumatology. Nat Rev Rheumatol. 2020;16(3):155–66.
45. The L. COVID-19: learning from experience. Lancet. 2020;395(10229):1011.
46. Fineberg HV. Ten weeks to crush the curve. N Engl J Med. 2020;382(17):e37.
47. Wei WE, Li Z, Chiew CJ, Yong SE, Toh MP, Lee VJ. Presymptomatic transmission of SARS-CoV-2 - Singapore, January 23–March 16, 2020. MMWR Morb Mortal Wkly Rep. 2020;69(14):411–5.
48. Klompas M, Morris CA, Shenoy ES. Universal masking in the Covid-19 era. N Engl J Med. 2020;383(2):e9.
49. Klompas M, Morris CA, Sinclair J, Pearson M, Shenoy ES. Universal masking in hospitals in the Covid-19 Era. N Engl J Med. 2020;382(21):e63.
50. Wilder-Smith A, Freedman DO. Isolation, quarantine, social distancing and community containment: pivotal role for old-style public health measures in the novel coronavirus (2019-nCoV) outbreak. J Travel Med. 2020;27(2):taaa020. https://doi.org/10.1093/jtm/taaa020.
51. Paton NI, Lee L, Xu Y, Ooi EE, Cheung YB, Archuleta S, et al. Chloroquine for influenza prevention: a randomised, double-blind, placebo controlled trial. Lancet Infect Dis. 2011;11(9):677–83.
52. Paton NI, Goodall RL, Dunn DT, Franzen S, Collaco-Moraes Y, Gazzard BG,

et al. Effects of hydroxychloroquine on immune activation and disease progression among HIV-infected patients not receiving antiretroviral therapy: a randomized controlled trial. JAMA. 2012;308(4):353–61.
53. Konig MF, Kim AH, Scheetz MH, Graef ER, Liew JW, Simard J, et al. Baseline use of hydroxychloroquine in systemic lupus erythematosus does not preclude SARS-CoV-2 infection and severe COVID-19. Ann Rheum Dis. 2020;79:1386–8.
54. Carmichael SJ, Charles B, Tett SE. Population pharmacokinetics of hydroxychloroquine in patients with rheumatoid arthritis. Ther Drug Monit. 2003;25(6):671–81.
55. Morita S, Takahashi T, Yoshida Y, Yokota N. Population pharmacokinetics of hydroxychloroquine in Japanese patients with cutaneous or systemic lupus erythematosus. Ther Drug Monit. 2016;38(2):259–67.
56. Cui C, Tu S, En VSJ, Li X, Yao X, Li H, et al. Review on the clinical pharmacology of hydroxychloroquine sulfate for the treatment of COVID-19. Curr Drug Metab. 2020;21:427–35.
57. Yao X, Ye F, Zhang M, Cui C, Huang B, Niu P, et al. In vitro antiviral activity and projection of optimized dosing design of hydroxychloroquine for the treatment of severe acute respiratory syndrome Coronavirus 2 (SARS CoV-2). Clin Infect Dis. 2020;71(15):732–9.
58. Calisher C, Carroll D, Colwell R, Corley RB, Daszak P, Drosten C, et al. Statement in support of the scientists, public health professionals, and medical professionals of China combatting COVID-19. Lancet. 2020;395(10226):e42–3.
59. Gao J, Hu S. Update on use of chloroquine/hydroxychloroquine to treat coronavirus disease 2019 (COVID-19). Biosci Trends. 2020;14(2):156–8.
60. Gao J, Tian Z, Yang X. Breakthrough: chloroquine phosphate has shown apparent efficacy in treatment of COVID-19 associated pneumonia in clinical studies. Biosci Trends. 2020;14(1):72–3.
61. Monti S, Balduzzi S, Delvino P, Bellis E, Quadrelli VS, Montecucco C. Clinical course of COVID-19 in a series of patients with chronic arthritis treated with immunosuppressive targeted therapies. Ann Rheum Dis. 2020;79(5):667–8.
62. Lahouati M, Meriglier E, Martin L, Bouchet S, Desclaux A, Bonnet F. COVID-19 infection also occurs in patients taking hydroxychloroquine. J Antimicrob Chemother. 2020;75(7):2014–5.
63. Wang C, Horby PW, Hayden FG, Gao GF. A novel coronavirus outbreak of global health concern. Lancet. 2020;395(10223):470–3.
64. Wu Z, McGoogan JM. Characteristics of and important lessons from the Coronavirus Disease 2019 (COVID-19) Outbreak in China: summary of a report of 72314 cases from the Chinese Center for Disease Control and Prevention. JAMA. 2020;323:1239–42.
65. WHO. Novel Coronavirus (2019-nCoV) situation report-22. 2020.
66. Jung JY, Yoon D, Choi Y, Kim HA, Suh CH. Associated clinical factors for serious infections in patients with systemic lupus erythematosus. Sci Rep. 2019;9(1):9704.
67. Ocampo-Piraquive V, Nieto-Aristizabal I, Canas CA, Tobon GJ. Mortality in systemic lupus erythematosus: causes, predictors and interventions. Expert Rev Clin Immunol. 2018;14(12):1043–53.
68. Jorge A, Wallace ZS, Zhang Y, Lu N, Costenbader KH, Choi HK. All-cause and cause-specific mortality trends of end-stage renal disease due to lupus nephritis from 1995 to 2014. Arthritis Rheumatol. 2019;71(3):403–10.
69. Li G, Fan Y, Lai Y, Han T, Li Z, Zhou P, et al. Coronavirus infections and immune responses. J Med Virol. 2020;92(4):424–32.
70. Wan S, Yi Q, Fan S, Lv J, Zhang X, Guo L, et al. Relationships among lymphocyte subsets, cytokines, and the pulmonary inflammation index in coronavirus (COVID-19) infected patients. Br J Haematol. 2020;189(3):428–37.
71. Matucci-Cerinic M, Bruni C, Allanore Y, Clementi M, Dagna L, Damjanov NS, et al. Systemic sclerosis and the COVID-19 pandemic: World Scleroderma Foundation preliminary advice for patient management. Ann Rheum Dis. 2020;79(6):724–6.
72. Orlandi M, Lepri G, Bruni C, Wang Y, Bartoloni A, Zammarchi L, et al. The systemic sclerosis patient in the COVID-19 era: the challenging crossroad between immunosuppression, differential diagnosis and long-term psychological distress. Clin Rheumatol. 2020;39(7):2043–7.
73. Minniti A, Maglione W, Pignataro F, Cappadona C, Caporali R, Del Papa N. Taking care of systemic sclerosis patients during COVID-19 pandemic: rethink the clinical activity. Clin Rheumatol. 2020;39(7):2063–5.
74. Lechien JR, Chiesa-Estomba CM, De Siati DR, Horoi M, Le Bon SD, Rodriguez A, et al. Olfactory and gustatory dysfunctions as a clinical presentation of mild-to-moderate forms of the coronavirus disease (COVID-19): a multicenter European study. Eur Arch Otorhinolaryngol. 2020;277(8):2251–61.
75. Furer V, Rondaan C, Heijstek MW, Agmon-Levin N, van Assen S, Bijl M, et al. 2019 update of EULAR recommendations for vaccination in adult patients with autoimmune inflammatory rheumatic diseases. Ann Rheum Dis. 2020;79(1):39–52.
76. Epidemiologists CoSaT. Interm-20-ID-01: standardized surveillance case definitions and national notification for 2019 novel coronavirus disease (COVID-19). 2020 2020.
77. Zhong J, Shen G, Yang H, Huang A, Chen X, Dong L, et al. COVID-19 in patients with rheumatic disease in Hubei province, China: a multicentre retrospective observational study. Lancet Rheumatol. 2020;2(9):e557–64.
78. Aouhab Z, Hong H, Felicelli C, Tarplin S, Ostrowski RA. Outcomes of systemic lupus erythematosus in patients who discontinue hydroxychloroquine. ACR Open Rheumatol. 2019;1(9):593–9.
79. Peschken CA. Possible consequences of a shortage of hydroxychloroquine for patients with systemic lupus erythematosus amid the COVID-19 Pandemic. J Rheumatol. 2020;47(6):787–90.
80. Jakhar D, Kaur I. Potential of chloroquine and hydroxychloroquine to treat COVID-19 causes fears of shortages among people with systemic lupus erythematosus. Nat Med. 2020;26(5):632.
81. Michaud K, Wipfler K, Shaw Y, Simon TA, Cornish A, England BR, et al. Experiences of patients with rheumatic diseases in the United States during early days of the COVID-19 pandemic. ACR Open Rheumatol. 2020;2(6):335–43.
82. Gomides A. Impact of chronic use of antimalarials on SARS-CoV-2 infection in patients with immune-mediated rheumatic diseases: protocol design for a multicentric observational cohort in Brazil. JMIR Res Protoc. 2020;9:e23532.

21

The effect of rehabilitation protocol using mobile health in overweight and obese patients with knee osteoarthritis

Muhammad Tariq Rafiq[1], Mohamad Shariff Abdul Hamid[2*] and Eliza Hafiz[3]

Abstract

Objective: The objective of this randomized controlled trial (RCT) was to investigate the effectiveness of the lower limb rehabilitation protocol (LLRP) combined with mobile health (mHealth) applications on knee pain, mobility, functional activity and activities of daily living (ADL) among knee osteoarthritis (OA) patients who were overweight and obese.

Methods: This study was a single-blind, RCT conducted at Teaching Bay of Rehmatul-Lil-Alameen Post Graduate Institute of Cardiology between February and November 2020. 114 knee OA patients who were overweight and obese were randomly divided by a computer-generated number into the rehabilitation group with mHealth (RGw-mHealth) to receive LLRP + instructions of daily care (IDC) combined with mHealth intervention, rehabilitation group without mHealth (RGwo-mHealth) to receive LLRP + IDC intervention and control group (CG) to receive IDC intervention. All three groups were also provided leaflets explaining about their intervention. The primary outcome measure was knee pain measured by the Western Ontario and McMaster Universities Osteoarthritis Index score. The secondary outcome measures were mobility measured by the Timed up and go (TUG) test, functional activity measured by the patient-specific functional scale (PSFS), and ADL measured by the Katz Index of independence in ADL scores.

Results: Among the 114 patients who were randomized (mean age, 53 years), 96 (84%) completed the trial. After 3-months of intervention, patients in all three groups had statistically significant knee pain reduction (RGw-mHealth: 2.54; RGwo-mHealth: 1.47; and CG: 0.37) within groups ($P < 0.05$). Furthermore, patients in the RGw-mHealth and RGwo-mHealth had statistically significant improvement in mobility, functional activity, and ADL within groups ($P < 0.05$), but no improvement was noted in the CG ($p > 0.05$). As indicated in the overall analysis of covariance, there were statistically significant differences in the mean knee pain, mobility, functional activity, and ADL changes between groups after 3-months ($p < 0.001$). The pairwise between-group comparisons (Bonferroni post hoc analysis) of the knee pain, mobility, functional activity, and ADL scores at 3-months revealed that patients in the RGw-mHealth had significantly higher mean change in the knee pain, TUG test, functional activity, and ADL scores compared to patients in the RGwo-mHealth or CG.

Conclusion: Reduction in knee pain, improvement in mobility, functional activity, and ADL were more among patients in the RGw-mHealth compared with the RGwo-mHealth or CG.

*Correspondence: ayip@um.edu.my
[2] Sports Medicine Department, University of Malaya Medical Centre, Kuala Lumpur, Malaysia

Keywords: Osteoarthritis, Knee, Overweight, Rehabilitation, Pain

Introduction

Osteoarthritis (OA) causes a considerable burden in the quality of life and medical treatment of patients [1]. In OA, the knee is the most commonly affected weight-bearing joint with the cardinal symptoms of pain and loss of function [2, 3]. In 2015, knee OA was the most frequent type of OA diagnosed and ranked the thirteenth leading cause of disability globally [4]. Knee OA is a joint destruction and active disease process driven by proinflammatory and biomechanical factors [5]. Knee OA is the most frequent cause of mobility dependency [6] and is highly prevalent in overweight and obese individuals [7].

Patients with knee OA possess 20–40% weaker relative strength of the quadriceps muscles compared to control subjects [8, 9]. The weakness of the quadriceps muscles precedes the onset of knee OA and therefore it could increase the risk of disease development, particularly in women [10]. The Ottawa Panel found evidence to support the use of therapeutic exercises, especially strengthening exercises and general physical activity, combined with manual therapy or separately for the improvement of pain and functional characteristics in OA patients [11]. The American College of Rheumatology Foundation reported a guideline in which physical activity is recommended as a core component of knee OA management [12]. There are different trials of exercise and physical activity-based interventions for the treatment of knee OA. These interventions reported improvement in knee pain, function, and other outcomes among knee OA patients [13]. A current systematic review on non-pharmacological interventions for treating symptoms of knee OA in overweight or obese patients concluded that strengthening exercise played a vital role in relieving knee pain and improving function [14]. Non-pharmacological interventions, primarily strengthening exercise and more recently strengthening exercises of the lower limb rehabilitation protocol (LLRP) in non-weight-bearing positions, are recommended as the first line of treatment among overweight or obese knee OA patients [15].

A current systematic review found that mobile health application (mHealth app) users were more satisfied to manage their health than those of conventional care. The mHealth app users have reported a positive impact on health outcomes and health-related behaviors [16]. Smart phone's mHealth apps have the potential to play an important role in supporting personal health management [17] and to increase access to healthcare services [18]. A study reported that consistent contact via phone can improve the clinical status of knee OA patients [19]. Effectiveness of rehabilitation combined with mHealth may provide more objective data than the standard rehabilitation approaches we are using today to treat overweight and obese knee OA patients. However, there is a gap in knowledge and a dearth of information regarding whether mHealth can improve the effects of LLRP among overweight and obese knee OA patients. Hence, the current randomized controlled trial (RCT) investigated the effects of LLRP combined with mHealth on knee pain, mobility, functional activity, and activities of daily living (ADL) among overweight and obese knee OA patients. The novelty of the current study could have been mediated by two factors, firstly it was provided as WhatsApp messages and secondly the researchers designed a LLRP to treat overweight and obese knee OA patients. The training sessions of LLRP are the strengthening exercises of the major muscle groups of the lower limbs in non-weight-bearing positions to reduce the mechanical load on the knee.

Methods

Study design and setting

The current study was a single-blind RCT of 3-month duration involving patients with knee OA who were overweight and obese. The study was conducted in the Teaching Bay of Rehmatul-Lil-Alameen Postgraduate Institute of Cardiology (RAIC), Punjab Employees Social Security Institution (PESSI) between February and November 2020. The study was approved by the Ethical Committee of RAIC PESSI with approval number RAIC PESSI/Estt/2020/33 and the trial was registered in the National Medical Research Registry, Malaysia, with ID NMRR-20-1094-52911. Pre-defined questionnaire of inclusion and exclusion criteria was used for screening of the patients. Written informed consent was obtained from all patients before participation in the study.

Sample size

Sample size estimation was performed using the G* Power 3.1.3 software. By assuming the medium effect size $f = 0.70$, setting $\alpha = 0.05$, power $(1 - B) = 0.90$, the total sample size estimated was 84 patients for the three groups. After considering 30% of drop-out or research mortality, the sample size of 114 patients for the three groups was decided (n = 38 per group).

Study patients' recruitment and selection

The inclusion criteria of the patients were as follows: both males and females, age between 45 and 60 years, overweight and obese, diagnosed with 2-mild or 3-moderate OA according to Kellgren and Lawrence radiographic [20] on one or both knees by an orthopaedic surgeon, symptoms of knee OA for more than 3-months, familiar with WhatsApp applications and residing in the Urban community of Lahore, Pakistan. Exclusion criteria were one or more of the following: diagnosed with flat foot or spinal deformities; history of cardiac or hormonal problems; previous surgery of the knee/s; corticosteroid injection of the knee/s for the last 6-months. Eligibility was determined using a predefined questionnaire of inclusion and exclusion criteria.

Patients were recruited using convenience sampling by active recruitment strategies through urban political and welfare organizations. The list of patients with knee OA in the studied area was obtained from the Welfare Organization upon explaining on the potential benefits of study participation. Two study coordinators prepared the list of potential patients in the recruitment area. After obtaining the list of potential patients, the researcher arranged a meeting with the potential patients through phone call. The meeting was held at the teaching bay of RAIC, PESSI, Lahore, Pakistan, in the presence of a medical specialist. Patients were screened for eligibility to participate in the study. Only patients fulfilling the inclusion and exclusion criteria of the study were invited to participate in this study. The experimental procedures, risks, and benefits associated with the study were explained (verbally and through participants' information sheets) to all patients prior to providing written informed consent.

Randomization

After completing the screening, the selected patients were randomized into three groups; Rehabilitation Group with mHealth (RGw-mHealth), Rehabilitation Group without mHealth (RGwo-mHealth) and the Control Group (CG) (Fig. 1), using a simple random technique

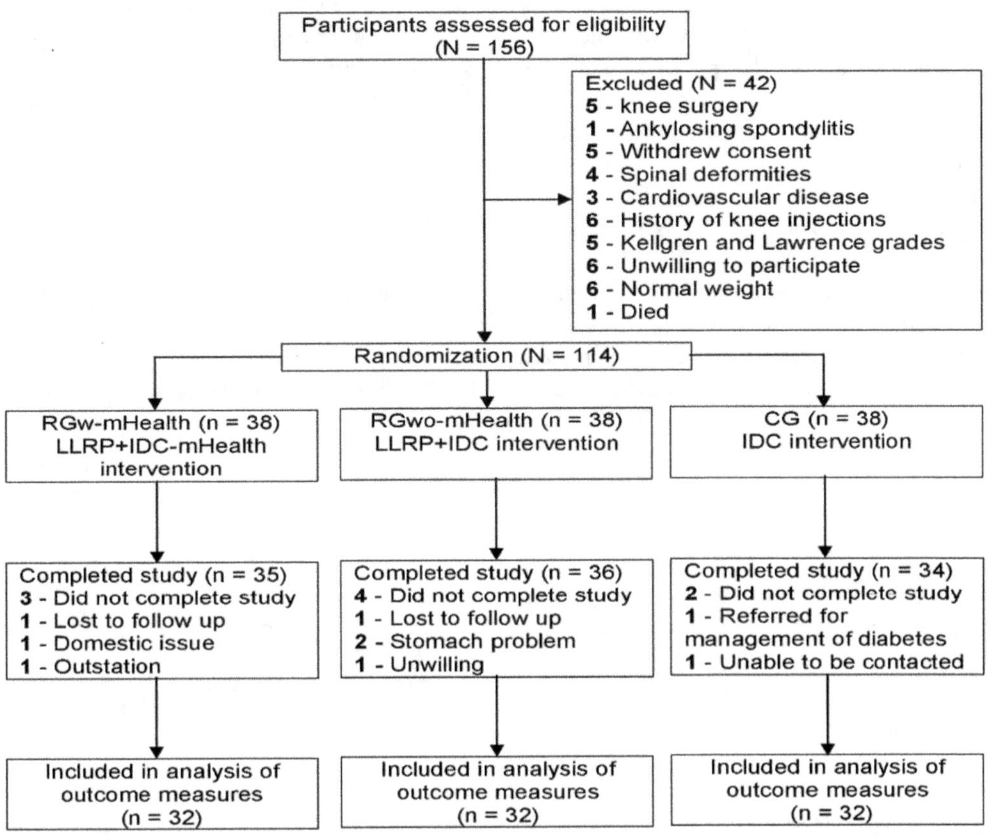

Fig. 1 Study flow diagram: RGw-mHealth = Rehabilitation group with mobile health; RGwo-mHealth = Rehabilitation group without mobile health; CG = Control group; LLRP = Lower limb rehabilitation protocol; IDC = Instructions of daily care; LLRP + IDC-mHealth = Lower limb rehabilitation protocol plus instructions of daily care combined with mobile health

(computer generated number). Each group consisted of 38 patients. All patients were also given a diary and asked to record the attendance of completion their interventions based on leaflets.

Blinding and allocation

The coordinators collecting data were independent individuals from the trials and were unaware of the group allocation. There were different coordinators at the baseline and post-test evaluation. Individuals performing the statistical analysis were kept blinded by labelling the groups with nonidentifying terms (such as X and Y).

Research procedures

Rehabilitation group with mHealth (RGw-mHealth)

Patients in the RGw-mHealth were prescribed with LLRP + IDC combined with mHealth (LLRP + IDC-mHealth) intervention. The LLRP focused on strengthening exercises for the lower limbs in non-weight bearing sitting or lying positions (Additional file 1) to reduce mechanical pressure on the knee. In the current study, the researcher with the help of several experts in the field of rehabilitation, designed a LLRP (Additional file 1) to be used in the RCT. The LLRP is designed to be a progressive exercise program that begins as a low intensity which gradually increases (frequency, intensity, and duration) to high intensity to ensure that patients could cope with the intervention.

The sequence of the training program started with ten minutes' warm-up with whole body range of motion (ROM) and dynamic stretching exercises. Patients performed ten repetitions of ROM of each muscle group and 5 repetitions of dynamic stretching of each muscle group as a part of warm-up. A study demonstrated that dynamic stretching is recommended for warm-up to avoid a decrease in strength and performance [21]. When static stretching is used as part of a warm-up immediately prior to exercise, then it causes harm to muscle strength [22]. After warm-up, the patients performed the strengthening exercises of the lower limbs for 3-months (Additional file 1).

Patients were advised to follow the IDC, which included advice on general guidelines of mobility and healthy eating (Table 1). The IDC was translated into Urdu language by two language experts to ensure better patients' understanding based on a recent pilot study [15]. After completing the strengthening exercises, the patients performed ten minutes cool-down with whole body ROM and static stretching exercises. Patients performed ten repetitions of ROM of each muscle group and 3 repetitions of static stretching of each muscle group as a part of cool-down. A study explained that after two to four repetitions of static stretching, there is no increase in muscle elongation [23].

Additionally, patients in the RGw-mHealth group receive regular reminders to carry out of the LLRP through mHealth in the form of WhatsApp messages. Two text messages per day for three days a week for a period of 3-months were sent to patients in the RGw-mHealth throughout the study period. Patients in the RGw-mHealth received a total 72 text messages. The text messages were sent between 7:00 to 9:00 a.m. and 5:00 to 7:00 p.m. during the days of Wednesday, Friday, and Sunday. A study reported that sending text messages in the morning was to ensure that the patients have enough time to plan and do exercise during the day [24]. In addition, every patient was actively followed by phone at least once a week to ensure that they read the messages and performed the intervention.

Rehabilitation group without mobile health (RGwo-mHealth)

Patients in RGwo-mHealth received LLRP + IDC intervention, but did not receive any reminders to carry out the LLRP exercises. Patients in the RGwo-mHealth were

Table 1 Instruction of daily care (IDC)

Activity name	IDC
Sitting	When there is option of sitting than standing, then prefer to sitting. Prefer your sitting on high stool or chair rather than low level
Standing from sitting	When you are standing from sitting position, and then initially sit at the edge of bed, chair or stool with the feet on the ground at the level of hips. Use the hands to push up from the bed, chair or stool
Walking	Do not walk, jog or run as an exercise plan. Walking stick can be used on the opposite hand of the affected knee OA. If both knees are affected, then walker can be used. Use of knee brace and jogging shoes with well cushioned soles during walking is highly recommended
Stair climbing	Avoid stair climbing. But if there is need of stair climbing then support the side rails with your hands by placing the affected foot first on a stair step then the unaffected foot on the same step
Working	Prefer working on a high stool or chair
Body weight	Try to reduce your weight by avoiding taking of sugary foods, drinks and high fat foods. Eat mostly plant-based foods. Add omega-3 fatty acids in your daily diet

IDC, instructions of daily care

trained on how to perform the LLRP 3-times a week and to adhere to the IDC for 3-months at home. Each training session started with ten minutes of warm-up, forty-five to sixty minutes of strengthening exercises for the lower limbs, and ten minutes of cool down at the end of the training protocol (Additional file 1).

Control group (CG)

Patients in the CG were only advised to follow the IDC intervention for the duration of 3-months (Table 1). No reminders through mHealth application (WhatsApp) were sent to patients in the CG. The feasibility and acceptability of the IDC among knee OA participants have been proved effective in a recent RCT [25].

Measurements and procedures

All patients were assessed at enrolment (baseline) and again at 3-months follow-up. Patients' assessment includes demographics, exercise adherence, primary and secondary outcome measures of interest. Patients demographic information gathered including age, gender, educational status, and marital status were recorded. The assessment of the patients' self-reported exercise adherence was collected after 3-months of intervention. A self-reported exercise adherence was measured using a numerical rating scale (NRS) ranging from zero = never performed intervention to 10 = always performed intervention. NRS have also been widely used in other trials [26, 27]. Outcome measures gathered were categorized into primary and secondary outcome measures.

Primary outcome measure

Primary outcome measure was knee pain symptoms assessed using the Western Ontario and McMaster Universities Osteoarthritis Index (WOMAC) that was already adapted and validated. The WOMAC score ranges from 0 to 4 on a Likert-type scale. The researcher used the section on pain of the WOMAC questionnaire. There were five items of WOMAC questionnaire for assessing knee pain. The total scores for the 5 items range from 0 to 20: the higher the score, the worse the pain [28].

Secondary outcome measures

The secondary outcome measures were mobility, functional activity, and ADL. Patients' mobility was assessed using the Timed Up and Go (TUG) test as described by Podsiadlo and Richardson [29]. The patients were observed and timed while they rose from an armchair, walked three meters, turned, walked back, and sat down again. Assessment was performed in accord with the technique as described in the literature [29].

The Patient-Specific Functional Scale (PSFS) was used for the measurement of functional activity. This is a valid and reliable tool that allows patients to report on their function at baseline and follow-up [30]. The patients were asked to identify up to three difficult activities to perform at enrolment. The patients were then asked to rate each of their identified activities on a numerical scale ranging from 0 = 'unable to perform an activity' to 10 = 'able to perform activities. After 12 weeks of intervention, the patients were again asked to rate their same difficult activities they had identified at baseline. The mean of the scores was used for the analysis of the nominated activities, with higher scores reflecting greater function.

The Katz Index of Independence in ADL was used to assess patients' ADL. In Katz ADL, six functions were assessed such as feeding, continence, toileting, dressing one self, bathing, and transferring. Each activity has a potential of either zero or one point. One point was used as independence with subheadings, no supervision, direction, or personal assistance. A score of zero is given to indicate that a participant is dependence on subheadings, supervision, direction, personal assistant, or total care in their daily activities. The overall score ranges from zero (patient very dependent) to six (patient fully independent) [31]. In Katz ADL, a total score of 2 or less indicates severe functional impairment, 4 indicates moderate impairment, and a score of 6 indicates full functional independence in ADL [32].

Statistical analysis

The Statistical Package for Social Sciences, version 22, Chicago, IL, was used to analyze the data. Continuous variables were presented as mean (standard deviation [SD]) based on data distribution. The Shapiro–Wilk test was used to assess the normality of all variables. Categorical variables were presented as frequencies (n) and percentages (%). For categorical demographic variables, the One-Way Analysis of Variance (ANOVA) was used to compare for differences between variables. Since all data was normally distributed; the Paired Samples t-test was used to analyze differences between the baseline and 3-months measurements within the groups.

The overall treatment effects on change in clinical outcome measures were estimated using the One Way ANOVA (unadjusted results) and Analyses of Covariance (ANCOVA, adjusted results) for mean changes (95% confidence interval [CI]) from baseline in the continuous outcome data. ANCOVA should be the preferred method for the analysis of pretest–posttest data. The use of ANCOVA in a randomized design is to reduce error variance, because the random assignment of subjects to groups guards against systematic bias [33]. The ANCOVA model included the changes as the dependent variable, with group as a main effect and the baseline scores as an additional covariate. The purpose of using the pretest (baseline) scores as a covariate in ANCOVA with a pretest–posttest design is to reduce the error variance and eliminate systematic bias [33]. The pairwise comparisons between groups were estimated using Bonferroni post hoc analysis. The value of $P < 0.05$ was considered statistically significant.

Results

There were 114 patients with knee OA enrolled in the 3-months trial. Patients were randomized into LLRP + IDC-mHealth intervention (n = 38), LLRP + IDC intervention (n = 38), and IDC intervention (n = 38). The retention rate in all groups was 84%. The safety coordinator determined that two serious adverse events were unrelated to the study. Both patients were in the RGw-mHealth, one patient had appendix surgery, and the other underwent gallbladder surgery. Patients in the CG had one nonserious adverse event of muscle spasm related to the study.

Figure 1 demonstrates the study flow chart. A total of 18 patients (6 LLRP + IDC-mHealth intervention, 6 LLRP + IDC intervention, and 6 IDC intervention) did not complete the study, resulting in 96 patients (32 LLRP + IDC-mHealth intervention, 32 LLRP + IDC intervention and 32 IDC intervention) included in the analysis of WOMAC pain for knee pain, TUG test for mobility, Katz Index of Independence for ADL and PSFS for functional activity scores. Figure 1 demonstrates the study flow chart including reasons given by patients who did not complete the study.

The patients' baseline demographics and clinical outcome measures are described in Table 2. No significant differences were observed in the baseline demographic characteristics between the three groups. No statistically significant difference in the Katz Index of Independence for ADL and the PSFS for functional activity scores between the groups. A significant difference in the WOMAC pain and TUG scores was observed at baseline. No significant differences were observed between patients who completed and those who withdrew on baseline demographic and clinical outcome measures (Table 3). Mean and 95% CI of WOMAC pain, TUG test, Katz ADL and PSFS scores at baseline and 3-month follow-up across the three groups are shown in Fig. 2.

After participation in 3-months of intervention, a statistically significant improvement compared to baseline was observed for knee pain, mobility, functional activity, and ADL scores ($p < 0.05$) in the RGw-mHealth, and RGwo-mHealth. In the CG, knee pain score was also significantly improved ($p < 0.05$) (Table 4).

Table 2 Baseline demographic and clinical outcome measures of patients

Demographic and clinical outcome measures	Overall (N = 114)	RGwo-mHealth (n = 38)	RGw-mHealth (n = 38)	CG (n = 38)	P
Age, mean (SD), y	52.92 (4.58)	51.73 (4.93)	53.97 (4.36)	52.94 (4.58)	*0.114*
Gender (M/F)	50/64	17/21	17/21	16/22	*0.966*
Educational status, No. (%)					
Matriculation	25 (21.90)	11 (9.60)	12 (10.50)	2 (1.80)	*0.071*
Intermediate	47 (41.20)	16 (14.00)	12 (10.50)	19 (16.70)	
Bachelor	24 (21.10)	6 (5.30)	9 (7.90)	9 (7.90)	
Master	18 (15.80)	5 (4.40)	5 (4.40)	8 (7.00)	
Marital status, No. (%)					
Single	7 (6.1)	4 (3.5)	3 (2.6)	0 (0)	*0.633*
Married	99 (86.8)	31 (27.2)	32 (28.1)	36 (31.6)	
Divorced	8 (7.0)	3 (2.6)	3 (2.6)	2 (1.8)	
Kellgren and Lawrence grade, No. (%)					
2 grade	69 (60.5)	25 (65.8)	20 (52.6)	24 (63.2)	*0.470*
3 grade	45 (39.5)	13 (34.2)	18 (47.4)	14 (36.8)	
BMI (kg/m^2)	32.17 (4.21)	31.98 (3.61)	33.06 (4.36)	32.02 (4.65)	*0.138*
WOMAC Pain score (0–20), mean (SD)	9.66 (2.54)	9.10 (2.32)	10.63 (2.46)	9.26 (2.62)	*0.015*
TUG score (seconds), mean (SD)	11.36 (2.81)	10.48 (2.08)	12.73 (3.47)	10.87 (2.17)	*0.001*
Katz ADL score (0–6), mean (SD)	4.12 (1.07)	4.26 (0.97)	3.89 (1.42)	4.21 (0.66)	*0.272*
PSFS (0–10), mean (SD)	4.57 (1.19)	4.61 (0.87)	4.68 (1.24)	4.42 (1.41)	*0.613*

RGw-mHealth, rehabilitation group with mobile health; RGwo-mHealth, rehabilitation group without mobile health; CG, control group; WOMAC, Western Ontario and McMaster Universities Osteoarthritis Index; BMI, body mass index; SD, standard deviation; TUG, timed up and go; ADL, activities of daily living; PSFS, patient specific functional scale; n, number

Table 3 Comparisons between patients who completed and withdrew by baseline demographic and clinical outcome measures

Demographic and clinical outcome measures	Completed (n = 96)	Withdrew (n = 18)	*P*
Age, mean (SD), year	52.96 (4.67)	52.72 (4.18)	*0.835*
Gender (M/F)	41/55	9/9	*0.540*
Educational status, No. (%)			
Matriculation	22 (22.9)	3 (16.7)	*0.911*
Intermediate	40 (41.7)	7 (38.9)	
Bachelor	20 (20.8)	4 (22.2)	
Master	14 (14.6)	4 (22.2)	
Marital status, No. (%)			
Single	6 (6.3)	1 (5.6)	*0.873*
Married	84 (87.5)	15 (83.3)	
Divorced	6 (6.3)	2 (11.1)	
Kellgren and Lawrence grade, No. (%)			
2 grade	58 (60.4)	11 (61.1)	*0.956*
3 grade	38 (39.6)	7 (38.9)	
BMI (kg/m^2)	32.14 (4.30)	32.32 (3.81)	*0.869*
WOMAC pain score (0–20), mean (SD)	9.61 (2.62)	9.94 (2.12)	*0.616*
TUG score (seconds), mean (SD)	11.47 (2.80)	10.80 (2.84)	*0.359*
Katz ADL score (0–6), mean (SD)	4.10 (1.05)	4.22 (1.21)	*0.671*
PSFS (0–10), mean (SD)	4.59 (1.17)	4.48 (1.32)	*0.742*

WOMAC, Western Ontario and McMaster Universities Osteoarthritis Index; SD, standard deviation; BMI, body mass index; TUG, timed up and go; ADL, activities of daily living; PSFS, patient specific functional scale; n, number

The mean changes in knee pain scores at 3-months from baseline were 2.54 (95% CI 1.99, 3.09), 1.47 (95% CI 0.93, 2.01) and 0.37 (95% CI −0.16, 0.90) for patients in the RGw-mHealth, RGwo-mHealth and CG, respectively (Table 5). The pairwise between-group comparisons of WOMAC Pain score at 3-months revealed that patients in the RGw-mHealth demonstrated a statistically significantly higher mean change in WOMAC pain score compared to the patients in the RGwo-mHealth ($p = 0.022$) and CG ($p < 0.001$). Additionally, there was also a statistically significant higher mean change in the WOMAC pain score in patients of the RGwo-mHealth compared to the CG ($p = 0.013$) (Table 6).

The mean changes in TUG test scores at 3-months from baseline were 2.64 s (95% CI 2.26, 3.02 s), 1.34 s (95% CI 0.97, 1.70 s), and 0.29 s (95% CI −0.06, 0.65 s) for patients in the RGw-mHealth, RGwo-mHealth and CG respectively (Table 5). As indicated by the overall ANCOVA, there was a statistically significant difference in the mean change in the TUG test scores between groups after 3-months interventions ($p < 0.001$). The pairwise between-group comparisons of the TUG test score at 3-months revealed that patients in the RGw-mHealth demonstrated a significantly higher mean change in the TUG test score compared to the RGwo-mHealth and CG ($p < 0.001$). Additionally, the mean change in the TUG test score among patients in the RGwo-mHealth was significantly higher compared to the CG ($p < 0.001$) (Table 6).

The mean changes in functional activity scores were −2.65 (95% CI −2.82, −2.48), −1.00 (95% CI −1.17, −0.83) and −0.06 (95% CI −0.22, 0.10) for patients in the RGw-mHealth, RGwo-mHealth and CG respectively (Table 5). The pairwise between-group comparisons of functional activity at 3-months revealed that patients in the RGw-mHealth had significantly higher mean change in the functional activity score relative to both RGwo-mHealth (difference, 1.65 [1.35, 1.94]; $p < 0.001$) and CG (difference, −2.59 [−2.89, −2.30]; $p < 0.001$). There was also a statistically significant difference in the mean change in the functional activity scores between the RGwo-mHealth and CG (difference, −0.94 [−1.24, −0.65]; $p < 0.001$) (Table 6).

Patients in the RGw-mHealth reported the greatest improvement in the ADL score of −1.13 (95% CI −1.36, −0.91) compared to baseline. Improvement in the ADL scores of −0.51 (95% CI −0.73, −0.29) and −0.12 (95% CI −0.38, 0.03) was noted in the RGwo-mHealth and CG respectively (Table 5). The pairwise between-group comparisons of the ADL score at 3-months revealed that patients in the RGw-mHealth had a significantly higher mean change in the ADL score compared to both RGwo-mHealth (difference, 0.62 [0.23, 1.01]; $p = 0.001$) and CG (difference, −0.94 [−1.33, −0.56]; $p < 0.001$). There

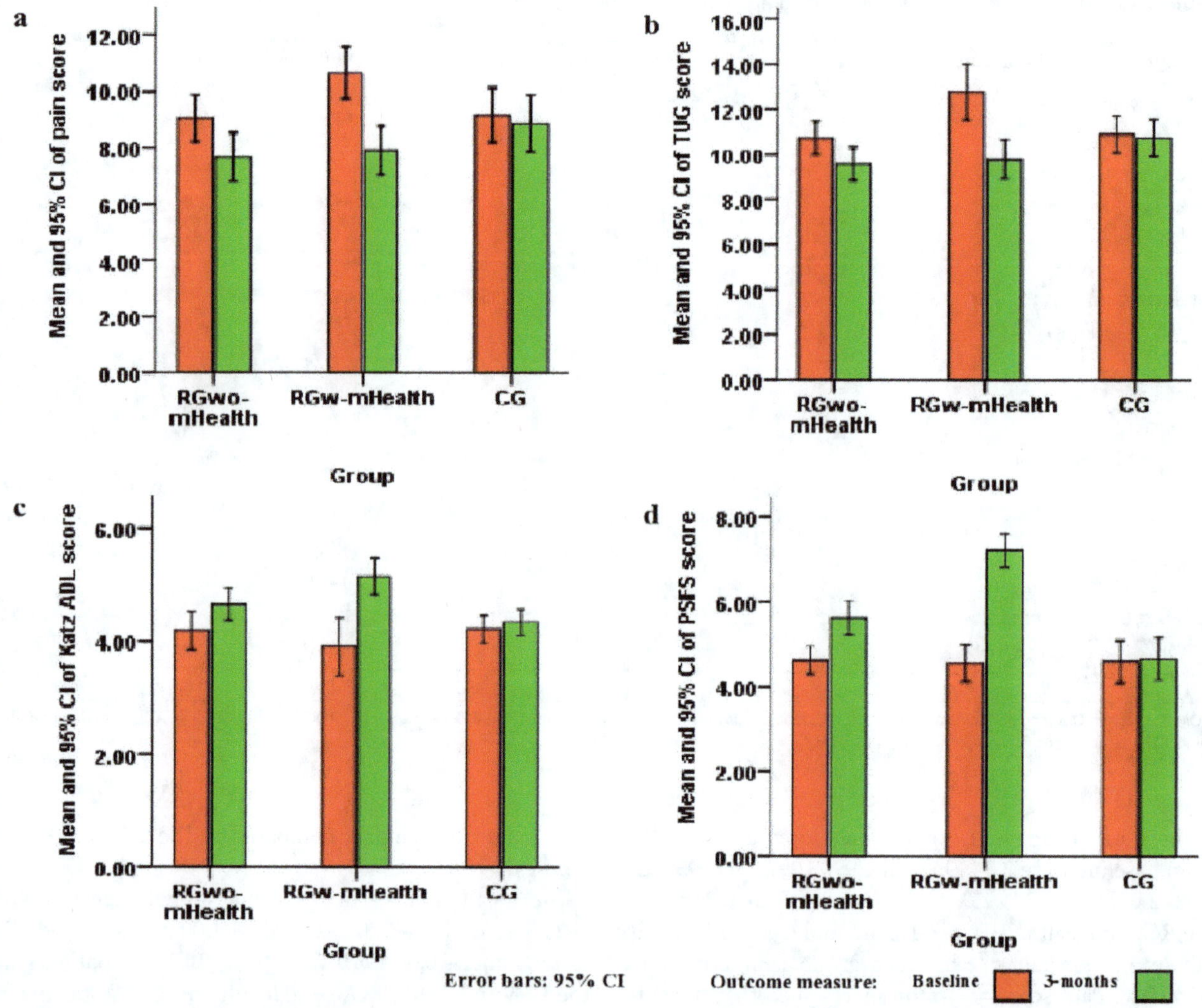

Fig. 2 Mean and 95% CI of the outcomes measures across the three groups. **a** mean and 95% CI of WOMAC pain score at baseline and 3-month follow-up, **b** mean and 95% CI of TUG test score at baseline and 3-month follow-up, **c** mean and 95% CI of Katz ADL score at baseline and 3-month follow-up, **d** mean and 95% CI of PSFS score at baseline and 3-month follow-up. WOMAC = Western Ontario and McMaster Universities Osteoarthritis Index; TUG = Timed Up and Go; ADL = Activities of daily living; PSFS = Patient specific functional scale; CI = Confidence interval

was not a statistically significant difference in the mean change in the ADL scores between the RGwo-mHealth and CG (difference, −0.32 [−0.71, 0.06]; $p = 0.127$) (Table 6).

As indicated by the ANOVA, there was a statistically significant difference in self-reported exercise adherence between the groups after 3-months of intervention ($p < 0.001$). The pairwise between-group comparisons of self-reported exercise adherence at 3-months revealed that patients in the RGw-mHealth had more self-reported adherence to their intervention relative to both patients in the RGwo-mHealth (difference, 0.79 [0.10, 1.47]; $p = 0.017$) and CG (difference, 3.00 [2.31, 3.68]; $p < 0.001$) in favour of the RGw-mHealth. There was also a statistically significant difference in self-reported exercise adherence between patients of the RGwo-mHealth and CG (difference, 2.20 [1.52, 2.89]; $p < 0.001$).

Discussion

To the best of our knowledge, this was the first RCT to investigate the effectiveness of LLRP combined with mHealth on knee pain, mobility, functional activity, and ADL among knee OA patients who were overweight and obese. In this study, patients who were assigned to the RGw-mHealth had significantly less pain, faster mobility, better functional activity, and better ADL scores over a 3-month period than patients in the RGwo-mHealth and CG. The results indicated that patients in

Table 4 Change in clinical outcome variables from baseline at 3-months within groups\

Variables	Group	Baseline, mean (SD)	3-months, Mean (SD)	Mean change (95% CI)	p
WOMAC pain score (0–20)	RGwo-mHealth	9.03 (2.33)	7.67 (2.36)	1.35 (0.45, 2.25)	*0.004*
	RG-mHealth	10.65 (2.58)	7.90 (2.42)	2.75 (2.43, 3.06)	*<0.001*
	CG	9.15 (2.70)	8.87 (2.80)	0.28 (0.01, 0.54)	0.037
TUG score (seconds)	RGwo-mHealth	10.72 (2.05)	9.58 (2.03)	1.14 (0.86, 1.43)	*<0.001*
	RG-mHealth	12.78 (3.47)	9.79 (2.39)	3.68 (2.98, 2.29)	*<0.001*
	CG	10.90 (2.27)	10.75 (2.23)	0.14 (−0.02, 0.32)	0.100
Katz ADL score (0–6)	RGwo-mHealth	4.18 (0.93)	4.65 (0.78)	−0.46 (−0.75, −0.17)	*0.002*
	RG-mHealth	3.90 (1.42)	5.15 (0.88)	−1.25 (−1.65, −0.84)	*<0.001*
	CG	4.21 (0.65)	4.34 (0.65)	−0.12 (−0.32, 0.07)	0.211
PS FS (0–10)	RGwo-mHealth	4.61 (0.90)	5.62 (1.15)	−1.00 (−1.18, −0.82)	*<0.001*
	RG-mHealth	4.55 (1.21)	7.21 (1.10)	−2.65 (−2.88, −2.43)	*<0.001*
	CG	4.59 (1.38)	4.65 (1.39)	−0.05 (−0.14, 0.02)	0.173

RGw-mHealth, rehabilitation group with mobile health; RGwo-mHealth, rehabilitation group without mobile health; CG, control group; WOMAC, Western Ontario and McMaster Universities Osteoarthritis Index; SD, standard deviation; TUG, timed up and go test; ADL, activities of daily living; PSFS, patient specific functional scale; CI, confidence interval; n, number

Table 5 Unadjusted and adjusted mean change in clinical outcome measures from baseline at 3-months

Change in outcome measures	RGwo-mHealth (n=32) Mean (95% CI)	RGw-mHealth (n=32) Mean (95% CI)	CG (n=32) Mean (95% CI)	p
Δ WOMAC pain (0–20)				
Unadjusted	1.35 (0.45, 2.25)	2.75 (2.43, 3.06)	0.28 (0.01, 0.54)	*<0.001*
Adjusted	1.47 (0.93, 2.01)	2.54 (1.99, 3.09)	0.37 (−0.16, 0.90)	*<0.001*
Δ TUG score (seconds)				
Unadjusted	1.14 (0.86, 1.43)	2.98 (2.29, 3.68)	0.14 (−0.02, 0.32)	*<0.001*
Adjusted	1.34 (0.97, 1.70)	2.64 (2.26, 3.02)	0.29 (−0.06, 0.65)	*<0.001*
Δ Katz ADL score (0–6)				
Unadjusted	−0.46 (−0.75, −0.17)	−1.25 (−1.65, −0.84)	−0.12 (−0.32, 0.07)	*<0.001*
Adjusted	−0.51 (−0.73, −0.29)	−1.13 (−1.36, −0.91)	−0.12 (0.41, 0.03)	*<0.001*
Δ PSFS (0–10)				
Unadjusted	−1.00 (−1.18, −0.82)	−2.65 (−2.88, −2.43)	−0.05 (−0.14, 0.02)	*<0.001*
Adjusted	−1.00 (−1.17, −0.83)	−2.65 (−2.82, −2.48)	−0.06 (−0.22, 0.10)	*<0.001*

RGw-mHealth, rehabilitation group with mobile health; RGwo-mHealth, rehabilitation group without mobile health; CG, control group; WOMAC, Western Ontario and McMaster Universities Osteoarthritis Index; SD, standard deviation; TUG, timed up and go; ADL, activities of daily living; PSFS, patient specific functional scale; CI, confidence interval; n, number

the RGw-mHealth who received additional reminders in the form of periodic manual WhatsApp messages showed greater improvements in reducing knee pain and improving mobility, functional activity and ADL than did patients in the RGwo-mHealth or CG. In the current study, the RGw-mHealth produced a clinically relevant reduction in knee pain and improvement in mobility, functional activity, and ADL, and this may explain why clinical improvement of outcome measures occurred. A potential reason why the RGw-mHealth had a significant result is that patient adherence to the LLRP combined with mHealth was good.

Two systematic reviews of randomized controlled trials reported that exercise therapy reduces pain for OA of the knee [34, 35]. In the current study, the pain score was significantly reduced in all three groups ($p<0.05$), but a marked reduction in pain score was reported by the patients in the RGw-mHealth ($p<0.001$). This may be due to the reminders of using mHealth that were sent to the patients of RGw-mHealth. The reminders of using mHealth stimulated the patients to follow their intervention more efficiently.

A randomized controlled trial reported significantly greater improvement in mobility scores following dietary

Table 6 Pairwise comparisons of clinical outcome measures between groups by Bonferroni test (post hoc)

Variables	Comparison between Groups	Mean difference (95% CI for difference)	*p*
WOMAC pain score (0–20)	RGw-mHealth and RGwo-mHealth	− 1.07 (− 2.02, − 0.11)	*0.022*
	RGwo-mHealth and CG	1.10 (0.18, 2.02)	*0.013*
	RGw-mHealth and CG	2.17 (1.22, 3.12)	*<0.001*
TUG test score (seconds)	RGw-mHealth and RGwo-mHealth	− 1.30 (− 1.96, − 0.64)	*<0.001*
	RGwo-mHealth and CG	1.04 (0.41, 1.67)	*<0.001*
	RGw-mHealth and CG	2.34 (1.69, 3.00)	*<0.001*
Katz ADL score (0–6)	RGw-mHealth and RGwo-mHealth	0.62 (0.23, 1.01)	*0.001*
	RGwo-mHealth and CG	− 0.32 (− 0.71, 0.06)	0.127
	RGw-mHealth and CG	− 0.94 (− 1.33, − 0.56)	*<0.001*
PSFS (0–10)	RGw-mHealth and RGwo-mHealth	1.65 (1.35, 1.94)	*<0.001*
	RGwo-mHealth and CG	− 0.94 (− 1.24, − 0.65)	*<0.001*
	RGw-mHealth and CG	− 2.59 (− 2.89, − 2.30)	*<0.001*

RGw-mHealth, rehabilitation group with mobile health; RGwo-mHealth, rehabilitation group without mobile health; CG, control group; WOMAC, Western Ontario and McMaster Universities Osteoarthritis Index; SD, standard deviation; TUG, timed up and go; ADL, activities of daily living; PSFS, patient specific functional scale; CI, confidence interval; N, number

intervention combined with an exercise program compared with either a dietary or exercise program [36]. Moreover, mobility improvement was also reported following dietary intervention combined with an exercise group of the arthritis, diet, and activity promotion trial [37]. The current study showed that the patients in all three groups reported a reduction in TUG test scores. However, statistically significant improvement in mobility score was only observed in patients of the RGw-mHealth and RGwo-mHealth. The rating of Katz ADL was recommended by the observation of health care professionals [38]. In the current study, a trained health professional recorded the score of Katz ADL. The patients in the RGw-mHealth and RGwo-mHealth reported statistically significant improvement in ADL score than the CG.

A current study demonstrated that a combination of dietary weight loss and exercise intervention was consistently better in improving a combination of performance and functional outcomes among participants with knee OA compared with exercise alone, diet alone, or a control group [37]. Many trials of different physical activity and exercise-based interventions reported improvement of function among knee OA patients [39]. The current study demonstrated a statistically significant improvement in functional activity in patients of RGw-mHealth and RGwo-mHealth, but not in the CG. It is noteworthy that the improvement in functional activity was greater among patients in the RGw-mHealth than the RGwo-mHealth and CG. This may be due to the reminders of using mHealth that were sent to the patients of RGw-mHealth.

Similarly, the results of the current study indicated that patients in the RGw-mHealth reported greater exercise adherence to their interventions compared to patients in the RGwo-mHealth or CG. The patients who got reminders by using mHealth to perform their intervention in the current study reported better adherence than those patients who received their intervention with home exercise programs with an app with remote support [13].

Clinically meaningful results of the outcome measures in the current study could have been mediated by a couple of factors. Apart from serving as mHealth appointment reminders, the LLRP helped to increase the clinical significant results of pain, mobility, functional activity, and ADL.

Based on these findings, this LLRP + IDC-mHealth intervention is expected to be more effective in terms of reducing pain, improving mobility, functional activity, and ADL than any other rehabilitation intervention among knee OA patients who are overweight and obese. In addition, this intervention is easy to use in the home care setting and can also be used for hemiplegia, paraplegia, or wheelchair patients with lower limb weakness.

Study limitations

This study has several limitations. Firstly, the current study was conducted in a single centre to recruit patients. Secondly, patients in the current study were followed up only until 3-months, hence the long-term effects of the interventions cannot be ascertain. Thus, further research across multiple centres and with long-term follow-up are required to confirm the results of LLRP + IDC-mHealth intervention. Thirdly, psychosocial, physical activity, and comorbidity factors may influence the outcomes. Therefore, further research considering these additional factors is required to confirm the findings of the study.

Conclusion

Among knee OA patients who were overweight and obese, after 3-months, patients in the RG-mHealth had less knee pain, better functional activity, faster mobility, and better improvement in ADL scores than those in the RGwo-mHealth and CG. The results of the current study suggest that less knee pain, faster mobility, better functional activity, and ADL score among knee OA patients who were overweight and obese, are augmented better by the implementation of the rehabilitation protocol by using mHealth for rehabilitation or general treatment without mHealth. In this study, the importance of mHealth was revealed in rehabilitation programs for overweight and obese knee OA patients.

Highlights

Knee osteoarthritis (OA) among patients who are overweight or obese has been shown to cause progressive changes in the muscles and articular cartilage of the joint that may not be sufficiently targeted with current rehabilitation approaches.

Using the strengthening exercises of LLRP combined with mHealth may have the potential to reduce pain, improve mobility, functional activity, and ADL among knee OA patients who are overweight or obese. The training sessions of the strength exercises of LLRP combined with mHealth may have the greatest contribution to the body of knowledge internationally because these strengthening exercises are performed in non-weight-bearing sitting or lying positions to reduce the mechanical load on the knee.

Abbreviations

RCT: randomized controlled trial; LLRP: lower limb rehabilitation protocol; mHealth: mobile health; Apps: applications; BMI: body mass index; OA: osteoarthritis; RGw-mHealth: rehabilitation group with mobile health; RGwo-mHealth: rehabilitation group without mobile health; CG: control group; WOMAC: Western Ontario and McMaster Universities Osteoarthritis Index; TUG: timed up and go; ADL: activities of daily living; PSFS: Patient Specific Functional Scale; IDC: instruction of daily care; ANOVA: one-way analysis of variance; ANCOVA: analysis of covariance; NMRR: National Medical Research Registry; RAIC: Rehmatul-Lil-Alameen Postgraduate Institute of Cardiology; PESSI: Punjab Employees Social Security Institution; ROM: range of motion; CI: confidence interval; SD: standard deviation; N: number; Kg: kilogram; M: meter; %: percentage.

Supplementary Information

Additional file 1. Lower limb rehabilitation protocol (LLRP).

Acknowledgements

We would like to thank Dr. Shariff for his invaluable feedback on an earlier draft for reviewing this article. This RCT was not supported by any grant. The sponsor of RAIC, PESSI had no role in the design of the study; data collection, analysis, and interpretation; review of the manuscript; approval and decision to submit the manuscript for publication.

Authors' contributions

MTR developed the design and protocol of the study, wrote the manuscript and original draft, under the supervision of EH and MSAH. MSAH reviewed the manuscript and corrected the draft twice. EH contributed with the literature search and revision of the article. All authors read and approved the final manuscript.

Author details

[1]Centre for Sport and Exercise Sciences, University of Malaya, Kuala Lumpur, Malaysia. [2]Sports Medicine Department, University of Malaya Medical Centre, Kuala Lumpur, Malaysia. [3]Sports Centre, Centre for Sport and Exercise Sciences, University of Malaya, Kuala Lumpur, Malaysia.

References

1. Maetzel A, Li LC, Pencharz J, Tomlinson G, Bombardier C, Community Hypertension and Arthritis Project Study Team. The economic burden associated with osteoarthritis, rheumatoid arthritis, and hypertension: a comparative study. Ann Rheum Dis. 2004;63(4):395–401. https://doi.org/10.1136/ard.2003.006031.
2. Felson DT. Clinical practice. Osteoarthritis of the knee. N Engl J Med. 2006;354(8):841–8. https://doi.org/10.1056/NEJMcp051726. Erratum in: N Engl J Med. 2006;354(23):2520.
3. Dieppe PA, Lohmander LS. Pathogenesis and management of pain in osteoarthritis. The Lancet. 2005;365(9463):965–73. https://doi.org/10.1016/S0140-6736(05)71086-2.
4. Vos T, Allen C, Arora M, Barber RM, Bhutta ZA, Brown A, et al. Global, regional, and national incidence, prevalence, and years lived with disability for 310 diseases and injuries, 1990–2015: a systematic analysis for the Global Burden of Disease Study 2015. The Lancet. 2016;388(10053):1545–602.
5. Griffin TM, Guilak F. The role of mechanical loading in the onset and progression of osteoarthritis. Exerc Sport Sci Rev. 2005;33(4):195–200. https://doi.org/10.1097/00003677-200510000-00008.
6. Helmick CG, Felson DT, Lawrence RC, Gabriel S, Hirsch R, Kwoh CK, National Arthritis Data Workgroup, et al. Estimates of the prevalence of arthritis and other rheumatic conditions in the United States. Part I. Arthritis Rheum. 2008;58(1):15–25. https://doi.org/10.1002/art.23177.
7. Martin KR, Kuh D, Harris TB, Guralnik JM, Coggon D, Wills AK. Body mass index, occupational activity, and leisure-time physical activity: an exploration of risk factors and modifiers for knee osteoarthritis in the 1946 British birth cohort. BMC Musculoskelet Disord. 2013;14:219. https://doi.org/10.1186/1471-2474-14-219.
8. Jamtvedt G, Dahm KT, Christie A, Moe RH, Haavardsholm E, Holm I, et al. Physical therapy interventions for patients with osteoarthritis of the knee: an overview of systematic reviews. Phys Ther. 2008;88(1):123–36. https://doi.org/10.2522/ptj.20070043.
9. Rutjes AW, Nüesch E, Sterchi R, Kalichman L, Hendriks E, Osiri M, et al. Transcutaneous electrostimulation for osteoarthritis of the knee. Cochrane Database Syst Rev. 2009;2009(4):CD002823. https://doi.org/10.1002/14651858.CD002823.pub2.
10. Bennell KL, Hunt MA, Wrigley TV, Lim BW, Hinman RS. Muscle and exercise in the prevention and management of knee osteoarthritis: an internal medicine specialist's guide. Med Clin N Am. 2009;93(1):161–77. https://doi.org/10.1016/j.mcna.2008.08.006.
11. Ottawa Panel Members, Ottawa Methods Group, Brosseau L, Wells GA, Tugwell P, Egan M, et al. Ottawa panel evidence-based clinical practice guidelines for therapeutic exercises and manual therapy in the manage ment of osteoarthritis. Phys Ther. 2005;85(9):907–71.
12. Kolasinski SL, Neogi T, Hochberg MC, Oatis C, Guyatt G, Block J, et al. 2019 American College of Rheumatology/arthritis foundation guideline for the management of osteoarthritis of the hand, hip, and knee. Arthritis Rheumatol. 2020;72(2):220–33. https://doi.org/10.1002/art.41142
13. Verhagen AP, Ferreira M, Reijneveld-van de Vendel EA, Teirlinck CH,

Runhaar J, van Middelkoop M, et al. Do we need another trial on exercise in patients with knee osteoarthritis? No new trials on exercise in knee OA. Osteoarthr Cartil. 2019;27(9):1266–9. https://doi.org/10.1016/j.joca.2019.04.020.
14. Rafiq MT, Hamid MSA, Hafiz E. Non-pharmacological interventions for treating symptoms of knee osteoarthritis in overweight or obese patients; A review. J Postgrad Med Inst. 2020;34(3):142–8.
15. Rafiq MT, Hamid MSA, Hafiz E, Amin S. Rehabilitation protocol with or without mobile health in overweight and obese knee osteoarthritis patients-a pilot study. Balneo Res J. 2019;10(4):580–4. https://doi.org/10.12680/balneo.2019.306.
16. Han M, Lee E. Effectiveness of mobile health application use to improve health behavior changes: a systematic review of randomized controlled trials. Healthc Inform Res. 2018;24(3):207–26. https://doi.org/10.4258/hir.2018.24.3.207.
17. Wantland DJ, Portillo CJ, Holzemer WL, Slaughter R, McGhee EM. The effectiveness of Web-based vs. non-Web-based interventions: a meta-analysis of behavioral change outcomes. J Med Internet Res. 2004;6(4):e40. https://doi.org/10.2196/jmir.6.4.e40.
18. World Health Organization (WHO). mHealth: new horizons for health through mobile technologies: based on the findings of the second global survey on eHealth. Geneva: WHO; 2011.
19. Zhang W, Nuki G, Moskowitz RW, Abramson S, Altman RD, Arden NK, et al. OARSI recommendations for the management of hip and knee osteoarthritis, part I: critical appraisal of existing treatment guidelines and systematic review of current research evidence. Osteoarthr Cartil. 2007;15(9):981–1000. https://doi.org/10.1016/j.joca.2007.06.014.
20. Kellgren JH, Lawrence JS. Radiological assessment of osteo-arthrosis. Ann Rheum Dis. 1957;16(4):494–502. https://doi.org/10.1136/ard.16.4.494.
21. Page P. Current concepts in muscle stretching for exercise and rehabilitation. Int J Sports Phys Ther. 2012;7(1):109–19.
22. McHugh MP, Nesse M. Effect of stretching on strength loss and pain after eccentric exercise. Med Sci Sports Exerc. 2008;40(3):566–73. https://doi.org/10.1249/MSS.0b013e31815d2f8c.
23. Taylor DC, Dalton JD Jr, Seaber AV, Garrett WE Jr. Viscoelastic properties of muscle-tendon units. The biomechanical effects of stretching. Am J Sports Med. 1990;18(3):300–9. https://doi.org/10.1177/036354659001800314.
24. Gell NM, Wadsworth DD. The use of text messaging to promote physical activity in working women: a randomized controlled trial. J Phys Act Health. 2015;12(6):756–63. https://doi.org/10.1123/jpah.2013-0144.
25. Rafiq MT, Hamid MSA, Hafiz E, et al. Feasibility and acceptability of instructions of daily care in overweight and obese knee osteoarthritis participants. Curr Rheumatol Rev. 2021. https://doi.org/10.2174/1573397117666210727095552.
26. Hjermstad MJ, Fayers PM, Haugen DF, Caraceni A, Hanks GW, Loge JH, et al. European Palliative Care Research Collaborative (EPCRC). Studies comparing Numerical Rating Scales, Verbal Rating Scales, and Visual Analogue Scales for assessment of pain intensity in adults: a systematic literature review. J Pain Symptom Manag. 2011;41(6):1073–93. https://doi.org/10.1016/j.jpainsymman.2010.08.016.
27. Williamson A, Hoggart B. Pain: a review of three commonly used pain rating scales. J Clin Nurs. 2005;14(7):798–804. https://doi.org/10.1111/j.1365-2702.2005.01121.x.
28. Alexandre Tda S, Cordeiro RC, Ramos LR. Factors associated to quality of life in active elderly. Rev Saude Publica. 2009;43(4):613–21. https://doi.org/10.1590/s0034-89102009005000030.
29. Podsiadlo D, Richardson S. The timed "Up & Go": a test of basic functional mobility for frail elderly persons. J Am Geriatr Soc. 1991;39(2):142–8. https://doi.org/10.1111/j.1532-5415.1991.tb01616.x.
30. Horn KK, Jennings S, Richardson G, Van Vliet D, Hefford C, Abbott JH. The patient-specific functional scale: psychometrics, clinimetrics, and application as a clinical outcome measure. J Orthop Sports Phys Ther. 2012;42(1):30–42.
31. Katz S, Ford AB, Moskowitz RW, Jackson BA, Jaffe MW. Studies of illness in the aged: the index of ADL: a standardized measure of biological and psychosocial function. JAMA. 1963;185(12):914–9. https://doi.org/10.1001/jama.1963.03060120024016.
32. Shelkey M, Wallace M. Katz Index of independence in activities of daily living. J Gerontol Nurs. 1999;25(3):8–9. https://doi.org/10.3928/0098-9134-19990301-05
33. Dimitrov DM, Rumrill PD Jr. Pretest–posttest designs and measurement of change. Work. 2003;20(2):159–65.
34. Fransen M, McConnell S, Harmer AR, Van der Esch M, Simic M, Bennell KL. Exercise for osteoarthritis of the knee: a cochrane systematic review. Br J Sports Med. 2015;49(24):1554–7. https://doi.org/10.1136/bjsports-2015-095424.
35. Juhl C, Christensen R, Roos EM, Zhang W, Lund H. Impact of exercise type and dose on pain and disability in knee osteoarthritis: a systematic review and meta-regression analysis of randomized controlled trials. Arthritis Rheumatol. 2014;66(3):622–36. https://doi.org/10.1002/art.38290.
36. Messier SP, Mihalko SL, Legault C, Miller GD, Nicklas BJ, DeVita P, et al. Effects of intensive diet and exercise on knee joint loads, inflammation, and clinical outcomes among overweight and obese adults with knee osteoarthritis: the IDEA randomized clinical trial. JAMA. 2013;310(12):1263–73. https://doi.org/10.1001/jama.2013.277669.
37. Messier SP, Loeser RF, Miller GD, Morgan TM, Rejeski WJ, Sevick MA, et al. Exercise and dietary weight loss in overweight and obese older adults with knee osteoarthritis: the arthritis, diet, and activity promotion trial. Arthritis Rheum. 2004;50(5):1501–10. https://doi.org/10.1002/art.20256.
38. Katz S, Ford AB, Moskowitz RW, Jackson BA, Jaffe MW. Studies of illness in the aged: the index of ADL: a standardized measure of biological and psychosocial function. JAMA. 1963;185:914–9. https://doi.org/10.1001/jama.1963.03060120024016.
39. Lambert TE, Harvey LA, Avdalis C, Chen LW, Jeyalingam S, Pratt CA, et al. An app with remote support achieves better adherence to home exercise programs than paper handouts in people with musculoskeletal conditions: a randomised trial. J Physiother. 2017;63(3):161–7. https://doi.org/10.1016/j.jphys.2017.05.015.

22

The impact of a low-calorie, low-glycemic diet on systemic lupus erythematosus

Aline Mizusaki Imoto[1*], Leila Bernarda Gottems[1], Ana Lúcia Salomon[2], Helbert Eustáquio Cardoso e Silva[1], Império Lombardi Júnior[3], Maria Stella Peccin[3], Fábio Ferreira Amorim[4,5] and Levy Aniceto Santana[1]

Abstract

Background: Diet plays a critical role in Systemic Lupus Erythematosus (SLE) patients, impacting on the microbiota composition and, consequently, on the immune response. The objective was to analyze and verify the diet effect on SLE patients.

Methods: This is a systematic review performed at the Evidences-based Health Lab, Escola Superior em Ciências da Saúde, Brasília (DF), Brazil. In March, 2021, five databases, and grey literature, through JSTOR, Open Grey, and Google Scholar were searched. Randomized Clinical Trials in which SLE patients with calorie restricted, low glycemic index or other diet involving the joint adequacy of these aspects, compared with placebo or different types of diet, were included.

Results: It was identified in the databases 758 articles; 132 were duplicated; 616 references were screened, and 604 were excluded. After reading the title and abstract, 12 articles were included for full-text reading. After the full-text reading, three studies were included for quantitative analysis. The diet improved the quality of life at 6 (MD 16.30; 5.91;26.69) and 12 weeks (MD 14.60; 0.88;28.32). The GRADE was used to evaluate the quality of evidence.

Conclusion: There is low evidence that the diet has a positive impact on the quality of life of SLE patients.

Trial registration PROSPERO—CRD42020122208.

Keywords: Evidence based nutrition, Nutrition intervention, Lupus erythematosus management

Introduction

Systemic lupus erythematosus (SLE) can be defined as a chronic autoimmune disease with varied, complex clinical manifestations [1]. According to the Lupus Commission of Brazilian Society of Rheumatology, it is an estimated prevalence of 65,000 people diagnosed with systemic lupus erythematosus in Brazil [2]. The incidence is higher in women, 1 in 1,700. In a systematic review (SR) of epidemiological studies by Rees et al. [3], the highest world incidence was verified in North America and the lowest in Africa. Furthermore, in most studies, European countries showed the lowest incidence, while Asia, Australia, and America showed the highest rates. It should be stressed that incidences may be associated with places where studies are more frequently conducted or more availability of treatment is confirmed.

Immune system activation in SLE is characterized by exaggerated B-cell and T-cell responses and loss of immune tolerance against self-antigens, contributing to

*Correspondence: alinem.imoto@gmail.com
[1] Evidences-Based Health Lab, Professional and Academic Master Program, Escola Superior em Ciências da Saúde, Brasília, DF, Brazil

several clinical manifestations, the most common are fatigue, loss of appetite and weight, skin lesions (mainly malar rash), arthritis, serositis (pleuritis and/or pericarditis), kidney or central nervous system involvement and hematological manifestations (cytopenias) associated with various autoantibodies, particularly antinuclear antibodies [4, 5].

Considering cardiovascular aspects, systemic lupus erythematosus patients have an increased risk of developing atherosclerosis, hypertension, dyslipidemia, and obesity [6, 7]. The characteristic of dyslipidemia is the increase in total cholesterol, low-density lipoprotein (LDL), and triglyceride, with a decrease in high-density lipoprotein (HDL) [8]. The continued use of corticosteroids is a contributing factor to increased cardiovascular risk [7].

There is an increasing number of studies, still inconclusive, that evaluate the antioxidant, anti-inflammatory, and immunomodulatory effect through dietary therapy in the prevention and management of symptoms and comorbidities of patients with SLE [9].

Environmental factors can influence and modulate the onset and progression of systemic lupus erythematosus. Among those, diet plays a critical role, impacting the microbiota composition and, consequently, the immune response. There are a degree and type variation of such immune response, which depends on genetic and additional factors, such as stress, lifestyle, and medication [10]. The objective of nutritional intervention is to provide bodyweight control and a decrease in calories, saturated fat, and total fat intake. The decision to perform the present systematic review was based on the high frequency of risk factors for cardiovascular involvement in systemic lupus erythematosus patients and on the importance of analyzing and verifying the diet effect on the disease activity, as well as on the lipid parameters.

Objective

To verify the diet impact on systemic lupus erythematosus patients.

Methods

Type of study

The present study consists of a systematic review of the literature. The research question was: "What is the diet effect on systemic lupus erythematosus patients?" This study's protocol was registered on the International Prospective Register of Systematic Reviews—PROSPERO (www.crd.york.ac.uk/PROSPERO/) under number CRD42020122089.

The basic protocol was defined in April 2019, and the search strategy, eligibility criteria, bias, and outcome assessment instrument were established. Subsequently, the systematic review was registered in PROSPERO, and due to the great demand for orders and required changes, the definitive answer came only in March 2020.

Inclusion criteria

Type of patient: systemic lupus erythematosus patients, with no age and gender restriction.

Type of intervention: Calorie restricted (Low Cal), low glycaemic index (Low GI) or other diet involving the joint adequacy of these aspects.

Control: Placebo or different types of diet.

Outcome: Questionnaires and scores to evaluate the disease activity, fatigue, quality of sleep, quality of life, and lipid profile parameters.

Type of study: Randomized clinical trials.

Exclusion criteria

Studies that investigate omega-3, calcium, or any other type of supplementation were not included in this research.

Searched databases

An extensive article search was conducted in March 2021 with no language and timeframe limitations. The databases searched were: The Cochrane Central Register of Controlled Trials (CENTRAL), ClinicalTrials.gov, EMBASE, PubMed, SCOPUS, Web of Science, LILACS, and grey literature, through JSTOR, Open Grey, and Google Scholar. The keywords provided in the Medical Subject Headings (MeSH) were used to develop the primary search strategy and applied in PubMed. When words allowing different spellings were found, the synonyms appearing in MeSH were used. This strategy was adapted for the other databases. In LILACS, the same keywords in Spanish and English were used. See Table 1 for the applied search strategy. Manual research on relevant articles reference list was also done.

Study selection

After the search was completed, the studies found were entered on COVIDENCE (https://www.covidence.org/home), and two independent reviewers performed the study selection (AMI and HES). The first selection filter was based on title and abstract and then on full text. There was no need for a third reviewer to resolve disagreements.

Data extraction and data analyses

For continuous data, the mean and standard deviation were extracted from the included studies. For the binary data, the number of events was extracted.

For the meta-analysis, the random-effects model would be used to estimate the effect of diet on the evaluated

Table 1 Database search strategy

Database	Search (December, 2020)	References
PubMed	#1 – ("Lupus Erythematosus, Systemic"[All Fields] OR "Systemic Lupus Erythematosus"[All Fields] OR "Lupus Erythematosus Disseminatus"[All Fields] OR "Libman-Sacks Disease"[All Fields] OR ("lupus erythematosus, systemic"[MeSH Terms] OR ("lupus"[All Fields] AND "erythematosus"[All Fields] AND "systemic"[All Fields]) OR "systemic lupus erythematosus"[All Fields] OR ("disease"[All Fields] AND "libman"[All Fields] AND "sacks"[All Fields])) OR "Libman Sacks Disease"[All Fields] OR "Lupus Vulgaris"[All Fields] OR "Central Nervous System Lupus Vasculitis"[All Fields] OR ("lupus vasculitis, central nervous system"[MeSH Terms] OR ("lupus"[All Fields] AND "vasculitis"[All Fields] AND "central"[All Fields] AND "nervous"[All Fields] AND "system"[All Fields]) OR "central nervous system lupus vasculitis"[All Fields] OR ("systemic"[All Fields] AND "lupus"[All Fields] AND "erythematosis"[All Fields] AND "central"[All Fields] AND "nervous"[All Fields] AND "system"[All Fields])) OR "Central Nervous System Lupus"[All Fields] OR ("lupus vasculitis, central nervous system"[MeSH Terms] OR ("lupus"[All Fields] AND "vasculitis"[All Fields] AND "central"[All Fields] AND "nervous"[All Fields] AND "system"[All Fields]) OR "central nervous system lupus vasculitis"[All Fields] OR ("central"[All Fields] AND "nervous"[All Fields] AND "system"[All Fields] AND "systemic"[All Fields] AND "lupus"[All Fields] AND "erythematosis"[All Fields])) OR "Neuropsychiatric Systemic Lupus Erythematosus"[All Fields] OR "Lupus Meningoencephalitis"[All Fields] OR ("lupus vasculitis, central nervous system"[MeSH Terms] OR ("lupus"[All Fields] AND "vasculitis"[All Fields] AND "central"[All Fields] AND "nervous"[All Fields] AND "system"[All Fields]) OR "central nervous system lupus vasculitis"[All Fields] OR ("lupus"[All Fields] AND "meningoencephalitides"[All Fields])) OR ("lupus vasculitis, central nervous system"[MeSH Terms] OR ("lupus"[All Fields] AND "vasculitis"[All Fields] AND "central"[All Fields] AND "nervous"[All Fields] AND "system"[All Fields]) OR "central nervous system lupus vasculitis"[All Fields] OR ("meningoencephalitides"[All Fields] AND "lupus"[All Fields])) OR ("lupus vasculitis, central nervous system"[MeSH Terms] OR ("lupus"[All Fields] AND "vasculitis"[All Fields] AND "central"[All Fields] AND "nervous"[All Fields] AND "system"[All Fields]) OR "central nervous system lupus vasculitis"[All Fields] OR ("meningoencephalitis"[All Fields] AND "lupus"[All Fields])) OR "Lupus Panniculitis"[All Fields] OR ("panniculitis, lupus erythematosus"[MeSH Terms] OR ("panniculitis"[All Fields] AND "lupus"[All Fields] AND "erythematosus"[All Fields]) OR "lupus erythematosus panniculitis"[All Fields] OR ("lupus"[All Fields] AND "panniculitides"[All Fields])) OR ("panniculitis, lupus erythematosus"[MeSH Terms] OR ("panniculitis"[All Fields] AND "lupus"[All Fields] AND "erythematosus"[All Fields]) OR "lupus erythematosus panniculitis"[All Fields] OR ("panniculitides"[All Fields] AND "lupus"[All Fields])) OR "Panniculitis, Lupus"[All Fields] OR "Lupus Erythematosus Panniculitis"[All Fields] OR ("panniculitis, lupus erythematosus"[MeSH Terms] OR ("panniculitis"[All Fields] AND "lupus"[All Fields] AND "erythematosus"[All Fields]) OR "lupus erythematosus panniculitis"[All Fields] OR ("lupus"[All Fields] AND "erythematosus"[All Fields] AND "panniculitides"[All Fields])) OR ("panniculitis, lupus erythematosus"[MeSH Terms] OR ("panniculitis"[All Fields] AND "lupus"[All Fields] AND "erythematosus"[All Fields]) OR "lupus erythematosus panniculitis"[All Fields] OR ("panniculitides"[All Fields] AND "lupus"[All Fields] AND "erythematosus"[All Fields])) OR "Lupus Erythematosus Profundus"[All Fields] OR "Lupus Profundus"[All Fields] OR "Discoid Lupus Erythematosus"[All Fields] OR ("lupus erythematosus, discoid"[MeSH Terms] OR ("lupus"[All Fields] AND "erythematosus"[All Fields] AND "discoid"[All Fields]) OR "discoid lupus erythematosus"[All Fields] OR ("lupus"[All Fields] AND "erythematosus"[All Fields] AND "chronic"[All Fields] AND "cutaneous"[All Fields])) OR ("lupus erythematosus, discoid"[MeSH Terms] OR ("lupus"[All Fields] AND "erythematosus"[All Fields] AND "discoid"[All Fields]) OR "discoid lupus erythematosus"[All Fields] OR ("lupus"[All Fields] AND "erythematosus"[All Fields] AND "cutaneous"[All Fields] AND "chronic"[All Fields])) OR "Cutaneous Lupus Erythematosus"[All Fields] OR "Lupus Erythematosus, Subacute Cutaneous"[All Fields] OR ("lupus erythematosus, cutaneous"[MeSH Terms] OR ("lupus"[All Fields] AND "erythematosus"[All Fields] AND "cutaneous"[All Fields]) OR "cutaneous lupus erythematosus"[All Fields] OR ("lupus"[All Fields] AND "erythematosus"[All Fields] AND "cutaneous"[All Fields] AND "subacute"[All Fields])) #2 – ("diet"[MeSH Terms] OR "diet"[All Fields]) OR ("diet"[MeSH Terms] OR "diet"[All Fields] OR "diets"[All Fields]) OR "nutritional management"[All Fields] OR "dietary management"[All Fields] OR "Diet, Healthy"[All Fields] OR "Diets, Healthy"[All Fields] OR "Healthy Diets"[All Fields] OR "Healthy Eating"[All Fields] OR "Eating, Healthy"[All Fields] OR "Healthy Eating Index"[All Fields] OR ("healthy diet"[MeSH Terms] OR ("healthy"[All Fields] AND "diet"[All Fields]) OR "healthy diet"[All Fields] OR ("eating"[All Fields] AND "index"[All Fields] AND "healthy"[All Fields])) OR ("healthy diet"[MeSH Terms] OR ("healthy"[All Fields] AND "diet"[All Fields]) OR "healthy diet"[All Fields] OR ("eating"[All Fields] AND "indices"[All Fields] AND "healthy"[All Fields])) OR "Healthy Eating Indices"[All Fields] OR ("healthy diet"[MeSH Terms] OR ("healthy"[All Fields] AND "diet"[All Fields]) OR "healthy diet"[All Fields] OR ("index"[All Fields] AND "healthy"[All Fields] AND "eating"[All Fields])) OR ("healthy diet"[MeSH Terms] OR ("healthy"[All Fields] AND "diet"[All Fields]) OR "healthy diet"[All Fields] OR ("indices"[All Fields] AND "healthy"[All Fields] AND "eating"[All Fields])) OR ("diet, carbohydrate loading"[MeSH Terms] OR ("diet"[All Fields] AND "carbohydrate"[All Fields] AND "loading"[All Fields]) OR "carbohydrate loading diet"[All Fields] OR ("carbohydrate"[All Fields] AND "loading"[All Fields] AND "diets"[All Fields])) OR "Carbohydrate Loading Diet"[All Fields] OR "Carbohydrate Loading"[All Fields] OR ("diet, vegan"[MeSH Terms] OR ("diet"[All Fields] AND "vegan"[All Fields]) OR "vegan diet"[All Fields] OR ("diets"[All Fields] AND "vegan"[All Fields])) OR "Vegan Diets"[All Fields] OR "Vegan Diet"[All Fields] OR "Veganism"[All Fields] OR "Diet, High Protein"[All Fields] OR ("diet, high-protein"[MeSH Terms] OR ("diet"[All Fields] AND "high-protein"[All Fields]) OR "high-protein diet"[All Fields] OR ("diets"[All Fields] AND "high"[All Fields] AND "protein"[All Fields])) OR "High-Protein Diets"[All Fields] OR "High-Protein Diet"[All Fields] OR "High Protein Diet"[All Fields] OR "Diet, High Protein Low Carbohydrate"[All Fields] OR ("diet, high-protein low-carbohydrate"[MeSH Terms] OR ("diet"[All Fields] AND "high-protein"[All Fields] AND "low-carbohydrate"[All Fields]) OR "high-protein low-carbohydrate diet"[All Fields] OR ("diets"[All Fields] AND "high"[All Fields] AND "protein"[All Fields] AND "low"[All Fields] AND "carbohydrate"[All Fields])) OR ("diet, high-protein low-carbohydrate"[MeSH Terms] OR ("diet"[All Fields] AND "high-protein"[All Fields] AND "low-carbohydrate"[All Fields]) OR "high-protein low-carbohydrate diet"[All Fields] OR ("low"[All Fields] AND "carbohydrate"[All Fields] AND "diet"[All Fields] AND "high"[All Fields] AND "protein"[All Fields])) OR ("diet, high-protein low-carbohydrate"[MeSH Terms] OR ("diet"[All Fields] AND "high-protein"[All Fields] AND "low-carbohydrate"[All Fields]) OR "high-protein low-carbohydrate diet"[All Fields] OR ("low"[All Fields] AND "carbohydrate"[All Fields] AND "diets"[All Fields] AND "high"[All Fields] AND "protein"[All Fields])) OR "Carbohydrate-Restricted High-Protein Diet"[All Fields] OR "Carbohydrate Restricted High Protein Diet"[All Fields] OR ("diet, high-protein low-carbohydrate"[MeSH Terms] OR ("diet"[All Fields] AND "high-protein"[All Fields] AND "low-carbohydrate"[All Fields]) OR "high-protein low-carbohydrate diet"[All Fields] OR ("diet"[All Fields] AND "carbohydrate"[All Fields] AND "restricted"[All Fields] AND "high"[All Fields] AND "protein"[All Fields])) OR ("diet, high-protein low-carbohydrate"[MeSH Terms] OR ("diet"[All Fields] AND "high-protein"[All Fields] AND "low-carbohydrate"[All Fields]) OR "high-protein low-carbohydrate diet"[All Fields] OR ("diets"[All Fields] AND "carbohydrate"[All Fields] AND "restricted"[All Fields] AND "high"[All Fields] AND "protein"[All Fields])) OR ("diet, high-protein low-carbohydrate"[MeSH Terms] OR ("diet"[All Fields] AND "high-protein"[All Fields] AND "low-carbohydrate"[All Fields]) OR "high-protein low-carbohydrate diet"[All Fields] OR ("high"[All Fields] AND "protein"[All Fields] AND "diet"[All Fields] AND "carbohydrate"[All Fields] AND "restricted"[All Fields])) OR ("diet, high-protein low-carbohydrate"[MeSH Terms] OR ("diet"[All Fields] AND "high-protein"[All Fields] AND "low-carbohydrate"[All Fields]) OR "high-protein low-carbohydrate diet"[All Fields] OR ("high"[All Fields] AND "protein"[All Fields] AND "diets"[All Fields] AND "carbohydrate"[All Fields] AND "restricted"[All Fields])) OR ("diet, high-protein low-carbohydrate"[MeSH Terms] OR ("diet"[All Fields] AND "high-protein"[All Fields] AND "low-carbohydrate"[All Fields]) OR "high-protein low-carbohydrate diet"[All Fields] OR ("carbohydrate"[All Fields] AND "restricted"[All Fields] AND "high"[All Fields] AND "protein"[All Fields] AND "diets"[All Fields])) OR ("diet, high-protein low-carbohydrate"[MeSH Terms] OR ("diet"[All Fields] AND "high-protein"[All Fields] AND "low-carbohydrate"[All Fields]) OR "high-protein low-carbohydrate diet"[All Fields] OR ("carbohydrate"[All Fields] AND "restricted"[All Fields] AND "high"[All Fields] AND "protein"[All Fields] AND "diets"[All Fields])) OR "Low-Carbohydrate High-Protein Diets"[All Fields] OR "Low Carbohydrate High Protein Diets"[All Fields] OR "High-Protein Low-Carbohydrate Diet"[All Fields] OR "High Protein LowCarbohydrate Diet"[All Fields] OR "High-Protein Low-Carbohydrate Diets"[All Fields] OR "High Protein Low Carbohydrate Diets"[All Fields] OR "Low-Carbohydrate High-Protein Diet"[All Fields] OR ("diet, high-protein low-carbohydrate"[MeSH Terms] OR ("diet"[All Fields] AND "high-protein"[All Fields] AND "low-carbohydrate"[All Fields]) OR "high-protein low-carbohydrate diet"[All Fields] OR ("diet"[All Fields]	11

Table 1 (continued)

Database	Search (December, 2020)	References
	AND "low"[All Fields] AND "carbohydrate"[All Fields] AND "high"[All Fields] AND "protein"[All Fields])) OR ("diet, high-protein low-carbohydrate"[MeSH Terms] OR ("diet"[All Fields] AND "high-protein"[All Fields] AND "low-carbohydrate"[All Fields]) OR "high-protein low-carbohydrate diet"[All Fields] OR ("diets"[All Fields] AND "low"[All Fields] AND "carbohydrate"[All Fields] AND "high"[All Fields] AND "protein"[All Fields])) OR ("diet, high-protein low-carbohydrate"[MeSH Terms] OR ("diet"[All Fields] AND "high-protein"[All Fields] AND "low-carbohydrate"[All Fields]) OR "high-protein low-carbohydrate diet"[All Fields] OR ("high"[All Fields] AND "protein"[All Fields] AND "diet"[All Fields] AND "low"[All Fields] AND "carbohydrate"[All Fields])) OR ("diet, high-protein low-carbohydrate"[MeSH Terms] OR ("diet"[All Fields] AND "high-protein"[All Fields] AND "low-carbohydrate"[All Fields]) OR "high-protein low-carbohydrate diet"[All Fields] OR ("high"[All Fields] AND "protein"[All Fields] AND "diets"[All Fields] AND "low"[All Fields] AND "carbohydrate"[All Fields])) OR "Low Carbohydrate High Protein Diet"[All Fields] OR ("diet, high-protein low-carbohydrate"[MeSH Terms] OR ("diet"[All Fields] AND "high-protein"[All Fields] AND "low-carbohydrate"[All Fields]) OR "high-protein low-carbohydrate diet"[All Fields] OR ("high"[All Fields] AND "protein"[All Fields] AND "carbohydrate"[All Fields] AND "restricted"[All Fields] AND "diets"[All Fields])) OR ("diet, high-protein low-carbohydrate"[MeSH Terms] OR ("diet"[All Fields] AND "high-protein"[All Fields] AND "low-carbohydrate"[All Fields]) OR "high-protein low-carbohydrate diet"[All Fields] OR ("carbohydrate"[All Fields] AND "restricted"[All Fields] AND "diet"[All Fields] AND "high"[All Fields] AND "protein"[All Fields])) OR ("diet, high-protein low-carbohydrate"[MeSH Terms] OR ("diet"[All Fields] AND "high-protein"[All Fields] AND "low-carbohydrate"[All Fields]) OR "high-protein low-carbohydrate diet"[All Fields] OR ("carbohydrate"[All Fields] AND "restricted"[All Fields] AND "diets"[All Fields] AND "high"[All Fields] AND "protein"[All Fields])) OR ("diet, high-protein low-carbohydrate"[MeSH Terms] OR ("diet"[All Fields] AND "high-protein"[All Fields] AND "low-carbohydrate"[All Fields]) OR "high-protein low-carbohydrate diet"[All Fields] OR ("diet"[All Fields] AND "high"[All Fields] AND "protein"[All Fields] AND "carbohydrate"[All Fields] AND "restricted"[All Fields])) OR ("diet, high-protein low-carbohydrate"[MeSH Terms] OR ("diet"[All Fields] AND "high-protein"[All Fields] AND "low-carbohydrate"[All Fields]) OR "high-protein low-carbohydrate diet"[All Fields] OR ("diets"[All Fields] AND "high"[All Fields] AND "protein"[All Fields] AND "carbohydrate"[All Fields] AND "restricted"[All Fields])) OR ("diet, high-protein low-carbohydrate"[MeSH Terms] OR ("diet"[All Fields] AND "high-protein"[All Fields] AND "low-carbohydrate"[All Fields]) OR "high-protein low-carbohydrate diet"[All Fields] OR ("high"[All Fields] AND "protein"[All Fields] AND "carbohydrate"[All Fields] AND "restricted"[All Fields] AND "diets"[All Fields])) OR ("diet, high-protein low-carbohydrate"[MeSH Terms] OR ("diet"[All Fields] AND "high-protein"[All Fields] AND "low-carbohydrate"[All Fields]) OR "high-protein low-carbohydrate diet"[All Fields] OR ("high"[All Fields] AND "protein"[All Fields] AND "carbohydrate"[All Fields] AND "restricted"[All Fields] AND "diet"[All Fields])) OR ("diet, high-protein low-carbohydrate"[MeSH Terms] OR ("diet"[All Fields] AND "high-protein"[All Fields] AND "low-carbohydrate"[All Fields]) OR "high-protein low-carbohydrate diet"[All Fields] OR ("high"[All Fields] AND "protein"[All Fields] AND "carbohydrate"[All Fields] AND "restricted"[All Fields] AND "diet"[All Fields])) OR "South Beach Diet"[All Fields] OR ("diet, high-protein low-carbohydrate"[MeSH Terms] OR ("diet"[All Fields] AND "high-protein"[All Fields] AND "low-carbohydrate"[All Fields]) OR "high-protein low-carbohydrate diet"[All Fields] OR ("diet"[All Fields] AND "south"[All Fields] AND "beach"[All Fields])) OR "Atkins Diet"[All Fields] OR "Diet, Atkins"[All Fields] OR "Diabetic Diets"[All Fields] OR ("diet, diabetic"[MeSH Terms] OR ("diet"[All Fields] AND "diabetic"[All Fields]) OR "diabetic diet"[All Fields] OR ("diets"[All Fields] AND "diabetic"[All Fields])) OR "Diabetic Diet"[All Fields] OR "Therapy, Diet"[All Fields] OR "Diet Therapies"[All Fields] OR ("diet therapy"[MeSH Terms] OR ("diet"[All Fields] AND "therapy"[All Fields]) OR "diet therapy"[All Fields] OR ("therapies"[All Fields] AND "diet"[All Fields])) OR "Dietary Modification"[All Fields] OR "Dietary Modifications"[All Fields] OR ("diet therapy"[MeSH Terms] OR ("diet"[All Fields] AND "therapy"[All Fields]) OR "diet therapy"[All Fields] OR ("modification"[All Fields] AND "dietary"[All Fields])) OR ("diet therapy"[MeSH Terms] OR ("diet"[All Fields] AND "therapy"[All Fields]) OR "diet therapy"[All Fields] OR ("modifications"[All Fields] AND "dietary"[All Fields])) OR "Diet Modification"[All Fields] OR "Diet Modifications"[All Fields] OR "Modification, Diet"[All Fields] OR "Modifications, Diet"[All Fields] OR "Atherogenic Diet"[All Fields] OR "Atherogenic Diets"[All Fields] OR ("diet, atherogenic"[MeSH Terms] OR ("diet"[All Fields] AND "atherogenic"[All Fields]) OR "atherogenic diet"[All Fields] OR ("diets"[All Fields] AND "atherogenic"[All Fields])) OR ("diet, vegetarian"[MeSH Terms] OR ("diet"[All Fields] AND "vegetarian"[All Fields]) OR "vegetarian diet"[All Fields] OR ("diets"[All Fields] AND "vegetarian"[All Fields])) OR "Vegetarian Diets"[All Fields] OR "Vegetarian Diet"[All Fields] OR "Vegetarianism"[All Fields] OR ("diet, macrobiotic"[MeSH Terms] OR ("diet"[All Fields] AND "macrobiotic"[All Fields]) OR "macrobiotic diet"[All Fields] OR ("diets"[All Fields] AND "macrobiotic"[All Fields])) OR "Macrobiotic Diet"[All Fields] OR "Macrobiotic Diets"[All Fields] OR "Diet, Fat Restricted"[All Fields] OR "Fat-Restricted Diet"[All Fields] OR ("diet, fat-restricted"[MeSH Terms] OR ("diet"[All Fields] AND "fat-restricted"[All Fields]) OR "fat-restricted diet"[All Fields] OR ("diets"[All Fields] AND "fat"[All Fields] AND "restricted"[All Fields])) OR "Fat Restricted Diet"[All Fields] OR "Fat-Restricted Diets"[All Fields] OR "Diet, Low-Fat"[All Fields] OR "Diet, Low Fat"[All Fields] OR ("diet, fat-restricted"[MeSH Terms] OR ("diet"[All Fields] AND "fat-restricted"[All Fields]) OR "fat-restricted diet"[All Fields] OR ("diets"[All Fields] AND "low"[All Fields] AND "fat"[All Fields])) OR "Low-Fat Diet"[All Fields] OR "Low-Fat Diets"[All Fields] OR ("diet, fat-restricted"[MeSH Terms] OR ("diet"[All Fields] AND "fat-restricted"[All Fields]) OR "fat-restricted diet"[All Fields] OR ("diet"[All Fields] AND "fat"[All Fields] AND "free"[All Fields])) OR ("diet, fat-restricted"[MeSH Terms] OR ("diet"[All Fields] AND "fat-restricted"[All Fields]) OR "fat-restricted diet"[All Fields] OR ("diet"[All Fields] AND "fat"[All Fields] AND "free"[All Fields])) OR ("diet, fat-restricted"[MeSH Terms] OR ("diet"[All Fields] AND "fat-restricted"[All Fields]) OR "fat-restricted diet"[All Fields] OR ("diets"[All Fields] AND "fat"[All Fields] AND "free"[All Fields])) OR "Fat-Free Diet"[All Fields] OR "Fat-Free Diets"[All Fields] OR "Diet, Protein Restricted"[All Fields] OR "Low-Protein Diet"[All Fields] OR "Low Protein Diet"[All Fields] OR "Protein-Restricted Diet"[All Fields] OR ("diet, protein-restricted"[MeSH Terms] OR ("diet"[All Fields] AND "protein-restricted"[All Fields]) OR "protein-restricted diet"[All Fields] OR ("diets"[All Fields] AND "protein"[All Fields] AND "restricted"[All Fields])) OR "Protein Restricted Diet"[All Fields] OR "Protein-Restricted Diets"[All Fields] OR ("diet, protein-restricted"[MeSH Terms] OR ("diet"[All Fields] AND "protein-restricted"[All Fields]) OR "protein-restricted diet"[All Fields] OR ("diet"[All Fields] AND "low"[All Fields] AND "protein"[All Fields])) OR ("diet, protein-restricted"[MeSH Terms] OR ("diet"[All Fields] AND "protein-restricted"[All Fields]) OR "protein-restricted diet"[All Fields] OR ("diet"[All Fields] AND "low"[All Fields] AND "protein"[All Fields])) OR ("diet, protein-restricted"[MeSH Terms] OR ("diet"[All Fields] AND "protein-restricted"[All Fields]) OR "protein-restricted diet"[All Fields] OR ("diets"[All Fields] AND "low"[All Fields] AND "protein"[All Fields])) OR "Low-Protein Diets"[All Fields] OR ("diet, protein-restricted"[MeSH Terms] OR ("diet"[All Fields] AND "protein-restricted"[All Fields]) OR "protein-restricted diet"[All Fields] OR ("diet"[All Fields] AND "protein"[All Fields] AND "free"[All Fields])) OR ("diet, protein-restricted"[MeSH Terms] OR ("diet"[All Fields] AND "protein-restricted"[All Fields]) OR "protein-restricted diet"[All Fields] OR ("diet"[All Fields] AND "protein"[All Fields] AND "free"[All Fields])) OR ("diet, protein-restricted"[MeSH Terms] OR ("diet"[All Fields] AND "protein-restricted"[All Fields]) OR "protein-restricted diet"[All Fields] OR ("diets"[All Fields] AND "protein"[All Fields] AND "free"[All Fields])) OR "Protein-Free Diet"[All Fields] OR "Protein-Free Diets"[All Fields] OR "Mediterranean Diet"[All Fields] OR ("diet, mediterranean"[MeSH Terms] OR ("diet"[All Fields] AND "mediterranean"[All Fields]) OR "mediterranean diet"[All Fields] OR ("diets"[All Fields] AND "mediterranean"[All Fields])) OR "Mediterranean Diets"[All Fields] OR "Diet, Carbohydrate Restricted"[All Fields] OR ("diet, carbohydrate-restricted"[MeSH Terms] OR ("diet"[All Fields] AND "carbohydrate-restricted"[All Fields]) OR "carbohydrate-restricted diet"[All Fields] OR ("diet"[All Fields] AND "low"[All Fields]	

Table 1 (continued)

Database	Search (December, 2020)	References
	AND "carbohydrate"[All Fields])) OR ("diet, carbohydrate-restricted"[MeSH Terms] OR ("diet"[All Fields] AND "carbohydrate-restricted"[All Fields]) OR"carbohydrate-restricted diet"[All Fields] OR ("carbohydrate"[All Fields] AND "diet"[All Fields] AND "low"[All Fields])) OR ("diet, carbohydrate-restricted"[MeSH Terms] OR ("diet"[All Fields] AND "carbohydrate-restricted"[All Fields]) OR "carbohydrate-restricted diet"[All Fields] OR ("carbohydrate"[All Fields] AND "diets"[All Fields] AND "low"[All Fields])) OR ("diet, carbohydrate-restricted"[MeSH Terms] OR ("diet"[All Fields] AND "carbohydrate-restricted"[All Fields]) OR "carbohydrate-restricted diet"[All Fields] OR ("diets"[All Fields] AND "low"[All Fields] AND "carbohydrate"[All Fields])) OR "Low Carbohydrate Diets"[All Fields] OR "Carbohydrate-Restricted Diet"[All Fields] OR "Carbohydrate Restricted Diet"[All Fields] OR "Carbohydrate-Restricted Diets"[All Fields] OR ("diet, carbohydrate-restricted"[MeSH Terms] OR ("diet"[All Fields] AND "carbohydrate-restricted"[All Fields]) OR "carbohydrate-restricted diet"[All Fields] OR ("diets"[All Fields] AND "carbohydrate"[All Fields] AND "restricted"[All Fields])) OR "Low-Carbohydrate Diet"[All Fields] OR ("diet, carbohydrate-restricted"[MeSH Terms] OR ("diet"[All Fields] AND "carbohydrate-restricted"[All Fields]) OR "carbohydrate-restricted diet"[All Fields] OR ("diet"[All Fields] AND "low"[All Fields] AND "carbohydrate"[All Fields])) OR ("diet, carbohydrate-restricted"[MeSH Terms] OR ("diet"[All Fields] AND "carbohydrate-restricted"[All Fields]) OR "carbohydrate-restricted diet"[All Fields] OR ("diets"[All Fields] AND "low"[All Fields] AND "carbohydrate"[All Fields])) OR "Low Carbohydrate Diet"[All Fields] OR "Low-Carbohydrate Diets"[All Fields] OR "Diet, Gluten Free"[All Fields] OR "Gluten-Free Diet"[All Fields] OR ("diet, gluten-free"[MeSH Terms] OR ("diet"[All Fields] AND "gluten-free"[All Fields]) OR "gluten-free diet"[All Fields] OR ("diets"[All Fields] AND "gluten"[All Fields] AND "free"[All Fields])) OR "Gluten Free Diet"[All Fields] OR "Gluten-Free Diets"[All Fields] OR "Ketogenic Diet"[All Fields] OR ("diet, ketogenic"[MeSH Terms] OR ("diet"[All Fields] AND "ketogenic"[All Fields]) OR "ketogenic diet"[All Fields] OR ("diets"[All Fields] AND "ketogenic"[All Fields])) OR "Ketogenic Diets"[All Fields] OR ("diet, high-fat"[MeSH Terms] OR ("diet"[All Fields] AND "high-fat"[All Fields]) OR "high-fat diet"[All Fields] OR ("diets"[All Fields] AND "high"[All Fields] AND "fat"[All Fields])) OR "High-Fat Diet"[All Fields] OR "High-Fat Diets"[All Fields] OR "Diet, High Fat"[All Fields] OR ("diet, high-fat"[MeSH Terms] OR ("diet"[All Fields] AND "high-fat"[All Fields]) OR "high-fat diet"[All Fields] OR ("diets"[All Fields] AND "high"[All Fields] AND "fat"[All Fields])) OR "High Fat Diet"[All Fields] OR "High Fat Diets"[All Fields] OR "Paleolithic Diet"[All Fields] OR ("diet, paleolithic"[MeSH Terms] OR ("diet"[All Fields] AND "paleolithic"[All Fields]) OR "paleolithic diet"[All Fields] OR ("diet"[All Fields] AND "stone"[All Fields] AND "age"[All Fields])) OR ("diet, paleolithic"[MeSH Terms] OR ("diet"[All Fields] AND "paleolithic"[All Fields]) OR "paleolithic diet"[All Fields] OR ("diets"[All Fields] AND "stone"[All Fields] AND "age"[All Fields])) OR "Stone Age Diet"[All Fields] OR "Stone Age Diets"[All Fields] OR ("diet, paleolithic"[MeSH Terms] OR ("diet"[All Fields] AND "paleolithic"[All Fields]) OR "paleolithic diet"[All Fields] OR ("diet"[All Fields] AND "paleo"[All Fields])) OR ("diet, paleolithic"[MeSH Terms] OR ("diet"[All Fields] AND "paleolithic"[All Fields]) OR "paleolithic diet"[All Fields] OR ("diets"[All Fields] AND "paleo"[All Fields])) OR "Paleo Diet"[All Fields] OR "Paleo Diets"[All Fields] OR ("diet, paleolithic"[MeSH Terms] OR ("diet"[All Fields] AND "paleolithic"[All Fields]) OR "paleolithic diet"[All Fields] OR ("diet"[All Fields] AND "caveman"[All Fields])) OR ("diet, paleolithic"[MeSH Terms] OR ("diet"[All Fields] AND "paleolithic"[All Fields]) OR "paleolithic diet"[All Fields] OR ("caveman"[All Fields] AND "diet"[All Fields])) OR ("diet, paleolithic"[MeSH Terms] OR ("diet"[All Fields] AND "paleolithic"[All Fields]) OR "paleolithic diet"[All Fields] OR ("caveman"[All Fields] AND "diets"[All Fields])) OR ("diet, paleolithic"[MeSH Terms] OR ("diet"[All Fields] AND "paleolithic"[All Fields]) OR "paleolithic diet"[All Fields] OR ("diets"[All Fields] AND "caveman"[All Fields])) OR ("diet, paleolithic"[MeSH Terms] OR ("diet"[All Fields] AND "paleolithic"[All Fields]) OR "paleolithic diet"[All Fields] OR ("diet"[All Fields] AND "hunter"[All Fields] AND "gatherer"[All Fields])) OR ("diet, paleolithic"[MeSH Terms] OR ("diet"[All Fields] AND "paleolithic"[All Fields]) OR "paleolithic diet"[All Fields] OR ("diet"[All Fields] AND "hunter"[All Fields] AND "gatherer"[All Fields])) OR ("diet, paleolithic"[MeSH Terms] OR ("diet"[All Fields] AND "paleolithic"[All Fields]) OR "paleolithic diet"[All Fields] OR ("diets"[All Fields] AND "hunter"[All Fields] AND "gatherer"[All Fields])) OR "Hunter-Gatherer Diet"[All Fields] OR "Hunter-Gatherer Diets"[All Fields] OR ("diet, western"[MeSH Terms] OR ("diet"[All Fields] AND "western"[All Fields]) OR "western diet"[All Fields] OR ("diets"[All Fields] AND "western"[All Fields])) OR "Western Diets"[All Fields] OR "Western Dietary Pattern"[All Fields] OR ("diet, western"[MeSH Terms] OR ("diet"[All Fields] AND "western"[All Fields]) OR "western diet"[All Fields] OR ("dietary"[All Fields] AND "pattern"[All Fields] AND "western"[All Fields])) OR ("diet, western"[MeSH Terms] OR ("diet"[All Fields] AND "western"[All Fields]) OR "western diet"[All Fields] OR ("dietary"[All Fields] AND "patterns"[All Fields] AND "western"[All Fields])) OR ("diet, western"[MeSH Terms] OR ("diet"[All Fields] AND "western"[All Fields]) OR "western diet"[All Fields] OR ("pattern"[All Fields] AND "western"[All Fields] AND "dietary"[All Fields])) OR ("diet, western"[MeSH Terms] OR ("diet"[All Fields] AND "western"[All Fields]) OR "western diet"[All Fields] OR ("patterns"[All Fields] AND "western"[All Fields] AND "dietary"[All Fields])) OR "Western Dietary Patterns"[All Fields] OR ("diet, western"[MeSH Terms] OR ("diet"[All Fields] AND "western"[All Fields]) OR "western diet"[All Fields] OR ("diet"[All Fields] AND "occidental"[All Fields])) OR ("diet, western"[MeSH Terms] OR ("diet"[All Fields] AND "western"[All Fields]) OR "western diet"[All Fields] OR ("diets"[All Fields] AND "occidental"[All Fields])) OR "Occidental Diet"[All Fields] OR "Occidental Diets"[All Fields] OR "Western Diet"[All Fields] OR ("diet, western"[MeSH Terms] OR ("diet"[All Fields] AND "western"[All Fields]) OR "western diet"[All Fields] OR ("meat"[All Fields] AND "sweet"[All Fields] AND "diet"[All Fields])) OR ("diet, western"[MeSH Terms] OR ("diet"[All Fields] AND "western"[All Fields]) OR "western diet"[All Fields] OR ("diet"[All Fields] AND "meat"[All Fields] AND "sweet"[All Fields])) OR ("diet, western"[MeSH Terms] OR ("diet"[All Fields] AND "western"[All Fields]) OR "western diet"[All Fields] OR ("diets"[All Fields] AND "meat"[All Fields] AND "sweet"[All Fields])) OR ("diet, western"[MeSH Terms] OR ("diet"[All Fields] AND "western"[All Fields]) OR "western diet"[All Fields] OR ("meat"[All Fields] AND "sweet"[All Fields] AND "diet"[All Fields])) OR ("diet, western"[MeSH Terms] OR ("diet"[All Fields] AND "western"[All Fields]) OR "western diet"[All Fields] OR ("meat"[All Fields] AND "sweet"[All Fields] AND "diets"[All Fields])) #3 – ("Clinical Trials, Randomized"[All Fields] OR "Trials, Randomized Clinical"[All Fields] OR "Controlled Clinical Trials, Randomized"[All Fields] OR "Randomized Controlled Trial"[All Fields]) #4 – (#1 AND #2 AND #3)	

Table 1 (continued)

Database	Search (December, 2020)	References
Scopus	(TITLE-ABS-KEY("Lupus Erythematosus, Systemic" OR "Systemic Lupus Erythematosus" OR "Lupus Erythematosus Disseminatus" OR "Libman-Sacks Disease" OR "Disease, Libman-Sacks" OR "Libman Sacks Disease" OR "Lupus Vulgaris" OR "Central Nervous System Lupus Vasculitis" OR "Systemic Lupus Erythematosis, Central Nervous System" OR "Central Nervous System Lupus" OR "Central Nervous System Systemic Lupus Erythematosis" OR "Neuropsychiatric Systemic Lupus Erythematosus" OR "Lupus Meningoencephalitis" OR "Lupus Meningoencephalitides" OR "Meningoencephalitides, Lupus" OR "Meningoencephalitis, Lupus" OR "Lupus Panniculitis" OR "Lupus Panniculitides" OR "Panniculitides, Lupus" OR "Panniculitis, Lupus" OR "Lupus Erythematosus Panniculitis" OR "Lupus Erythematosus Panniculitides" OR "Panniculitides, Lupus Erythematosus" OR "Lupus Erythematosus Profundus" OR "Lupus Profundus" OR "Discoid Lupus Erythematosus" OR "Lupus Erythematosus, Chronic Cutaneous" OR "Lupus Erythematosus, Cutaneous, Chronic" OR "Cutaneous Lupus Erythematosus" OR "Lupus Erythematosus, Subacute Cutaneous" OR "Lupus Erythematosus, Cutaneous, Subacute") AND (Diet OR Diets OR "nutritional management" OR "dietary management" OR "Diet, Healthy" OR "Diets, Healthy" OR "Healthy Diets" OR "Healthy Eating" OR "Eating, Healthy" OR "Healthy Eating Index" OR "Eating Index, Healthy" OR "Eating Indices, Healthy" OR "Healthy Eating Indices" OR "Index, Healthy Eating" OR "Indices, Healthy Eating" OR "Carbohydrate Loading Diets" OR "Carbohydrate Loading Diet" OR "Carbohydrate Loading" OR "Diets, Vegan" OR "Vegan Diets" OR "Vegan Diet" OR "Veganism" OR "Diet, High Protein" OR "Diets, High-Protein" OR "High-Protein Diets" OR "High-Protein Diet" OR "High Protein Diet" OR "Diet, High Protein Low Carbohydrate" OR "Diets, High-Protein Low-Carbohydrate" OR "Low-Carbohydrate Diet, High-Protein" OR "Low-Carbohydrate Diets, High-Protein" OR "Carbohydrate-Restricted High-Protein Diet" OR "Carbohydrate Restricted High Protein Diet" OR "Diet, Carbohydrate-Restricted High-Protein" OR "Diets, Carbohydrate-Restricted High-Protein" OR "High-Protein Diet, Carbohydrate-Restricted" OR "High-Protein Diets, Carbohydrate-Restricted" OR "Carbohydrate-Restricted High-Protein Diets" OR "Carbohydrate Restricted High Protein Diets" OR "Low-Carbohydrate High-Protein Diets" OR "Low Carbohydrate High Protein Diets" OR "High-Protein Low-Carbohydrate Diet" OR "High Protein Low Carbohydrate Diet" OR "High-Protein Low-Carbohydrate Diets" OR "High Protein Low Carbohydrate Diets" OR "Low-Carbohydrate High-Protein Diet" OR "Diet, Low-Carbohydrate High-Protein" OR "Diets, Low-Carbohydrate High-Protein" OR "High-Protein Diet, Low-Carbohydrate" OR "High-Protein Diets, Low-Carbohydrate" OR "Low Carbohydrate High Protein Diet" OR "High-Protein Carbohydrate-Restricted Diets" OR "Carbohydrate-Restricted Diet, High-Protein" OR "Carbohydrate-Restricted Diets, High-Protein" OR "Diet, High-Protein Carbohydrate-Restricted" OR "Diets, High-Protein Carbohydrate-Restricted" OR "High Protein Carbohydrate Restricted Diets" OR "High-Protein Carbohydrate-Restricted Diet" OR "High Protein Carbohydrate Restricted Diet" OR "South Beach Diet" OR "Diet, South Beach" OR "Atkins Diet" OR "Diet, Atkins" OR "Diabetic Diets" OR "Diets, Diabetic" OR "Diabetic Diet" OR "Therapy, Diet" OR "Diet Therapies" OR "Therapies, Diet" OR "Dietary Modification" OR "Dietary Modifications" OR "Modification, Dietary" OR "Modifications, Dietary" OR "Diet Modification" OR "Diet Modifications" OR "Modification, Diet" OR "Modifications, Diet" OR "Atherogenic Diet" OR "Atherogenic Diets" OR "Diets, Atherogenic" OR "Diets, Vegetarian" OR "Vegetarian Diets" OR "Vegetarian Diet" OR "Vegetarianism" OR "Diets, Macrobiotic" OR "Macrobiotic Diet" OR "Macrobiotic Diets" OR "Diet, Fat Restricted" OR "Fat-Restricted Diet" OR "Diets, Fat-Restricted" OR "Fat Restricted Diet" OR "Fat-Restricted Diets" OR "Diet, Low-Fat" OR "Diet, Low Fat" OR "Diets, Low-Fat" OR "Low-Fat Diet" OR "Low-Fat Diets" OR "Diet, Fat-Free" OR "Diet, Fat Free" OR "Diets, Fat-Free" OR "Fat-Free Diet" OR "Fat-Free Diets" OR "Diet, Protein Restricted" OR "Low-Protein Diet" OR "Low Protein Diet" OR "Protein-Restricted Diet" OR "Diets, Protein-Restricted" OR "Protein Restricted Diet" OR "Protein-Restricted Diets" OR "Diet, Low-Protein" OR "Diet, Low Protein" OR "Diets, Low-Protein" OR "Low-Protein Diets" OR "Diet, Protein-Free" OR "Diet, Protein Free" OR "Diets, Protein-Free" OR "Protein-Free Diet" OR "Protein-Free Diets" OR "Mediterranean Diet" OR "Diets, Mediterranean" OR "Mediterranean Diets" OR "Diet, Carbohydrate Restricted" OR "Diet, Low Carbohydrate" OR "Carbohydrate Diet, Low" OR "Carbohydrate Diets, Low" OR "Diets, Low Carbohydrate" OR "Low Carbohydrate Diets" OR "Carbohydrate-Restricted Diet" OR "Carbohydrate Restricted Diet" OR "Carbohydrate-Restricted Diets" OR "Diets, Carbohydrate-Restricted" OR "Low-Carbohydrate Diet" OR "Diet, Low-Carbohydrate" OR "Diets, Low-Carbohydrate" OR "Low Carbohydrate Diet" OR "Low-Carbohydrate Diets" OR "Diet, Gluten Free" OR "Gluten-Free Diet" OR "Diets, Gluten-Free" OR "Gluten Free Diet" OR "Gluten-Free Diets" OR "Ketogenic Diet" OR "Diets, Ketogenic" OR "Ketogenic Diets" OR "Diets, High-Fat" OR "High-Fat Diet" OR "High-Fat Diets" OR "Diet, High Fat" OR "Diets, High Fat" OR "High Fat Diet" OR "High Fat Diets" OR "Paleolithic Diet" OR "Diet, Stone Age" OR "Diets, Stone Age" OR "Stone Age Diet" OR "Stone Age Diets" OR "Diet, Paleo" OR "Diets, Paleo" OR "Paleo Diet" OR "Paleo Diets" OR "Diet, Caveman" OR "Caveman Diet" OR "Caveman Diets" OR "Diets, Caveman" OR "Diet, Hunter-Gatherer" OR "Diet, Hunter Gatherer" OR "Diets, Hunter-Gatherer" OR "Hunter-Gatherer Diet" OR "Hunter-Gatherer Diets" OR "Diets, Western" OR "Western Diets" OR "Western Dietary Pattern" OR "Dietary Pattern, Western" OR "Dietary Patterns, Western" OR "Pattern, Western Dietary" OR "Patterns, Western Dietary" OR "Western Dietary Patterns" OR "Diet, Occidental" OR "Diets, Occidental" OR "Occidental Diet" OR "Occidental Diets" OR "Western Diet" OR "Meat-Sweet Diet" OR "Diet, Meat-Sweet" OR "Diets, Meat-Sweet" OR "Meat Sweet Diet" OR "Meat-Sweet Diets") AND ("Clinical Trials, Randomized" OR "Trials, Randomized Clinical" OR "Controlled Clinical Trials, Randomized" OR "Randomized Controlled Trial"))	400

Table 1 (continued)

Database	Search (December, 2020)	References
Web of Science	Tópico: ("Lupus Erythematosus, Systemic" OR "Systemic Lupus Erythematosus" OR "Lupus Erythematosus Disseminatus" OR "Libman-Sacks Disease" OR "Disease, Libman-Sacks" OR "Libman Sacks Disease" OR "Lupus Vulgaris" OR "Central Nervous System Lupus Vasculitis" OR "Systemic Lupus Erythematosis, Central Nervous System" OR "Central Nervous System Lupus" OR "Central Nervous System Systemic Lupus Erythematosis" OR "Neuropsychiatric Systemic Lupus Erythematosus" OR "Lupus Meningoencephalitis" OR "Lupus Meningoencephalitides" OR "Meningoencephalitides, Lupus" OR "Meningoencephalitis, Lupus" OR "Lupus Panniculitis" OR "Lupus Panniculitides" OR "Panniculitides, Lupus" OR "Panniculitis, Lupus" OR "Lupus Erythematosus Panniculitis" OR "Lupus Erythematosus Panniculitides" OR "Panniculitides, Lupus Erythematosus" OR "Lupus Erythematosus Profundus" OR "Lupus Profundus" OR "Discoid Lupus Erythematosus" OR "Lupus Erythematosus, Chronic Cutaneous" OR "Lupus Erythematosus, Cutaneous, Chronic" OR "Cutaneous Lupus Erythematosus" OR "Lupus Erythematosus, Subacute Cutaneous" OR "Lupus Erythematosus, Cutaneous, Subacute") AND Tópico: (Diet OR Diets OR "nutritional management" OR "dietary management" OR "Diet, Healthy" OR "Diets, Healthy" OR "Healthy Diets" OR "Healthy Eating" OR "Eating, Healthy" OR "Healthy Eating Index" OR "Eating Index, Healthy" OR "Eating Indices, Healthy" OR "Healthy Eating Indices" OR "Index, Healthy Eating" OR "Indices, Healthy Eating" OR "Carbohydrate Loading Diets" OR "Carbohydrate Loading Diet" OR "Carbohydrate Loading" OR "Diets, Vegan" OR "Vegan Diets" OR "Vegan Diet" OR "Veganism" OR "Diet, High Protein" OR "Diets, High-Protein" OR "High-Protein Diets" OR "High-Protein Diet" OR "High Protein Diet" OR "Diet, High Protein Low Carbohydrate" OR "Diets, High-Protein Low-Carbohydrate" OR "Low-Carbohydrate Diet, High-Protein" OR "Low-Carbohydrate Diets, High-Protein" OR "Carbohydrate-Restricted High-Protein Diet" OR "Carbohydrate Restricted High Protein Diet" OR "Diet, Carbohydrate-Restricted High-Protein" OR "Diets, Carbohydrate-Restricted High-Protein" OR "High-Protein Diet, Carbohydrate-Restricted" OR "High-Protein Diets, Carbohydrate-Restricted" OR "Carbohydrate-Restricted High-Protein Diets" OR "Carbohydrate Restricted High Protein Diets" OR "Low-Carbohydrate High-Protein Diets" OR "Low Carbohydrate High Protein Diets" OR "High-Protein Low-Carbohydrate Diet" OR "High Protein Low Carbohydrate Diet" OR "High-Protein Low-Carbohydrate Diets" OR "High Protein Low Carbohydrate Diets" OR "Low-Carbohydrate High-Protein Diet" OR "Diet, Low-Carbohydrate High-Protein" OR "Diets, Low-Carbohydrate High-Protein" OR "High-Protein Diet, Low-Carbohydrate" OR "High-Protein Diets, Low-Carbohydrate" OR "Low Carbohydrate High Protein Diet" OR "High-Protein Carbohydrate-Restricted Diets" OR "Carbohydrate-Restricted Diet, High-Protein" OR "Carbohydrate-Restricted Diets, High-Protein" OR "Diet, High-Protein Carbohydrate-Restricted" OR "Diets, High-Protein Carbohydrate-Restricted" OR "High Protein Carbohydrate Restricted Diets" OR "High-Protein Carbohydrate-Restricted Diet" OR "High Protein Carbohydrate Restricted Diet" OR "South Beach Diet" OR "Diet, South Beach" OR "Atkins Diet" OR "Diet, Atkins" OR "Diabetic Diets" OR "Diets, Diabetic" OR "Diabetic Diet" OR "Therapy, Diet" OR "Diet Therapies" OR "Therapies, Diet" OR "Dietary Modification" OR "Dietary Modifications" OR "Modification, Dietary" OR "Modifications, Dietary" OR "Diet Modification" OR "Diet Modifications" OR "Modification, Diet" OR "Modifications, Diet" OR "Atherogenic Diet" OR "Atherogenic Diets" OR "Diets, Atherogenic" OR "Diets, Vegetarian" OR "Vegetarian Diets" OR "Vegetarian Diet" OR "Vegetarianism" OR "Diets, Macrobiotic" OR "Macrobiotic Diet" OR "Macrobiotic Diets" OR "Diet, Fat Restricted" OR "Fat-Restricted Diet" OR "Diets, Fat-Restricted" OR "Fat Restricted Diet" OR "Fat-Restricted Diets" OR "Diet, Low-Fat" OR "Diet, Low Fat" OR "Diets, Low-Fat" OR "Low-Fat Diet" OR "Low-Fat Diets" OR "Diet, Fat-Free" OR "Diet, Fat Free" OR "Diets, Fat-Free" OR "Fat-Free Diet" OR "Fat-Free Diets" OR "Diet, Protein Restricted" OR "Low-Protein Diet" OR "Low Protein Diet" OR "Protein-Restricted Diet" OR "Diets, Protein-Restricted" OR "Protein Restricted Diet" OR "Protein-Restricted Diets" OR "Diet, Low-Protein" OR "Diet, Low Protein" OR "Diets, Low-Protein" OR "Low-Protein Diets" OR "Diet, Protein-Free" OR "Diet, Protein Free" OR "Diets, Protein-Free" OR "Protein-Free Diet" OR "Protein-Free Diets" OR "Mediterranean Diet" OR "Diets, Mediterranean" OR "Mediterranean Diets" OR "Diet, Carbohydrate Restricted" OR "Diet, Low Carbohydrate" OR "Carbohydrate Diet, Low" OR "Carbohydrate Diets, Low" OR "Diets, Low Carbohydrate" OR "Low Carbohydrate Diets" OR "Carbohydrate-Restricted Diet" OR "Carbohydrate Restricted Diet" OR "Carbohydrate-Restricted Diets" OR "Diets, Carbohydrate-Restricted" OR "Low-Carbohydrate Diet" OR "Diet, Low-Carbohydrate" OR "Diets, Low-Carbohydrate" OR "Low Carbohydrate Diet" OR "Low-Carbohydrate Diets" OR "Diet, Gluten Free" OR "Gluten-Free Diet" OR "Diets, Gluten-Free" OR "Gluten Free Diet" OR "Gluten-Free Diets" OR "Ketogenic Diet" OR "Diets, Ketogenic" OR "Ketogenic Diets" OR "Diets, High-Fat" OR "High-Fat Diet" OR "High-Fat Diets" OR "Diet, High Fat" OR "Diets, High Fat" OR "High Fat Diet" OR "High Fat Diets" OR "Paleolithic Diet" OR "Diet, Stone Age" OR "Diets, Stone Age" OR "Stone Age Diet" OR "Stone Age Diets" OR "Diet, Paleo" OR "Diets, Paleo" OR "Paleo Diet" OR "Paleo Diets" OR "Diet, Caveman" OR "Caveman Diet" OR "Caveman Diets" OR "Diets, Caveman" OR "Diet, Hunter-Gatherer" OR "Diet, Hunter Gatherer" OR "Diets, Hunter-Gatherer" OR "Hunter-Gatherer Diet" OR "Hunter-Gatherer Diets" OR "Diets, Western" OR "Western Diets" OR "Western Dietary Pattern" OR "Dietary Pattern, Western" OR "Dietary Patterns, Western" OR "Pattern, Western Dietary" OR "Patterns, Western Dietary" OR "Western Dietary Patterns" OR "Diet, Occidental" OR "Diets, Occidental" OR "Occidental Diet" OR "Occidental Diets" OR "Western Diet" OR "Meat-Sweet Diet" OR "Diet, Meat-Sweet" OR "Diets, Meat-Sweet" OR "Meat Sweet Diet" OR "Meat-Sweet Diets") AND Tópico: ("Clinical Trials, Randomized" OR "Trials, Randomized Clinical" OR "Controlled Clinical Trials, Randomized" OR "Randomized Controlled Trial")	05

Table 1 (continued)

Database	Search (December, 2020)	References
Cochrane	#1 – ""("Lupus Erythematosus, Systemic""" OR """Systemic Lupus Erythematosus""" OR """Lupus Erythematosus Disseminatus""" OR """Libman-Sacks Disease""" OR """Disease, Libman-Sacks""" OR """Libman Sacks Disease""" OR """Lupus Vulgaris""" OR """Central Nervous System Lupus Vasculitis""" OR """Systemic Lupus Erythematosis, Central Nervous System""" OR """Central Nervous System Lupus""" OR """Central Nervous System Systemic Lupus Erythematosis""" OR """Neuropsychiatric Systemic Lupus Erythematosus""" OR """Lupus Meningoencephalitis""" OR """Lupus Meningoencephalitides""" OR """Meningoencephalitides, Lupus""" OR """Meningoencephalitis, Lupus""" OR """Lupus Panniculitis""" OR """Lupus Panniculitides""" OR """Panniculitides, Lupus""" OR """Panniculitis, Lupus""" OR """Lupus Erythematosus Panniculitis""" OR """Lupus Erythematosus Panniculitides""" OR """Panniculitides, Lupus Erythematosus""" OR """Lupus Erythematosus Profundus""" OR """Lupus Profundus""" OR """Discoid Lupus Erythematosus""" OR """Lupus Erythematosus, Chronic Cutaneous""" OR """Lupus Erythematosus, Cutaneous, Chronic""" OR """Cutaneous Lupus Erythematosus""" OR """Lupus Erythematosus, Subacute Cutaneous""" OR """Lupus Erythematosus, Cutaneous, Subacute""") #2 – (Diet OR Diets OR "nutritional management" OR "dietary management" OR "Diet, Healthy" OR "Diets, Healthy" OR "Healthy Diets" OR "Healthy Eating" OR "Eating, Healthy" OR "Healthy Eating Index" OR "Eating Index, Healthy" OR "Eating Indices, Healthy" OR "Healthy Eating Indices" OR "Index, Healthy Eating" OR "Indices, Healthy Eating" OR "Carbohydrate Loading Diets" OR "Carbohydrate Loading Diet" OR "Carbohydrate Loading" OR "Diets, Vegan" OR "Vegan Diets" OR "Vegan Diet" OR "Veganism" OR "Diet, High Protein" OR "Diets, High-Protein" OR "High-Protein Diets" OR "High-Protein Diet" OR "High Protein Diet" OR "Diet, High Protein Low Carbohydrate" OR "Diets, High-Protein Low-Carbohydrate" OR "Low-Carbohydrate Diet, High-Protein" OR "Low-Carbohydrate Diets, High-Protein" OR "Carbohydrate-Restricted High-Protein Diet" OR "Carbohydrate Restricted High Protein Diet" OR "Diet, Carbohydrate-Restricted High-Protein" OR "Diets, Carbohydrate-Restricted High-Protein" OR "High-Protein Diet, Carbohydrate-Restricted" OR "High-Protein Diets, Carbohydrate-Restricted" OR "Carbohydrate-Restricted High-Protein Diets" OR "Carbohydrate Restricted High Protein Diets" OR "Low-Carbohydrate High-Protein Diets" OR "Low Carbohydrate High Protein Diets" OR "High-Protein Low-Carbohydrate Diet" OR "High Protein Low Carbohydrate Diet" OR "High-Protein Low-Carbohydrate Diets" OR "High Protein Low Carbohydrate Diets" OR "Low-Carbohydrate High-Protein Diet" OR "Diet, Low-Carbohydrate High-Protein" OR "Diets, Low-Carbohydrate High-Protein" OR "High-Protein Diet, Low-Carbohydrate" OR "High-Protein Diets, Low-Carbohydrate" OR "Low Carbohydrate High Protein Diet" OR "High-Protein Carbohydrate-Restricted Diets" OR "Carbohydrate-Restricted Diet, High-Protein" OR "Carbohydrate-Restricted Diets, High-Protein" OR "Diet, High-Protein Carbohydrate-Restricted" OR "Diets, High-Protein Carbohydrate-Restricted" OR "High Protein Carbohydrate Restricted Diets" OR "High-Protein Carbohydrate-Restricted Diet" OR "High Protein Carbohydrate Restricted Diet" OR "South Beach Diet" OR "Diet, South Beach" OR "Atkins Diet" OR "Diet, Atkins" OR "Diabetic Diets" OR "Diets, Diabetic" OR "Diabetic Diet" OR "Therapy, Diet" OR "Diet Therapies" OR "Therapies, Diet" OR "Dietary Modification" OR "Dietary Modifications" OR "Modification, Dietary" OR "Modifications, Dietary" OR "Diet Modification" OR "Diet Modifications" OR "Modification, Diet" OR "Modifications, Diet" OR "Atherogenic Diet" OR "Atherogenic Diets" OR "Diets, Atherogenic" OR "Diets, Vegetarian" OR "Vegetarian Diets" OR "Vegetarian Diet" OR "Vegetarianism" OR "Diets, Macrobiotic" OR "Macrobiotic Diet" OR "Macrobiotic Diets" OR "Diet, Fat Restricted" OR "Fat-Restricted Diet" OR "Diets, Fat-Restricted" OR "Fat Restricted Diet" OR "Fat-Restricted Diets" OR "Diet, Low-Fat" OR "Diet, Low Fat" OR "Diets, Low-Fat" OR "Low-Fat Diet" OR "Low-Fat Diets" OR "Diet, Fat-Free" OR "Diet, Fat Free" OR "Diets, Fat-Free" OR "Fat-Free Diet" OR "Fat-Free Diets" OR "Diet, Protein Restricted" OR "Low-Protein Diet" OR "Low Protein Diet" OR "Protein-Restricted Diet" OR "Diets, Protein-Restricted" OR "Protein Restricted Diet" OR "Protein-Restricted Diets" OR "Diet, Low-Protein" OR "Diet, Low Protein" OR "Diets, Low-Protein" OR "Low-Protein Diets" OR "Diet, Protein-Free" OR "Diet, Protein Free" OR "Diets, Protein-Free" OR "Protein-Free Diet" OR "Protein-Free Diets" OR "Mediterranean Diet" OR "Diets, Mediterranean" OR "Mediterranean Diets" OR "Diet, Carbohydrate Restricted" OR "Diet, Low Carbohydrate" OR "Carbohydrate Diet, Low" OR "Carbohydrate Diets, Low" OR "Diets, Low Carbohydrate" OR "Low Carbohydrate Diets" OR "Carbohydrate-Restricted Diet" OR "Carbohydrate Restricted Diet" OR "Carbohydrate-Restricted Diets" OR "Diets, Carbohydrate-Restricted" OR "Low-Carbohydrate Diet" OR "Diet, Low-Carbohydrate" OR "Diets, Low-Carbohydrate" OR "Low Carbohydrate Diet" OR "Low-Carbohydrate Diets" OR "Diet, Gluten Free" OR "Gluten-Free Diet" OR "Diets, Gluten-Free" OR "Gluten Free Diet" OR "Gluten-Free Diets" OR "Ketogenic Diet" OR "Diets, Ketogenic" OR "Ketogenic Diets" OR "Diets, High-Fat" OR "High-Fat Diet" OR "High-Fat Diets" OR "Diet, High Fat" OR "Diets, High Fat" OR "High Fat Diet" OR "High Fat Diets" OR "Paleolithic Diet" OR "Diet, Stone Age" OR "Diets, Stone Age" OR "Stone Age Diet" OR "Stone Age Diets" OR "Diet, Paleo" OR "Diets, Paleo" OR "Paleo Diet" OR "Paleo Diets" OR "Diet, Caveman" OR "Caveman Diet" OR "Caveman Diets" OR "Diets, Caveman" OR "Diet, Hunter-Gatherer" OR "Diet, Hunter Gatherer" OR "Diets, Hunter-Gatherer" OR "Hunter-Gatherer Diet" OR "Hunter-Gatherer Diets" OR "Diets, Western" OR "Western Diets" OR "Western Dietary Pattern" OR "Dietary Pattern, Western" OR "Dietary Patterns, Western" OR "Pattern, Western Dietary" OR "Patterns, Western Dietary" OR "Western Dietary Patterns" OR "Diet, Occidental" OR "Diets, Occidental" OR "Occidental Diet" OR "Occidental Diets" OR "Western Diet" OR "Meat-Sweet Diet" OR "Diet, Meat-Sweet" OR "Diets, Meat-Sweet" OR "Meat Sweet Diet" OR "Meat-Sweet Diets") #3 – (#1 AND #2) in trials	29

Table 1 (continued)

Database	Search (December, 2020)	References
ClinicalTrials.gov	#1 – ""("Lupus Erythematosus, Systemic""" OR """Systemic Lupus Erythematosus""" OR """Lupus Erythematosus Disseminatus""" OR """Libman-Sacks Disease""" OR """Disease, Libman-Sacks""" OR """Libman Sacks Disease""" OR """Lupus Vulgaris""" OR """Central Nervous System Lupus Vasculitis""" OR """Systemic Lupus Erythematosis, Central Nervous System""" OR """Central Nervous System Lupus""" OR """Central Nervous System Systemic Lupus Erythematosis""" OR """Neuropsychiatric Systemic Lupus Erythematosus""" OR """Lupus Meningoencephalitis""" OR """Lupus Meningoencephalitides""" OR """Meningoencephalitides, Lupus""" OR """Meningoencephalitis, Lupus""" OR """Lupus Panniculitis""" OR """Lupus Panniculitides""" OR """Panniculitides, Lupus""" OR """Panniculitis, Lupus""" OR """Lupus Erythematosus Panniculitis""" OR """Lupus Erythematosus Panniculitides""" OR """Panniculitides, Lupus Erythematosus""" OR """Lupus Erythematosus Profundus""" OR """Lupus Profundus""" OR """Discoid Lupus Erythematosus""" OR """Lupus Erythematosus, Chronic Cutaneous""" OR """Lupus Erythematosus, Cutaneous, Chronic""" OR """Cutaneous Lupus Erythematosus""" OR """Lupus Erythematosus, Subacute Cutaneous""" OR """Lupus Erythematosus, Cutaneous, Subacute""") #2 – (Diet OR Diets OR “nutritional management” OR “dietary management” OR “Diet, Healthy” OR “Diets, Healthy” OR “Healthy Diets” OR “Healthy Eating” OR “Eating, Healthy” OR “Healthy Eating Index” OR “Eating Index, Healthy” OR “Eating Indices, Healthy” OR “Healthy Eating Indices” OR “Index, Healthy Eating” OR “Indices, Healthy Eating” OR “Carbohydrate Loading Diets” OR “Carbohydrate Loading Diet” OR “Carbohydrate Loading” OR “Diets, Vegan” OR “Vegan Diets” OR “Vegan Diet” OR “Veganism” OR “Diet, High Protein” OR “Diets, High-Protein” OR “High-Protein Diets” OR “High-Protein Diet” OR “High Protein Diet” OR “Diet, High Protein Low Carbohydrate” OR “Diets, High-Protein Low-Carbohydrate” OR “Low-Carbohydrate Diet, High-Protein” OR “Low-Carbohydrate Diets, High-Protein” OR “Carbohydrate-Restricted High-Protein Diet” OR “Carbohydrate Restricted High Protein Diet” OR “Diet, Carbohydrate-Restricted High-Protein” OR “Diets, Carbohydrate-Restricted High-Protein” OR “High-Protein Diet, Carbohydrate-Restricted” OR “High-Protein Diets, Carbohydrate-Restricted” OR “Carbohydrate-Restricted High-Protein Diets” OR “Carbohydrate Restricted High Protein Diets” OR “Low-Carbohydrate High-Protein Diets” OR “Low Carbohydrate High Protein Diets” OR “High-Protein Low-Carbohydrate Diet” OR “High Protein Low Carbohydrate Diet” OR “High-Protein Low-Carbohydrate Diets” OR “High Protein Low Carbohydrate Diets” OR “Low-Carbohydrate High-Protein Diet” OR “Diet, Low-Carbohydrate High-Protein” OR “Diets, Low-Carbohydrate High-Protein” OR “High-Protein Diet, Low-Carbohydrate” OR “High-Protein Diets, Low-Carbohydrate” OR “Low Carbohydrate High Protein Diet” OR “High-Protein Carbohydrate-Restricted Diets” OR “Carbohydrate-Restricted Diet, High-Protein” OR “Carbohydrate-Restricted Diets, High-Protein” OR “Diet, High-Protein Carbohydrate-Restricted” OR “Diets, High-Protein Carbohydrate-Restricted” OR “High Protein Carbohydrate Restricted Diets” OR “High-Protein Carbohydrate-Restricted Diet” OR “High Protein Carbohydrate Restricted Diet” OR “South Beach Diet” OR “Diet, South Beach” OR “Atkins Diet” OR “Diet, Atkins” OR “Diabetic Diets” OR “Diets, Diabetic” OR “Diabetic Diet” OR “Therapy, Diet” OR “Diet Therapies” OR “Therapies, Diet” OR “Dietary Modification” OR “Dietary Modifications” OR “Modification, Dietary” OR “Modifications, Dietary” OR “Diet Modification” OR “Diet Modifications” OR “Modification, Diet” OR “Modifications, Diet” OR “Atherogenic Diet” OR “Atherogenic Diets” OR “Diets, Atherogenic” OR “Diets, Vegetarian” OR “Vegetarian Diets” OR “Vegetarian Diet” OR “Vegetarianism” OR “Diets, Macrobiotic” OR “Macrobiotic Diet” OR “Macrobiotic Diets” OR “Diet, Fat Restricted” OR “Fat-Restricted Diet” OR “Diets, Fat-Restricted” OR “Fat Restricted Diet” OR “Fat-Restricted Diets” OR “Diet, Low-Fat” OR “Diet, Low Fat” OR “Diets, Low-Fat” OR “Low-Fat Diet” OR “Low-Fat Diets” OR “Diet, Fat-Free” OR “Diet, Fat Free” OR “Diets, Fat-Free” OR “Fat-Free Diet” OR “Fat-Free Diets” OR “Diet, Protein Restricted” OR “Low-Protein Diet” OR “Low Protein Diet” OR “Protein-Restricted Diet” OR “Diets, Protein-Restricted” OR “Protein Restricted Diet” OR “Protein-Restricted Diets” OR “Diet, Low-Protein” OR “Diet, Low Protein” OR “Diets, Low-Protein” OR “Low-Protein Diets” OR “Diet, Protein-Free” OR “Diet, Protein Free” OR “Diets, Protein-Free” OR “Protein-Free Diet” OR “Protein-Free Diets” OR “Mediterranean Diet” OR “Diets, Mediterranean” OR “Mediterranean Diets” OR “Diet, Carbohydrate Restricted” OR “Diet, Low Carbohydrate” OR “Carbohydrate Diet, Low” OR “Carbohydrate Diets, Low” OR “Diets, Low Carbohydrate” OR “Low Carbohydrate Diets” OR “Carbohydrate-Restricted Diet” OR “Carbohydrate Restricted Diet” OR “Carbohydrate-Restricted Diets” OR “Diets, Carbohydrate-Restricted” OR “Low-Carbohydrate Diet” OR “Diet, Low-Carbohydrate” OR “Diets, Low-Carbohydrate” OR “Low Carbohydrate Diet” OR “Low-Carbohydrate Diets” OR “Diet, Gluten Free” OR “Gluten-Free Diet” OR “Diets, Gluten-Free” OR “Gluten Free Diet” OR “Gluten-Free Diets” OR “Ketogenic Diet” OR “Diets, Ketogenic” OR “Ketogenic Diets” OR “Diets, High-Fat” OR “High-Fat Diet” OR “High-Fat Diets” OR “Diet, High Fat” OR “Diets, High Fat” OR “High Fat Diet” OR “High Fat Diets” OR “Paleolithic Diet” OR “Diet, Stone Age” OR “Diets, Stone Age” OR “Stone Age Diet” OR “Stone Age Diets” OR “Diet, Paleo” OR “Diets, Paleo” OR “Paleo Diet” OR “Paleo Diets” OR “Diet, Caveman” OR “Caveman Diet” OR “Caveman Diets” OR “Diets, Caveman” OR “Diet, Hunter-Gatherer” OR “Diet, Hunter Gatherer” OR “Diets, Hunter-Gatherer” OR “Hunter-Gatherer Diet” OR “Hunter-Gatherer Diets” OR “Diets, Western” OR “Western Diets” OR “Western Dietary Pattern” OR “Dietary Pattern, Western” OR “Dietary Patterns, Western” OR “Pattern, Western Dietary” OR “Patterns, Western Dietary” OR “Western Dietary Patterns” OR “Diet, Occidental” OR “Diets, Occidental” OR “Occidental Diet” OR “Occidental Diets” OR “Western Diet” OR “Meat-Sweet Diet” OR “Diet, Meat-Sweet” OR “Diets, Meat-Sweet” OR “Meat Sweet Diet” OR “Meat-Sweet Diets”) #3 – (#1 AND #2) in trials	7
Lilacs (Portuguese)	(tw:(“Lúpus Eritematoso Sistêmico” OU “Lúpus Eritematoso Sistêmico” OU “Lúpus Eritematoso Disseminado” OU “Doença de Libman-Sacks” OU “Lupus Vulgaris” OU “Lúpus do Sistema Nervoso Central” OU “Lúpus Eritematoso Sistêmico do Sistema Nervoso Central” OU “Lúpus Eritematoso Sistêmico Neuropsiquiátrico” OU “Meningoencefalite Lúpica” OU “Meningoencefalites Lúpicas” OU "Paniculite Lúpica" OU "Paniculite Lúpicas" OU "Paniculite Lúpica Eritematosa" OU "Paniculite Lúpicas Eritematosas" OU “Lúpus Eritematoso Profundus” OU “Lupus Profundus” OU “Lúpus Eritematoso Discóide” OU “Lupus Eritematoso Crônico Cutâneo” OU “Lúpus Eritematoso Cutâneo Crônico” OU “Lúpus Eritematoso Cutâneo” OU “Lúpus Eritematoso Subcutâneo Cutâneo” OU “Lúpus Eritematoso Cutâneo Subagudo”)) AND (tw:(Dieta OU Dietas)) AND (tw:(“Ensaios Clínicos Randomizados” OU “Ensaio Clínico Controlado Aleatório”)) AND (db:("LILACS"))	0
EMBASE	(lupus OR ’lupus erythematosus’/exp OR ’lupus erythematosus’ OR ’systemic lupus erythematosus’/exp OR ’systemic lupus erythematosus’) AND (’nutrition’/exp OR nutrition OR ’diet, food, and nutrition’ OR ’nutrition’ OR ’nutrition council’ OR ’nutrition phenomena’ OR ’nutrition physiology’ OR ’nutrition processes’ OR ’nutrition research’ OR ’nutrition research center’ OR ’nutrition study’ OR ’nutrition survey’ OR ’nutrition surveys’ OR ’nutritional physiological phenomena’ OR ’nutritional physiology’ OR ’nutritive solution’ OR ’sports nutritional physiological phenomena’ OR ’diet therapy’/exp OR ’diet intervention’ OR ’diet therapy’ OR ’diet treatment’ OR ’dietary intervention’ OR ’dietary therapy’ OR ’dietary treatment’ OR ’nutrition therapy’ OR ’diet’/exp OR diet OR ’diet’ OR ’diet influence’ OR ’diet regimen’ OR ’diet surveys’ OR ’dietary effect’ OR ’dietary influence’ OR ’dietary survey’ OR ’dietary surveys’ OR ’dieting’) AND (’controlled clinical trial’/exp OR ’clinical trial, controlled’ OR ’controlled clinical comparison’ OR ’controlled clinical drug trial’ OR ’controlled clinical experiment’ OR ’controlled clinical study’ OR ’controlled clinical test’ OR ’controlled clinical trial’ OR ’randomized controlled trial’/exp OR ’controlled trial, randomized’ OR ’randomised controlled study’ OR ’randomised controlled trial’ OR ’randomized controlled study’ OR ’randomized controlled trial’ OR ’trial, randomized controlled’)	255
Open Grey	""("Lupus Erythematosus, Systemic""" OR """Systemic Lupus Erythematogemsus""" OR """Lupus Erythematosus Disseminatus""") AND Search (Diet OR Diets OR """nutritional management""" OR """dietary manaent""") AND ""("Clinical Trials, Randomized""" OR """Trials, Randomized Clinical""" OR """Controlled Clinical Trials, Randomized""" OR """Randomized Controlled Trial	0
Google Scholar	With all words ""("Systemic Lupus Erythematosus""" AND """Diet""" AND "Randomized Controlled Trial" With the exact term ""("Systemic Lupus Erythematosus""" AND """Diet""")	60
JSTOR	((("Lupus Erythematosus, Systemic") AND (Diet OR Diets)) AND ("Clinical Trials, Randomized" OR "Trials, Randomized Clinical" OR "Controlled Clinical Trials, Randomized" OR "Randomized Controlled Trial"))	0

outcomes. For binary data, a risk ratio (RR) with a 95% confidence interval (CI) was used to assess the effect size. The risk difference between the intervention and control groups was calculated according to the Cochrane Collaboration handbook through the following calculus: $100 \times (1 - RR)\%$. Continuous data were evaluated through mean with a 95% CI. Due to the data heterogeneity, the meta-analysis was not possible to be performed; however, the effect size of the collected data was estimated with a 95% CI and are presented in Table 2. Based on the Cochrane Collaboration handbook, for data interpretation, not only the statistical significance was considered, but also the change in the outcomes, which may not be relevant to the statistical aspect, but is relevant to the clinical aspect.

Unit of analysis issues

The unit of analysis was individual patients.

Dealing with missing data

In case of missing data, the authors of the studies would be consulted. However, it was not necessary, as the studies provided quantitative data.

Studies summary

The studies were summarized per author, publishing date, country, and place of study, intervention performed and results obtained.

Risk of bias assessment and GRADE approach

Through the Cochrane Collaboration risk-of-bias tool, the following domains were evaluated: random sequence generation, allocation sequence concealment, blinding of participants and personnel, blinding of reviewer, missing data, outcome selection, and other biases. Biases in texts included in the studies selection were identified. The risk of bias was evaluated by two independent reviewers (AMI and HES). There was no need for a third reviewer to resolve disagreements. The data was extracted from the selected articles, and the answers were classified using parameters of "yes", for low risk of bias; "no", for high risk of bias; and "unclear", for unknown or obscure risk of bias. The GRADE approach three domains and other considerations were used to grade the evidence for the main outcomes.

Outcomes

The potential significant outcomes were the evaluation of:

- Lipid profile parameters: High-density lipoprotein, Low-density lipoprotein, Triglyceride, Glycemic index)
- Disease activity, assessed with the Global activity by Systemic Lupus Erythematosus Disease Activity Index (SLEDAI), British Isles Lupus Assessment Group (BILAG), and European Community Lupus Activity Measure (ECLAM).
- Quality of life assessed with Lupus Quality of Life (LupusQoL), SLE-specific Quality of Life questionnaire (SLEQoL), SLE Quality of Life Questionnaire (L-QoL)), or another questionnaire with the same purpose.
- Quality and efficiency of sleep
- Fatigue with Fatigue Severity Scale (FSS).

The potential minor outcome was adherence to the diet.

Results

It was identified in the databases 758 articles; 132 were duplicated (Fig. 1); 616 references were screened, and 604 were excluded. After reading the title and abstract, 12 articles were included for full-text reading. After the full-text reading, three studies were included for quantitative analysis. The reasons for the exclusion of nine articles from the study were: Alternative Treatments – antiseptics, antibiotics, supplementation (n = 7); Cross-sectional, case–control, cohort studies, or any interventional design other than randomized clinical trials (n = 2).

The three articles included for the quantitative analysis were written in the United States (n = 1), in Brazil (n = 1), and in the United Kingdom (n = 1) in 2002, 2012, and 2018, respectively. The sample size varied between 17 and 31 people diagnosed with systemic lupus erythematosus. The description of these studies is shown in Table 3.

Sample characteristics

Silva et al [11]. included adolescents diagnosed with systemic lupus erythematosus for at least six months, with any clinical manifestation and disease activity. Shah et al. [8] and Davies et al. [7] included only women diagnosed with systemic lupus erythematosus for at least six months. In the study by Davies et al. [7] there was no difference between the groups in the number of patients with hypertension and hyperlipidemia, nor was the number of caucasians and non-caucasians similar between the groups. Shah et al. [8] found that African American were 60% of both groups and the remainder, predominantly of Hispanic origin.

Table 2 Summary of descriptive characteristics of included articles (n = 3)

Author, year, country	Participants (n, inclusion criteria)	Intervention	Outcomes	Risk of bias assessment						
				Random sequence generation	Allocation concealment	Blinding of participants and personnel	Blinding of outcome assessment	Incomplete outcome data	Selective reporting	Other bias
Davies et al., 2012, United Kingdom [4]	23 women diagnosed with SLE and classified according to the ACR criteria. Aged 18–65 years, with mild and stable disease, body mass index (BMI) > 25 kg/m^2 and stable prednisolone doses 5–20 mg/day	All patients were advised on dietary treatment by the same dietician - 11 subjects were assigned to the Low GI diet, whereby carbohydrate intake was limited to 45 g per day of low GI food, without restricting the consumption of fat and protein 12 subjects were assigned to a conventional Low Cal diet with calorie restriction of 2000 kcal per day, approximately 50% of calories from carbohydrate, 15% from protein and 30% from fat Dietetic support was given in the form of a weekly telephone call	At baseline and at 6 weeks Disease activity: British Isles Lupus Assessment Group (BILAG) index, the SLE Disease Activity Index (SLEDAI), the European Community Lupus Activity Measure (ECLAM) and Systemic Lupus International Collaborating Clinics/American College of Rheumatology (SLICC/ACR) damage scores Fatigue and sleep quality: Fatigue Severity Scale (FSS) and the Pittsburgh Sleep Quality Index (PSQI) Fasting blood Samples: low-density lipoprotein (LDL) cholesterol, high-density lipoprotein (HDL) cholesterol, triglyceride level, serum lipoprotein A, homocysteine, fibrinogen, high sensitivity C-reactive protein (hsCRP) and uric acid; oral glucose tolerance test; urine was dip-tested for ketones, blood and protein at baseline and on follow-up	Low risk	High risk	High risk	High risk	Low risk	Unclear	Low risk

Table 2 (continued)

Author, year, country	Participants (n, inclusion criteria)	Intervention	Outcomes	Risk of bias assessment						
				Random sequence generation	Allocation concealment	Blinding of participants and personnel	Blinding of outcome assessment	Incomplete outcome data	Selective reporting	Other bias
Shah et al., 2002, United States [5]	17 women diagnosed with SLE for at least six months, have an LDL cholesterol level ≥ 100 mg/dl, and be able to read	Diet intervention group:counselled to follow the National Cholesterol Education Program Step 2 diet Duration: 12 weeks; weekly sessions during the first 6 weeks, followed by telephone counselling sessions every 2 weeks for the next 6 weeks Control group: any dietary advice. Both groups were asked to maintain their usual level of physical activity	Lipid and lipoproteins, body weight, physical activity day food record and quality of life at baseline and 6 and 12 weeks	Low risk	High risk	High risk	High risk	Low risk	Unclear	Low risk

Table 2 (continued)

Author, year, country	Participants (n, inclusion criteria)	Intervention	Outcomes	Risk of bias assessment						
				Random sequence generation	Allocation concealment	Blinding of participants and personnel	Blinding of outcome assessment	Incomplete outcome data	Selective reporting	Other bias
Silva et al., 2018, Brazil [7]	31 adolescents with JSLE for at least six months with any clinical manifestation or any degree of disease activity	The nutritional intervention: six steps at monthly intervals and three reinforcement visits (1) general orientation on dietary behaviour; (2) notions of healthy eating based on food rotation; (3) emphases on adequate carbohydrate and fat intake; (4) orientation on adequate salt, sugar, sweetener; (5) qualitative changes emphasizing fruit and vegetable; (6) orientation on lifestyle, sedentary, leisure activities, parties and other events	BMI Height for age Day food record SLEDAI-2 K SLICC-ACR/DI	Low risk	Low risk	High risk	High risk	Low risk	Unclear	Unclear

SLE = systemic lupus erythematosus; ACR = American College of Rheumatology; GI = glycaemic index; BILAG = British Isles Lupus Assessment Group; SLEDAI = Systemic Lupus Erythematosus Disease Activity Index 2000; ECLAM = European Community Lupus Activity Measure; SLICC/ACR/DI = Systemic Lupus International Collaborating Clinics/American College of Rheumatology/Damage index; FSS = Fatigue Severity Scale; PSQIP = Pittsburgh Sleep Quality Index; LDL = low-density lipoprotein; JSLE = juvenile systemic lupus erythematosus; BMI = body mass index; SLEDAI-2K = Systemic Lupus Erythematosus Disease Activity Index-2000

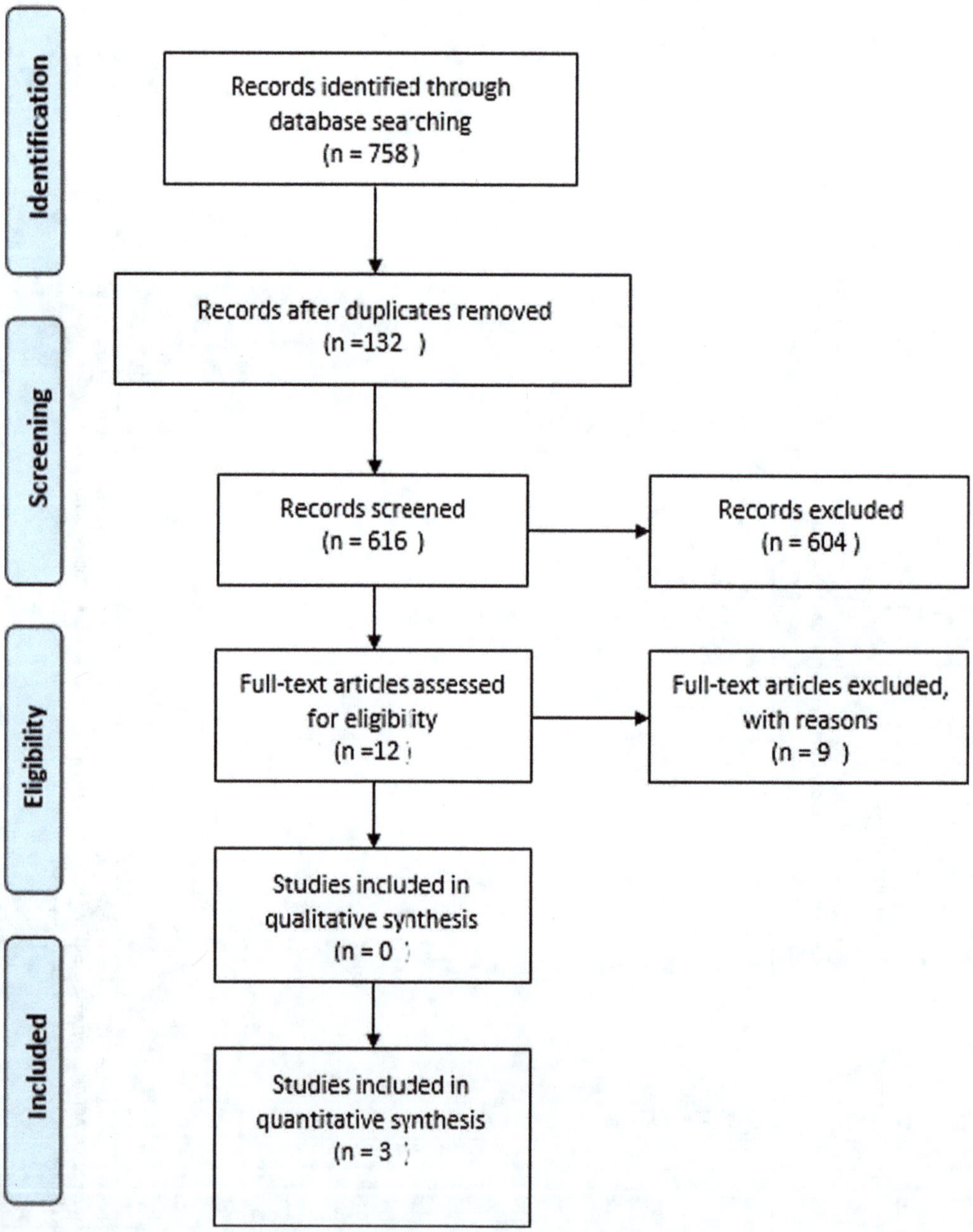

Fig. 1 PRISMA Flow diagram of literature searched and selection criteria

Medication used by patients

Regarding the use of medication, in the studies by Davies et al. [7] and Silva et al. [11], there was no significant difference between the groups in terms of prednisolone dosage and hydroxychloroquine users. Shah et al. [8] found that prednisolone use was slightly higher in the control group but without significant difference. In addition, four patients in the diet group and five patients in the control group were using cholesterol-lowering medication.

Diet types

The study conducted by Silva et al. [11] researched diet based on general behavioural guidelines, healthy eating, food diversity, balanced intake of fat and carbohydrate, and adequate intake of salt, fruit, vegetables, omega-3, and fibres. Additionally, orientations on lifestyle, frequency of meals, and physical activities were also analyzed. The controlled nutritional intervention study lasted nine months.

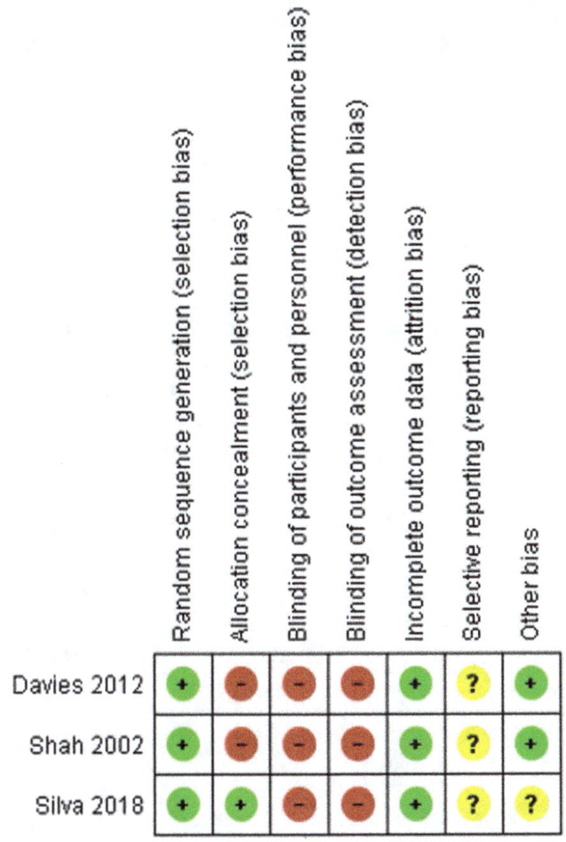

Fig. 2 Risk of bias assessment of included studies

Shah et al. [8] followed the National Cholesterol Education Program Step 2 diet: 30% or less calories from fat (7% from saturated fat, 13% from monounsaturated fat, and 10% from polyunsaturated fat), and < 200 mg of cholesterol per day. The diet intervention lasted for 12 weeks.

Davies et al. [7] compared two diet types. One diet type limited the carbohydrate intake to 45 g per day, without restricting the consumption of fat and protein. The composition of this diet was 10–15% of daily calories from carbohydrate, 25% from protein, and 60% from both saturated and unsaturated fat. The other was a calorie-restricted diet with limitation of 2000 kcal per day, approximately 50% from carbohydrates, 15% from protein, and 30% from fat.

Diet effects compared to control

Quality of life

Shah et al. [8] evaluated the quality of life using a self-administered questionnaire. The diet produced a small contribution to the quality of life improvement at six weeks (mean difference (MD) 16.30; 95% confidence interval (CI) 5.91; 26.69) and 12 weeks (MD 14.60; 95% CI 0.88; 28.32). There was statistically significant difference in both times of evaluation.

Disease activity

Silva et al. [11] evaluated the disease activity through Systemic Lupus Erythematosus Disease Activity Index (SLEDAI) 2 K>4. There was no relevant difference between both groups (RR 1.07; 95% CI – 0.32–3.52). There was no statistically significant difference.

Lipid profile at six weeks

Shah et al. [8] evaluated the lipid profile at six weeks. Although the diet caused a small improvement in the lipid profile of high-density lipoprotein (MD – 5.50; 95% CI – 18.21; 7.21), low-density lipoprotein (MD 5.70; 95% CI – 16.72; 28.12), and triglyceride (MD – 2.50; 95% CI – 70.67; 65.67), there was no statistically significant difference.

Lipid profile at 12 weeks

Shah et al. [8] evaluated the lipid profile at 12 weeks. The diet caused an improvement in the lipid profile of high-density lipoprotein (MD – 3.90; 95% CI – 17.54; 9.74), low-density lipoprotein (MD 15.30; 95% CI – 8.12; 38.72), and triglyceride (MD – 13.40; 95% CI – 50.27; 23.47), however, there was no statistically significant difference.

Lipid profile at nine months

Silva et al. [11] evaluated the lipid profile at nine months. The low calorie diet was favorable for the improvement in high-density lipoprotein (MD 4.30; 95% CI – 6.96; 15.56 P = 0.45), low-density lipoprotein (MD – 13.15; 95% CI – 29.38; 3.08 P = 0.11), and triglyceride (MD 11.30; 95% CI – 16.90; 39.50 P = 0.43), however, there was no statistically significant difference.

Comparison between the low glycemic index diet and the calorie-restricted diet

Evaluation of disease activity, fatigue, and quality of sleep

Davies et al. [7] evaluated the lipid profile at six weeks. The diet type did not affect the evaluation of fatigue, through the Fatigue Severity Scale (FSS) (MD 0.00; 95% CI – 1.20; 1.20 P = 0.00); disease activity, through the British Isles Lupus Assessment Group (BILAG) (MD 0.00; 95% CI – 3.52; 3.52 P = 1.00); and quality of sleep, case on which it had small impact (MD 0.00; 95% CI – 3.52; 3.52 P = 1.00). Although there was no statistically significant difference, by evaluating the disease activity through the European Community

Table 3 Post-intervention values of estimated effects for all outcomes evaluated

Outcome	Studies	N	MD	Lower 95%	Higher 95%
Diet effects compared to control					
Quality of life					
6 weeks	1	16	16.30	5.91	26.69
12 weeks	1	16	14.60	0.88	28.32
Lipid profile – 6 weeks					
HDL	1	16	5.50	− 7.21	18.21
LDL	1	16	5.70	16.72	28.12
Triglyceride	1	16	− 2.50	− 70.67	65.67
Lipid profile – 12 weeks					
HDL	1	16	3.90	17.54	9.74
LDL	1	16	15.30	− 8.12	38.72
Triglyceride	1	16	− 13.40	− 50.27	23.47
Lipid profile – 9 months					
HDL	1	31	4.30	− 6.96	15.56
LDL	1	31	− 13.15	− 29.38	3.08
Triglyceride	1	31	11.30	− 16.90	39.50
			RR	Lower 95%	Higher 95%
Disease activity (SLEDAI 2 K > 4) – 6 weeks	1	31	1.07	0.32	3.52
Outcome	**Studies**	**N**	**MD**	**Lower 95%**	**Higher 95%**
Comparison between the low glycemic index diet and the calorie-restricted diet					
Fatigue, quality of sleep, disease activity – 6 weeks					
Fatigue Severity Scale	1	23	0.00	− 1.20	1.20
Pittsburgh Sleep/Quality Index	1	23	0.50	− 3.14	4.14
British Isles Lupus Assessment Group	1	23	0.00	− 3.52	3.52
European Consensus Lupus Activity Measurement	1	23	− 0.90	− 1.94	0.14
Lipid profile – 6 weeks					
HDL	1	23	− 0.24	− 0.48	− 0.00
LDL	1	23	− 1.00	− 1.60	− 0.40
Triglyceride	1	23	− 0.35	− 0.89	0.19

MD = mean difference; RR = relative risk; HDL = high-density lipoprotein; LDL = low-density lipoprotein; SLEDAI = Systemic Lupus Erythematosus Disease Activity Index

Lupus Activity Measure (ECLAM), the low glycemic index diet showed a favourable effect (MD 0.90; 95% CI – 1.94; 0.14 P = 0.09).

Lipid profile analyses

Silva et al. [11] evaluated the lipid profile at six weeks. The low glycemic index diet was favorable for the improvement in high-density lipoprotein (MD – 0.24; 95% CI – 0.48; – 0.00 P = 0.05), low-density lipoprotein (MD – 1; 95% CI -1.60; – 0.40 P = 0.001), and triglyceride (MD – 0.35; 95% CI – 0.89; 0.19 P = 0.20). There was no statistically significant difference in the low-density lipoprotein evaluation (P = 0.0001).

Risk of bias and quality of evidence

None of the studies met all methodological quality criteria. Two studies did not describe the concealment of the allocation sequence [7, 8], and none of the studies described the blinding of participants and personnel as determined by the Risk of Bias instrument used.

Three studies were considered to have a low risk of bias for incomplete outcomes and did not report the main predetermined result [7, 10]. However, they were deemed to be free of other problems that could lead to a high risk of bias.

Quality of life, disease activity, and lipid profile outcomes at both 12 weeks and 9 months were selected and described as main outcomes in Table 4. Based on the risk of bias assessment and the GRADE approach three domains, it was found that through the evaluated outcomes, the level of evidence for the impact of diet on systemic lupus erythematosus patients is low (Fig. 2).

Discussion

The present study verified that the diet had a positive impact on the quality of life, and lipid profile of systemic lupus erythematosus patients. Three randomized controlled trials (RCTs) were included; however, due to the heterogeneity of the studies in relation to the control group and the moment of evaluation, it was not possible to perform the data meta-analysis. Nonetheless, to verify the effect size of interventions and compare it among the groups, the data presentation of choice was by effect size estimation.

According to Shah et al. [8], the diet intervention presented a small effect on the quality of life improvement. The questionnaire used by the authors assessed the general energy level, ability to perform specific tasks, quality of sleep, satisfaction with food eaten, satisfaction with personal life, relationships, etc. According to Chaigne et al. [12], musculoskeletal involvement, sociodemographic factors, fatigue, and comorbidities are directly related to the quality of life of systemic lupus erythematosus patients and can be modified when subjected to a controlled diet.

The European League Against Rheumatism (EULAR) stated that the quality of life-related to health is an important parameter and should be continuously evaluated in the clinical routine. Regarding the quality of life, the authors did not attribute a slight improvement to the diet itself, but the intensity of counselling received by patients in the intervention group.

The disease activity assessed by Systemic Lupus Erythematosus Disease Activity Index 2 K > 4 at the end of the study conducted by Silva et al. [11], which lasted for six months, did not show any relevant difference between the group submitted to the diet and the control group. According to the authors, the groups did not differ regarding the corticoid dose used throughout the study. The authors observed that there was a significant change in the intervention group, with a reduction in the carbohydrate, saturated fat, trans and total fat, and calories intake. There was no change in the body mass index among participants in the intervention group, but when compared to the control group, these participants presented a weight gain. As the adipose tissue secretes pro-inflammatory cytokines, the increased adipose mass may contribute to the inflammation worsening, which may justify the disease activity worsening in the control group [13].

The subject is still controversial, but there is a suggestion that obesity and a high-fat diet are related to SLE, with the frequency of obesity being higher in SLE patients than in the general population. Vitamin D deficiency and increased adipokines, such as leptin and adiponectin, may explain the relationship between obesity and SLE [14].

Regarding the lipid profile, the study conducted by Shah et al. [8] showed that the diet improved the high-density lipoprotein, low-density lipoprotein, and triglyceride levels at both 6 and 12 weeks, which was more accentuated at 12 weeks. Silva et al. [11] showed an improvement in high-density lipoprotein, low-density lipoprotein, and triglyceride levels in adolescents at the 9-month evaluation. The results of both studies prove the effectiveness of protecting the cardiovascular system through diet and that adults and adolescents adhered to the proposed diet. For involving adolescents, the study conducted by Silva et al. [11] proves that the diet can be effective even among groups that are usually resistant to changing habits [15]. According to the Update of the Brazilian Guideline on Dyslipidemias and Prevention of Atherosclerosis, the control of saturated fat intake and its substitution with polyunsaturated fatty acids, precepts followed in both studies, are associated with cholesterol total and low-density lipoprotein cholesterol decrease, as well as with a decrease in cardiovascular events and death [16].

The comparison between the diets was also enabled by Davies et al. study [7], which compared the low glycemic index and calorie-restricted diets. As for the lipid profile, Davies et al. [7] verified that none of the groups presented a significant index reduction when compared to the initial evaluation. However, when the data was inserted in the forest plot, it shows that the low glycemic index diet was more favourable for high-density lipoprotein, low-density lipoprotein, and triglyceride improvement than the calorie-restricted diet. The type of diet did not affect the fatigue, quality of sleep, and disease activity as assessed through the British Isles Lupus Assessment Group. However, when the European Community Lupus Activity Measure evaluated the low glycemic index diet, its effect was favourable on fatigue. The study conducted by Davies et al. [7] shows that the low glycemic index diet redresses the postprandial hyperglycemia and hyperinsulinemia and the late postprandial hypoglycemia, which increases the risk of obesity, diabetes, and cardiovascular disease. The Update of the Brazilian Guideline on Dyslipidemias and Prevention of Atherosclerosis indicates as an adequate strategy for handling dyslipidemia diets such as the Mediterranean diet, emphasizing the importance of keeping a moderate-fat quantity, eliminating trans fatty acids, controlling the consumption of saturated fats, prioritizing polyunsaturated and monounsaturated

Table 4 Summary of findings

Question: What is the diet effect on systemic lupus erythematosus (SLE) patients?

Patients or population: Patients diagnosed with SLE
Setting: Ambulatory care
Intervention: Diet
Comparison: No diet

Outcomes	Illustrative comparative risk (96%CI) Assumed risk Corresponding risk Control Diet		Relative effect	No of participants (studies)	Quality of Evidence (GRADE)	Comments
Quality of life:12 weeks **Range: 0-100** **An increased score reflects improved QOL**	The mean quality of life in the control groups was 53.8.	The mean quality of life in the intervention groups was MD 14.6 higher (0.88 higher to 28.32 higher)	---------------------	16 (1 study)	⊕⊕◯◯ LOW[a,b]	Risk of bias: serious Imprecision: serious The author of the study named didn't specify the tool used to evaluate the quality of life
Disease activity (SLEDAI 2K>4): **six weeks** **Range: 0-105.** **higher value higher disease activity.** **a value above 6 indicates a significant clinical change sufficient to change the management**	**266 per 1000**	**278 per 1000** (83 to 915)	RR 1.07 (0.32 to 3.52)	31 (1 study)	⊕⊕◯◯ LOW[c,d]	Risk of bias: serious Imprecision: serious
HDL: 12 weeks **Higher is better**	The mean HDL leve in the control groups was 49.4	The mean HDL level in the intervention groups was MD 3.9 higher (9.74 lower to 17.54 higher)	---------------------	16 (1 study)	⊕⊕◯◯ LOW[a,b]	Risk of bias: serious Imprecision: serious
Total cholesterol: 12 weeks **Higher is worse**	The mean total cholesterol in the control groups was 194.3.	The mean total cholesterol level in the intervention groups was MD 15.8 higher (8.46 lower to 40.06 higher)	---------------------	16 (1 study)	⊕⊕◯◯ LOW[a,e]	Risk of bias: serious Imprecision: serious
Triglyceride: 12 weeks **Higher is worse**	The mean triglyceride level in the control groups was 128.	The mean triglyceride level in the intervention groups was MD 13.4 lower (50.27 lower to 23.47 higher)	---------------------	16 (1 study)	⊕⊕◯◯ LOW[a,e]	Risk of bias: serious Imprecision: serious
LDL: 12 weeks **Higher is worse**	The mean LDL level in the control groups was 128.	The mean LDL level in the intervention groups was MD 15.3 higher (8.12 lower to 38.72 higher)	---------------------	16 (1 study)	⊕⊕◯◯ LOW [a,e]	Risk of bias: serious Imprecision: serious
Total cholesterol: nine months **Higher is worse**	The mean total cholesterol level in the control groups was 160.2	The mean total cholesterol at nine months in the intervention groups was MD 15.3 lower (36.35 lower to 5.75 higher)	---------------------	31 (1 study)	⊕⊕◯◯ LOW [a,b]	Risk of bias: serious Imprecision: serious
LDL: nine months **Higher is worse**	The mean LDl level in the control groups was 87.75	The mean LDL level at nine months in the intervention groups was MD 13.15 lower (29.38 lower to 3.08 higher)	---------------------	31 (1 study)	⊕⊕◯◯ LOW[c,b]	Risk of bias: serious Imprecision: serious
Triglyceride: nine months **Higher is worse**	The mean triglyceride level in the control groups was 87.2	The mean triglyceride level at nine months in the intervention groups was MD 11.3 higher (16.9 lower to 39.5 higher)	---------------------	31 (1 study)	⊕⊕◯◯ LOW[c,b]	Risk of bias: serious Imprecision: serious
HDL: nine months **Higher is worse**	The mean HDL level in the control groups was 54	The mean HDL level at nine months in the intervention groups was MD 4.3 lower (15.56 lower to 6.96 higher)	---------------------	31 (1 study)	⊕⊕◯◯ LOW[c,b]	Risk of bias: serious Imprecision: serious

Table 4 (continued)

The basis for the assumed risk (e.g. the median control group risk across studies) is provided in footnotes. The corresponding risk (and its 95% confidence interval) is based on the assumed risk in the comparison group and the relative effect of the intervention (and its 95% CI)

CI = confidence interval; MD = mean difference; RR = risk ratio; SLEDAI = Systemic Lupus Erythematosus Disease Activity Index; HDL = high-density lipoprotein; LDL = low-density lipoprotein; a = There is a selection and detection bias; b = Small sample size; c = Detection bias; d = Small sample size and small number of events; e = Few patients and very large confidence interval (> 0.5)

fats, reducing sugars, and including lean meats, fruits, grains, and vegetables in the diet [16]. It further stresses that high carbohydrate intake increases glycemia, which generates hyperinsulinemia. In turn, this condition activates the transcription factors that promote the synthesis of fatty acids and triglycerides. There is still no substantial evidence proving the effectiveness of the low carbohydrate diet on lipid profile, mainly because the studies diverge significantly on the low carbohydrate diet definition. The 2018 United Kingdom guidelines on diabetes show that long-term adherence to low carbohydrate diets is low [17].

It has been demonstrated in studies that medications such as hydroxychloroquine and prednisone may affect the lipid profile [18, 19]. Hydroxychloroquine seems to have a beneficial effect due to the reduction of atherogenic lipoproteins and prednisone is associated with a worsening in the lipid profile of patients with lupus activity [18]. The studies included in this review did not differ between groups regarding the use of hydroxychloroquine and prednisone. It is important to note that the review evaluated patients with inactive disease and, probably, with low doses of these drugs.

Medeiros et al. [] published a systematic review investigating the effects of nutritional supplements such as omega-3 and vitamin D, as well as the study by Islam et al. who recommends intake of Omega 3 and 6; vitamins A, B, C, D, and E; minerals (calcium, zinc, selenium, iron, and copper) and polyphenol-containing foods to produce an immunomodulatory effect in SLE patients [21], differing from the present study because the objective of the latter was to evaluate the nutritional diet impact, not a specific nutritional supplement. Regarding methodological aspects, the review by Medeiros et al. [] restricted the search to the period from 2006 to 2016, and the exclusion criteria evaluated nutrients or diet analyses only. Furthermore, the systematic review did not describe the results regarding the effectiveness of the interventions.

Supplementation of macronutrients and micronutrients produces immunomodulatory effects in SLE patients, so the intake of Omega 3 and 6, vitamins A, B, C, D, and E, minerals such as calcium, zinc, selenium, iron, and copper, and polyphenol-containing foods are recommended.

Because dietary supplementation of various macro and micronutrients have exhibited immunomodulatory effects, including maintenance of homeostasis and improved physical and mental well-being in SLE patients, it is recommended that these patients consume a balanced diet that is low in calories and protein but contains plenty of fiber, PUFAs (ω3 and ω-6), vitamins (A, B, C, D, and E), minerals (calcium, zinc, selenium, iron, and copper), and polyphenol-containing foods.

The present systematic review is the first study about the nutritional diet impact on systemic lupus erythematosus patients and followed the methodological principles considered essential to conduct and report a systematic review, which includes conducting searches in several databases without date and language restriction, evaluating and selecting articles independently, and registering the protocol on PROSPERO.

Some limitations were found in this review. The small number of included studies and the small number of patients included can lead to a conclusion that does not correspond to reality. The different types of diets evaluated makes it difficult to standardize the studied intervention. This problem can be overcome by conducting studies with the involvement of several centres in a multicenter way. Also, the heterogeneity of the data makes it impossible to carry out a meta-analysis. Due to these limitations, further studies are needed to confirm the association between the impact of diet on patients with systemic lupus erythematosus.

Conclusions

Regarding its implication for the practice, studies such as the present systematic review help to promote public policies focusing on the population with rare and chronic diseases such as systemic lupus erythematosus. As for its implication for research, being the proposed interventions safe and effective, it should encourage researches aimed at verifying the outcome of the specific nutritional diet implementation in systemic lupus erythematosus patients.

The diet had a positive impact on the quality of life and a possible clinical relevance on lipid profile (high-density lipoprotein, low-density lipoprotein, triglyceride levels) of systemic lupus erythematosus patients. Both types of diet, calorie-restricted and low glycemic index did not influence disease activity, fatigue and quality of sleep outcomes. Based on GRADE approach, the evidence level for all outcomes was considered low.

Acknowledgements

Not applicable.

Authors' contributions

Conceptua Imoto AM lization (lead), data curation (lead), formal analysis (lead), funding acquisition (lead), methodology (lead), project administration (lead), supervision (lead), validation (lead), visualization (lead), writing-original draft (lead), writing-review and editing (lead); Gottems L: funding acquisition (supporting), writing-original draft (supporting), writing-review and editing (supporting); Salomon AL: conceptualization (supporting), data curation (sup porting), writing-original draft (supporting), writing-review and editing (sup porting); Silva HEC: conceptualization (supporting), data curation (supporting), funding acquisition (supporting), methodology (supporting), writing-original draft (supporting); Lombardi Júnior I: writing-review and editing (supporting); Peccin MS: writing-review and editing (supporting); Amorim FF: writing-original draft (supporting), writing-review and editing (supporting); Santana LA: writing-review and editing (supporting). All authors read and approved the final manuscript.

Author details

[1]Evidences-Based Health Lab, Professional and Academic Master Program, Escola Superior em Ciências da Saúde, Brasília, DF, Brazil. [2]Professional and Aca demic Master Program, Escola Superior em Ciências da Saúde, Brasília, DF, Brazil. [3]Human Movement Sciences Department, Interdisciplinary Post-Graduation Program in Health Sciences, Universidade Federal de São Paulo (UNIFESP), Santos, SP, Brazil. [4]Medicine Graduation Course, Escola Superior em Ciências da Saúde, Brasília, DF, Brazil. [5]Family Health Master Program (ProfSaúde), Escola Superior em Ciências da Saúde, Brasília, DF, Brazil.

References

1. Zucchi D, Elefante E, Calabresi E, et al. One year in review 2019: systemic lupus erythematosus. Clin Exp Rheumatol. 2019;37(5):715–22.
2. Lupus Commission. Systemic lupus erythematosus (SLE): BSR primer. Brazilian Society of Rheumatology. 2011. http://reumatologia.org.br/orientacoes-ao-paciente/lupus-eritematoso-sistemico-les-cartilha-da-sbr. Accessed 08 Oct 2020.
3. Rees F, Doherty M, Grainge MJ, Lanyon P, Zhang W. The worldwide incidence and prevalence of systemic lupus erythematosus: a systematic review of epidemiological studies. Rheumatology (Oxford). 2017;56(11):1945–61. https://doi.org/10.1093/rheumatology/kex260.
4. Kiriakidou M, Ching CL. Systemic lupus erythematosus. Ann Intern Med. 2020;172(11):ITC81–96. https://doi.org/10.7326/AITC202006020.
5. Petri M, Orbai AM, Alarcón GS, et al. Derivation and validation of the Systemic Lupus International Collaborating Clinics classification criteria for systemic lupus erythematosus. Arthritis Rheum. 2012;64(8):2677–86. https://doi.org/10.1002/art.34473.
6. Klack K, Bonfa E, Borba Neto EF. Diet and nutritional aspects in systemic lupus erythematosus. Rev Bras Reumatol. 2012;52(3):384–408. https://doi.org/10.1590/S0482-50042012000300009.
7. Davies RJ, Lomer MC, Yeo SI, et al. Weight loss and improvements in fatigue in systemic lupus erythematosus: a controlled trial of a low glycaemic index diet versus a calorie restricted diet in patients treated with corticosteroids. Lupus. 2012;21(6):649–55. https://doi.org/10.1177/09612.03312436854.
8. Shah M, Kavanaugh A, Coyle Y, Adams-Huet B, Lipsky PE. Effect of a culturally sensitive cholesterol lowering diet program on lipid and lipoproteins, body weight, nutrient intakes, and quality of life in patients with systemic lupus erythematosus. J Rheumatol. 2002;29(10):2122–8.
9. Aparicio-Soto M, Sánchez-Hidalgo M, Alarcón-de-la-Lastra C. An update on diet and nutritional factors in systemic lupus erythematosus management. Nutr Res Rev. 2017;30(1):118–37. https://doi.org/10.1017/S0954422417000026
10. La Cava A. The influence of diet and obesity on gene expression in SLE. Genes (Basel). 2019;10(5):405. https://doi.org/10.3390/genes10050405.
11. da Silva SGL, Terreri MT, Abad TTO, et al. The effect of nutritional intervention on the lipid profile and dietary intake of adolescents with juvenile systemic lupus erythematosus: a randomized, controlled trial. Lupus. 2018;27(5):820–7. https://doi.org/10.1177/0961203317751851.
12. Chaigne B, Chizzolini C, Perneger T, et al. Impact of disease activity on health-related quality of life in systemic lupus erythematosus—a cross-sectional analysis of the Swiss Systemic Lupus Erythematosus Cohort Study (SSCS). BMC Immunol. 2017;18(1):17. https://doi.org/10.1186/s12865-017-0200-5.
13. Coppack SW. Pro-inflammatory cytokines and adipose tissue. Proc Nutr Soc. 2001;60(3):349–56. https://doi.org/10.1079/pns2001110.
14. Kono M, Nagafuchi Y, Shoda H, et al. The impact of obesity and a high-fat diet on clinical and immunological features in systemic lupus erythematosus. Nutrients. 2021;13(2):504. https://doi.org/10.3390/nu13020504.
15. Ho M, Garnett SP, Baur L, et al. Effectiveness of lifestyle interventions in child obesity: systematic review with meta-analysis. Pediatrics. 2012;130(6):e1647–71. https://doi.org/10.1542/peds.2012-1176.
16. Faludi AA, Izar MCO, Saraiva JFK, et al. Atualização da Diretriz Brasileira de Dislipidemias e Prevenção da Aterosclerose – 2017. Arq Bras Cardiol. 2017;109(2 Supl 1):1–76. https://doi.org/10.5935/abc.20170121.
17. Dyson PA, Twenefour D, Breen C, et al. Diabetes UK evidence-based nutrition guidelines for the prevention and management of diabetes. Diabet Med. 2018;35(5):541–7. https://doi.org/10.1111/dme.13603.
18. Cairoli E, Rebella M, Danese N, Garra V, Borba EF. Hydroxychloroquine reduces low-density lipoprotein cholesterol levels in systemic lupus erythematosus: a longitudinal evaluation of the lipid-lowering effect. Lupus. 2012;21(11):1178–82. https://doi.org/10.1177/0961203312450084.
19. Sarkissian T, Beyene J, Feldman B, McCrindle B, Silverman ED. Longitudinal examination of lipid profiles in pediatric systemic lupus erythematosus. Arthritis Rheum. 2007;56(2):631–8. https://doi.org/10.1002/art.22332.
20. Durcan L, Winegar DA, Connelly MA, et al. Longitudinal evaluation of lipoprotein variables in systemic lupus erythematosus reveals adverse changes with disease activity and prednisone and more favorable profiles with hydroxychloroquine therapy. J Rheumatol. 2016;43(4):745–50. https://doi.org/10.3899/jrheum.150437.
21. Islam MA, Khandker SS, Kotyla PJ, Hassan R. Immunomodulatory effects of diet and nutrients in systemic lupus erythematosus (SLE): a systematic review. Front Immunol. 2020;11:1477. https://doi.org/10.3389/fimmu.2020.01477.

Permissions

All chapters in this book were first published by BioMed Central; hereby published with permission under the Creative Commons Attribution License or equivalent. Every chapter published in this book has been scrutinized by our experts. Their significance has been extensively debated. The topics covered herein carry significant findings which will fuel the growth of the discipline. They may even be implemented as practical applications or may be referred to as a beginning point for another development.

The contributors of this book come from diverse backgrounds, making this book a truly international effort. This book will bring forth new frontiers with its revolutionizing research information and detailed analysis of the nascent developments around the world.

We would like to thank all the contributing authors for lending their expertise to make the book truly unique. They have played a crucial role in the development of this book. Without their invaluable contributions this book wouldn't have been possible. They have made vital efforts to compile up to date information on the varied aspects of this subject to make this book a valuable addition to the collection of many professionals and students.

This book was conceptualized with the vision of imparting up-to-date information and advanced data in this field. To ensure the same, a matchless editorial board was set up. Every individual on the board went through rigorous rounds of assessment to prove their worth. After which they invested a large part of their time researching and compiling the most relevant data for our readers.

The editorial board has been involved in producing this book since its inception. They have spent rigorous hours researching and exploring the diverse topics which have resulted in the successful publishing of this book. They have passed on their knowledge of decades through this book. To expedite this challenging task, the publisher supported the team at every step. A small team of assistant editors was also appointed to further simplify the editing procedure and attain best results for the readers.

Apart from the editorial board, the designing team has also invested a significant amount of their time in understanding the subject and creating the most relevant covers. They scrutinized every image to scout for the most suitable representation of the subject and create an appropriate cover for the book.

The publishing team has been an ardent support to the editorial, designing and production team. Their endless efforts to recruit the best for this project, has resulted in the accomplishment of this book. They are a veteran in the field of academics and their pool of knowledge is as vast as their experience in printing. Their expertise and guidance has proved useful at every step. Their uncompromising quality standards have made this book an exceptional effort. Their encouragement from time to time has been an inspiration for everyone.

The publisher and the editorial board hope that this book will prove to be a valuable piece of knowledge for researchers, students, practitioners and scholars across the globe.

List of Contributors

Vinícius Alexandre de Souza Almeida, Carlos Henrique Fernandes, Lia Miyamoto Meireles, Flavio Faloppa, Benno Ejnisman and Moises Cohen
Trauma and Orthopaedics Department, Federal University of Sao Paulo, São Paulo, Brazil

Carina M. F. Gomes
Rheumatology Division, Universidade Federal de Sao Paulo (Unifesp/EPM), São Paulo, Brazil

Maria Teresa Terreri
Pediatric Rheumatology Unit, Department of Pediatrics, Universidade Federal de Sao Paulo (Unifesp/EPM), São Paulo, Brazil

Maria Isabel Moraes-Pinto
Pediatric Infectious Diseases Division, Department of Pediatrics, Universidade Federal de Sao Paulo (Unifesp/EPM), São Paulo, Brazil

Marcelo M. Pinheiro
Head of the Spondyloarthritis and Immunobiological Therapy Section, Rheumatology Division, Universidade Federal de Sao Paulo (Unifesp/EPM), Rua Leandro Dupré, 204, Conj. 74, Vila Clementino, São Paulo, SP CEP 04025-010, Brazil

Karina Rossi Bonfiglioli and Ana Cristina de Medeiros Ribeiro
Disciplina Reumatologia do Hospital das Clínicas, Faculdade de Medicina, Universidade de São Paulo (HC-FMUSP), Av. Dr. Arnaldo, 455 - 3° andar - Reumatologia, São Paulo, SP, CEP 01246-903, Brasil

Licia Maria Henrique da Mota and Cleandro Pires de Albuquerque
Serviço de Reumatologia do Hospital, Universitário de Brasília (HUB/UnB), Brasília, Brazil

Maria Raquel da Costa Pinto
Serviço de Reumatologia, Universidade Federal de Minas Gerais (UFMG), Belo Horizonte, Brazil

Ieda Maria Magalhães Laurindo
Disciplina de Reumatologia, Universidade Nove de Julho (UNINOVE), São Paulo, Brazil

Rina Dalva Neubarth Giorgi
Serviço de Reumatologia, Hospital do Servidor Público Estadual de São Paulo (HSPE-IAMSPE), São Paulo, Brazil

Angela Luzia Branco Pinto Duarte
Universidade Federal de Pernambuco (UFPE), Recife, Brazil

Mariana Peixoto Guimarães Ubirajara e Silva de Souza
Santa Casa de Belo Horizonte (MG), Belo Horizonte, Brazil

Claiton Viegas Brenol and Odirlei Monticielo
Hospital de Clínicas de Porto Alegre, Universidade Federal do Rio Grande do Sul (HCPA/UFRGS), Porto Alegre, Brazil

Geraldo da Rocha Castelar Pinheiro
Universidade do Estado do Rio de Janeiro (UERJ), Rio de Janeiro, Brazil

Charlles Heldan de Moura Castro
Escola Paulista de Medicina, Universidade Federal de São Paulo, São Paulo, Brazil

Gustavo Luiz Behrens Pinto
Universidade Federal da Bahia (UFBA), Salvador, Brazil

Jose Fernando Verztman
Hospital Federal dos Servidores do Estado do RJ, Rio de Janeiro, Brazil

Luciana Feitosa Muniz
Hospital Regional de Sobradinho (DF), Brasília, Brazil

Manoel Barros Bertolo
Disciplina de Reumatologia, Faculdade de Ciências Médicas, Universidade Estadual de Campinas, Campinas, Brazil

Paulo Louzada Júnior
Disciplina de Reumatologia, Faculdade de Medicina de Ribeirão Preto, Universidade de São Paulo (USP-RP), Ribeirão Preto, Brazil

Vitor Alves Cruz16,
16 Disciplina de Reumatologia, Faculdade de Medicina, Universidade Federal de Goiás, Goiânia, Brazil

Ivanio Alves Pereira
Serviço de Reumatologia do Hospital Universitário, Universidade Federal de Santa Catarina- UFSC, Florianópolis, Brazil

Max Vitor Carioca de Freitas
Universidade de Fortaleza - UNIFOR, Fortaleza, Brazil

Bóris Afonso Cruz
Pulsus - Belo Horizonte (MG), Belo Horizonte, Brazil

Eduardo Paiva
Disciplina de Reumatologia, Universidade Federal do Paraná (UFPR), Curitiba, Brazil

José Roberto Provenza
Disciplina de Reumatologia da Pontificia, Universidade Católica de Campinas, PUC-Campinas, Campinas, Brazil

Sueli Carneiro
Universidade Federal do Rio de Janeiro (UFRJ), Rua Farme de Amoedo, 140/601. Ipanema, Rio de Janeiro, RJ CEP 22420-020, Brazil

Penelope Esther Palominos and Charles Lubianca Kohem
Universidade Federal Do Rio Grande Do Sul (UFRS), Porto Alegre, Brazil

Sônia Maria Alvarenga Anti
Hospital Do Servidor Público Do Estado de São Paulo, São Paulo, Brazil

Rodrigo Luppino Assad
Universidade de São Paulo (USP), Ribeirão Preto, São Paulo, Brazil.

Rafaela Silva Guimarães Gonçalves and Cláudia Diniz Lopes Marques
Universidade Federal de Pernambuco (UFPE), Recife, Brazil

Adriano Chiereghin
Pontifícia Universidade Católica de Sorocaba (PUC), Sorocaba, Brazil

Andre Marun Lyrio and Rubens Bonfiglioli
Pontifícia Universidade Católica de Campinas (PUC), Campinas, Brazil

Antônio Carlos Ximenes
Hospital Estadual Geral de Goiania (HGG), Goiânia, Brazil

Carla Gonçalves Saad, Célio Roberto Gonçalves, Cláudia Goldenstein Schainberg, Eduardo de Souza Meirelles, Percival Degrava Sampaio-Barros and Wanderley Marques Bernardo
Universidade de São Paulo (USP), São Paulo, Brazil

Gustavo Gomes Resende and Ricardo da Cruz Lage
Universidade Federal de Minas Gerais (UFMG), Belo Horizonte, MG, Brazil

Lenise Brandao Pieruccetti
Hospital Heliópolis, São Paulo, Brazil

Mauro Waldemar Keiserman
Pontifícia Universidade Católica de Porto Alegre (PUC), Porto Alegre, Brazil

Michel Alexandre Yazbek
Universidade Estadual de Campinas (UNICAMP), Campinas, Brazil

Marcelo de Medeiros Pinheiro and Thauana Luíza Oliveira
Universidade Federal de São Paulo (UNIFESP), São Paulo, Brazil

Valderílio Feijó Azevedo
Universidade Federal do Paraná (UFPR), Curitiba, Paraná, Brazil

Washington Alves Bianchi
Santa Casa de Misericórdia do Rio de Janeiro (SCM), Rio de Janeiro, Brazil

Ricardo dos Santos Simões
Associação Médica Brasileira, Conselho Federal de Medicina (AMB/CFM), São Paulo, Brazil

Cristiano Barbosa Campanholo
Santa Casa de Misericórdia de São Paulo (SCM), São Paulo, Brazil

Gerardo Quintana-López
Reumavance Group, Rheumatology Section, Department of Internal Medicine, Fundación Santa Fe de Bogotá University Hospital, Carrera 7 No. 117-15, 110111 Bogota, Colombia
Department of Internal Medicine, School of Medicine, Universidad Nacional de Colombia, Bogota, Colombia
Department of Internal Medicine, School of Medicine, Universidad de Los Andes, Bogota, Colombia

Kevin Maldonado-Cañón and Jorge Bruce Flórez-Suárez
Reumavance Group, Rheumatology Section, Department of Internal Medicine, Fundación Santa Fe de Bogotá University Hospital, Carrera 7 No. 117-15, 110111 Bogota, Colombia

Paul Méndez-Patarroyo and Paola Coral-Alvarado
Reumavance Group, Rheumatology Section, Department of Internal Medicine, Fundación Santa Fe de Bogotá University Hospital, Carrera 7 No. 117-15, 110111 Bogota, Colombia
Department of Internal Medicine, School of Medicine, Universidad de Los Andes, Bogota, Colombia

Enrique Calvo
Department of Radiology, School of Medicine, Universidad Nacional de Colombia, Bogota, Colombia

Sandeep Surendran, C. B. Mithun and Arun Tiwari
Department of Rheumatology, Amrita Institute of Medical Sciences, Amrita Vishwa Vidyapeetham, Kochi, Kerala, India

Merlin Moni
Department of General Medicine, Amrita Institute of Medical Sciences, Amrita Vishwa Vidyapeetham, Kochi, Kerala, India

Manu Pradeep
Department of Pharmacology, Amrita Institute of Medical Sciences, Amrita Vishwa Vidyapeetham, Kochi, Kerala, India

Ali A. Ahmed, Samar Tharwat and Dina A. Shahin
Rheumatology and Immunology Unit, Internal Medicine Department, Faculty of Medicine, Mansoura University Hospital, Mansoura University, El Gomhouria St, Mansoura, Dakahlia Governorate, Egypt

Nihal M. Batouty and Ahmed M. Tawfik
Diagnostic and Interventional Radiology Department, Faculty of Medicine, Mansoura University, Mansoura, Dakahlia Governorate, Egypt

Ahmed El Bahy
Mansoura University Nephrology and Dialysis Unit, Internal Medicine Department, Faculty of Medicine, Mansoura University, Mansoura, Dakahlia Governorate, Egypt

Fabiola Reis Oliveira
Hospital das Clínicas da Faculdade de Medicina de Ribeirão Preto (HCFMRPUSP), Av. Bandeirantes, 3900, Vila Monte Alegre, Ribeirão Preto, SP CEP: 14049-900, Brazil

Valeria Valim
Serviço de Reumatologia, Hospital Universitário Cassiano Antônio de Moraes, Universidade Federal do Espírito Santo, Av. Marechal Campos, 1468, Maruípe, Vitória, ES CEP: 29075-910, Brazil

Sandra Gofinet Pasoto and Lissiane Karine Noronha Guedes
Disciplina de Reumatologia, Laboratório de Autoimunidade (DLC + LIM17), Hospital das Clínicas da Faculdade de Medicina da USP (HCFMUSP), R. Dr. Ovídio Pires de Campos, 225 - Cerqueira César, São Paulo, SP CEP: 05403-010, Brazil

Marilena Leal Mesquita Silvestre Fernandes
Disciplina de Reumatologia, Hospital Federal dos Servidores do Estado do Rio de Janeiro,, R. Sacadura Cabral, 178, Saúde, Rio de Janeiro, RJ CEP: 20221-903, Brazil

Maria Lucia Lemos Lopes
Disciplina de Reumatologia Departamento de Clínica Médica, Universidade Federal de Ciências da Saúde de Porto Alegre (UFCSPA),, R. Sarmento Leite, 245 - Centro Histórico de Porto Alegre, Porto Alegre, RS CEP: 90050-170, Brazil

Sonia Cristina de Magalhães Souza Fialho
Serviço de Reumatologia, Universidade Federal de Santa Catarina, R. Profa. Maria Flora Pausewang, s/n - Trindade, Florianópolis, SC CEP: 88036-800, Brazil

Aysa César Pinheiro
Disciplina de Reumatologia, Departamento de Clínica Médica, Universidade Federal de Pernambuco, Av. Prof. Moraes Rego, 1235, Cidade Universitária, Recife, PE CEP: 50670-901, Brazil

Laura Caldas dos Santos and Tania Fidelix
Departamento de Oftalmologia, Escola Paulista de Medicina-Universidade Federal de São Paulo (EPM-UNIFESP), Rua Botucatu, 820, Vila Clementino, Sao Paulo, SP CEP: 04023-062, Brazil

Alisson Pugliesi and Simone Appenzeller
Departamento de Ortopedia, Reumatologia e Traumatologia da Faculdade de Ciências Médicas da Universidade Estadual de Campinas (UNICAMP), R. Tessália Vieira de Camargo, 126 - Cidade Universitária, Campinas, SP CEP: 13083-887, Brazil

Sandra Lucia Euzébio Ribeiro and Tatiana Libório
Disciplina de Reumatologia, Universidade Federal do Amazonas, Rua Afonso Pena, 1053, Manaus, AM CEP: 69020-160, Brazil

Danielle Christinne Soares Egypto de Brito
Disciplina de Reumatologia, Departamento de Medicina Interna, Centro de Ciências Médicas, Universidade Federal de Paraíba (UFPB), Campus I - Lot. Cidade Universitária, Paraíba, PB CEP: 58051-900, Brazil

Maria Carmen Lopes Ferreira Silva Santos
Departamento de Patologia, Hospital Universitário Cassiano Antônio de Moraes, Universidade Federal do Espírito Santo, Av. Marechal Campos, 1468, Maruípe, Vitória, ES CEP: 29075-910, Brazil

Leandro Tanure
Disciplina de Reumatologia, Universidade Federal de Minas Gerais, Av. Pres. Antônio Carlos, 6627, Pampulha, Belo Horizonte, MG CEP: 31270-901, Brazil

Juliana DAgostino Gennari
Serviço de Reumatologia da Santa Casa de São Paulo, R. Dr. Cesário Mota Júnior, 112, Vila Buarque, São Paulo, SP CEP: 01221-020, Brazil

Vinicius Tassoni Civile, Ana Carolina Pereira Nunes Pinto and César Ramos Rocha-Filho
Disciplina de Medicina de Urgência e Medicina Baseada em Evidências, Escola Paulista de Medicina-Universidade Federal de São Paulo (EPM-UNIFESP), Rua Botucatu 740 Vila Clementino, São Paulo, SP CEP: 04023-062, Brazil

Samira Tatiyama Miyamoto
Departamento de Educação Integrada em Saúde, Universidade Federal do Espírito Santo (UFES), Av. Marechal Campos, 1468, Maruípe, Vitória, ES CEP: 29040-090, Brazil

Virginia Fernandes Moça Trevisani
Disciplina de Medicina de Urgência e Medicina Baseada em Evidências, Escola Paulista de Medicina-Universidade Federal de São Paulo (EPM-UNIFESP), Rua Botucatu 740 Vila Clementino, São Paulo, SP CEP: 04023-062, Brazil
Disciplina de Reumatologia, Universidade de Santo Amaro, Rua Enéas Siqueira Neto, Jardim das Imbuias, São Paulo, SP CEP: 04829-300, Brazil

Belkıs Nihan Coskun, Yavuz Pehlivan and Ediz Dalkilic
Division of Rheumatology, Uludağ University Faculty of Medicine (Uludağ Üniversitesi Tıp Fakültesi Romatoloji Bilim Dalı), Görükle, Nilüfer, Bursa 16059, Turkey

Burcu Yagiz
Division of Rheumatology, Afyonkarahisar State Hospital, Afyon, Turkey

Goran Radunović, Zoran Veličković, Melanija Rašić and Saša Janjić
Institute of Rheumatology, Faculty of Medicine, University of Belgrade, Resavska 69, Belgrade, Serbia

Vladana Marković
Neurology Clinic, Faculty of Medicine, University of Belgrade, Dr Subotića 6, Belgrade, Serbia

Saša Radovanović
Institute for Medical Research, University of Belgrade, Dr Subotića 4, 11129 Belgrade, Serbia

Sara Pezzato, Cristian Caimmi, Ilaria Montanari, Maurizio Rossini, Antonio Carletto and Elena Fracassi
Rheumatology Unit, University of Verona, Policlinico G.B. Rossi, Piazzale Scuro, 10, 37134 Verona, VR, Italy

Chiara Bonetto, Simona Tomassi, Maria Giulia Gnatta, Doriana Cristofalo and Sarah Tosato
Department of Neuroscience, Biomedicine and Movement Sciences, Section of Psychiatry, University of Verona, Verona, Italy

Marina Carvalho Arruda Barreto
Department of Public Health, Universidade Federal do Ceará, Ceará, Fortaleza, Brazil

Fabianna Resende Jesus Moraleida, Camila Ferreira Leite, Shamyr Sulyvan Castro and Ana Carla Lima Nunes
Department of Physical Therapy, Federal University of Ceará, Major Weyne Street, 1440, Fortaleza, CE 60430-450, Brazil

Cristiane Vitaliano Graminha
Department of Physical Therapy, Universidade Federal do Triângulo Mineiro, Ceará, Uberaba, Brazil

Patricia Gabrielli Vassão and Ana Claudia Muniz Renno
Department of Biosciences, Federal University of São Paulo, Campus Baixada Santista, Rua Silva Jardim, 136, Santos, SP 11015-020, Brazil

Ana Carolina Flygare de Souza and Helga Tatiana Tucci
Department of Human Movement Science, Federal University of São Paulo, Campus Baixada Santista, Rua Silva Jardim, 136, Santos, SP 11015-020, Brazil

Raquel Munhoz da Silveira Campos
Department of Biosciences, Federal University of São Paulo, Campus Baixada Santista, Rua Silva Jardim, 136, Santos, SP 11015-020, Brazil
Post Graduate Program of Interdisciplinary Health Sciences, Federal University of São Paulo, Campus Baixada Santista, Rua Silva Jardim, 136, Santos, SP 11015-020, Brazil

Livia Assis Garcia
Scientific Institute and Technological Department -University Brazil, São Paulo-Itaquera, SP, Brazil

Miyabi Uda, Mie Torii and Kazuko Nin
Department of Human Health Sciences, Kyoto University Graduate School of Medicine, 53 Shogoin Kawahara-cho, Sakyo-ku, Kyoto 606-8507, Japan

Motomu Hashimoto
Department of Advanced Medicine for Rheumatic Diseases, Kyoto University Graduate School of Medicine, Kyoto, Japan
Department of Clinical Immunology, Graduate School of Medicine, Osaka City University, Osaka, Japan

Masao Tanaka, Moritoshi Furu and Hiromu Ito
Department of Advanced Medicine for Rheumatic Diseases, Kyoto University Graduate School of Medicine, Kyoto, Japan

Ryuji Uozumi
Department of Biomedical Statistics and Bioinformatics, Kyoto University Graduate School of Medicine, Kyoto, Japan

Takao Fujii
Department of Rheumatology and Clinical Immunology, Wakayama Medical University, Wakayama, Japan

Chikashi Terao
Department of Rheumatology and Clinical Immunology, Graduate School of Medicine, Kyoto University, Kyoto, Japan
Laboratory for Statistical and Translational Genetics, RIKEN Center for Integrative Medical Sciences, Yokohama, Japan
Clinical Research Center, Shizuoka General Hospital, Shizuoka, Japan
The Department of Applied Genetics, The School of Pharmaceutical Sciences, University of Shizuoka, Shizuoka, Japan

Wataru Yamamoto
Department of Health Information Management, Kurashiki Sweet Hospital, Okayama, Japan

Genichi Sugihara
Department of Psychiatry, Kyoto University Graduate School of Medicine, Kyoto, Japan

Yukako Nakagami
Department of Psychiatry, Kyoto University Graduate School of Medicine, Kyoto, Japan
Kyoto University Health Service, Kyoto, Japan

Tsuneyo Mimori
Department of Rheumatology and Clinical Immunology, Kyoto University Graduate School of Medicine, Kyoto, Japan
Ijinkai Takeda General Hospital, Kyoto, Japan

Uğur Güngör Demir
Department of Physical Therapy and Rehabilitation, University of Health Sciences, Antalya Training and Research Hospital, 07100 Muratpaşa, Antalya, Turkey

Ali Nail Demir
Department of Physical Medicine and Rehabilitation Rheumatology Clinic, Faculty of Medicine, Akdeniz University, 07100 Antalya, Turkey

Naciye Füsun Toraman
Department of Physical Therapy and Rehabilitation, University of Health Sciences, Antalya Training and Research Hospital, 07100 Antalya, Turkey

Francisco Paulin
Interstitial Lung Disease Clinic, Hospital General de Agudos Juan A. Fernández, Mansilla, 2838, 1425 Buenos Aires, Argentina

Anastasia Secco, Federico Benavidez, Agustina Cáceres, Patricia Sasaki, Augusto Riopedre and María Celina de la Vega
CEIM Investigaciones Médicas, Buenos Aires, Argentina

Juan José Rodríguez Moncalvo, Martin Eduardo Fernández, Fabian Caro and María Laura Alberti
Hospital María Ferrer, Buenos Aires, Argentina

Orlando Gabriel Carballo and Fernanda Ingenito
Hospital General de Agudos Carlos G. Durand, Buenos Aires, Argentina

Paola Orausclio and Santiago Rossi
Centro Diagnostico Rossi, Buenos Aires, Argentina

Maria de la Vega
CEIM Investigaciones Médicas, Laprida 1307, Ciudad De Buenos Aires, 1425 Buenos Aires, Argentina

Generoso Guerra Bautista
Centro de Investigación Marbella, Paitilla Panamá, Panamá

César Pacheco-Tena
Universidad Autónoma de Chihuahua, Chihuahua, Mexico

Gastón Solano
Pfizer, San José, Costa Rica

Ronald D. Pedersen and Bonnie Vlahos
Pfizer, Collegeville, PA, USA

Annette Eva Szumski
Syneos Health, Princeton, NJ, USA

Cecilia Borlenghi
Pfizer, Buenos Aires, Argentina

Karina Santana
Pfizer, Ciudad de México, Mexico

Yu Fu
College of Pharmaceutical Sciences, Southwest University, Chongqing 400715, China
Key Laboratory of Drug Targeting and Drug Delivery System of the Education Ministry, Sichuan Engineering Laboratory for Plant-Sourced Drug and Sichuan Research Center for Drug Precision Industrial Technology, West China School of Pharmacy, Sichuan University, Chengdu 610064, China

Qing Lin and Zhi-rong Zhang
Key Laboratory of Drug Targeting and Drug Delivery System of the Education Ministry, Sichuan Engineering Laboratory for Plant-Sourced Drug and Sichuan Research Center for Drug Precision Industrial Technology, West China School of Pharmacy, Sichuan University, Chengdu 610064, China

Sevinç Külekçioğlu
Physical Medicine and Rehabilitation, City Hospital, Bursa, Turkey

Alp Çetin
Faculty of Medicine, Physical Medicine and Rehabilitation, Hacettepe University, Ankara, Turkey

Gecilmara Salviato Pileggi and Ana Beatriz Bacchiega
Rheumatology Unit of Escola Paulista de Medicina (Unifesp/ EPM), São Paulo, SP, Brazil

Gilda Aparecida Ferreira, Adriana Maria Kakehasi and Cristina Costa Duarte Lanna
Hospital das Clínicas, Universidade Federal de Minas Gerais (UFMG), Belo Horizonte, MG, Brazil

Ana Paula Monteiro Gomides Reis, Cleandro Pires Albuquerque and Licia Maria Henrique Mota
Hospital Universitário de Brasília da Universidade de Brasília, EBSERH (HUB-UnB), Brasília, DF, Brazil

Edgard Torres Reis-Neto, Emília Inoue Sato and Marcelo Medeiros Pinheiro
Hospital São Paulo da Universidade Federal de São Paulo, Escola Paulista de Medicina (Unifesp/ EPM), São Paulo, SP, Brazil

Mirhelen Mendes Abreu and Blanca Bica
Hospital Universitário Clementino Fraga Filho, Universidade Federal Do Rio de Janeiro (UFRJ), Rio de Janeiro, RJ, Brazil

Nafice Costa Araújo
Hospital Do Servidor Público Estadual, Instituto de Assistência Médica Ao Servidor Público Estadual (IAMSPE), São Paulo, SP, Brazil

Dante Valdetaro Bianchi
Santa Casa de Misericórdia Do Rio de Janeiro (HGSCMRJ), Rio de Janeiro, RJ, Brazil

Eloisa Duarte Bonfa and Eduardo Ferreira Borba
Rheumatology Division, Hospital das Clínicas HCFMUSP, Faculdade de Medicina, Universidade de São Paulo, São Paulo, SP, Brazil

Danielle Christinne Soares Egypto Brito
Hospital Universitário Lauro Wanderley, Universidade Federal da Paraíba (UFPB), João Pessoa, PB, Brazil

Ângela Luzia Branco Pinto Duarte and Claudia Diniz Lopes Marques
Hospital das Clínicas da Universidade Federal de Pernambuco (UFPE), Recife, PE, Brazil

Rafaela Cavalheiro Espírito Santo, Odirlei André Monticielo and Ricardo Machado Xavier
Hospital de Clínicas de Porto Alegre, Universidade Federal Do Rio Grande Do Sul (UFRGS), Porto Alegre, RS, Brazil

Paula Reale Fernandes and Viviane Angelina de Souza
Hospital Universitário da Universidade Federal de Juiz de Fora (UFJF), Juiz de Fora, MG, Brazil

Mariana Peixoto Guimarães
Santa Casa de Misericórdia de Belo Horizonte, Belo Horizonte, MG, Brazil

Kirla Wagner Poti Gomes
Hospital Geral de Fortaleza (HGF), Fortaleza, CE, Brazil

Evandro Mendes Klumb
Hospital Universitário Pedro Ernesto, Universidade Do Estado Do Rio de Janeiro (UERJ), Rio de Janeiro, RJ, Brazil

Gabriela Araújo Munhoz
Irmandade da Santa Casa de Misericórdia de São Paulo (ISCMSP), São Paulo, SP, Brazil

Eduardo Santos Paiva
Universidade Federal Do Paraná (UFPR), Curitiba, PR, Brazil

Helena Lucia Alves Pereira
Hospital Universitário Getúlio Vargas Universidade Federal Do Amazonas, Manaus, AM, Brazil

Laurindo Ferreira Rocha Junior
Instituto de Medicina Integral Professor Fernando Figueira (IMIP/ PE), Recife, PE, Brazil

Camila Santana Justo Cintra Sampaio
Instituto de Ensino E Pesquisa No Sírio Libanês, São Paulo, SP, Brazil

Vanderson Souza Sampaio and Marcus Vinícius Guimarães Lacerda
Fundação de Vigilância Em Saúde Do Amazonas, Manaus, AM, Brazil
Instituto Leônidas and Maria Deane, Fiocruz, Manaus, AM, Brazil
Fundação de Medicina Tropical Dr. Heitor Vieira Dourado, Manaus, AM, Brazil

Thelma Skare
Hospital Universitário Evangélico Mackenzie (HUEM), Curitiba, PR, Brazil

Muhammad Tariq Rafiq
Centre for Sport and Exercise Sciences, University of Malaya, Kuala Lumpur, Malaysia

Mohamad Shariff Abdul Hamid
Sports Medicine Department, University of Malaya Medical Centre, Kuala Lumpur, Malaysia

Eliza Hafiz
Sports Centre, Centre for Sport and Exercise Sciences, University of Malaya, Kuala Lumpur, Malaysia

Aline Mizusaki Imoto, Leila Bernarda Gottems, Helbert Eustáquio Cardoso e Silva and Levy Aniceto Santana
Evidences-Based Health Lab, Professional and Academic Master Program, Escola Superior em Ciências da Saúde, Brasília, DF, Brazil

Ana Lúcia Salomon
Professional and Academic Master Program, Escola Superior em Ciências da Saúde, Brasília, DF, Brazil

Império Lombardi Júnior and Maria Stella Peccin
Human Movement Sciences Department, Interdisciplinary Post-Graduation Program in Health Sciences, Universidade Federal de São Paulo (UNIFESP), Santos, SP, Brazil

Fábio Ferreira Amorim
Medicine Graduation Course, Escola Superior em Ciências da Saúde, Brasília, DF, Brazil
Family Health Master Program (ProfSaúde), Escola Superior em Ciências da Saúde, Brasília, DF, Brazil

Index

www.ingramcontent.com/pod-product-compliance
Lightning Source LLC
LaVergne TN
LVHW081025210926
848485LV00004B/948